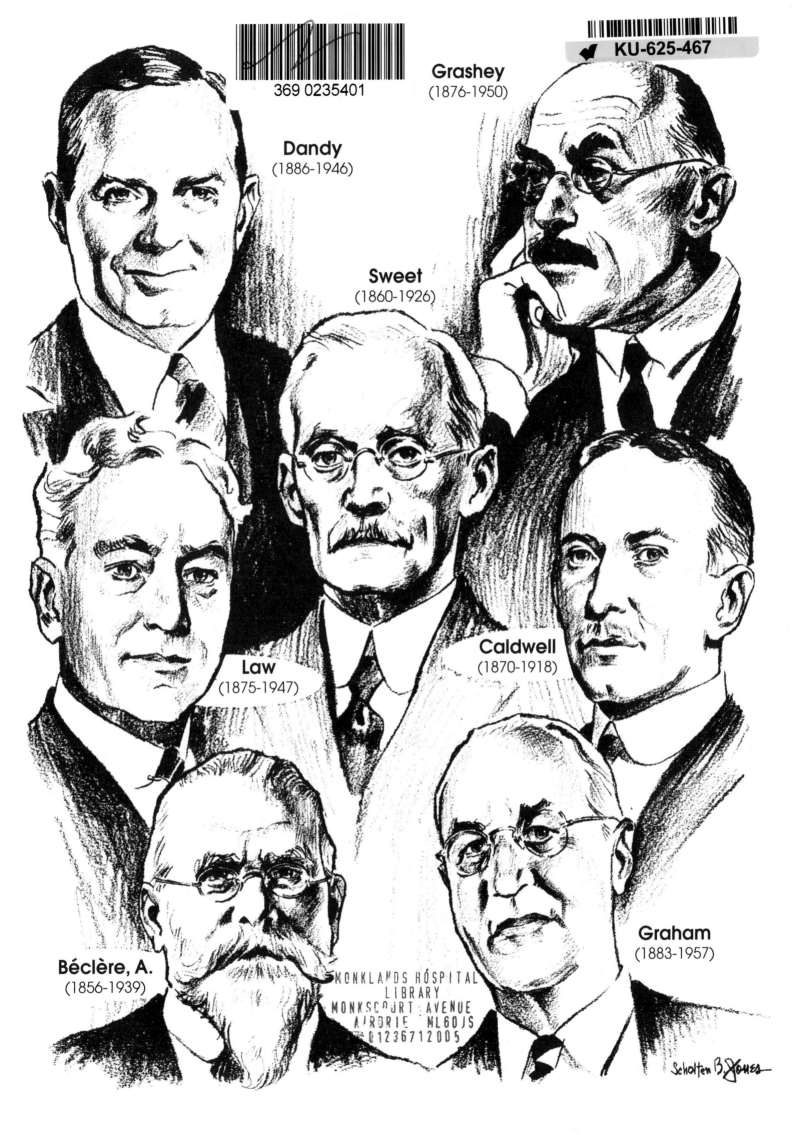

Dandy
(1886-1946)

Grashey
(1876-1950)

Sweet
(1860-1926)

Law
(1875-1947)

Caldwell
(1870-1918)

Béclère, A.
(1856-1939)

Graham
(1883-1957)

Scholten B. Jones

MERRILL'S ATLAS OF

RADIOGRAPHIC POSITIONING & PROCEDURES

THIRTEENTH EDITION | VOLUME TWO

MERRILL'S ATLAS OF
RADIOGRAPHIC POSITIONING & PROCEDURES

Bruce W. Long, MS, RT(R)(CV), FASRT, FAEIRS
Director and Associate Professor
Radiologic Imaging and Sciences Programs
Indiana University School of Medicine
Indianapolis, Indiana

Jeannean Hall Rollins, MRC, BSRT(R)(CV)
Associate Professor
Medical Imaging and Radiation Sciences Department
Arkansas State University
Jonesboro, Arkansas

Barbara J. Smith, MS, RT(R)(QM), FASRT, FAEIRS
Instructor, Radiologic Technology
Medical Imaging Department
Portland Community College
Portland, Oregon

ELSEVIER

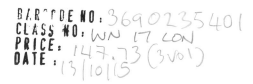

ELSEVIER
MOSBY

3251 Riverport Lane
St. Louis, Missouri 63043

MERRILL'S ATLAS OF RADIOGRAPHIC POSITIONING
& PROCEDURES, THIRTEENTH EDITION

ISBN: 978-0-323-26342-9 (vol 1)
ISBN: 978-0-323-26343-6 (vol 2)
ISBN: 978-0-323-26344-3 (vol 3)
ISBN: 978-0-323-26341-2 (set)

Notices

Knowledge and best practice in this field are constantly changing. As new research and experience broaden our understanding, changes in research methods, professional practices, or medical treatment may become necessary.

Practitioners and researchers must always rely on their own experience and knowledge in evaluating and using any information, methods, compounds, or experiments described herein. In using such information or methods, they should be mindful of their own safety and the safety of others, including parties for whom they have a professional responsibility.

With respect to any drug or pharmaceutical products identified, readers are advised to check the most current information provided (i) on procedures featured or (ii) by the manufacturer of each product to be administered, to verify the recommended dose or formula, the method and duration of administration, and contraindications. It is the responsibility of practitioners, relying on their own experience and knowledge of their patients, to make diagnoses, to determine dosages and the best treatment for each individual patient, and to take all appropriate safety precautions.

To the fullest extent of the law, neither the Publisher nor the authors, contributors, or editors assume any liability for any injury and/or damage to persons or property as a matter of product liability, negligence, or otherwise, or from any use or operation of any methods, products, instructions, or ideas contained in the material herein.

The Publisher

Previous editions copyrighted 2012, 2007, 2003, 1999, 1995, 1991, 1986, 1982, 1975, 1967, 1959, 1949

International Standard Book Numbers:
978-0-323-26342-9 (vol 1)
978-0-323-26343-6 (vol 2)
978-0-323-26344-3 (vol 3)
978-0-323-26341-2 (set)

Executive Content Strategist: Sonya Seigafuse
Content Development Manager: Billie Sharp
Content Development Specialist: Betsy McCormac
Publishing Services Manager: Julie Eddy
Senior Project Manager: Richard Barber
Designer: Margaret Reid

Printed in the United States of America

Last digit is the print number: 9 8 7 6 5 4 3 2 1

**Working together
to grow libraries in
developing countries**

www.elsevier.com • www.bookaid.org

PREVIOUS AUTHORS

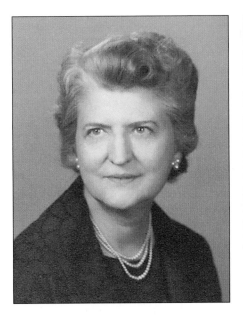

Vinita Merrill
1905-1977

Vinita Merrill was born in Oklahoma in 1905 and died in New York City in 1977. Vinita began compilation of Merrill's in 1936, while she worked as Technical Director and Chief Technologist in the Department of Radiology, and Instructor in the School of Radiography at the New York Hospital. In 1949, while employed as Director of the Educational Department of Picker X-ray Corporation, she wrote the first edition of the *Atlas of Roentgenographic Positions*. She completed three more editions from 1959 to 1975. Sixty-six years later, Vinita's work lives on in the thirteenth edition of *Merrill's Atlas of Radiographic Positioning & Procedures*.

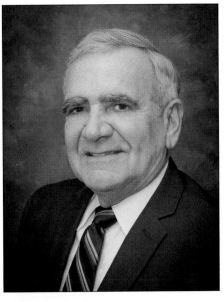

Philip W. Ballinger, PhD, RT(R), FASRT, FAEIRS, became the author of *Merrill's Atlas* in its fifth edition, which published in 1982. He served as author through the tenth edition, helping to launch successful careers for thousands of students who have learned radiographic positioning from *Merrill's*. Phil currently serves as Professor Emeritus in the Radiologic Sciences and Therapy, Division of the School of Health and Rehabilitation Sciences, at The Ohio State University. In 1995, he retired after a 25-year career as Radiography Program Director and, after ably guiding *Merrill's Atlas* through six editions, he retired as *Merrill's* author. Phil continues to be involved in professional activities, such as speaking engagements at state, national, and international meetings.

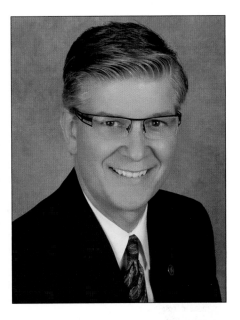

Eugene D. Frank, MA, RT(R), FASRT, FAEIRS, began working with Phil Ballinger on the eighth edition of *Merrill's Atlas* in 1995. He became the coauthor in its ninth and 50th-anniversary edition, published in 1999. He served as lead author for the eleventh and twelfth editions and mentored three coauthors. Gene retired from the Mayo Clinic/Foundation in Rochester, Minnesota, in 2001, after 31 years of employment. He was Associate Professor of Radiology in the College of Medicine and Director of the Radiography Program. He also served as Director of the Radiography Program at Riverland Community College, Austin, Minnesota, for 6 years before fully retiring in 2007. He is a Fellow of the ASRT and AEIRS. In addition to *Merrill's*, he is the coauthor of two radiography textbooks, *Quality Control in Diagnostic Imaging* and *Radiography Essentials for Limited Practice*. He now works in hospice through Christian Hospice Care and helps design and equip x-ray departments in underdeveloped countries.

THE MERRILL'S TEAM

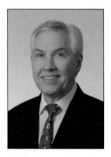

Bruce W. Long, MS, RT(R)(CV), FASRT, FAEIRS, is Director and Associate Professor of the Indiana University Radiologic and Imaging Sciences Programs, where he has taught for 29 years. A Life Member of the Indiana Society of Radiologic Technologists, he frequently presents at state and national professional meetings. His publication activities include 28 articles in national professional journals and two books, *Orthopaedic Radiography* and *Radiography Essentials for Limited Practice,* in addition to being coauthor of the *Atlas.* The thirteenth edition is Bruce's third on the Merrill's team and first as lead author.

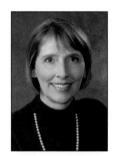

Barbara J. Smith, MS, RT(R)(QM), FASRT, FAEIRS, is an instructor in the Radiologic Technology program at Portland Community College, where she has taught for 30 years. The Oregon Society of Radiologic Technologists inducted her as a Life Member in 2003. She presents at state, regional, national, and international meetings, is a trustee with the ARRT, and is involved in professional activities at these levels. Her publication activities include articles, book reviews, and chapter contributions. As coauthor, her primary role on the Merrill's team is working with the contributing authors and editing Volume 3. The thirteenth edition is Barb's third on the Merrill's team.

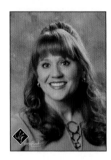

Jeannean Hall Rollins, MRC, BSRT(R) (CV), is an Associate Professor in the Medical Imaging and Radiation Sciences department at Arkansas State University, where she has taught for 22 years. She is involved in the imaging profession at local, state, and national levels. Her publication activities include articles, book reviews, and chapter contributions. Jeannean's first contribution to *Merrill's Atlas* was on the tenth edition as coauthor of the trauma radiography chapter. The thirteenth edition is Jeannean's third on the Merrill's team and first as a coauthor. Her previous role was writing the workbook, Mosby's Radiography Online, and the Instructor Resources that accompany *Merrill's Atlas.*

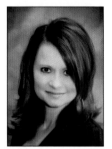

Tammy Curtis, PhD, RT(R)(CT)(CHES), is an associate professor at Northwestern State University, where she has taught for 14 years. She presents on state, regional, and national levels and is involved in professional activities on state level. Her publication activities include articles, book reviews, and book contributions. Previously, Tammy served on the advisory board and contributed the updated photo for Vinita Merrill, as well as other projects submitted to the *Atlas.* Her primary role on the Merrill's team is writing the workbook. The thirteenth edition is Tammy's first on the Merrill's team.

ADVISORY BOARD

This edition of *Merrill's Atlas* benefits from the expertise of a special advisory board. The following board members have provided professional input and advice and have helped the authors make decisions about Atlas content throughout the preparation of the thirteenth edition:

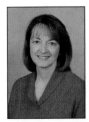

Andrea J. Cornuelle, MS, RT(R)
Professor, Radiologic Technology
Director, Health Science Program
Northern Kentucky University
Highland Heights, Kentucky

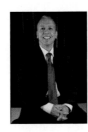

Joe A. Garza, MS, RT(R)
Associate Professor, Radiography Program
Lone Star College—Montgomery
Conroe, Texas

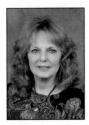

Patricia J. (Finocchiaro) Duffy, MPS, RT(R)(CT)
Clinical Education Coordinator/Assistant Professor
Medical Imaging Sciences Department
College of Health Professions
SUNY Upstate Medical University
Syracuse, New York

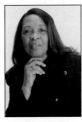

Parsha Y. Hobson, MPA, RT(R)
Associate Professor, Radiography
Passaic County Community College
Paterson, New Jersey

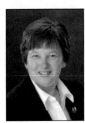

Lynn M. Foss, RT(R), ACR, DipEd, BHS
Instructor, Saint John School of Radiological Technology
Horizon Health Network
Saint John, New Brunswick, Canada

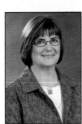

Robin J. Jones, MS, RT(R)
Associate Professor and Clinical Coordinator
Radiologic Sciences Program
Indiana University Northwest
Gary, Indiana

CHAPTER CONTENT EXPERTS

Valerie F. Andolina, RT(R)(M)
Senior Technologist
Elizabeth Wende Breast Care, LLC
Rochester, New York

Dennis Bowman, AS, RT(R)
Clinical Instructor
Community Hospital of the Monterey
  Peninsula
Monterey, California

Terri Bruckner, PhD, RT(R)(CV)
Instructor and Clinical Coordinator,
  Retired
Radiologic Sciences and Therapy
  Division
The Ohio State University
Columbus, Ohio

**Leila A. Bussman-Yeakel, MEd,
RT(R)(T)**
Director, Radiation Therapy Program
Mayo School of Health Sciences
Mayo Clinic College of Medicine
Rochester, Minnesota

Derek Carver, MEd, RT(R)(MR)
Clinical Instructor
Manager of Education and Training
Department of Radiology
Boston Children's Hospital
Boston, Massachusetts

Kim Chandler, MEdL, CNMT, PET
Program Director
Nuclear Medicine Technology Program
Mayo School of Health Sciences
Rochester, Minnesota

**Cheryl DuBose, EdD, RT(R)(MR)
(CT)(QM)**
Assistant Professor
Program Director, MRI Program
Department of Medical Imaging and
  Radiation Sciences
Arkansas State University
Jonesboro, Arkansas

**Angela M. Franceschi, MEd,
CCLS**
Certified Child Life Specialist
Department of Radiology
Boston Children's Hospital
Boston, Massachusetts

Joe A. Garza, MS, RT(R)
Professor, Radiologic Science
Lone Star College—Montgomery
Conroe, Texas

**Nancy Johnson, MEd, RT(R)(CV)
(CT)(QM)**
Faculty Diagnostic Medical Imaging
GateWay Community College
Phoenix, Arizona

**Sara A. Kaderlik, RT(R)(VI), RCIS,
CEPS**
Special Procedures Radiographer
St. Charles Medical Center
Bend, Oregon

Lois J. Layne, MSHA, RT(R)(CV)
Covenant Health
Centralized Privacy
Knoxville, Tennessee

**Cheryl Morgan-Duncan, MAS,
RT(R)(M)**
Radiographer Lab Coordinator/Adjunct
  Instructor
Passaic County Community College
Paterson, New Jersey

Susanna L. Ovel, RT(R), RDMS, RVT
Sonographer, Clinical Instructor
Sutter Medical Foundation
Sacramento, California

**Paula Pate-Schloder, MS, RT(R)
(CV)(CT)(VI)**
Associate Professor, Medical Imaging
  Department
Misericordia University
Dallas, Pennsylvania

**Bartram J. Pierce, BS, RT(R)(MR),
FASRT**
MRI Supervisor
Good Samaritan Regional Medical
  Center
Corvallis, Oregon

Jessica L. Saunders, RT(R)(M)
Technologist
Elizabeth Wende Breast Care, LLC
Rochester, New York

**Sandra Sellner-Wee, MS,
RT(R)(M)**
Program Director, Radiography
Riverland Community College
Austin, Minnesota

Raymond Thies, BS, RT(R)
Department of Radiology
Boston Children's Hospital
Boston, Massachusetts

Jerry G. Tyree, MS, RT(R)
Program Coordinator
Columbus State Community College
Columbus, Ohio

**Sharon R. Wartenbee, RT(R)(BD),
CBDT, FASRT**
Senior Diagnostic and Bone
  Densitometry Technologist
Avera Medical Group McGreevy
Sioux Falls, South Dakota

Kari J. Wetterlin, MA, RT(R)
Lead Technologist, General and
  Surgical Radiology
Mayo Clinic/Foundation
Rochester, Minnesota

Gayle K. Wright, BS, RT(R)(MR)(CT)
Instructor, Radiography Program
CT & MRI Program Coordinator
Medical Imaging Department
Portland Community College
Portland, Oregon

PREFACE

Welcome to the thirteenth edition of *Merrill's Atlas of Radiographic Positioning & Procedures*. This edition continues the tradition of excellence begun in 1949, when Vinita Merrill wrote the first edition of what has become a classic text. Over the past 66 years, *Merrill's Atlas* has provided a strong foundation in anatomy and positioning for thousands of students around the world who have gone on to successful careers as imaging technologists. *Merrill's Atlas* is also a mainstay for everyday reference in imaging departments all over the world. As the coauthors of the thirteenth edition, we are honored to follow in Vinita Merrill's footsteps.

Learning and Perfecting Positioning Skills

Merrill's Atlas has an established tradition of helping students learn and perfect their positioning skills. After covering preliminary steps in radiography, radiation protection, and terminology in introductory chapters, the first two volumes of *Merrill's* teach anatomy and positioning in separate chapters for each bone group or organ system. The student learns to position the patient properly so that the resulting radiograph provides the information the physician needs to correctly diagnose the patient's problem. The atlas presents this information for commonly requested projections, as well as for those less commonly requested, making it the only reference of its kind in the world.

The third volume of the atlas provides basic information about a variety of special imaging modalities, such as mobile and surgical imaging, pediatrics, geriatrics, computed tomography (CT), vascular radiology, magnetic resonance imaging (MRI), sonography, nuclear medicine technology, bone densitometry, and radiation therapy.

Merrill's Atlas is not only a comprehensive resource to help students learn, but also an indispensable reference as they move into the clinical environment and ultimately into practice as imaging professionals.

New to This Edition

Since the first edition of *Merrill's Atlas* in 1949, many changes have occurred. This new edition incorporates many significant changes designed not only to reflect the technologic progress and advancements in the profession, but also to meet the needs of today's radiography students. The major changes in this edition are highlighted as follows.

NEW PATIENT PHOTOGRAPHY

All patient positioning photographs have been replaced in Chapters 4 and 8. The new photographs show positioning detail to a greater extent and in some cases from a more realistic perspective. In addition, the equipment in these photos is the most modern available, and computed radiography plates are used. The use of electronic central ray angles enables a better understanding of where the central ray should enter the patient.

REVISED IMAGE EVALUATION CRITERIA

All image evaluation criteria have been revised and reorganized to improve the student's ability to learn what constitutes a quality image. In addition, the criteria are presented in a way that improves the ability to correct positioning errors.

WORKING WITH THE OBESE PATIENT

Many in the profession, especially students, requested that we include material on how to work with obese and morbidly obese patients. *Joe Garza*, of our advisory

board, assisted in the creation of this new section. For this edition, new information and illustrations have been added related to equipment, transportation, communication, and technical considerations specific to this patient population. This was accomplished with input from a wide variety of educators and practitioners with expertise working with obese patients.

FULLY REVISED PEDIATRIC CHAPTER

The pediatric chapter has been completely reorganized, with new photos, images, and illustrations. Time-tested techniques and current technologies are covered. New material has been added addressing the needs of patients with autism spectrum disorders.

UPDATED GERIATRIC CHAPTER

To meet the need of imaging professionals to provide quality care for all elderly patients, material has been added, addressing elder abuse and Alzheimer's disease. Imaging aspects, in addition to patient care challenges, are included.

CONSOLIDATED CRANIAL CHAPTERS

The chapters on the skull, facial bones, and paranasal sinuses have been combined. This facilitates learning by placing the introductory and anatomy material closer to the positioning details for the facial bones and sinuses.

DIGITAL RADIOGRAPHY COLLIMATION

With the expanding use of digital radiography (DR) and the decline in the use of cassettes in Bucky mechanisms, concern was raised regarding the collimation sizes for the various projections. Because collimation is considered one of the critical aspects of obtaining an optimal image, especially with computed radiography

(CR) and DR, this edition contains the specific collimation sizes that students and radiographers should use when using manual collimation with DR in-room and DR mobile systems. The correct collimation size for projections is now included as a separate heading.

ENGLISH/METRIC IR SIZES

English and metric sizes for image receptors (IRs) continue to challenge radiographers and authors in the absence of a standardized national system. With film/screen technology, the trend was toward the use of metric measurements for most of the cassette sizes. However, with CR and DR, the trend has moved back toward English sizes. Most of the DR x-ray systems use English for collimator settings. Because of this trend, the IR sizes and collimation settings for all projections are stated in English, and the metric equivalents are provided in parentheses.

INTEGRATION OF CT AND MRI

In the past three editions, both CT and MRI images have been included in the anatomy and projection pages. This edition continues the practice of having students learn cross-section anatomy with regular anatomy.

NEW ILLUSTRATIONS

Many who use *Merrill's* in teaching and learning have stated that the line art is one of the most useful aspects in learning new projections. New illustrations have been added to this edition to enable the user to comprehend bone position, central ray (CR) direction, and body angulations.

DIGITAL RADIOGRAPHY UPDATED

Because of the rapid expansion and acceptance of CR and direct DR, either selected positioning considerations and modifications or special instructions are indicated where necessary. A special icon alerts the reader to digital notes. The icon is shown here:

COMPUTED RADIOGRAPHY

OBSOLETE PROJECTIONS DELETED

Projections identified as obsolete by the authors and the advisory board continue to be deleted. A summary is provided at the beginning of any chapter containing deleted projections so that the reader may refer to previous editions for information. Continued advances in CT,

MRI, and ultrasound have prompted these deletions. The projections that have been removed appear on the Evolve site at evolve.elsevier.com.

NEW RADIOGRAPHS

Nearly every chapter contains updated, optimum radiographs, including many that demonstrate pathology. With the addition of updated radiographic images, the thirteenth edition has the most comprehensive collection of high-quality radiographs available to students and practitioners.

Learning Aids for the Student
POCKET GUIDE TO RADIOGRAPHY

The new edition of *Merrill's Pocket Guide to Radiography* complements the revision of *Merrill's Atlas*. Instructions for positioning the patient and the body part for all the essential projections are presented in a complete yet concise manner. Tabs are included to help the user locate the beginning of each section. Space is provided for the user to write in specifics of department techniques.

RADIOGRAPHIC ANATOMY, POSITIONING, AND PROCEDURES WORKBOOK

The new edition of this workbook features extensive review and self-assessment exercises that cover the first 29 chapters in *Merrill's Atlas* in one convenient volume. The features of the previous editions, including anatomy labeling exercises, positioning exercises, and self-tests, are still available. However, this edition features more image evaluations to give students additional opportunities to evaluate radiographs for proper positioning and more positioning questions to complement the workbook's strong anatomy review. The comprehensive multiple-choice tests at the end of each chapter help students assess their comprehension of the whole chapter. New exercises in this edition focus on improved understanding of essential projections and the need for appropriate collimated field sizes for digital imaging. Additionally, review and assessment exercises in this edition have been expanded for the chapters on pediatrics, geriatrics, vascular and interventional radiography, sectional anatomy, and computed tomography in Volume 3. Exercises in these chapters help students learn the theory and concepts of these spe-

cial techniques with greater ease. Answers to the workbook questions are found on the Evolve website.

Teaching Aids for the Instructor
EVOLVE INSTRUCTOR ELECTRONIC RESOURCES

This comprehensive resource provides valuable tools, such as lesson plans, PowerPoint slides, and an electronic test bank for teaching an anatomy and positioning class. The test bank includes more than 1,500 questions, each coded by category and level of difficulty. Four exams are already compiled in the test bank to be used "as is" at the instructor's discretion. The instructor also has the option of building new tests as often as desired by pulling questions from the ExamView pool or using a combination of questions from the test bank and questions that the instructor adds.

Evolve may be used to publish the class syllabus, outlines, and lecture notes; set up "virtual office hours" and e-mail communication; share important dates and information through the online class Calendar; and encourage student participation through Chat Rooms and Discussion Boards. Evolve allows instructors to post exams and manage their grade books online. For more information, visit *www.evolve.elsevier.com* or contact an Elsevier sales representative.

MOSBY'S RADIOGRAPHY ONLINE

Mosby's Radiography Online: Merrill's Atlas of Radiographic Positioning & Procedures is a well-developed online course companion for the textbook and workbook. This online course includes animations with narrated interactive activities and exercises, in addition to multiple-choice assessments that can be tailored to meet the learning objectives of your program or course. The addition of this online course to your teaching resources offers greater learning opportunities while accommodating diverse learning styles and circumstances. This unique program promotes problem-based learning with the goal of developing critical thinking skills that will be needed in the clinical setting.

EVOLVE—ONLINE COURSE MANAGEMENT

Evolve is an interactive learning environment designed to work in coordination with

Merrill's Atlas. Instructors may use Evolve to provide an Internet-based course component that reinforces and expands on the concepts delivered in class.

We hope you will find this edition of *Merrill's Atlas of Radiographic Positioning &Procedures* the best ever. Input from generations of readers has helped to keep the atlas strong through 10 editions, and we welcome your comments and suggestions. We are constantly striving to build on Vinita Merrill's work, and we trust that she would be proud and pleased to know that the work she began 66 years ago is still so appreciated and valued by the imaging sciences community.

Bruce W. Long
Jeannean Hall Rollins
Barbara J. Smith
Tammy Curtis

ACKNOWLEDGMENTS

In preparing for the thirteenth edition, our advisory board continually provided professional expertise and aid in decision making on the revision of this edition. The advisory board members are listed on p. vii. We are most grateful for their input and contributions to this edition of the *Atlas*.

Scott Slinkard, a radiography student from the College of Nursing and Health Sciences in Cape Girardeau, Missouri, and a professional photographer, provided many of the new photographs seen throughout the *Atlas*.

Contributors

The group of radiography professionals listed below contributed to this edition of the *Atlas* and made many insightful suggestions. We are most appreciative of their willingness to lend their expertise.

Special recognition and appreciation to the imaging staff of St. Vincent Hospital, Carmel, Indiana, for sharing their extensive experience and expertise in imaging obese and morbidly obese patients, as a Bariatric Center of Excellence. We especially thank Carolyn McCutcheon, RT(R), director of Medical Imaging; Todd Judy, BS, RT(R), team leader of Medical Imaging; and Lindsay Black, BS, RT(R), clinical instructor. Thanks also to Mark Adkins, MSEd, RT(R)(QM), Radiography Program director, for his assistance.

Special recognition and appreciation to the imaging professionals at NEA Baptist Hospital and St. Bernard's Medical Center in Jonesboro, Arkansas. The time, expertise, and efforts of Gena Morris, RT(R), RDMS, PACS administrator, and Loisey Wortham, RT(R), at NEA Baptist Hospital, and also to Mitzi Pierce, MSHS, RT(R)(M), radiology educator at St. Bernard's Medical Center, have been essential to this revision.

Suzie Crago, AS, RT(R)
Senior Staff Technologist
Riley Hospital for Children
Indianapolis, Indiana

Dan Ferlic, RT(R)
Ferlic Filters
White Bear Lake, Minnesota

Susan Herron, AS, RT(R)
Ezkenazi Health
Indianapolis, Indiana

Joy Menser, MSM, RT(R)(T)
Radiography Program Director
Owensboro Community & Technical
    College
Owensboro, Kentucky

Michael Mial
Student Radiographer
Indiana University Radiography Program
Indianapolis, Indiana
(Patient model for Chapter 8)

Kate Richmond, BS, RT(R)
Radiographer
Indianapolis, Indiana
(Patient model for Chapter 4)

Susan Robinson, MS, RT(R)
Associate Professor of Clinical
    Radiologic and Imaging Sciences
Clinical Instructor at Riley Hospital
    for Children
Indiana University School of Medicine
Indianapolis, Indiana

**Andrew Woodward MA,
RT(R)(CT)(QM)**
Assistant Professor and Clinical
    Coordinator
University of North Carolina at
    Chapel Hill
Chapel Hill, North Carolina

CONTENTS

11

LONG BONE MEASUREMENT

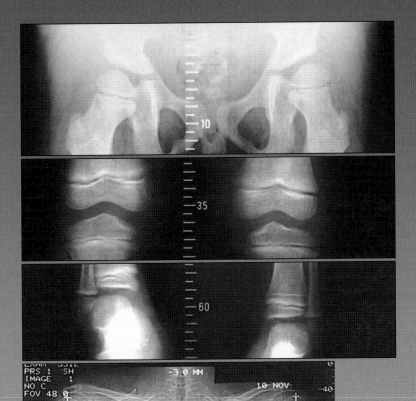

Imaging Methods

Long bone measurement to evaluate for limb length discrepancy may be accomplished by radiography, microdose digital radiography, ultrasonography (US), computed tomography (CT), and magnetic resonance imaging (MRI).[1] Radiographic methods are the orthoroentgenogram, scanogram, and teleoroentgenogram. Both the orthoroentgenogram and the scanogram require three precisely centered exposures at the hip, knee, and ankle joints and include the use of a radiopaque ruler taped to the table between the limbs. The image receptor (IR) size is the primary difference, with the orthoroentgenogram using a single IR that remains stationary while the table and the x-ray tube move to an unexposed section. The scanogram technique uses three separate IRs. The teleoroentgenogram is a single upright AP exposure of both limbs on a special long IR at an SID of at least 6 ft (180 cm). Digital imaging usually employs a hybrid of these traditional techniques by obtaining the three exposures centered at the hip, knee, and ankle joints with the patient standing upright. Digital postprocessing "stitches" the three images together for equally accurate measurements of the entire lower limbs with lower radiation dose than is used in the film-screen methods.[1,2] Although studies are occasionally made of the upper limbs, radiography is most frequently applied to the lower limbs. This chapter explains patient positioning for the three joint exposures, as well as for CT scanograms.

ABBREVIATIONS USED IN CHAPTER 11

AP	Anteroposterior
CT	Computed tomography
IR	Image receptor
MRI	Magnetic resonance imaging
US	Ultrasonography

See Addendum B for a summary of all abbreviations used in Volume 2.

[1]Sabharwal S, Kumar A: Methods for assessing leg length discrepancy, *Clin Orthop Relat Res* 466:12, 2008.

[2]Khakharia S et al: Comparison of PACS and hardcopy 51-inch radiographs for measuring leg length and deformity, *Clin Orthop Relat Res* 469:244, 2011.

Radiation Protection

Differences in limb length are common in children and may occur in association with various disorders. Patients with unequal limb growth may require yearly imaging evaluations. More frequent examinations may be necessary in patients who have undergone surgical procedures to equalize limb length. For these reasons, radiation protection is a primary consideration in imaging for long bone measurement. Gonad shielding is necessary, as are careful patient positioning, secure immobilization, and accurate centering of a closely collimated beam of radiation to prevent unnecessary repeat exposures. Microdose digital radiography yields the lowest dose but requires specialized equipment, which can be cost-prohibitive. MRI and US have promise as means to safely image for long bone measurement, with recent research demonstrating 99% accuracy and reliability for MRI measurements.[1,3]

Position of Patient

Three exposures of each limb are made, with the accuracy of the examination depending on the patient not moving the limb or limbs even slightly. Small children must be carefully immobilized to prevent motion. If movement of the limb occurs before the examination is completed, all images may need to be repeated.

- Place the patient in the supine position for orthoroentgenography and scanography.
- Stand the patient upright backed up closely to the vertical Bucky device for a digital teleoroentgenogram.
- Both sides are examined for comparison either separately or simultaneously for all techniques.
- When a soft tissue abnormality (swelling or atrophy) is causing rotation of the pelvis, elevate the low side on a radiolucent support to overcome the rotation, if necessary.

Position of Part

The limb to be examined should be positioned as follows:

[3]Doyle A, Winsor S: Magnetic resonance imaging (MRI) lower limb length measurement, *J Med Imaging Radiat Oncol* 55:191, 2011.

- Adjust and immobilize the limb for an AP projection.
- If the two lower limbs are examined simultaneously, separate the ankles 5 to 6 inches (13 to 15 cm) and place the specialized ruler under the pelvis and extended down between the legs.
- If the limbs are examined separately, position the patient with a special ruler beneath each limb.
- When the knee of the patient's abnormal side cannot be fully extended, flex the normal knee to the same degree and support each knee on one of a pair of supports of *identical size* to ensure that the joints are flexed to the same degree and are equidistant from the image receptor (IR).

Localization of Joints

For methods that require centering of the central ray above the joints, the following steps should be taken:

- Localize each joint accurately, and use a skin-marking pencil to indicate the central ray centering point.
- Because both sides are examined for comparison and a discrepancy in bone length usually exists, mark the joints of each side after the patient is in the required position.
- With the upper limb, place the marks as follows: for the *shoulder joint,* over the superior margin of the head of the humerus; for the *elbow joint,* ½ to ¾ inch (1.3 to 1.9 cm) below the plane of the epicondyles of the humerus (depending on the size of the patient); and for the wrist, midway between the styloid processes of the radius and ulna.
- With the lower limb, locate the *hip joint* by placing a mark 1 to 1¼ inches (2.5 to 3.2 cm) (depending on the size of the patient) laterodistally and at a right angle to the midpoint of an imaginary line extending from the anterior superior iliac spine to the pubic symphysis.
- Locate the *knee joint* just below the apex of the patella at the level of the depression between the femoral and tibial condyles.
- Locate the *ankle joint* directly below the depression midway between the malleoli.

In all images made by a single x-ray exposure, the image is larger than the actual body part because the x-ray photons start at a small area on the target of the x-ray tube and diverge as they travel in straight lines through the body to the IR (Fig. 11-1). This magnification can be decreased by putting the body part as close to the IR as possible and using the maximum SID allowed by the equipment. For orthoroentgenography, a metal measurement ruler is placed between the patient's lower limbs, and three exposures are made on the same x-ray IR. The following steps are taken:

- Using narrow collimation and careful centering of limb parts to the upper, middle, and lower thirds of the IR, make three exposures on one IR.
- For all three exposures, place the central ray perpendicular to and passing directly through the specified joint (hence the term *orthoroentgenology,* from the Greek word *orthos,* meaning "straight").
- Do not move the limb between exposures. Because the IR is in the Bucky tray for all exposures including exposure of the ankle, exposure factors must be modified accordingly.
- Position the x-ray tube directly over the patient's hip, and make the first exposure (Fig. 11-2, *A*).
- Move the x-ray tube directly over the patient's knee joint, and make a second exposure (Fig. 11-2, *B*).
- Move the x-ray tube directly over the patient's ankle joint, and make a third exposure (Fig. 11-2, *C*).

If the child holds the leg perfectly still while the three exposures are made, the true distance from the proximal end of the femur to the distal end of the tibia can be directly measured on the image, as follows:

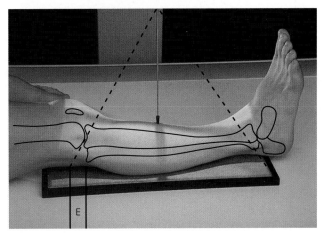

Fig. 11-1 Conventional radiographic images are magnified (elongated) images. Proximal elongation in this example is equal to the distance (*E*). Similar elongation occurs distally.

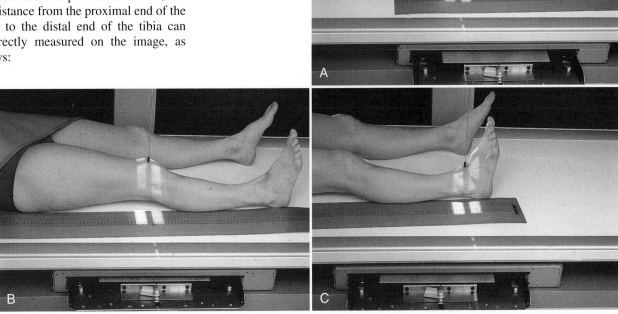

Fig. 11-2 Patient positioned for orthoroentgenographic measurement of lower limb. **A-C,** Central ray is centered over hip joint (**A**), knee joint (**B**), and ankle joint (**C**). A metal ruler was placed near lateral aspect of leg for photographic purposes. Ruler is normally placed between limbs (see Fig. 11-4).

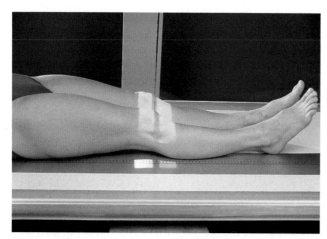

Fig. 11-3 Bilateral leg length measurement, with metal ruler placed beside leg for photographic purposes. (Proper placement of ruler is shown in Fig. 11-4.)

- Place a special metal ruler (engraved with radiopaque ½-inch [1.3-cm] marks that show when an image is made) under the leg and on top of the table (see Fig. 11-2).
- If the IR is placed in the Bucky tray and then is moved between exposures, as for a scanogram (see Fig. 11-2), calculate the length of the femur and tibia by subtracting the numeric values projected over the two joints obtained by simultaneously exposing the patient and the metal ruler.

Another method of measuring the length of the femurs and tibias is to examine both limbs simultaneously (Figs. 11-3 and 11-4):

- Center the midsagittal plane of the patient's body to the midline of the grid.
- Adjust the patient's lower limbs in the anatomic position (i.e., slight medial rotation).
- Tape the special metal ruler to the top of the table so that part of it is included in each of the exposure fields. This records the position of each joint.
- Place an IR in the Bucky tray, and shift it for centering at the three joint levels without moving the patient.

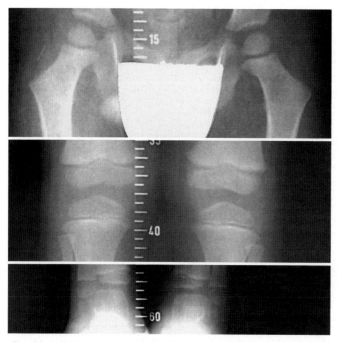

Fig. 11-4 Orthoroentgenogram for measurement of leg length.

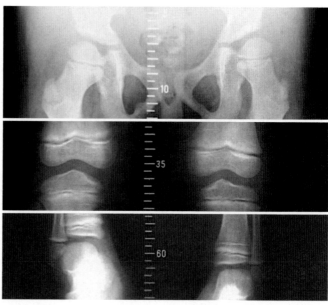

Fig. 11-5 Leg measurement showing that right leg is shorter than left leg.

- Center the IR and the tube successively at the previously marked level of the hip joints, the knee joints, and the ankle joints for simultaneous bilateral projections.
- When a difference in level exists between the contralateral joints, center the tube midway between the two levels.
- Digital imaging typically requires three exposures on three separate 14 × 17-inch (35 × 43-cm) IRs with a minimum 6-ft (180-cm) SID. The computer postprocesses the three images into a single image of the entire limb through a process termed "stitching." Limb length can then be quickly calculated by the computer.[1,2]

The bilateral orthoroentgenographic method is reasonably accurate if the limbs are of almost the same length. When more than a slight discrepancy in limb length exists (Fig. 11-5), it is impossible to place the center of the x-ray tube exactly over both knee joints and make a single exposure or exactly over both ankle joints and make a single exposure. In such cases, the tube is centered midway between the two joints; however, this results in bilateral distortion because of the diverging x-ray beam. In Fig. 11-5, the measurement obtained for the right femur is less than the actual length of the bone, whereas the measurement of the left femur is greater than the true length. The following measure can be taken to correct this problem:

- Examine each limb separately (Fig. 11-6).
- Center the limb being examined on the grid, and place the special ruler beneath the limb.
- Make a closely collimated exposure over each joint. This restriction of the exposure field not only increases the accuracy of the procedure but considerably reduces radiation exposure (most important, to the gonads).
- After making joint localization marks, position the patient and apply local gonad shielding.
- Adjust the collimator to limit the exposure field as much as possible.
- With successive centering to the localization marks, make exposures of the hip, knee, and ankle.
- Repeat the procedure for the opposite limb.
- Use the same approach to measure lengths of the long bones in the upper limbs (Fig. 11-7).

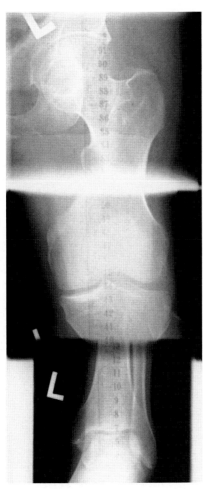

Fig. 11-6 Unilateral leg measurement.

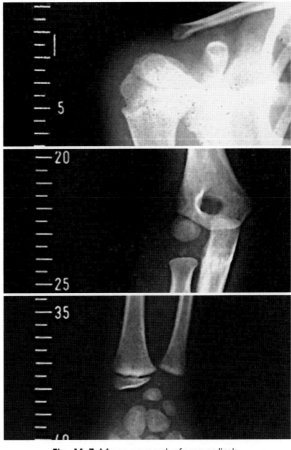

Fig. 11-7 Measurement of upper limb.

5

Computed Tomography Technique

Helms and McCarthy[4] reported a method for using computed tomography (CT) to measure discrepancies in leg length. Temme et al[5] compared conventional orthoroentgenograms with CT scans for long bone measurements. Both sets of investigators concluded that the CT scanogram is more consistently reproduced and that it causes less radiation exposure to the patient than the conventional radiographic approach. The CT approach is as follows:

- Take CT localizer or "scout" images of the femurs and tibias.

- Place cursors over the respective hip, knee, and ankle joints, as described earlier in this chapter. To study the upper limb similarly, obtain scout images of the humerus, radius, and ulna.

- Place CT cursors over the shoulder, elbow, and wrist joints, and obtain the measurements. These measurements are displayed on the cathode ray tube (Figs. 11-8 to 11-10).

The accuracy of the CT examination depends on proper placement of the cursor. Helms and McCarthy[4] found that accuracy improved when the cursors were placed three times and the values obtained were averaged. These authors also reported that CT examinations used radiation doses that were 50 to 200 times less than those used with conventional radiography, while Sabharwal and Kumar[1] reported the CT dose as 80% less than that of orthoroentgenograms. CT examination requires about the same amount of time as conventional radiography, and the costs are comparable.[1]

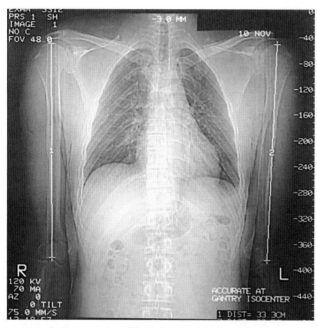

Fig. 11-8 Measurement of arms using CT. Note arm labels and measurements in right lower corner.

[4]Helms CA, McCarthy S: CT scanograms for measuring leg length discrepancy, *Radiology* 252:802, 1984.
[5]Temme JB et al: CT scanograms compared with conventional orthoroentgenograms in long bone measurement, *Radiol Technol* 59:65, 1987.

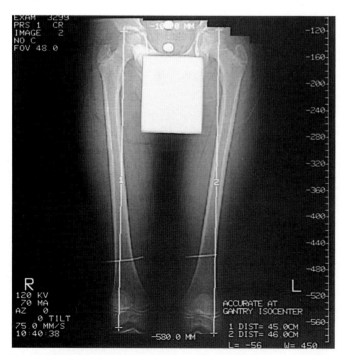

Fig. 11-9 CT measurements of femurs. Right femur is 1 cm shorter than left femur in the same patient as in Fig. 11-8.

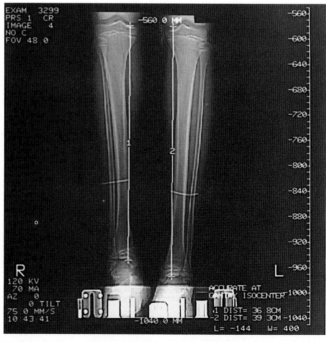

Fig. 11-10 CT measurement of legs in the same patient as in Figs. 11-8 and 11-9.

12
CONTRAST ARTHROGRAPHY

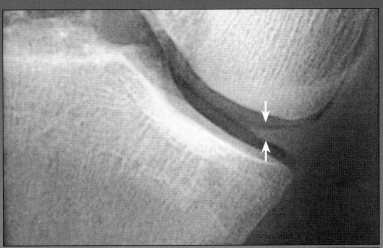

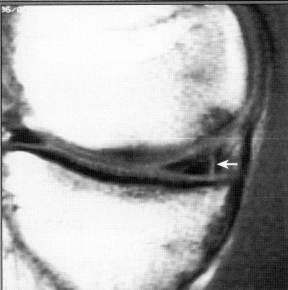

Overview

Contrast computed tomography (CT), shoulder magnetic resonance imaging (MRI) with and without contrast, and ultrasound (US) have drastically reduced the need for radiographic contrast arthrography (Fig. 12-1). Radiography of joints is still recommended as the initial imaging for many of the joints once imaged using contrast arthrography, yet the most recent recommendations by the American College of Radiology (ACR) rank radiographic contrast arthrography from very low or not at all as an appropriate diagnostic tool. Exceptions include the following:

- Contraindications for administration of gadolinium or lack of expertise for US exams[1]
- Aspiration in suspected septic or inflammatory arthropathies of the shoulder[1]
- After knee arthroplasty as a routine follow-up or for complications[2]
- To rule out the hip as the referred pain source after other negative imaging[3]

---

[1]ACR Appropriateness Criteria®: Acute shoulder pain, 2010.

[2]ACR Appropriateness Criteria®: Imaging after total knee arthroplasty, 2011.

[3]ACR Appropriateness Criteria®: Chronic hip pain, 2011.

Arthrography (Greek *arthron*, meaning "joint") is radiography of a joint or joints. *Pneumoarthrography, opaque arthrography,* and *double-contrast arthrography* are terms used to denote radiologic examinations of the soft tissue structures of joints (menisci, ligaments, articular cartilage, bursae) after injection of one or two contrast agents into the capsular space. A gaseous medium is used in pneumoarthrography, a water-soluble iodinated medium is used in opaque arthrography (Fig. 12-2), and a combination of gaseous and water-soluble iodinated media is used in double-contrast arthrography. Although contrast studies may be made on any

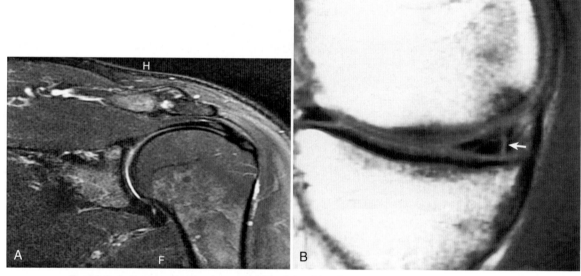

Fig. 12-1 A, Non–contrast-enhanced MRI of shoulder. **B,** Non–contrast-enhanced MRI of knee, showing torn medial meniscus (*arrow*).

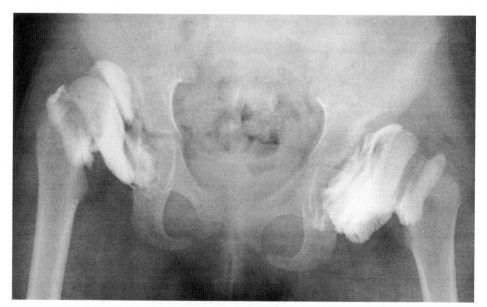

Fig. 12-2 Bilateral opaque arthrogram of bilateral congenital hip dislocations.

encapsulated joint, the shoulder is the most frequent site of investigation. The joints discussed in this chapter—shoulder, knee, and hip—are the ones most likely to be imaged using radiographic contrast arthrography. Other joints may be imaged occasionally with arthrography. As noted previously, MRI, CT, and US are the modalities most likely to be used to demonstrate pathologies of the joints and associated soft tissues.

Arthrogram examinations are usually performed with a local anesthetic. The injection is made under careful aseptic conditions, usually in a combination fluoroscopic-radiographic examining room that has been carefully prepared in advance. The sterile items required, particularly the length and gauge of the needles, vary according to the part being examined. The sterile tray and the nonsterile items should be set up on a conveniently placed instrument cart or a small two-shelf table (Fig. 12-3).

After aspirating any effusion, the radiologist injects the contrast agent or agents and manipulates the joint to ensure proper distribution of the contrast material. The examination is usually performed by fluoroscopy and spot images. Conventional radiographic images may be obtained when special images, such as an axial projection of the shoulder or an intercondyloid fossa position of the knee, are desired.

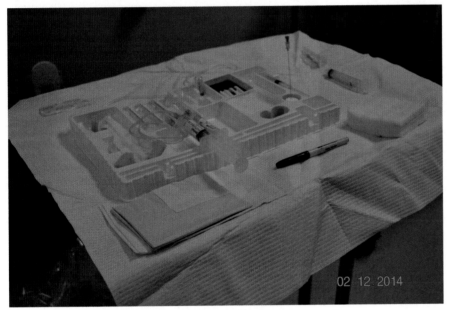

Fig. 12-3 Sterile arthrogram tray.

CONTRAST ARTHROGRAPHY PROCEDURES REMOVED

Based on review of the most recent ACR Appropriateness Criteria® available at the time of publication of this edition, contrast arthrography of the following joint has been removed from this edition. This procedure may be reviewed in the twelfth and all previous editions.

• Temporomandibular joint arthrography

SUMMARY OF PATHOLOGY

Condition	Definition
Developmental dysplasia of the hip	Denotes a wide spectrum of congenital hip abnormalities, ranging from acetabular dysplasia, joint laxity, and subluxation to complete dislocation
Dislocation	Displacement of a bone from a joint
Joint capsule tear	Rupture of the joint capsule
Ligament tear	Rupture of the ligament
Meniscus tear	Rupture of the meniscus
Rotator cuff tear	Rupture of any muscle of the rotator cuff

ABBREVIATIONS USED IN CHAPTER 12

ACR	American College of Radiology
DDH	Developmental dysplasia of the hip
MRI	Magnetic resonance imaging
PA	Posteroanterior

See Addendum B for a summary of all abbreviations used in Volume 2.

Shoulder Arthrography

Arthrography of the shoulder is performed primarily for the evaluation of partial or complete tears in the rotator cuff or glenoid labrum, persistent pain or weakness, and frozen shoulder. A single-contrast technique (Fig. 12-4) or a double-contrast technique (Fig. 12-5) may be used.

The usual injection site is approximately ½ inch (1.3 cm) inferior and lateral to the coracoid process. Because the joint capsule is usually deep, use of a spinal needle is recommended.

For a single-contrast arthrogram (Fig. 12-6), approximately 10 to 12 mL of positive contrast medium is injected into the shoulder. For double-contrast examinations, approximately 3 to 4 mL of positive contrast medium and 10 to 12 mL of air are injected into the shoulder.

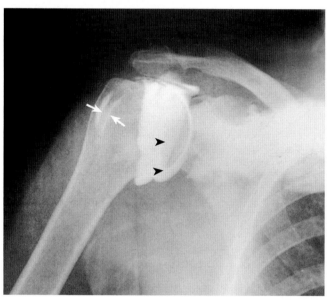

Fig. 12-4 Normal AP single-contrast shoulder arthrogram with contrast medium surrounding biceps tendon sleeve and lying in intertubercular (bicipital) groove (*arrows*). Axillary recess is filled but has normal medial filling defect (*arrowheads*), created by glenoid labrum.

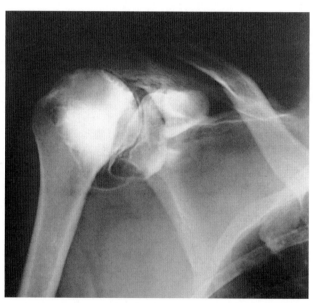

Fig. 12-5 Normal AP double-contrast shoulder arthrogram.

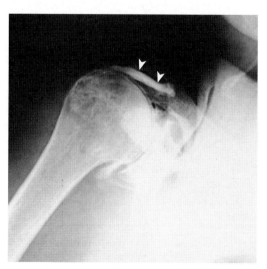

Fig. 12-6 Single-contrast arthrogram showing rotator cuff tear (*arrowheads*).

The projections most often used are the AP (internal and external rotation), 30-degree AP oblique, axillary (Figs. 12-7 and 12-8), and tangential. (See Volume 1, Chapter 5, for a description of patient and part positioning.)

After double-contrast shoulder arthrography is performed, computed tomography (CT) may be used to examine some patients. CT images may be obtained at approximately 5-mm intervals through the shoulder joint. In shoulder arthrography, CT has been found to be sensitive and reliable in diagnosis. Radiographs and CT scans of the same patient are presented in Figs. 12-5 and 12-9. Shoulder arthrography is increasingly performed with MRI, with injection of gadolinium contrast media into the joint capsule (Fig. 12-9, B).

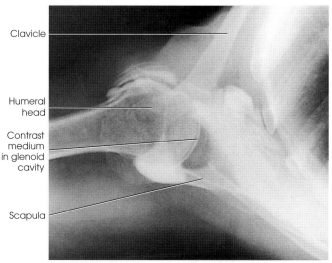

Fig. 12-7 Normal axillary single-contrast shoulder arthrogram.

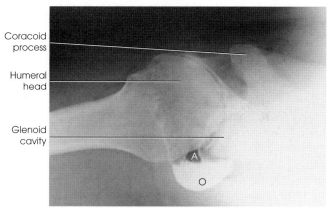

Fig. 12-8 Normal axillary double-contrast shoulder arthrogram projection of patient in supine position. Opaque medium (*O*) and air-created (*A*) density are seen anteriorly.

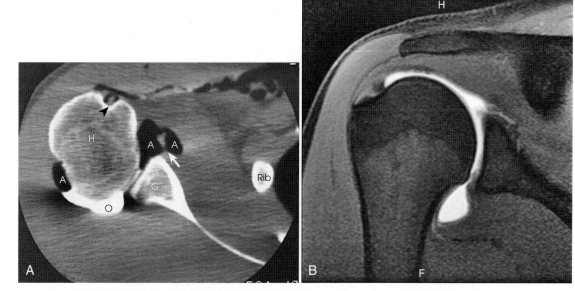

Fig. 12-9 A, CT shoulder arthrogram. Radiographic arthrogram in this patient was normal (see Fig. 12-5). CT shoulder arthrogram shows small chip fracture (*arrow*) on anterior surface of glenoid cavity. Head of humerus (*H*), air surrounding biceps tendon (*arrowhead*), air contrast medium (*A*), opaque contrast medium (*O*), and glenoid portion of scapula (*G*) are evident. **B,** MRI arthrogram of shoulder with injection of gadolinium contrast medium.

Contrast Arthrography of the Knee
VERTICAL RAY METHOD

Contrast arthrography of the knee by the vertical ray method requires the use of a stress device. The following steps are taken:

- Place the limb in the frame to widen or "open up" the side of the joint space under investigation. This widening, or spreading, of the intrastructural spaces

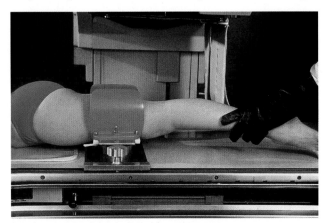

Fig. 12-10 Patient lying on lead rubber for gonad shielding and positioned in stress device on fluoroscopic table.

permits better distribution of the contrast material around the meniscus.
- After the contrast material is injected, place the limb into the stress device (Fig. 12-10). To delineate the medial side of the joint, place the stress device just above the knee and then laterally stress the lower leg.
- When contrast arthrograms are to be made by conventional radiography, turn the patient to the prone position, and fluoroscopically localize the centering

point for each side of the joint. The mark ensures accurate centering for closely collimated studies of each side of the joint and permits multiple exposures to be made on one IR. The images obtained of each side of the joint usually consist of an AP projection and a 20-degree right and left AP oblique projection.
- Obtain the oblique position by leg rotation or by central ray angulation (Fig. 12-11).
- On completion of these studies, remove the frame and perform lateral and intercondyloid fossa projections.

NOTE: Anderson and Maslin[1] recommended that tomography be used in knee arthrography. In addition, the technique frequently can be used for other contrast-filled joint capsules.

---

[1]Anderson PW, Maslin P: Tomography applied to knee arthrography, *Radiology* 110:271, 1974.

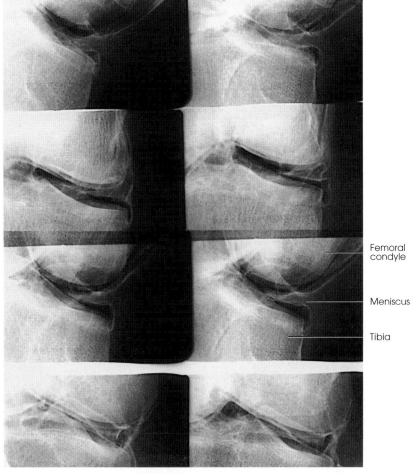

Femoral condyle

Meniscus

Tibia

Fig. 12-11 Vertical ray double-contrast knee arthrogram.

Double-Contrast Arthrography of the Knee
HORIZONTAL RAY METHOD

The horizontal central ray method of performing double-contrast arthrography of the knee was described first by Andrén and Wehlin[2] and later by Freiberger et al.[3] These investigators found that using a horizontal x-ray beam position and a comparatively small amount of each of the two contrast agents (gaseous medium and water-soluble iodinated medium) improved double-contrast delineation of the knee joint structures. With this technique, the excess of the heavy iodinated solutions drains into the dependent part of the joint, leaving only the desired thin opaque coating on the gas-enveloped uppermost part—the part under investigation.

[2]Andrén L, Wehlin L: Double-contrast arthrography of knee with horizontal roentgen ray beam, *Acta Orthop Scand* 29:307, 1960.
[3]Freiberger RH et al: Arthrography of the knee by double contrast method, *AJR Am J Roentgenol* 97:736, 1966.

Medial meniscus

- Adjust the patient in a semiprone position that places the posterior aspect of the medial meniscus uppermost (Fig. 12-12).
- To widen the joint space, manually stress the knee.
- Draw a line on the medial side of the knee, and direct the central ray along the line and centered to the meniscus.
- With rotation toward the supine position, turn the leg 30 degrees for each of the succeeding five exposures.
- Direct the central ray along the localization line for each exposure, ensuring that it is centered to the meniscus.

Lateral meniscus

- Adjust the patient in a semiprone position that places the posterior aspect of the lateral meniscus uppermost (Fig. 12-13).
- To widen the joint space, manually stress the knee.
- As with the medial meniscus, make six images on one IR.
- With movement toward the supine position, rotate the leg 30 degrees for each of the consecutive exposures, from the initial prone oblique position to the supine oblique position.
- Adjust the central ray angulation as required to direct it along the localization line and center it to the meniscus.

NOTE: To show the cruciate ligaments after filming of the menisci is completed,[1] the patient sits with the knee flexed 90 degrees over the side of the radiographic table. A firm cotton pillow is placed under the knee and is adjusted so that some forward pressure can be applied to the leg. With the patient holding a grid IR in position, a closely collimated and slightly overexposed lateral projection is made.

[1]Mittler S et al: A method of improving cruciate ligament visualization in double-contrast arthrography, *Radiology* 102:441, 1972.

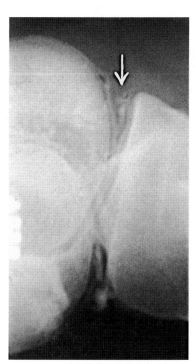

Fig. 12-12 Image showing tear (*arrow*) in medial meniscus.

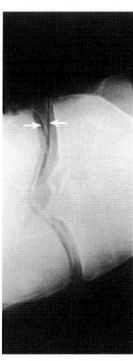

Fig. 12-13 Normal lateral meniscus (*arrows*).

Hip Arthrography

Hip arthrography is most often performed on children in a surgery suite by an orthopedic surgeon. Arthrography is used to evaluate lateral femoral head displacement and after closed reduction to ensure that there is no folding or impingement of soft tissues (see Fig. 12-2, pretreatment) (Figs. 12-14 and 12-15, post-treatment). In adults, the primary use of hip arthrography is to detect a loose hip prosthesis or to confirm the presence of infection. The cement used to fasten hip prosthesis components has barium sulfate added to make the cement and the cement-bone interface radiographically visible (Fig. 12-16). Although the addition of barium sulfate to cement is helpful in confirming proper seating of the prosthesis, it makes evaluation of the same joint by arthrography difficult.

Because cement and contrast material produce the same approximate radiographic brightness, a subtraction technique is recommended—either photographic subtraction, as shown in Figs. 12-17 and 12-18, or digital subtraction, as shown in Figs. 12-19 and 12-20 (see Chapter 23). A common puncture site for hip arthrography is ¾ inch (1.9 cm) distal to the inguinal crease and ¾ inch (1.9 cm) lateral to the palpated femoral pulse. A spinal needle is useful for reaching the joint capsule.

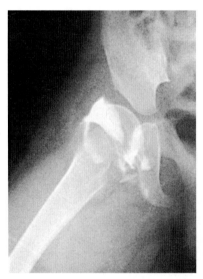

Fig. 12-14 AP opaque arthrogram showing treated congenital right hip dislocation in the same patient as in Fig. 12-2.

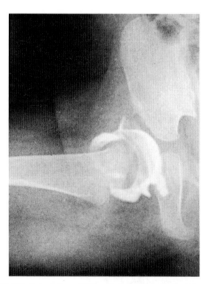

Fig. 12-15 Axiolateral "frog" right hip of patient treated for congenital dislocation of the hip.

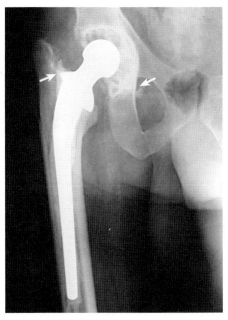

Fig. 12-16 AP hip radiograph showing radiopaque cement (*arrows*) used to secure hip prosthesis.

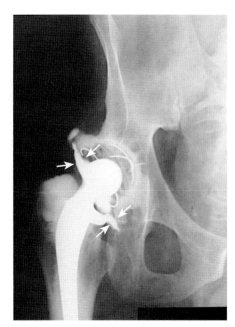

Fig. 12-17 AP hip arthrogram showing hip prosthesis in proper position. Cement with radiopaque additive is difficult to distinguish from contrast medium used to perform arthrography (*arrows*).

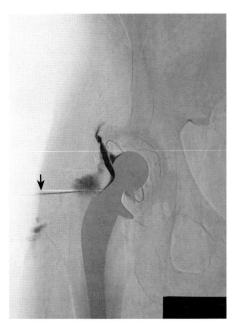

Fig. 12-18 Normal photographic subtraction AP hip arthrogram in the same patient as in Fig. 12-16. Contrast medium (*black image*) is readily distinguished from hip prosthesis by subtraction technique. Contrast medium does not extend inferiorly below level of injection needle (*arrow*). (See Chapter 23 for a description of subtraction technique.)

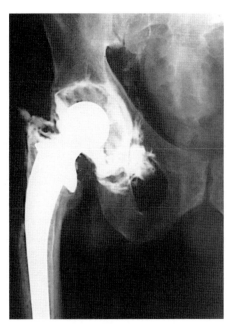

Fig. 12-19 AP hip radiograph after injection of contrast medium.

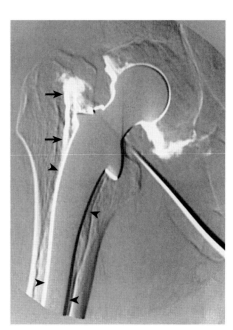

Fig. 12-20 Digital subtraction hip arthrogram in the same patient as in Fig. 12-19. Contrast medium around prosthesis in proximal lateral femoral shaft (*arrows*) indicates loose prosthesis. Lines on medial and lateral aspect of femur (*arrowheads*) are a subtraction registration artifact caused by slight patient movement during injection of contrast medium. (See Chapter 23 for a description of subtraction technique.)

Other Joints

Essentially any joint *can* be evaluated by arthrography. A wrist arthrogram is included here as an example (Fig. 12-21).

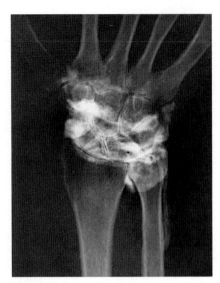

Fig. 12-21 Opaque arthrogram of wrist, showing rheumatoid arthritis.

13

TRAUMA RADIOGRAPHY

JOE A. GARZA

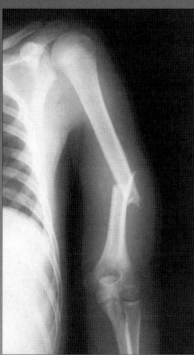

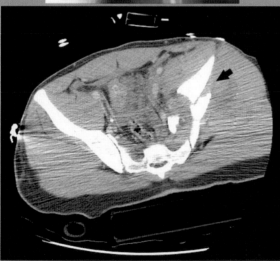

Introduction

Trauma is defined as severe injury or damage to the body caused by an accident or violence. Victims of trauma require immediate and specialized care, which is commonly provided in larger hospitals within a specialized unit, termed the *emergency department* (ED). Physicians and many nurses specialize in trauma care. Imaging professionals are essential to the diagnosis of injuries sustained during traumatic events, so extra study in this area of imaging is necessary. Trauma radiography can be an exciting and challenging environment for a properly prepared imaging professional. These procedures can be intimidating and stressful for individuals unprepared for the innumerable injuries seen in the ED. The essential key to quality imaging procedures for trauma patients is proper study and preparation for imaging professionals.

Preparation for the trauma environment requires an understanding of the following: the most common traumatic injuries, the most commonly affected populations, types of trauma care facilities, specialized imaging equipment designed for imaging of trauma patients, the role of the imaging technologist as part of the ED team, and imaging procedures commonly performed on trauma patients. This chapter provides the information necessary to improve the skills and confidence of all imaging professionals caring for trauma patients.

Trauma Statistics

Trauma-related injuries affect persons in all age ranges. Fig. 13-1 shows trauma incidence by age and gender, as reported by the American College of Surgeons' National Trauma Database (NTDB) 2012 annual report. The database contains more than 5 million records from more than 744 hospitals and has received information from across the United States. These data show that trauma patients most commonly are male and range in age from teenagers to early adults. Fig. 13-2 shows the distribution of trauma injuries by cause; the most common are falls, followed by motor vehicle accidents (MVAs). Firearms rank last as a cause of injury; however, the 2012 NTDB report also shows that

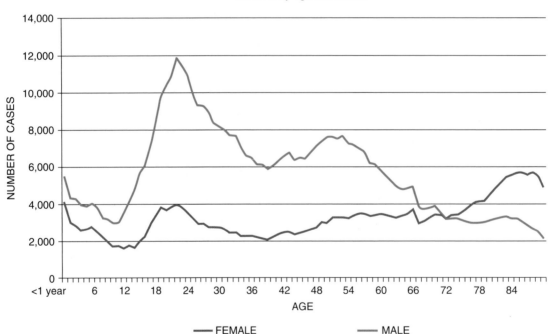

Fig. 13-1 NTDB annual report, 2012, table showing number of trauma incidents by age and gender.

(Reprinted by permission of the American College of Surgeons.)

firearms have the highest fatality rate. The data show the most common trauma patients and mechanisms of injury, but the imaging professional who chooses to work in the ED must be prepared to care for patients of every age exhibiting a vast array of injuries.

Many types of facilities provide emergency medical care, ranging from major medical centers to small outpatient clinics in rural areas. The term *trauma center* denotes a specific level of emergency medical care as defined by the American College of Surgeons Commission on Trauma. Four levels of care are defined. Level I is the most comprehensive, and Level IV is the most basic. A *Level I* trauma center is usually a university-based center, research facility, or large medical center. It provides the most comprehensive emergency medical care available with complete imaging capabilities and all types of specialty physicians available on site 24 hours per day. Imaging professionals are also available 24 hours per day. A *Level II* trauma center probably has all of the same specialized care available but is not a research or teaching hospital, and some specialty physicians may not be available on site. *Level III* trauma centers are usually located in smaller communities where Level I or Level II care is unavailable. Level III centers generally do not have all specialists available but can resuscitate, stabilize, assess, and prepare a patient for transfer to a larger trauma center. A *Level IV trauma* center may not be a hospital at all, but rather a clinic or other outpatient setting. These facilities usually provide care for minor injuries and offer stabilization and arrange for transfer of patients with more serious injuries to a larger trauma center.

Trauma injuries can occur by several types of forces, including *blunt, penetrating, explosive,* and *heat.* Examples of blunt trauma are MVAs, which include motorcycle accidents, collisions with pedestrians, falls, and aggravated assaults. Penetrating trauma events include gunshot wounds (GSWs), stab wounds, impalement injuries, and foreign body ingestion or aspiration. Explosive trauma causes injury by several mechanisms including pressure shock waves, high-velocity projectiles, and burns. Heat trauma includes burn injuries, which may be caused by numerous agents including fire, steam, hot water, chemicals, electricity, and frostbite.

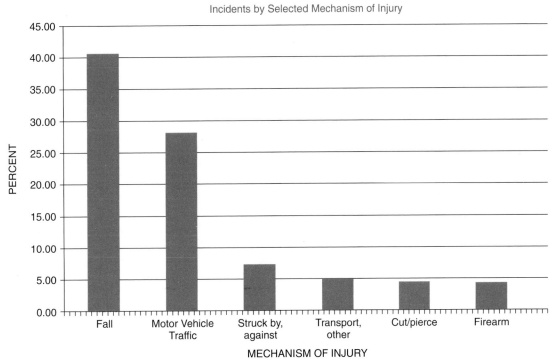

Fig. 13-2 NTDB annual report, 2012, table showing number of patients injured by each mechanism.

(Reprinted by permission of the American College of Surgeons.)

Preliminary Considerations

SPECIALIZED EQUIPMENT

Time is a crucial element in the care of a trauma patient. To minimize the time needed to acquire diagnostic x-ray images, many EDs have dedicated radiographic equipment located in the department or immediately adjacent to the department. Trauma radiographs must be taken with minimal patient movement, requiring more maneuvering of the tube and image receptor (IR). Specialized trauma radiographic systems are available and are designed to provide greater flexibility in x-ray tube and IR maneuverability (Fig. 13-3). These specialized systems help to minimize movement of the injured patient while imaging procedures are performed. Additionally, some EDs are equipped with specialized beds or stretchers that have a movable tray to hold the IR. This type of stretcher allows the use of a mobile radiographic unit and eliminates the requirement for and risk of transferring an injured patient to the radiographic table.

Computed tomography (CT) is widely used for imaging of trauma patients. In many cases, CT is the first imaging modality used, now that image acquisition has become almost instantaneous. (Refer to Chapter 29 in Volume 3 for a detailed explanation and description of CT.) The only major concern with CT imaging compared with radiography is the radiation dose. The debate centers on the exclusive use of CT, when lower-dose radiographs may be sufficient for a diagnosis. Patients who are at high risk and who are not good candidates for quality radiographs based on their injuries may be referred to CT first.

Mobile radiography is often a necessity in the emergency department. Many patients have injuries that prohibit transfer to a radiographic table, or their condition may be too critical to interrupt treatment. Trauma radiographers must be competent in performing mobile radiography on almost any part of the body and must be able to use accessory devices (e.g., grids, air-gap technique) to produce quality mobile images.

Mobile fluoroscopic units, usually referred to as *C-arms* because of their shape, are becoming more commonplace in EDs. C-arms are used for fracture reduction procedures, foreign body localization in limbs, and reduction of joint dislocations (Fig. 13-4).

An emerging imaging technology has the potential to have a significant effect on trauma radiography. The Statscan (Lodox Systems [Pty.], Ltd., Johannesburg, South Africa) is a relatively new imaging device that produces full-body imaging scans in approximately 13 seconds without the need to move the patient (Figs. 13-5 to 13-7). At present approximately 17 of these systems are available worldwide. At a cost of approximately $450,000, this technology is an expensive addition to a trauma imaging department.

Positioning aids are essential for quality imaging in trauma radiography. Sponges, sandbags, and tape used creatively are often the trauma radiographer's most useful tools. Most patients who are injured cannot hold the required positions because of pain or impaired consciousness. Other patients cannot be moved into the proper position because to do so would exacerbate their injury. Proper use of positioning aids assists in quick adaptation of procedures to accommodate the patient's condition.

Grids and IR holders are also an important part of trauma radiography because many projections require the use of a horizontal central ray. Grids should be inspected regularly because a damaged grid often causes image artifacts. IR holders enable the radiographer to perform cross-table lateral projections (dorsal decubitus position) on numerous body parts with minimal distortion. To prevent unnecessary exposure, ED personnel should not hold the IR.

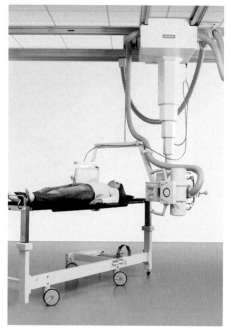

Fig. 13-3 Dedicated C-arm–type trauma radiographic room with patient on the table.

(Courtesy Siemens Healthcare.)

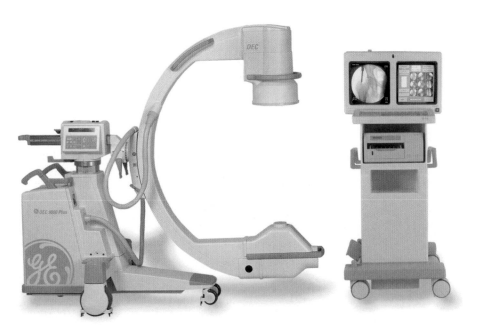

Fig. 13-4 Mobile fluoroscopic C-arm.

(Courtesy OEC Diasonics, Inc.)

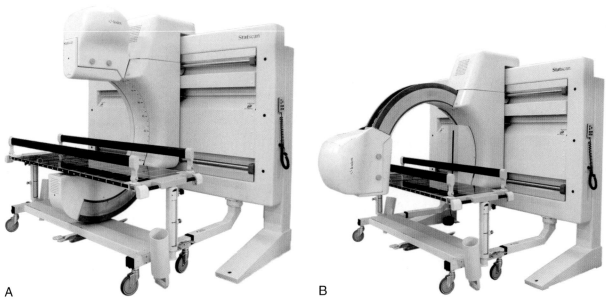

A   B

Fig. 13-5 A, Statscan system configured for AP projection. **B,** Statscan system configured for lateral projection.

(Courtesy Lodox Systems (Pty.), Ltd.)

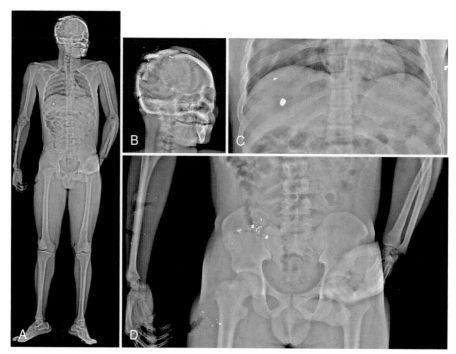

Fig. 13-6 Statscan of patient with multiple GSWs. **A,** AP full-body scan—13 seconds required for acquisition. Shrapnel and projectile pathways identified by zooming in on areas of full-body scan. **B,** Skull. **C,** Diaphragm area. **D,** Pelvis.

(Courtesy Lodox Systems (Pty.), Ltd.)

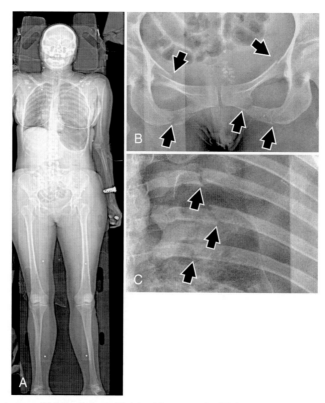

Fig. 13-7 Statscan of MVA victim with blunt trauma. **A,** AP full-body scan. Tension pneumothorax shown without additional processing. **B,** Zoomed lower pelvis showing multiple fractures (*arrows*). **C,** Zoomed bony thorax showing rib fractures (*arrows*).

(Courtesy Lodox Systems (Pty.), Ltd.)

EXPOSURE FACTORS

Patient motion is always a consideration in trauma radiography. The shortest possible exposure time that can be set should be used in all procedures, except when a breathing technique is desired. Unconscious patients cannot suspend respiration for the exposure. Conscious patients are often in extreme pain and unable to cooperate for the procedure.

Radiographic exposure factor compensation may be required when exposures are made through immobilization devices such as a spine board or backboard. Most trauma patients arrive at the hospital with some type of immobilization device (Fig. 13-8). Pathologic changes should also be considered when technical factors are set. Internal bleeding in the abdominal cavity would absorb a greater amount of radiation than a bowel obstruction.

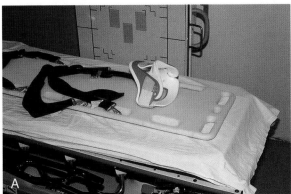
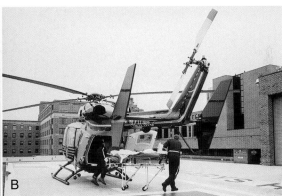
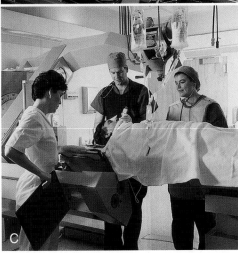

Fig. 13-8 A, Typical backboard and neck brace used for trauma patients. **B,** Backboard, brace, and other restraints are used on the patient throughout transport. **C,** All restraints remain with and on the patient until all x-ray examinations are completed.

POSITIONING OF THE PATIENT

The primary challenge of the trauma radiographer is to obtain a high-quality, diagnostic image on the first attempt when the patient is unable to move into the desired position. Many methods are available to adapt a routine projection and obtain the desired image of the anatomic part. To minimize the risk of aggravating the patient's condition, the x-ray tube and IR should be positioned, rather than the patient or the part. The stretcher can be positioned adjacent to the vertical Bucky or upright table as the patient's condition allows (Fig. 13-9). This location enables accurate positioning with minimal patient movement for cross-table lateral images (dorsal decubitus positions) on numerous parts of the body. Additionally, the grid in the table or vertical Bucky is usually of a higher ratio than grids used for mobile radiography, so image contrast is improved. Another technique to increase efficiency while minimizing patient movement is to take all of the AP projections of the requested examinations while moving superiorly to inferiorly. All lateral projections of the requested examinations are then performed while moving inferiorly to superiorly. This method moves the x-ray tube in the most expeditious manner.

When radiographs are taken to localize a penetrating foreign object, such as metal, glass fragments, or bullets, entrance and exit wounds should be marked with a radiopaque marker that is visible on all projections (Fig. 13-10). Two exposures at right angles to each other will demonstrate the depth and path of the projectile.

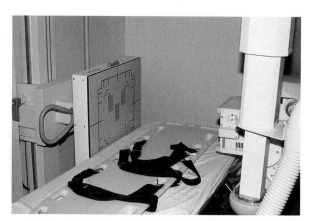

Fig. 13-9 Stretcher positioned adjacent to vertical Bucky to expedite positioning. Note x-ray tube in position for lateral projections.

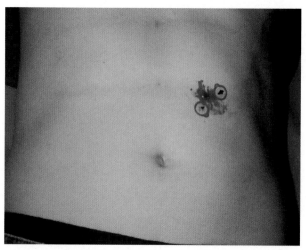

Fig. 13-10 Proper placement of radiopaque markers (*inside red circles*) on each side of bullet entrance wound. Red circles are "stickies" that contain radiopaque marker.

Radiographer's Role as Part of the Trauma Team

The role of the radiographer within the ED ultimately depends on the department protocol and staffing and the extent of emergency care provided at the facility. Regardless of the size of the facility, the primary responsibilities of a radiographer in an emergency situation include the following:

- Perform quality diagnostic imaging procedures as requested
- Practice ethical radiation protection for self, patient, and other personnel
- Provide competent patient care

Ranking these responsibilities is impossible because they occur simultaneously, and all are vital to quality care in the ED.

DIAGNOSTIC IMAGING PROCEDURES

Producing a high-quality diagnostic image is an obvious role of any radiographer; a radiographer in the trauma environment has the added responsibility to perform that task efficiently. Efficiency and productivity are common and practical goals for the radiology department. In the ED, efficiency is often crucial to saving the patient's life. Diagnostic imaging in the ED is paramount to an accurate, timely, and often lifesaving diagnosis.

RADIATION PROTECTION

One of the most important duties and ethical responsibilities of the trauma radiographer is radiation protection of the patient, members of the trauma team, and the radiographer himself or herself. In critical care situations, members of the trauma team cannot leave the patient while imaging procedures are being performed. The trauma radiographer must ensure that the other team members are protected from unnecessary radiation exposure. Common practices should minimally include the following:

- Close collimation to the anatomy of interest to reduce scatter
- Gonadal shielding for patients of child-bearing age (when doing so does not interfere with the anatomy of interest)
- Lead aprons for all personnel that remain in the room during the procedure
- Exposure factors that minimize patient dose and scattered radiation
- Announcement of impending exposure to allow unnecessary personnel to exit the room

Consideration must also be given to patients on nearby stretchers. If these patients are less than 6 feet away from the x-ray tube, appropriate shielding should be provided. Some of the greatest exposures to patients and medical personnel result from fluoroscopic procedures. If the C-arm fluoroscopic unit is used in the ED, special precautions should be in place to ensure that fluoroscopic exposure time is kept to a minimum and that all personnel are wearing protective aprons.

PATIENT CARE

As with all imaging procedures, trauma procedures require a patient history. The patient may provide this history, if he or she is conscious, or the attending physician may inform the radiographer of the injury and the patient's status. If the patient is conscious, the radiographer should explain what he or she is doing in detail and in terms the patient can understand. The radiographer should listen to the patient's rate and manner of speech, which may provide insight into the patient's mental and emotional status. The radiographer should make eye contact with the patient to provide comfort and reassurance. A trip to the ED is an emotionally stressful event, regardless of the severity of injury or illness.

Radiographers are often responsible for the total care of the trauma patient while performing diagnostic imaging proce-dures. It is crucial that the radiographer constantly assess the patient's condition, recognize any signs of deterioration or distress, and report any change in the status of the patient's condition to the attending physician. The trauma radiographer must be knowledgeable in taking vital signs as well as knowing normal ranges and must be competent in performing cardiopulmonary resuscitation (CPR), administering oxygen, and dealing with all types of medical emergencies. The radiographer must be prepared to perform these procedures when covered by a standing physician's order or as departmental policy allows. The radiographer should also be familiar with the location and contents of the adult and pediatric crash carts and should understand how to use the suctioning devices.

The CAB *(compressions, airway, and breathing)* of basic life support techniques must be constantly assessed during radiographic procedures. Visual inspection and verbal questioning enable the radiographer to determine whether the status of the patient changes during the procedure. Table 13-1 provides a guide for the trauma radiographer regarding changes in status that should be reported immediately to the attending physician. Table 13-1 includes only the *common* injuries in which the radiographer may be the sole health care professional with the patient during the imaging procedure. Patients with multiple trauma injuries and patients in respiratory or cardiac arrest usually are imaged with a mobile radiographic unit while ED personnel are present in the room. In these situations, the primary responsibility of the trauma radiographer is to produce quality images in an efficient manner while practicing ethical radiation protection measures.

TABLE 13-1
Guide for reporting patient status change

Noted symptom	Possible cause	When to report to physician immediately
Cool, clammy skin	Shock* Vasovagal reaction†	Other symptoms of shock present
Excessive sweating (*diaphoresis*)	Shock*	Other symptoms of shock present
Slurred speech	Head injury Stroke (cerebrovascular accident‡) Drug or ethanol influence§	Accompanied by vomiting, especially if vomiting stops when patient is moved to different position
Agitation or confusion	Head injury Drug or ethanol influence§	Accompanied by vomiting, especially if vomiting stops when patient is moved to different position
Vomiting (without abdominal complaints) (*hyperemesis*)	Head injury Hyperglycemia‖ Drug or ethanol overdose	Position of patient abruptly stimulates vomiting or abruptly stops vomiting
Increased drowsiness (*lethargy*)	Shock* Head injury Hyperglycemia‖	Other symptoms of shock present or accompanied by vomiting
Loss of consciousness (unresponsive to voice or touch)	Shock* Head injury Hyperglycemia‖	Immediately
Pale or bluish skin pallor (*cyanosis*)	Airway compromise Hypovolemic shock	Immediately
Bluish nail beds	Circulatory compromise	Immediately
Patient complains of thirst	Shock* Hyperglycemia‖ Hypoglycemia	Other symptoms of shock present
Patient complains of tingling or numbness (*paresthesia*) or inability to move a limb	Spinal cord injury Peripheral nerve impairment	Accompanied by any symptoms of shock or altered consciousness
Seizures	Head injury	Immediately
Patient states that he or she cannot feel your touch (*paralysis*)	Spinal cord injury Peripheral nerve impairment	Accompanied by any symptoms of shock or altered consciousness
Extreme eversion of foot	Fracture of proximal femur or hip joint	Report only if x-ray request specifies "frog leg" lateral projection of hip. This movement would exacerbate patient's injury and cause intense pain. Surgical lateral position should be substituted. Watch for changes in abdominal size and firmness
Increasing abdominal distention and firmness to palpation	Internal bleeding from pelvic fracture¶ or organ laceration	Immediately

Hypovolemic or *hemorrhagic shock* is a medical condition in which levels of blood plasma in the body are abnormally low, such that the body cannot properly maintain blood pressure, cardiac output of blood, and normal amounts of fluid in the tissues. It is the most common type of shock in trauma patients. Symptoms include diaphoresis, cool and clammy skin, decrease in venous pressure, decrease in urine output, thirst, and altered state of consciousness.

†*Vasovagal reaction* is also called a vasovagal attack, situational syncope, and vasovagal syncope. It is a reflex of the involuntary nervous system or a normal physiologic response to emotional stress. Patients may complain of nausea, feeling flushed (warm), and feeling light-headed. They may appear pale before they lose consciousness for several seconds.

‡*Cerebrovascular accident* (CVA) is commonly called a stroke and may be caused by thrombosis, embolism, or hemorrhage in the vessels of the brain.

§*Drugs or alcohol*. Patients under the influence of drugs or alcohol or both commonly present in the ED. In this situation, the usual symptoms of shock and head injury are unreliable. Be on guard for aggressive physical behaviors and abusive language.

‖*Hyperglycemia* is also known as diabetic ketoacidosis. The cause is increased blood glucose levels. The patient may exhibit any combination of symptoms noted and has fruity-smelling breath.

¶*Pelvic fractures* have a high mortality rate (mortality with open fractures may be 50%). Hemorrhage and shock are often associated with this type of injury.

Best Practices in Trauma Radiography

Radiography of the trauma patient seldom allows the use of "routine" positions and projections. Additionally, the trauma patient requires special attention to patient care techniques while difficult imaging procedures are performed. The following best practices provide some universal guidelines for the trauma radiographer.

1. *Speed:* Trauma radiographers must produce quality images in the shortest amount of time. Speed in performing a diagnostic examination is crucial to saving the patient's life. Many practical methods that increase examination efficiency without sacrificing image quality are introduced in this chapter.

2. *Accuracy:* Trauma radiographers must provide accurate images with a minimal amount of distortion and with the maximum amount of recorded detail. Alignment of the central ray, the part, and the IR is imperative in trauma radiography. Using the shortest exposure time minimizes the possibility of involuntary and uncontrollable patient motion on the image.

3. *Quality:* Quality does not have to be sacrificed to produce an image quickly. The patient's condition should not be used as an excuse for careless positioning and accepting less than high-quality images.

4. *Positioning:* Careful precautions must be taken to ensure that performance of the imaging procedure does not worsen the patient's injuries. The "golden rule" of two projections at right angles from one another still applies. As often as possible, the radiographer should position the tube and the IR, rather than the patient, to obtain the desired projections.

5. *Practice standard precautions:* Exposure to blood and body fluids should be expected in trauma radiography. The radiographer should wear gloves, mask, eye shields, and gown when appropriate. IR and sponges should be placed in nonporous plastic to protect them from body fluids. Hand hygiene should be performed frequently, especially between patients. All equipment and accessory devices should be kept clean and ready for use.

6. *Immobilization:* The radiographer should *never* remove any immobilization device without physician's orders. The radiographer should provide proper immobilization and support to increase patient comfort and to minimize risk of motion.

7. *Anticipation:* Anticipating required special projections or diagnostic procedures for certain injuries makes the radiographer a vital part of the ED team. Patients requiring surgery generally require an x-ray of the chest. In facilities where CT is not readily available for emergency patients, fractures of the pelvis may require a cystogram to determine the status of the urinary bladder. The radiographer should know which procedures are often referred to CT first or for additional images. Being prepared for and understanding the necessity of these additional procedures and images instills confidence in, and creates an appreciation for, the role of the radiographer in the emergency setting.

8. *Attention to detail:* The radiographer should *never* leave a trauma patient (or any patient) unattended during imaging procedures. The patient's condition may change at any time, and it is the radiographer's responsibility to note these changes and report them immediately to the attending physician. If the radiographer cannot process images while maintaining eye contact with the patient, he or she should call for help. Someone must be with the injured patient at all times.

9. *Attention to department protocol and scope of practice:* The radiographer should know department protocols and practice only within his or her own competence and abilities. The scope of practice for radiographers varies from state to state and from country to country. The radiographer should study and understand the scope of his or her role in the emergency setting. The radiographer should not provide or offer a patient anything by mouth. The radiographer should always ask the attending physician before giving the patient anything to eat or drink, no matter how persistent the patient may be.

10. *Professionalism:* Ethical conduct and professionalism in all situations and with every person is a requirement of all health care professionals, but the conditions encountered in the ED can be particularly complicated. The radiographer should adhere to the Code of Ethics for Radiologic Technologists (see Chapter 1) and the Radiography Practice Standards. The radiographer should be aware of the people present or nearby at all times when discussing a patient's care. The ED radiographer is exposed to countless tragic conditions. Emotional reactions are common and expected but must be controlled until emergency care of the patient is complete.

Radiographic Procedures in Trauma

The projections included in this chapter result from a telephone survey of Level I trauma centers. The results indicate that common radiographic projections ordered for initial trauma surveys are as follows[1]:

- Cervical spine, dorsal decubitus position (cross-table lateral)
- Chest, AP (mobile)
- Abdomen, AP (kidneys, ureter, and bladder [KUB] and acute abdominal series)
- Pelvis, AP
- Cervical spine, AP and obliques
- Lumbar spine
- Lower limb
- Upper limb

Skull radiographs did not rank as one of the most common imaging procedures performed in the ED of Level I trauma centers. Most Level I trauma centers have replaced conventional trauma skull radiographs (e.g., AP, lateral, Towne, reverse Waters) with CT scan of the head (Fig. 13-11). Research articles continue to delineate the advantages of CT over radiography, and the results indicate that certain types of head trauma should be referred to CT first. However, because smaller facilities may not have CT readily available, trauma skull positioning remains valuable knowledge for the radiographer.

[1]Thomas Wolfe, Methodist Medical Center, Memphis, TN, conducted the survey as a part of his graduate practicum for Midwestern State University.

This section provides trauma positioning instructions for radiography projections of the following body areas:

- Cervical spine
  Lateral (dorsal decubitus position)
  Cervicothoracic (dorsal decubitus position)
  AP axial
  AP axial oblique
- Thoracic and lumbar spine
  Lateral (dorsal decubitus position)
- Chest
  AP
- Abdomen
  AP
  AP (left lateral decubitus position)
- Pelvis
  AP
- Skull
  Lateral (dorsal decubitus position)
  AP or PA
  AP axial (Towne method)
- Facial bones
  Acanthioparietal (reverse Waters method)
- Limbs
- Other imaging procedures

In addition to the dorsal decubitus positions, AP projections of the thoracic and lumbar spine are usually required for trauma radiographic surveys. AP projections of this anatomy vary minimally in the trauma setting and are not discussed in detail. Critical study and clinical practice of these procedures should adequately prepare a radiographer for work in the ED. Certain criteria that apply in all trauma imaging procedures are explained next and are not included on each procedure in detail.

PATIENT PREPARATION

Remembering that the patient has endured an emotionally disturbing and distressing event in addition to the physical injuries he or she may have sustained is important. If the patient is conscious, speak calmly and look directly into the patient's eyes while explaining the procedures that have been ordered. Do not assume that the patient cannot hear you, even if he or she cannot or will not respond. Check the patient thoroughly for items that might cause an artifact on the images. Explain what you are removing from the patient and why. Place all removed personal effects, especially valuables, in the proper container used by the facility (i.e., plastic bag) or in the designated secure area. Each facility has a procedure regarding proper storage of a patient's personal belongings. Know the procedure and follow it carefully.

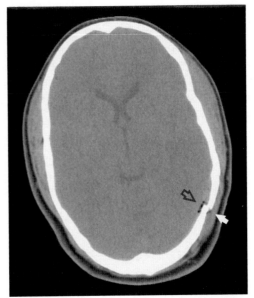

Fig. 13-11 CT scan of skull showing displaced fracture (*white arrow*). Intracranial air is present (*black open arrow*).

(Courtesy Sunie Grossman, RT(R), St. Bernard's Medical Center, Jonesboro, AR.)

BREATHING INSTRUCTIONS

Most injured patients have difficulty following the recommended breathing instructions for routine projections. For these patients, exposure factors should be set using the shortest possible exposure time to minimize motion on the radiograph, necessitating use of the large focal spot. The decrease in resolution from using a large focal spot is minimal compared with the significant loss of resolution due to patient motion. If a breathing technique is desired, this can be explained to a conscious trauma patient in the usual manner. If the patient is unconscious or unresponsive, careful attention should be paid to the rate and degree of chest wall movement. If inspiration is desired on the image, the exposure should be timed to correspond to the highest point of chest expansion. Conversely, if the routine projection calls for exposure on expiration, the exposure should be made when the patient's chest wall falls to its lowest point.

IMMOBILIZATION DEVICES

A wide variety of immobilization devices are used to stabilize injured patients. Standard protocol is to perform radiographic images without removing immobilization devices. After injuries have been diagnosed or ruled out, the attending physician gives the order for immobilization devices to be removed or changed, or to remain in place.

Many procedures necessitate the use of some sort of immobilization to prevent involuntary and voluntary motion. Many patient care textbooks discuss prudent use of such immobilization devices. The key issues in the use of immobilization in trauma are to avoid exacerbating the patient's injury and to avoid increasing his or her discomfort.

IMAGE RECEPTOR SIZE AND COLLIMATED FIELD

The IR sizes (film-screen and CR imaging plates) used in trauma procedures are the same as those specified for the routine projection of the anatomy of interest. Occasionally, the physician may request that more of a part be included, and then a larger IR or field size is acceptable. When using the large flat panel digital radiography (DR) detectors, use the recommended IR size as a reference; it is important to collimate to the anatomy of interest to provide optimal quality images and ethical radiation protection for the patient and other personnel who may be required to be in the room during the imaging procedures. Exposure of unnecessary tissue generates excessive scatter, which is a primary source of radiation exposure for radiographers and other health care professionals.

CENTRAL RAY, PART, AND IMAGE RECEPTOR ALIGNMENT

Unless otherwise indicated for the procedure, the central ray should be directed perpendicular to the midpoint of the grid or IR or both. Tips for minimizing distortion are detailed in the procedures in which distortion is a potential threat to image quality.

IMAGE EVALUATION

Ideally, trauma images should be of optimal quality to ensure prompt and accurate diagnosis of the patient's injuries. Evaluate images for proper positioning and technique as indicated in the routine projections. Allowances can be made when true right-angle projections (AP, PA, and lateral) must be altered as a result of the patient's condition.

DOCUMENTATION

Deviation from routine projections is necessary in many instances. Documenting the alterations in routine projections for the attending physician and radiologist is important, so that they can interpret the images properly. Additionally, the radiographer often has to determine whether the anatomy of interest has been adequately shown and perform additional projections (within the scope of the ordered examination) on an injured part to aid in proper diagnosis. Notations concerning additional projections are extremely helpful for the interpreting physicians.

ABBREVIATIONS USED IN CHAPTER 13	
CPR	Cardiopulmonary resuscitation
CR	Central ray
CVA	Cerebrovascular accident
EAM	External acoustic meatus
ED	Emergency department
GSW	Gunshot wound
IOML	Infraorbitomeatal line
IVU	Intravenous urography
KUB	Kidneys, ureters, and bladder
MML	Mentomeatal line
MVA	Motor vehicle accident
OML	Orbitomeatal line
SID	Source–to–image receptor distance

See Addendum B for a summary of all abbreviations used in Volume 2.

LATERAL PROJECTION[1]
Dorsal decubitus position
Trauma positioning tips

- *Always* perform this projection first, before any other projections. Level I centers may refer patients with indications for cervical spine imaging to CT first, depending on concomitant injuries.
- The *attending physician* or radiologist must review this image to rule out vertebral fracture or dislocation before other projections are performed.
- Use a 72-inch (183-cm) SID whenever attainable.
- Move the patient's head and neck as little as possible.
- *Shield gonads and other personnel in the room.*

---

[1]See mobile lateral projection in Volume 3, p. 207.

Patient position considerations

- The patient is generally immobilized on a backboard and in a cervical collar.
- The patient should relax the shoulders as much as possible.
- The patient should look straight ahead without any rotation of the head or neck.
- Place IR in a holder at the top of the shoulder (Fig. 13-12). For DR, the collimated field should include the sella turcica (located 2 inches [5 cm] anterior and superior to the external acoustic meatus [EAM]) to T1, located 2 inches (5 cm) above the jugular notch. The anteroposterior field margins should extend about 1 inch (2.5 cm) beyond the skin shadow.
- Check that the IR is perfectly vertical.
- Ensure that the central ray is *horizontal* and is centered to the midpoint of the IR.

Structures shown

The entire cervical spine, from sella turcica to the top of T1, must be shown in profile with minimal rotation and distortion (Fig. 13-13). Evidence of proper collimation should be visible.

NOTE: If all seven cervical vertebrae including the spinous process of C7 and the C7-T1 interspace are not clearly visible, a lateral projection of the cervicothoracic region must be performed.

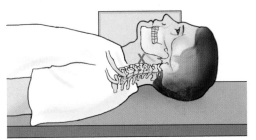

Horizontal CR to C4

Fig. 13-12 Patient and IR positioned for trauma lateral projection of cervical spine using dorsal decubitus position. The X marks the CR entrance point.

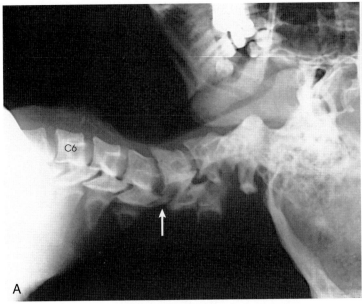
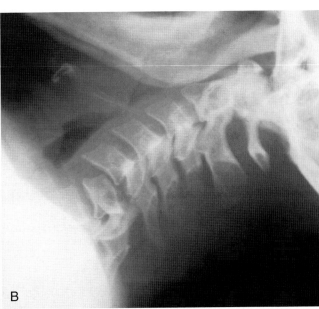

Fig. 13-13 Dorsal decubitus position lateral projection of cervical spine performed on a trauma patient. **A,** Dislocation of C3 and C4 articular processes (*arrow*). C7 is not well shown, so lateral projection of cervicothoracic vertebrae should also be performed. **B,** Fracture of pedicles with dislocation of C5 and C6. Note superior portion of C7 shown on this image.

Cervical Spine

LATERAL PROJECTION
Dorsal decubitus position

This projection is often called the *swimmer's technique.* (See Chapter 8, Vol. 1, p. 402-403, for a complete description.)

Trauma positioning tips

- *This projection should be performed if the entire cervical spine including C7 and the interspace between C7 and T1 is not shown on the dorsal decubitus lateral projection. The patient must be able to move both arms. Do not move the patient's arms without permission from the attending physician and review of the lateral projection.*
- Collimate the width of the x-ray beam closely, to approximately 10 × 12 inches (24 × 30 cm) or less, to reduce scatter radiation.
- If required and the patient is in stable condition, position the stretcher adjacent to a vertical Bucky to increase efficiency and obtain optimal image quality.
- *Shield gonads and other personnel in the room.*

Patient position considerations

- Position the patient supine, usually on a backboard and in a cervical collar.
- Have the patient depress the shoulder closest to the tube as much as possible. *Do not push on the patient's shoulder.*
- Instruct the patient to raise the arm opposite the tube over his or her head. Assist the patient as needed, but *do not use force or move the limb too quickly* (Fig. 13-14).
- Ensure that the patient is looking straight ahead without any rotation of the head or neck.
- The central ray is *horizontal* and perpendicular to the IR entering the side of the neck just above the clavicle, passing through the C7-T1 interspace.
- Instruct the patient to breathe normally, if he or she is conscious.
- If possible, use a long exposure time technique to blur the rib shadows.

Structures shown

The lower cervical and upper thoracic vertebral bodies and spinous processes should be seen in profile between the shoulders. Contrast and density should show bony cortical margins and trabeculation (Fig. 13-15). Evidence of proper collimation should be visible.

▼ COMPENSATING FILTER

The use of a compensating filter can improve image quality owing to the extreme difference in thickness between the upper thorax and the lower cervical spine.

NOTE: A grid is required to improve image contrast. If a breathing technique cannot be used, make the exposure with respiration suspended.

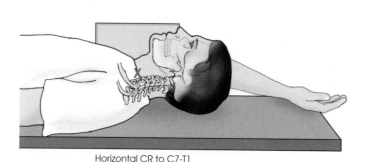

Horizontal CR to C7-T1

Fig. 13-14 Patient and IR positioned for trauma lateral projection of cervicothoracic vertebrae using dorsal decubitus position.

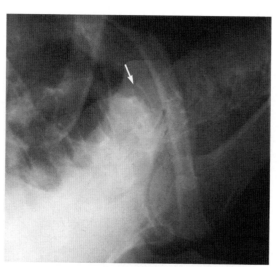

Fig. 13-15 Dorsal decubitus position lateral projection of cervicothoracic region performed on a trauma patient. Negative examination. Note excellent image of C7-T1 joint with use of Ferlic swimmer's filter (*arrow*).

AP AXIAL PROJECTION[1]

Trauma positioning tips

- *Do not perform this projection until the attending physician has reviewed the lateral projection.*
- This projection is usually performed after the lateral projection.
- If the patient is on a backboard, either on a stretcher or on an x-ray table, gently and slowly lift the backboard and place the IR in position under the patient's neck.
- Move the patient's head and neck as little as possible.
- Collimate the width of the x-ray beam to 1 inch (2.5 cm) beyond the skin to reduce scatter radiation. Use 12-inch (30.5-cm) lengthwise collimation.
- *Shield gonads and other personnel in the room.*

---

[1]See standard projection, Volume 1, p. 387-388.

Patient position considerations

- Position the patient supine, usually on a backboard and in a cervical collar.
- Have the patient relax the shoulders as much as possible.
- Ensure that the patient is looking straight ahead without any rotation of the head or neck.
- Place the IR under the backboard, if present, centered to approximately C4 (Fig. 13-16).
- The central ray is directed 15 to 20 degrees cephalad to the center of the IR and entering at C4.

Structures shown

C3 through T1 or T2 including interspaces and surrounding soft tissues should be shown with minimal rotation and distortion. Density and contrast should show cortical margins and soft tissue shadows (Fig. 13-17). Evidence of proper collimation should be visible.

NOTE: If the patient is not on a backboard or an x-ray table, preferably the attending physician should lift the patient's head and neck while the radiographer positions the IR under the patient.

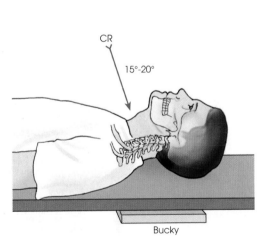

Fig. 13-16 Patient and IR positioned for trauma AP axial projection of cervical vertebrae.

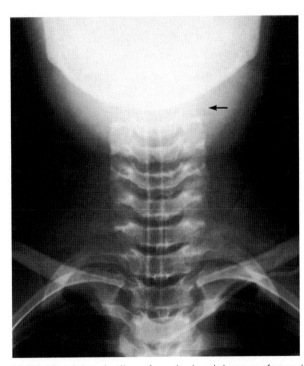

Fig. 13-17 AP axial projection of cervical vertebrae performed on an 11-year-old trauma patient. Cervical spine is completely dislocated between C2 and C3 (*arrow*). The patient died on the x-ray table after x-ray examinations were performed.

AP AXIAL OBLIQUE PROJECTION
Trauma positioning tips

- *Do not perform this projection until the attending physician has reviewed the lateral projection.*
- If the patient is on a backboard, gently and slowly lift the board and place the IR in position.
- Move the patient's head and neck as little as possible.
- Do not use a grid IR because the compound central ray angle results in grid cutoff. Many radiography machines do not allow the x-ray tube head to move in a compound angle, however. On these machines, only the 45-degree angle is used, and a grid IR may be used to improve contrast.
- Collimate the width of the x-ray beam to 1 inch (2.5 cm) of the skin lines to reduce scatter radiation. Use 12-inch (30.5-cm) lengthwise collimation.
- *Shield gonads and other personnel in the room.*

Patient position considerations

- Position the patient supine, usually on a backboard and in a cervical collar.
- Have the patient relax the shoulders as much as possible.
- Ensure that the patient is looking straight ahead without any rotation of the head or neck.
- Place the IR under the immobilization device, if present, centered at the level of C4 and the adjacent mastoid process (about 3 inches [7.6 cm] lateral to midsagittal plane of neck) (Fig. 13-18). If a grid IR is used with one central ray angle, the grid lines should be perpendicular to the long axis of the spine.
- The central ray is directed 45 degrees lateromedially. When a double angle is used, angle 15 to 20 degrees cephalad.
- The central ray enters slightly lateral to the midsagittal plane at the level of the thyroid cartilage and passing through C4.
- The central ray exit point should coincide with the center of the IR.

Structures shown

Cervical and upper thoracic vertebral bodies, pedicles, open intervertebral disk spaces, and open intervertebral foramina of the side that the central ray enters are shown. This projection provides excellent detail of the facet joints, and it is important in detecting subluxations and dislocations (Fig. 13-19). If the 15-degree cephalic angle is not used, the intervertebral foramina are foreshortened. Evidence of proper collimation should be visible.

NOTE: If the patient is not on a backboard or an x-ray table, preferably the attending physician should lift the patient's head and neck while the radiographer positions the IR under the patient.

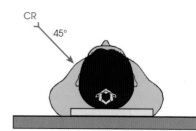

Fig. 13-18 Patient and IR positioned for trauma AP axial oblique projection of cervical vertebrae. Central ray (*CR*) is positioned 45 degrees mediolaterally and, if possible, 15 to 20 degrees cephalad.

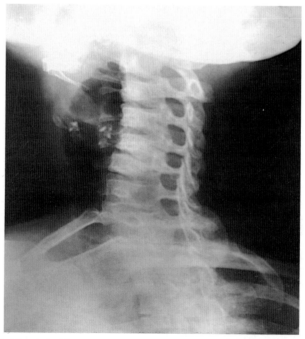

Fig. 13-19 AP axial oblique projection of cervical vertebrae performed on a trauma patient using 45-degree angle. Radiograph was made using non–grid exposure technique. Negative image. Note excellent alignment of vertebral bodies and intervertebral foramen.

LATERAL PROJECTIONS
Dorsal decubitus positions
Trauma positioning tips

- *Always* perform dorsal decubitus positions before AP projections of the spine because the *attending physician* should review the dorsal decubitus lateral projections *to rule out vertebral fracture or dislocation* before other *projections are performed.*
- Move the patient as little as possible.
- Use of a grid is necessary to improve image contrast. Use a vertical Bucky, if not working with a C-arm configured unit, to maximize positioning and for optimal image quality.
- *Shield gonads and other personnel in the room.*

Patient position considerations

- The patient is generally immobilized and on a backboard.
- Have the patient cross the arms over the chest to remove them from the anatomy of interest.
- *Thoracic spine:* Place the top of the IR 1½ to 2 inches (3.8 to 5 cm) above the patient's relaxed shoulders. DR field projected size is from the jugular notch to the inferior costal margin and 7 inches (18 cm) in anteroposterior width, centered at the level of the midcoronal plane.

- *Lumbar spine:* Center the IR at the level of the iliac crests (Fig. 13-20). DR field projected size extends from the xiphoid to the midsacrum and 8 inches (20 cm) in anteroposterior width, centered at the level of the midcoronal plane.
- Ensure that the IR is perfectly vertical.
- The central ray is *horizontal,* perpendicular to the longitudinal center of the IR, and going through the spine.
- Collimate closely to the spine to reduce scattered radiation and patient dose.

Structures shown

For the thoracic spine, the image should include T3 or T4-L1. The lumbar spine image should, at a minimum, include T12 to the sacrum. The vertebral bodies should be seen in profile with minimal rotation and distortion. Density and contrast should be sufficient to show cortical margins and bony trabeculation (Fig. 13-21). Evidence of proper collimation should be visible.

NOTE: A lateral projection of the cervicothoracic spine must be performed to allow visualization of the upper thoracic spine in profile.

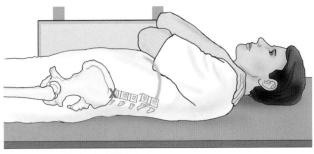

Horizontal CR to top
of iliac crest

Fig. 13-20 Patient and IR positioned for trauma lateral projection of lumbar spine using dorsal decubitus position and vertical Bucky device.

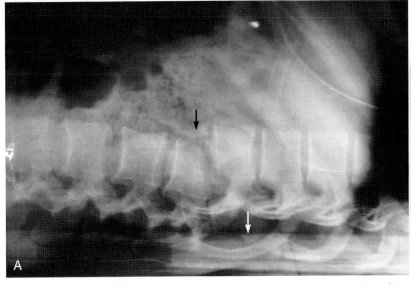

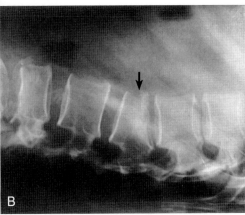

Fig. 13-21 Dorsal decubitus position lateral projection of lumbar spine performed on a trauma patient. **A,** Fracture and dislocation of L2 (*black arrow*). Note backboard (*white arrow*). **B,** Compression fracture of body of L2 (*arrow*). This coned-down image provides better detail of fracture area.

AP PROJECTION[1,2]

Trauma positioning tips

- Most trauma patients must be imaged in the supine position. If it is necessary to see air-fluid levels, a cross-table lateral x-ray beam (dorsal decubitus position) can be performed. (*Note:* Patients with chest trauma with suspected vascular injury may be referred to CT first.)
- Obtain help in lifting the patient to position the IR if the stretcher is not equipped with an IR tray or a C-arm configured trauma unit is not being used.
- Check for signs of respiratory distress or changes in level of consciousness during radiographic examination, and *report any changes to the attending physician immediately.*

[1]See standard projection, Volume 1.
[2]See mobile projection, Volume 3.

- Assess the patient's ability to follow breathing instructions.
- Use the maximum SID possible to minimize magnification of the heart shadow.
- Use universal precautions if wounds or bleeding or both are present, and protect the IR with plastic covering.
- Mark entrance and exit wounds with radiopaque indicators if evaluating a penetrating injury.
- Use of a grid improves image contrast.
- *Shield gonads and other personnel in the room.*

Patient position considerations

- Position the top of the IR about $1\frac{1}{2}$ to 2 inches (3.8 to 5 cm) above the patient's shoulders. DR field size should measure approximately 14×17 inches (35×43 cm) oriented to accommodate the patient's body habitus.
- Move the patient's arms away from the thorax and out of the collimated field.
- Ensure that the patient is looking straight ahead with the chin extended out of the collimated field.
- Check for rotation by determining whether the shoulders are equidistant to the IR or stretcher. This position places the midcoronal plane parallel to the IR, minimizing image distortion.
- The central ray should be directed perpendicular to the center of the IR at a point 3 inches (7.6 cm) below the jugular notch (Fig. 13-22).

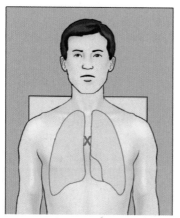

CR to center of IR

Fig. 13-22 Patient and IR positioned for trauma AP projection of chest.

Structures shown

AP projection of the thorax is shown. The lung fields should be included in their entirety, with minimal rotation and distortion present. Adequate aeration of the lungs must be imaged to show the lung parenchyma (Fig. 13-23). Evidence of proper collimation should be visible.

NOTE: Ribs are visible on an AP projection, necessitating the use of a grid IR to increase image contrast. Use proper breathing instructions and techniques to ensure adequate visualization of ribs of interest.

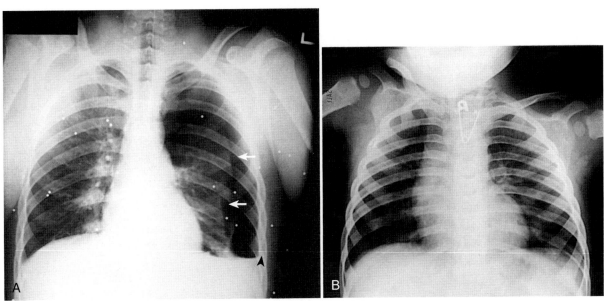

Fig. 13-23 AP upright projection of chest performed on a trauma patient. **A,** Multiple buckshot in chest caused hemopneumothorax. *Arrows* show margin of collapsed lung with free air laterally. *Arrowhead* shows fluid level at costophrenic angle, left lung. **B,** Open safety pin lodged in esophagus of a 13-month-old infant.

AP PROJECTION[1,2]

Trauma positioning tips

- *Note:* Sonography is often used to evaluate abdominal trauma.
- Use of a grid provides optimal image quality. If not working with a C-arm configured unit, verify transfer to a standard x-ray table with the attending physician before moving the patient.
- Determine the possibility of fluid accumulation within the abdominal cavity to establish appropriate exposure factors.
- For patients with blunt force or projectile injuries, check for signs of internal bleeding during radiographic examination and *report any changes to the attending physician immediately.*

---

[1]See standard projection, Volume 2.
[2]See mobile projection, Volume 3.

- Mark entrance and exit wounds with radiopaque markers if evaluating projectile injuries.
- Assess the ability of the patient to follow breathing instructions.
- Use standard precautions if wounds or bleeding or both are present, and protect the IR with plastic covering if it is to come in contact with the patient.
- *Shield gonads, if possible, and other personnel in the room.*

Patient position considerations

- Ask ED personnel to assist in transferring the patient to the radiographic table, if possible.
- If not working with a C-arm configured trauma unit and transfer is not advisable, obtain assistance to lift the patient carefully to position the grid IR under the patient, centered to the level of iliac crest (Fig. 13-24). (On patients with a long torso, a second AP projection of the upper abdomen may be required to show the diaphragm and lower ribs.)
- If the patient is on a stretcher, check that the grid IR is parallel with the patient's midcoronal plane. Correct tilting with sponges, sandbags, or rolled towels. The grid IR must be perfectly horizontal to prevent grid cutoff and image distortion. If you are unable to correct tilt on grid IR, angle the central ray to maintain part–IR–central ray alignment.
- The central ray is directed to the center of the IR. The DR collimated field should be approximately 17 inches (43 cm) in length on adult sthenic patients, and the width should be approximately 1 inch (2.5 cm) beyond the skin margin.

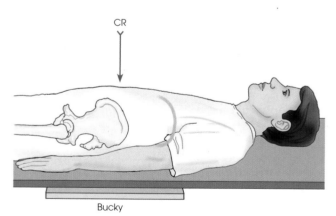

Fig. 13-24 Patient and IR positioned for trauma AP projection of abdomen.

Structures shown

AP projection of the abdomen is shown. The entire abdomen including the pubic symphysis and diaphragm should be included without distortion or rotation. Density and contrast should be adequate to show tissue interfaces, such as the lower margin of the liver, kidney shadows, psoas muscles, and cortical margins of bones (Fig. 13-25). Evidence of proper collimation should be visible.

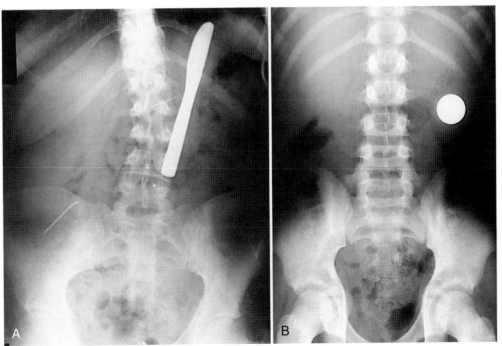

Fig. 13-25 AP projection of abdomen performed on a trauma patient. **A,** Table knife in stomach along with other small metallic foreign bodies swallowed by the patient. **B,** Coin in stomach swallowed by the patient.

AP PROJECTION[1,2]

Left lateral decubitus position

Trauma positioning tips

- *If not using a C-arm configured unit,* a vertical Bucky provides optimal image quality. If the patient must be imaged using a mobile radiographic unit, a grid IR is required.
- Verify with the *attending physician* that patient movement is possible and whether the image is necessary to assess fluid accumulation or free air in the abdominal cavity.
- The *left lateral* decubitus position shows free air in the abdominal cavity because the density of the liver provides good contrast for visualization of any free air.
- If fluid accumulation is of primary interest, the side down, or dependent side, must be elevated off the stretcher or table to be completely shown.
- Check for signs of internal bleeding during the radiographic examination, and *report any changes to the attending physician immediately.*

---

[1]See standard projection, Volume 2.
[2]See mobile projection, Volume 3.

- Use universal precautions if wounds or bleeding or both are present, and protect the IR with plastic covering. Mark all entrance and exit wounds with radiopaque markers when imaging for penetrating injuries.
- *Shield gonads, if possible, and personnel in the room.*

Patient position considerations

- Carefully and slowly turn the patient into the recumbent left lateral position. Flex the knees to provide stability.
- If the image is being taken for visualization of fluid, carefully place a block under the length of the abdomen to ensure that the entire right side is visualized.
- Ensure that the midcoronal plane is vertical to prevent image distortion.
- Center the IR 2 inches (5 cm) above the iliac crests to include the diaphragm (Fig. 13-26). DR field size should be approximately 17 inches (43 cm) in length, and the width should be 1 inch (2.5 cm) beyond the skin margins.

- The patient should be in the lateral position at least 5 minutes before the exposure to allow any free air to rise and be visualized.
- The central ray is directed *horizontal* and perpendicular to the center of the IR.

Structures shown

Air and fluid levels within the abdominal cavity are shown. This projection is especially helpful in assessing free air in the abdomen when an upright position cannot be used. Density and contrast should be adequate to show tissue interfaces, such as the lower margin of the liver, kidney shadows, psoas muscles, and cortical margins of bones (Fig. 13-27). Evidence of proper collimation should be visible.

NOTE: A lateral projection using the dorsal decubitus position may be substituted for this projection if the patient is too ill or injured to be positioned properly in a left lateral position. (The position is identical to the dorsal decubitus position, lateral projection of the lumbar spine. See Fig. 13-20.)

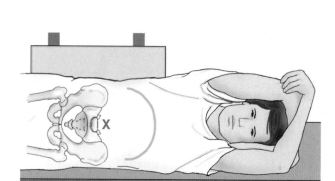

Horizontal CR to center of IR

Fig. 13-26 Patient and IR positioned for trauma AP projection of abdomen using left lateral decubitus position and using vertical Bucky device.

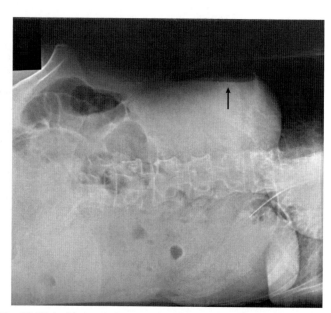

Fig. 13-27 Left lateral decubitus position AP projection of abdomen performed on a trauma patient. Free intraperitoneal air is seen on upper right side of abdomen (*arrow*). Radiograph is slightly underexposed to show free air more easily.

AP PROJECTION[1,2]

Trauma positioning tips

- *Note:* Level I centers often refer patients with pelvic trauma to CT first because research has shown that CT is superior in showing fracture extent and associated visceral and vascular damage.
- Up to 50% of pelvic fractures are fatal as a result of vascular damage and shock. The mortality risk increases with the energy of the force and according to the health of the victim.
- Pelvic fractures have a high incidence of internal hemorrhage. *Alert the attending physician immediately if the abdomen becomes distended and firm.*
- Hemorrhagic shock is common with pelvic and abdominal injuries. *Reassess the patient's level of consciousness repeatedly while performing radiographic examinations.*
- *Do not* attempt internal rotation of the limbs for true AP projection of proximal femora on this projection.
- Collimate closely to reduce scatter radiation.
- *Shield gonads, if possible, and other personnel in the room.*

[1]See standard projection, Volume 1.
[2]See mobile projection, Volume 3.

Patient position considerations

- The patient is supine, possibly on a backboard or in trauma pants.
- Carefully and slowly transfer the patient to the radiographic table to allow the use of a Bucky, if not working with a C-arm configured unit.
- If unable to transfer the patient, use a grid IR positioned under the immobilization device or patient. Ensure that the grid is horizontal and parallel to the patient's midcoronal plane to minimize distortion and rotation. Carefully align it to the central ray to minimize distortion and rotation.
- Position the IR so that the center is 2 inches (5 cm) inferior to the anterior superior iliac spine or 2 inches (5 cm) superior to the pubic symphysis.
- The central ray is directed perpendicular to the center of the IR (Fig. 13-28).

- The DR field size should be approximately 14 × 17 inches (35 × 43 cm). Check the collimated field to ensure that the iliac crests and the hip joints are included.

Structures shown

The pelvis and proximal femora should be shown in their entirety with minimal rotation and distortion. Femoral necks are foreshortened, and lesser trochanters are seen. Optimal density and contrast should show bony trabeculation and soft tissue shadows (Fig. 13-29). Evidence of proper collimation should be visible.

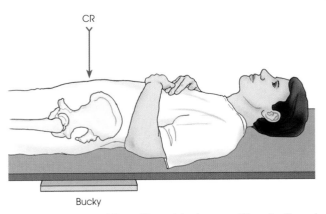

Fig. 13-28 Patient and IR positioned for trauma AP projection of pelvis.

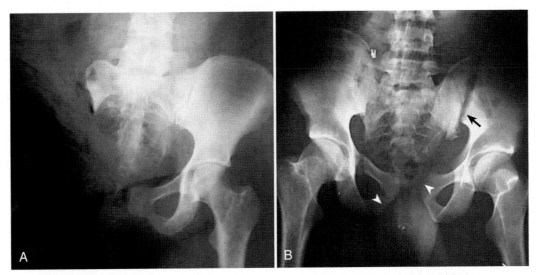

Fig. 13-29 AP projection of pelvis performed on a trauma patient. **A,** Entire right limb torn off after being hit by a car. Pelvic bone was disarticulated at pubic symphysis and sacroiliac joint. The patient survived. **B,** Separation of pubic bones (*arrowheads*) anteriorly and associated fracture of left ilium (*arrow*).

LATERAL PROJECTION[1]
Dorsal decubitus position
Trauma positioning tips

- *Note:* Patients with head injuries are often referred to CT imaging first because of its superiority in showing associated soft tissue and vascular damage.
- Because the scalp and face are vascular, these areas tend to bleed profusely. Protect IRs with plastic covering and practice universal precautions.
- A grid IR is used for this projection. Elevate the patient's head on a radiolucent sponge *only after cervical injury, such as fracture or dislocation, has been ruled out.*

[1]See standard projection, Volume 2.

- Vomiting is a symptom of intracranial injury. *If a patient begins to vomit, logroll him or her to a lateral position to prevent aspiration, and alert the attending physician immediately.*
- *Alert the attending physician immediately if there is any change in the patient's level of consciousness or if the pupils are unequal.*
- Collimate closely to reduce scatter radiation.
- *Shield gonads and other personnel in the room.*

Patient position considerations

- Have the patient relax the shoulders.
- After cervical spine injury has been ruled out, the patient's head may be positioned to align the interpupillary line perpendicular to the IR and the midsagittal plane vertical.
- If the patient is wearing a cervical collar, carefully minimize rotation and tilt of the cranium.
- Ensure that the IR is vertical.
- Direct the central ray *horizontal* entering perpendicular to a point 2 inches (5 cm) above the EAM (Fig. 13-30). The DR field should be set to 12 inches (30 cm) in the anteroposterior dimension and 10 inches (24 cm) in the superoinferior dimension.

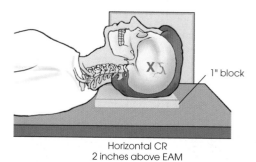

Horizontal CR
2 inches above EAM

Fig. 13-30 Patient and IR positioned for trauma lateral projection of cranium using dorsal decubitus position. Note sponge in place to raise head to show posterior cranium (after checking lateral cervical spine radiograph).

Structures shown

A profile image of the superimposed halves of the cranium is seen with detail of the side closer to the IR shown (Fig. 13-31). With some injuries, air-fluid levels can be shown in the sphenoid sinuses. Evidence of proper collimation should be visible.

NOTE: The supine lateral position may be used on a patient without a cervical spine injury. See Volume 2, p. 294-295.

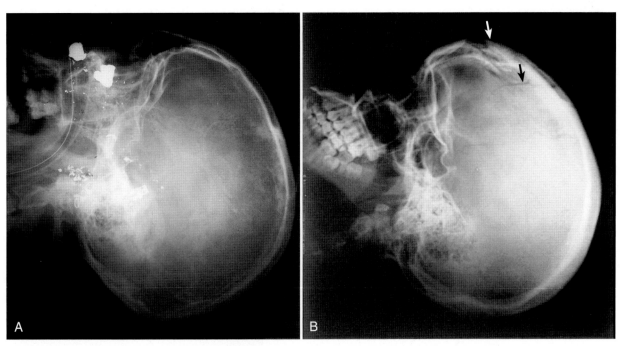

Fig. 13-31 Dorsal decubitus position lateral projection of cranium performed on a trauma patient. **A,** Two GSWs entering at level of C1 and traveling forward to face and lodging in area of zygomas. Note bullet fragments in EAM area. **B,** Multiple frontal skull fractures (*arrows*) caused by hitting windshield during MVA.

AP PROJECTION[1]
AP AXIAL PROJECTION—TOWNE METHOD[2]

Trauma positioning tips

- Profuse bleeding should be anticipated with head and facial injuries. Use universal precautions and protect IRs and sponges with plastic.
- *Cervical spine injury should be ruled out before attempting to position the head.*
- AP projection is used for injury to the anterior cranium. The AP axial projection, Towne method, shows the posterior cranium.

---

[1]See standard projection, Volume 2.
[2]See standard projection, Volume 2.

- Vomiting is a symptom of an intracranial injury. *If a patient begins to vomit, logroll him or her to a lateral position to prevent aspiration and alert the attending physician immediately.*
- *Alert the attending physician if the patient's level of consciousness decreases or if pupils are unequal.*
- Collimate closely to 1 inch (2.5 cm) beyond projected skin shadows on all sides of the cranium to reduce scatter radiation.
- A grid IR or Bucky should be used to ensure proper image contrast.
- *Shield gonads and other personnel in the room.*

Patient position considerations

- If not using a C-arm configured unit, and if the patient's condition allows, carefully and slowly transfer the patient to the x-ray table using the immobilization device and proper transfer techniques. Transfer allows the use of the Bucky and minimizes risk of injury to the patient when positioning the IR.

- If the patient is not transferred to the radiographic table, the grid IR should be placed under the immobilization device. If no such device is present, the *attending physician* should carefully lift the patient's head and neck while the radiographer positions the grid IR under the patient.
- After a cervical spine injury has been ruled out, the patient's head may be positioned to place the orbitomeatal line (OML) or infraorbitomeatal line (IOML) and midsagittal plane perpendicular to the IR.
- If the patient is wearing a cervical collar, the OML or IOML cannot be positioned perpendicularly. For the AP axial projection, Towne method, the central ray angle may have to be increased 60 degrees caudad, while a 30-degree angle to the OML is maintained.

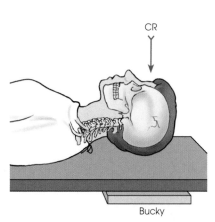

Fig. 13-32 Patient and IR positioned for trauma AP projection of cranium.

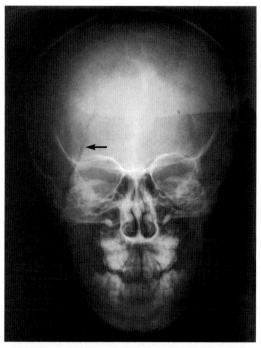

Fig. 13-33 AP projection of cranium performed on a trauma patient. Fracture of occipital bone (*arrow*).

- For an AP projection, the central ray enters perpendicular to the nasion (Fig. 13-32). An AP axial projection with the central ray directed 15 degrees cephalad is sometimes performed in place of, or to accompany, the AP projection.
- For AP axial projection, Towne method, position the top of the IR at the level of the cranial vertex. The central ray is directed 30 degrees caudad to the OML or 37 degrees to the IOML (Fig. 13-33). The central ray passes through the EAM and exits the foramen magnum.
- The DR field should be set at 10 inches (24 cm) wide and 12 inches (30 cm) in the inferosuperior dimension, centered the same as for an imaging plate, as specified previously.

Structures shown

AP projection shows the anterior cranium (Fig. 13-34). AP axial projection, Towne method, shows the posterior cranium and foramen magnum (Fig. 13-35). Evidence of proper collimation should be visible.

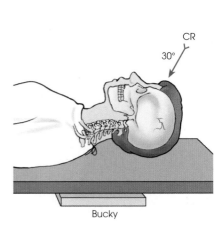

Fig. 13-34 Patient and IR positioned for trauma AP axial projection, Towne method, of cranium using 30-degree central ray (CR) angulation.

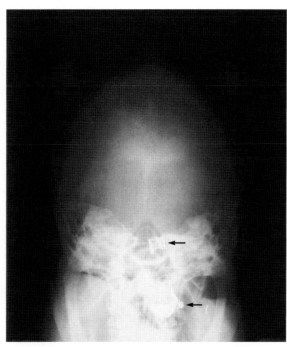

Fig. 13-35 AP axial projection, Towne method, performed on a trauma patient with GSW to the head. Metal clip (*upper arrow*) indicates entrance of bullet on anterior cranium. Flattened bullet and fragments (*lower arrow*) are lodged in area of C2.

ACANTHIOPARIETAL PROJECTION[1]
REVERSE WATERS METHOD

Trauma positioning tips

- Anticipate profuse bleeding with facial trauma. Protect IRs with plastic covering and practice universal precautions.
- Cervical spine injury should be ruled out before positioning of the head is attempted.
- *Alert the attending physician if the patient's level of consciousness decreases or if pupils are unequal.*
- A grid IR or Bucky is used to ensure proper image contrast.
- Collimate closely to the facial bones to reduce scatter radiation. The DR field should be set at approximately 10 inches (24 cm) wide and 12 inches (30 cm) in the inferosuperior dimension.
- *Shield gonads and other personnel in the room.*

[1]See standard projection, Volume 2.

Patient position considerations

- If required and if the patient's condition allows, carefully and slowly transfer the patient to the x-ray table using the immobilization device and proper transfer techniques. Transfer allows use of the Bucky and minimizes risk of injury to the patient when the IR is positioned.
- If mobile radiography must be used, the grid IR should be placed under the immobilization device. If no such device is present, the *attending physician* should carefully lift the patient's head and neck while the radiographer positions the grid IR under the patient.
- Trauma patients are often unable to hyperextend the neck far enough to allow placement of the OML 37 degrees to the IR and the MML perpendicular to the plane of the IR. In these patients, the acanthioparietal projection, or the reverse Waters projection, can be achieved by adjusting the central ray so that it enters the acanthion while remaining parallel with the MML.
- The midsagittal plane should be perpendicular to prevent rotation.
- The central ray is angled cephalad until it is parallel with the MML. The central ray enters the acanthion (Fig. 13-36).
- Center the IR to the central ray.

Structures shown

The superior facial bones are shown (Fig. 13-37). The image should be similar to the parietoacanthial projection or routine Waters method and should show symmetry of the face. Evidence of proper collimation should be visible.

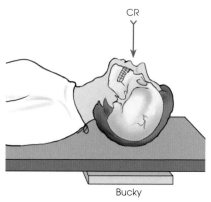

Fig. 13-36 Central ray aligned parallel to MML for trauma acanthioparietal projection, reverse Waters method, of cranium.

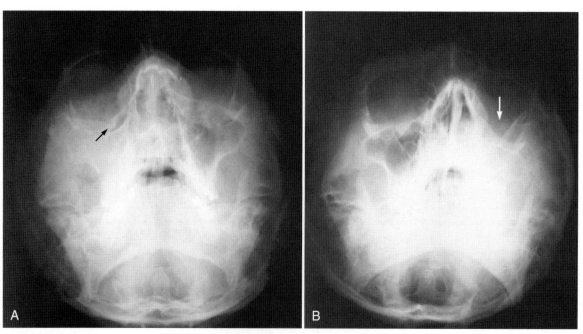

Fig. 13-37 Acanthioparietal projections, reverse Waters method, performed on trauma patients to show facial bones. **A,** Fracture of right orbital floor (*arrow*) with blood-filled maxillary sinus (note no air is in sinus). The patient hit face on steering wheel during MVA. **B,** Blowout fracture of left orbital floor (*arrow*) with blood-filled maxillary sinus (note no air is in sinus). Patient was hit with a fist.

Trauma positioning tips

- Use standard precautions, and cover IRs and positioning aids in plastic if wounds are present.
- When lifting an injured limb, *support it at both joints and lift slowly. Lift only enough to place the IR under the part—sometimes only 1 to 2 inches (2.5 to 5 cm).* Always obtain help in lifting injured limbs and positioning the IRs to minimize patient discomfort.
- If the limb is severely injured, *do not* attempt to position for true AP or lateral projections. Expose the two projections, 90 degrees apart, while moving the injured limb as little as possible.

- Check the patient's status during radiographic examination. Shock can occur from crushing injuries to extremities.
- Long bone radiographs must include both joints on the image.
- Separate examinations of the adjacent joints *may be required* if injury indicates. Do not attempt to "short cut" by performing only one projection of the long bone.
- *Shield gonads and other personnel in the room.*

Patient position considerations

- If possible, demonstrate the desired position for a conscious patient. Assist the patient in attempting to assume the position, rather than moving the injured limb.
- If the patient is unable to position the limb close to that required, move the IR and x-ray tube to obtain the desired projection (Figs. 13-38 to 13-41).

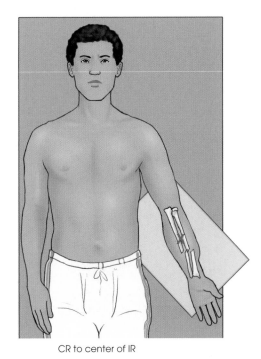

CR to center of IR

Fig. 13-38 Patient and IR positioned for trauma AP projection of forearm.

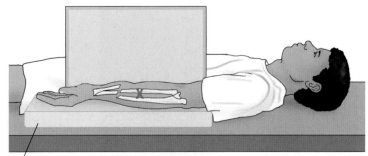

2-inch block   Horizontal CR to center of IR

Fig. 13-39 Patient and IR positioned for trauma cross-table lateral projection of forearm.

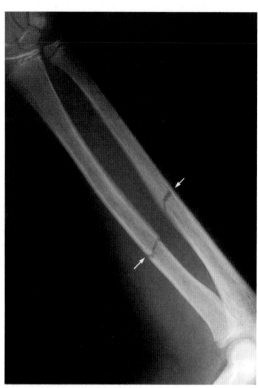

Fig. 13-40 AP projection of forearm performed on a trauma patient. Fracture of midportion of radius and ulna (*arrows*).

- Shoulder injuries should be initially imaged "as is" without rotating the limb. The "reverse" PA oblique projection of the scapular Y (an AP oblique) is useful in showing dislocation of the glenohumeral joint with minimal patient movement. The patient is turned up 45 degrees and is supported in position (Figs. 13-42 and 13-43).
- If imaging while the patient is still on a stretcher, check to ensure that the IR is perfectly horizontal to minimize image distortion.
- The central ray must be directed perpendicular to the IR to minimize distortion.
- Immobilization techniques for the IR and upper limb are useful in obtaining an optimal image with minimal patient discomfort.

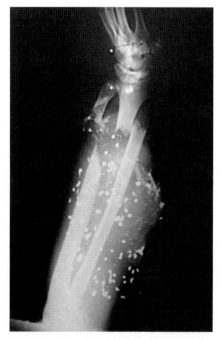

Fig. 13-41 Cross-table lateral projection of forearm performed on a trauma patient. GSW to forearm with fracture of radius and ulna and extensive soft tissue damage.

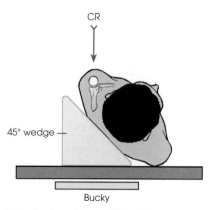

Fig. 13-42 Patient and IR positioned for trauma AP oblique projection of shoulder to show scapular Y. (Reverse of PA oblique, scapular Y—see Chapter 5.)

Structures shown

Images of the anatomy of interest, 90 degrees from one another, should be shown. Density and contrast should be sufficient to visualize cortical margins, bony trabeculation, and surrounding soft tissues. Both joints should be included in projections of long bones. Projections of adjacent joints must be centered to the joint to show the articular ends properly (Figs. 13-44 and 13-45). Evidence of proper collimation should be visible.

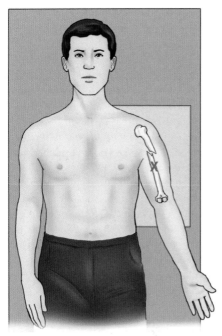

CR to center of IR

Fig. 13-44 Patient and IR positioned for trauma AP projection of humerus.

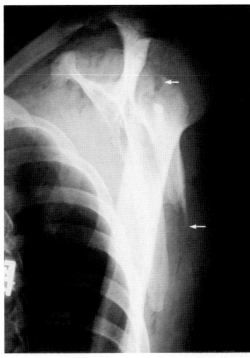

Fig. 13-43 AP oblique projection of shoulder (reverse of PA oblique, scapular Y) performed on a trauma patient. Several fractures of scapula (*arrows*) with significant displacement.

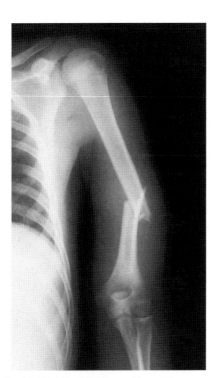

Fig. 13-45 AP projection of humerus performed on a trauma patient. Fracture of midshaft of humerus.

Trauma Radiography

Trauma positioning tips

- Use standard precautions, and cover IRs and positioning aids in plastic if open wounds are present.
- Immobilization devices are often present with injuries to the lower limbs, especially in cases with suspected femoral fractures. *Perform image procedures with immobilization in place, unless directed to remove them by the attending physician.*
- When lifting an injured limb, *support at both joints and lift slowly. Lift only enough to place the IR under the part—sometimes only 1 to 2 inches (2.5 to 5 cm).* Always obtain help in lifting injured limbs and in positioning IRs to minimize patient discomfort (Fig. 13-46).

- If the limb is severely injured, *do not attempt to position it for true AP and lateral projections.* Take two projections, 90 degrees apart, moving the injured limb as little as possible.
- Long bone examinations must include both joints. Separate images may be required.
- Examinations of adjacent joints may be required if the condition indicates. The central ray and IR must be properly centered to the joint of interest to show the anatomy properly.
- Check on patient status during radiographic examination. Shock can occur with severe injuries to the lower extremities.
- A grid IR should be used on thicker anatomic parts, such as the femur.
- *Shield gonads and other personnel in the room.*

Patient position considerations

- Demonstrate or describe the desired position for the patient and allow him or her to attempt to assume the position, rather than moving the injured limb. Assist the patient as needed.
- If the patient is unable to position the limb close to the required true position, move the IR and x-ray tube to obtain projection (Figs. 13-47 and 13-48).
- If imaging while the patient is still on a stretcher, check to ensure that the IR is perfectly horizontal to minimize image distortion.
- The central ray must be directed perpendicular to the IR to minimize distortion.
- Immobilization techniques for the IR and lower limb are extremely useful in obtaining optimal quality with minimal patient discomfort.

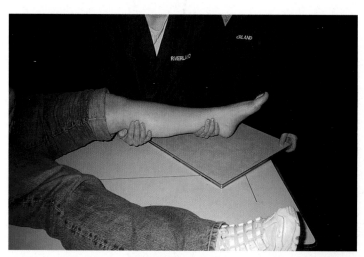

Fig. 13-46 Proper method of lifting lower limb for placement of IR (for AP projection) or placement of elevation blocks (for cross-table lateral). Lift only high enough to place IR or blocks underneath. Note that two hands are used to lift this patient with a broken leg gently.

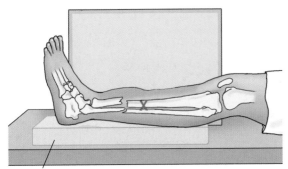

2-inch block   Horizontal CR to center of IR

Fig. 13-47 Patient and IR positioned for trauma cross-table lateral projection of lower leg. IR and central ray (CR) may be moved superiorly or inferiorly to center for other portions of lower limb. Note positioning blocks placed under limb to elevate it so that all anatomy of interest is seen.

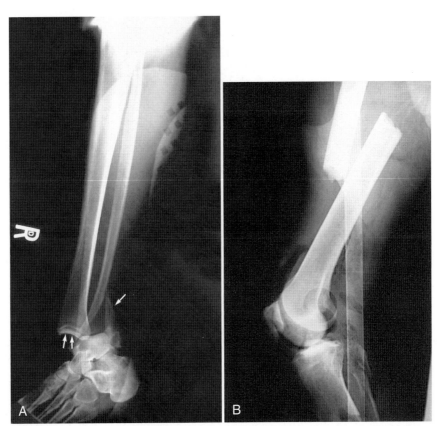

Fig. 13-48 Cross-table lateral projection of lower limb performed on a trauma patient.
A, Dislocation of tibia from talus (*double arrows*) and fracture of fibula (*arrow*).
B, Complete fracture and displacement of femur. Proximal femur is seen in AP projection, and distal femur is rotated 90 degrees at fracture point, resulting in lateral projection. Note artifacts caused by immobilization devices.

Trauma Radiography

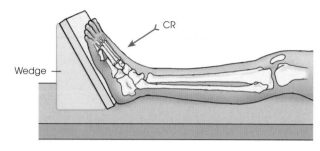

Fig. 13-49 Patient and IR positioned for trauma AP projection of foot or toes. IR is supported with sandbags for positioning against foot.

Structures shown

Images of the anatomy of interest, 90 degrees from each other, should be shown. Density and contrast should be sufficient to visualize cortical margins, bony trabeculation, and surrounding soft tissues. Both joints should be included in examinations of long bones. Images of articulations must be properly centered to show anatomy properly (Figs. 13-49 and 13-50). Evidence of proper collimation should be visible.

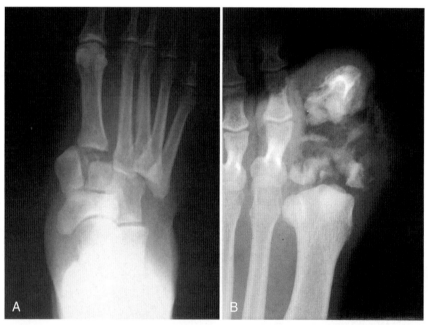

Fig. 13-50 AP projection of foot performed on a trauma patient. **A,** Fracture and dislocation of tarsal bones with exposure technique adjusted for optimal image of this area. **B,** GSW to great toe.

Follow-up imaging procedures by other modalities are often warranted when radiography reveals a traumatic injury. In many instances, however, radiography is *not* the modality used first for detection of injuries sustained in a trauma. Because of this fact, most trauma centers have CT readily available or a dedicated unit for trauma cases (Figs. 13-51 to 13-54). The role of sonography in trauma imaging has increased significantly, and it provides the advantage of yielding a great deal of diagnostic information without radiation exposure. Magnetic resonance imaging (MRI) has also increased in its utility in trauma imaging, primarily owing to decreased scan times provided by newer scan protocols and techniques.

Computed Tomography

In many major trauma centers, CT is readily available for emergency imaging. This fact has influenced the decision-making policies associated with diagnostic imaging of trauma. CT is the first imaging modality used for trauma to the following parts of the body:

- Head and brain
- Cervical spine
- Thorax
- Pelvis

The Glasgow Coma Scale (GCS) is often the diagnostic indicator for the necessity of a head CT scan. The GCS is used to provide an objective and consistent neurologic evaluation. The highest possible score is 15, and the lowest

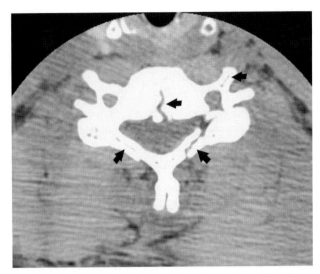

Fig. 13-51 CT scan of C5 showing multiple fractures (*arrows*) resulting from a fall from a tree. (Courtesy Sunie Grossman, RT(R), St. Bernard's Medical Center, Jonesboro, AR.)

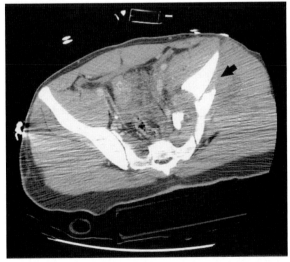

Fig. 13-52 CT scan of pelvis showing fracture of left ilium (*arrow*) with fragment displacement. Clothing and backboard artifacts are evident.

(Courtesy St. Bernard's Medical Center, Jonesboro, AR.)

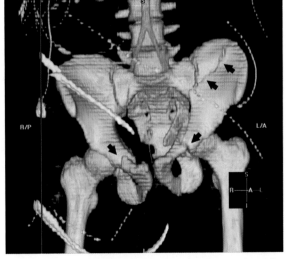

Fig. 13-53 Three-dimensional reconstruction of pelvis from the patient in Fig. 13-52. Multiple pelvic fractures are well visualized (*arrows*).

(Courtesy St. Bernard's Medical Center, Jonesboro, AR.)

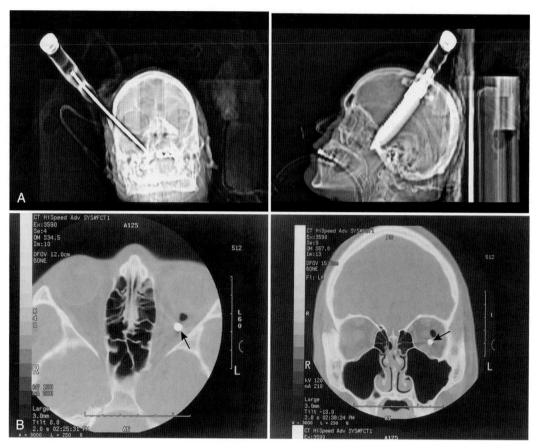

Fig. 13-54 A, AP and lateral CT scout images of cranium. Note knife placement in cranium. Conventional cranium radiographs were not obtained on this trauma patient. The patient was sent directly to CT scanner for these images and sectional images before going to surgery. The patient recovered and returned home. **B,** Axial and coronal CT sectional images of cranium at level of the eye. The patient was shot in the left eye with a BB gun. Note BB *(arrow)*. Adjacent black area is air. The patient now has monocular vision.

(**A,** Courtesy Tony Hofmann, RT(R)(CT), Shands Hospital School of Radiologic Technology, Jacksonville, FL; **B,** courtesy Mark H. Layne, RT(R).)

possible score is 3. The GCS score and other head injury signs and symptoms, such as headache, loss of consciousness, post-traumatic amnesia, and seizure, are used to determine whether a head CT scan is required. Patients with cervical spine injuries are often referred to CT first, especially patients with multiple injuries and associated symptoms of cord injury. CT of the thorax is often the first imaging modality used in cases of suspected aortic dissection. Chest radiography is still the gold standard for many emergency cases involving the thorax, but because of time factors, patients with certain types of force trauma are sent directly to the CT scanner.

CT of the pelvis is often performed in place of radiography because CT shows the extent of pelvic fractures better than radiography and offers the advantage of showing injuries to the pelvic organs and vasculature simultaneously.

Diagnostic Medical Sonography

The role of sonography in emergency imaging is evolving and increasing rapidly. Focused abdominal sonography in trauma (FAST) has been recognized as a valuable trauma diagnostic imaging tool. Research continues to assess the role of sonography in trauma imaging, and a wide variety of procedures have been studied so far, such as pediatric fracture reduction; chest and thoracic trauma, specifically pneumothorax and hemorrhage in the abdomen and pelvis; cranial trauma in infants; and superficial musculoskeletal sprains and tears. Advantages of sonography in trauma include lack of radiation exposure and improved efficiency of image access. The disadvantage is that sonography image quality is critically operator-dependent, and the ED physician may be uncomfortable with image interpretation, requiring the presence of a radiologist.

Selected bibliography

American College of Emergency Physicians: Policy statement: emergency ultrasound guidelines, *Ann Emerg Med* 53:550, 2009.

American College of Surgeons: *National trauma databank annual report*, 2012, Available at: http://www.facs.org/trauma/ntdb/docpub.html. Accessed August 29, 2013.

Bagley L: Imaging of spinal trauma, *Radiol Clin North Am* 44:1, 2006.

Centers for Disease Control and Prevention: Guidelines for field triage of injured patients: recommendations of the national expert panel on field triage, *MMWR Morb Mortal Wkly Rep*, Available at: http://www.cdc.gov/mmwr/preview/mmwrhtml/rr5801a1.htm. Accessed August 4, 2009.

Jagoda A et al: Clinical policy: neuroimaging and decision making in adult mild traumatic brain injury in the acute setting, *Ann Emerg Med* 52:714, 2008.

Kool D, Blickman J: Advanced trauma life support. ABCDE from a radiological point of view, *Emerg Radiol* 14:135, 2007.

Shanmuganathan K, Matsumoto J: Imaging of penetrating chest trauma, *Radiol Clin North Am* 44:225, 2006.

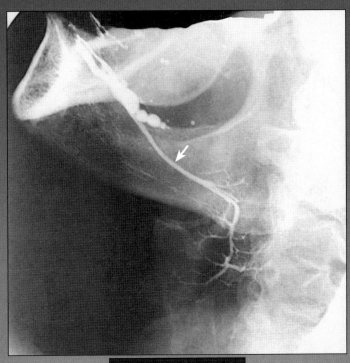

14

MOUTH AND SALIVARY GLANDS

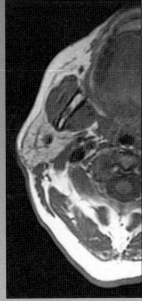

SUMMARY OF PROJECTIONS

PROJECTIONS, POSITIONS, AND METHODS

Page	Essential	Anatomy	Projection	Position	Method
64		Parotid gland	Tangential		
66		Parotid and submandibular glands	Lateral	R or L	

Mouth

The *mouth*, or *oral cavity*, is the first division of the digestive system (Fig. 14-1). It encloses the dental arches and receives the saliva secreted by the salivary glands. The cavity of the mouth is divided into (1) the *oral vestibule*, the space between the teeth and the cheeks, and (2) the *oral cavity*, or mouth proper, the space within the dental arches. The roof of the oral cavity is formed by the hard and soft palates. The floor is formed principally by the tongue, and it communicates with the pharynx posteriorly via the *oropharynx*.

The *hard palate* is the anteriormost portion of the roof of the oral cavity. The hard palate is formed by the horizontal plates of the maxillae and palatine bones. The anterior and lateral boundaries are formed by the inner wall of the maxillary alveolar processes, which extend superiorly and medially to blend with the horizontal processes. The height of the hard palate varies considerably, and it determines the angulation of the inner surface of the alveolar process. The angle is less when the palate is high and is greater when the palate is low.

The *soft palate* begins behind the last molar and is suspended from the posterior border of the hard palate. Highly sensitive to touch, the soft palate is a movable musculomembranous structure that functions chiefly as a partial septum between the mouth and the pharynx. At the center of the inferior border, the soft palate is prolonged into a small, pendulous process called the *uvula*. On each side of the uvula, two arched folds extend laterally and inferiorly. The *anterior arches* project forward to the sides of the base of the tongue. The *posterior arches* project posteriorly to blend with the posterolateral walls of the pharynx. The triangular space between the anterior and posterior arches is occupied by the palatine *tonsil*.

The *tongue* is situated in the floor of the oral cavity, with its base directed posteriorly and its *apex* directed anteriorly (Fig. 14-2; see Fig. 14-1). The tongue is freely movable. The tongue is composed of numerous muscles and is covered with a mucous membrane that varies in complexity in the different regions of the organ. The extrinsic muscles of the tongue form the greater part of the oral floor. The

mucous membrane covering the undersurface of the tongue is reflected laterally over the remainder of the floor to the gums. This part of the floor lies under the free anterior and lateral portions of the tongue and is called the *sublingual space*. Posterior movement of the free anterior part of the tongue is restricted by a median vertical band, or fold, of mucous membrane called the *frenulum of the tongue*, which extends between the undersurface of the tongue and the sublingual space. On each side of the frenulum, extending around the outer limits of the sublingual space and over the underlying salivary glands, the mucous membrane is elevated into a crestlike ridge called the *sublingual fold*. In the relaxed state, the two folds are quite prominent and are in contact with the gums.

The *teeth* serve the function of *mastication*, the process of chewing and grinding food into small pieces. During mastication, the teeth cut, grind, and tear food, which is then mixed with saliva and swallowed, and later digested. The saliva softens the food, keeps the mouth moist, and contributes digestive enzymes.

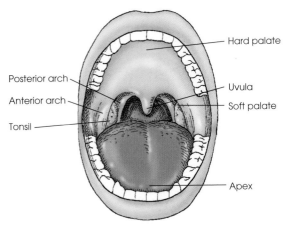

Fig. 14-1 Anterior view of oral cavity.

Hard palate
Posterior arch
Anterior arch
Tonsil
Uvula
Soft palate
Apex

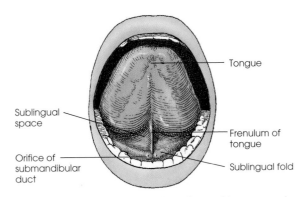

Fig. 14-2 Anterior view of undersurface of tongue and floor of mouth.

Tongue
Sublingual space
Frenulum of tongue
Orifice of submandibular duct
Sublingual fold

Salivary Glands

The three pairs of salivary glands produce approximately 1 L of saliva each day. The glands are named the *parotid, submandibular,* and *sublingual* (Fig. 14-3). Each gland is composed of numerous lobes, and each lobe contains small lobules. The whole gland is held together by connective tissue and a fine network of blood vessels and ducts. The minute ducts of the lobules merge into larger tributaries, which unite and form the large efferent duct that conveys the saliva from the gland to the mouth.

Each of the *parotid glands,* the largest of the salivary glands, consists of a flattened superficial portion and a wedge-shaped deep portion (Fig. 14-4). The superficial part lies immediately anterior to the external ear and extends inferiorly to the mandibular ramus and posteriorly to the mastoid process. The deep, or retromandibular, portion extends medially toward the pharynx. The *parotid duct* runs anteriorly and medially to open into the oral vestibule opposite the second upper molar.

The *submandibular glands* are large, irregularly shaped glands. On each side, a submandibular gland extends posteriorly from a point below the first molar almost to the angle of the mandible (Fig. 14-5). Although the upper part of the gland rests against the inner surface of the mandibular body, its greater portion projects below the mandible. The *submandibular duct* extends anteriorly and superiorly to open into the mouth on a small papilla at the side of the frenulum of the tongue.

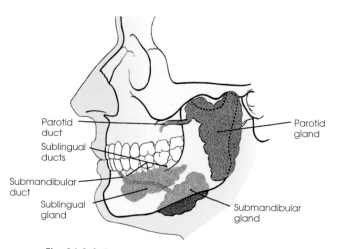

Parotid duct

Sublingual ducts

Submandibular duct

Sublingual gland

Parotid gland

Submandibular gland

Fig. 14-3 Salivary glands from left lateral aspect.

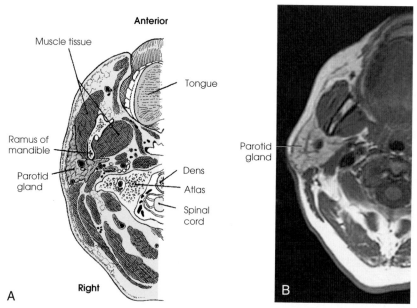

Anterior

Muscle tissue

Tongue

Ramus of mandible

Parotid gland

Dens

Atlas

Spinal cord

A

Right

Parotid gland

B

Fig. 14-4 A, Horizontal section of face, showing relationship of parotid gland to mandibular ramus. Auricle is not shown. **B,** Axial MRI of parotid gland.

(**B,** Courtesy J. Louis Rankin, BS, RT(R)(MR).)

The *sublingual glands,* the smallest pair, are narrow and elongated in form (see Fig. 14-5). These glands are located in the floor of the mouth beneath the sublingual fold. Each is in contact with the mandible laterally and extends posteriorly from the side of the frenulum of the tongue to the submandibular gland. Numerous small *sublingual ducts* exist. Some of these ducts open into the floor of the mouth along the crest of the sublingual fold, and others open into the submandibular duct. The main sublingual duct opens beside the orifice of the submandibular duct.

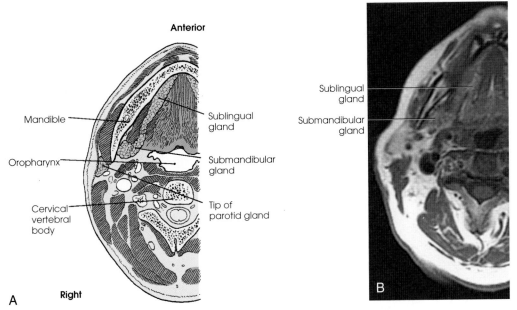

Fig. 14-5 A, Horizontal section of face, showing relationship of submandibular and sublingual glands to surrounding structures. Auricle is not shown. **B,** Axial MRI of submandibular and sublingual glands.

(**B,** Courtesy J. Louis Rankin, BS, RT(R)(MR).)

SUMMARY OF ANATOMY

Mouth	Salivary glands
Oral vestibule	Parotid glands
Oral cavity	Parotid ducts
Oropharynx	Submandibular glands
Hard palate	Submandibular ducts
Soft palate	Sublingual glands
Uvula	Sublingual ducts
Anterior arches	
Posterior arches	
Tonsil	
Tongue	
Apex	
Sublingual space	
Frenulum of the tongue	
Sublingual fold	
Teeth	

Mouth and Salivary Glands

SUMMARY OF PATHOLOGY

Condition	Definition
Calculus	Abnormal concretion of mineral salts, often called a *stone*
Fistula	Abnormal connection between two internal organs or between an organ and the body surface
Foreign body	Foreign material in the airway
Salivary duct	Condition that prevents passage of saliva through the duct obstruction
Stenosis	Narrowing or contraction of a passage
Tumor	New tissue growth where cell proliferation is uncontrolled

Sialography

Sialography is the term applied to radiologic examination of the salivary glands and ducts with the use of a contrast material, usually one of the water-soluble iodinated media. Because of improvements in computed tomography (CT) and magnetic resonance imaging (MRI) techniques, sialography is rarely performed. When the presence of a salivary stone or lesion is suspected, CT or MRI is often the modality of choice. Sialography remains a viable tool, however, when a definitive diagnosis is necessary for a problem related to one of the salivary ducts.

Sialography is used to show such conditions as inflammatory lesions and tumors; to determine the extent of salivary fistulae; and to localize diverticula, strictures, and calculi. Because the glands are paired and the pairs are in such close proximity, only one gland at a time can be examined by the sialographic method (Fig. 14-6).

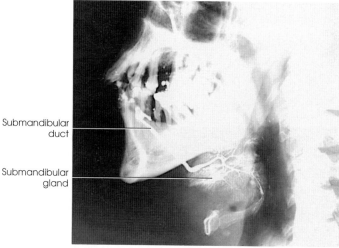

Submandibular duct

Submandibular gland

Fig. 14-6 Sialogram showing opacified submandibular gland.

Sialography is performed as follows:
- Inject the radiopaque medium into the main duct. From there, the contrast material flows into the intraglandular ductules, making it possible to show the surrounding glandular parenchyma and the duct system (Fig. 14-7).
- Obtain preliminary images to detect any condition demonstrable without the use of a contrast medium and to establish the optimal exposure technique.

- About 2 or 3 minutes before the sialographic procedure, give the patient a secretory stimulant to open the duct for ready identification of its orifice and for easier passage of a cannula or catheter. For this purpose, have the patient suck on a wedge of fresh lemon. On completion of the examination, have the patient suck on another lemon wedge to stimulate rapid evacuation of the contrast medium.
- Take an image about 10 minutes after the procedure to verify clearance of the contrast medium, if necessary.

Most physicians inject the contrast medium by manual pressure (i.e., with a syringe attached to the cannula or catheter). Other physicians advocate delivery of the medium by hydrostatic pressure only. The latter method requires the use of a water-soluble iodinated medium, with the contrast solution container (usually a syringe barrel with the plunger removed) attached to a drip stand and set at a distance of 28 inches (70 cm) above the level of the patient's mouth. Some physicians perform the filling procedure under fluoroscopic guidance and obtain spot images.

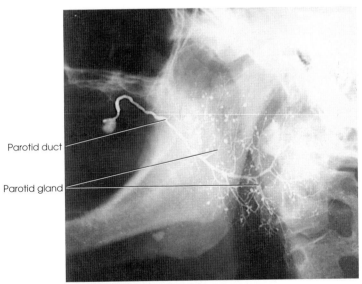

Fig. 14-7 Sialogram showing parotid gland in a patient without teeth.

Parotid duct

Parotid gland

Mouth and Salivary Glands

TANGENTIAL PROJECTION

Image receptor: 8 × 10 inch (18 × 24 cm) lengthwise

Position of patient
• Place the patient in a recumbent or a seated position.
• Because the parotid gland lies midway between the anterior and posterior surfaces of the skull, obtain the tangential projection of the glandular region from the posterior or the anterior direction.

Position of part
Supine body position
• With the patient supine, rotate the head slightly toward the side being examined so that the parotid area is perpendicular to the plane of the IR.
• Center the IR to the parotid area.
• With the patient's head resting on the occiput, adjust the head so that the mandibular ramus is parallel with the longitudinal axis of the IR (Fig. 14-8).

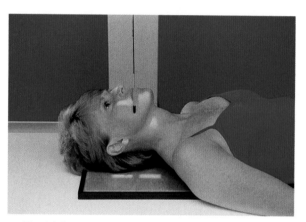

Fig. 14-8 Tangential parotid gland, supine position.

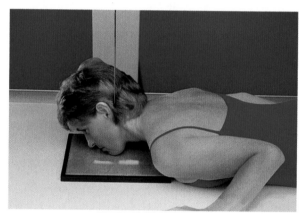

Fig. 14-9 Tangential parotid gland, prone position.

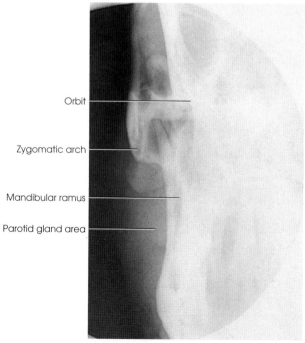

Orbit

Zygomatic arch

Mandibular ramus

Parotid gland area

Fig. 14-10 Tangential parotid gland. Examination of right cheek area to rule out tumor reveals soft tissue fullness and no calcification.

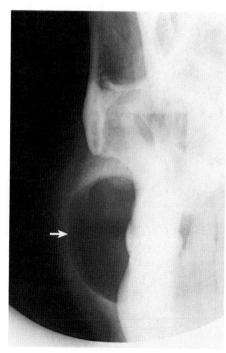

Fig. 14-11 Right cheek (*arrow*) distended with air in mouth (same patient as in Fig. 14-10). No abnormal finding in region of parotid gland.

Prone body position

- With the patient prone, rotate the head so that the parotid area being examined is perpendicular to the plane of the IR.
- Center the IR to the parotid region.
- With the patient's head resting on the chin, adjust the flexion of the head so that the mandibular ramus is parallel with the longitudinal axis of the IR (Fig. 14-9).
- When the parotid (Stensen) duct does not have to be shown, rest the patient's head on the forehead and nose.
- *Shield gonads.*
- *Respiration:* Improved radiographic quality can be obtained, particularly to show calculi, by having the patient fill the mouth with air and then puff the cheeks out as much as possible. When this cannot be done, ask the patient to suspend respiration for the exposure.

Central ray

- Perpendicular to the plane of the IR, directed along the lateral surface of the mandibular ramus

Structures shown

A tangential projection shows the region of the parotid gland and duct. These structures are clearly outlined when an opaque medium is used (Figs. 14-10 to 14-14).

EVALUATION CRITERIA

The following should be clearly shown:

- Exposure technique demonstrating soft tissues
- Most of the parotid gland lateral to and clear of the mandibular ramus
- Mastoid overlapping only the upper portion of the parotid gland

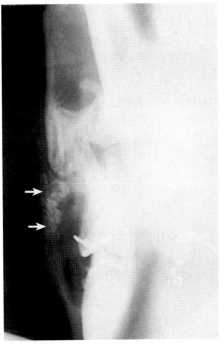

Fig. 14-12 Tangential parotid gland, with right cheek distended with air. Considerable calcification is seen in region of parotid gland (*arrows*).

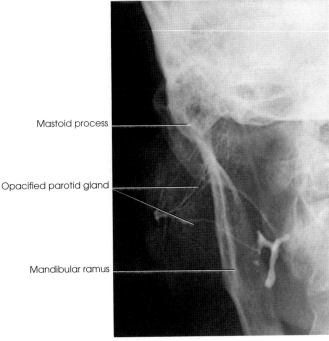

Mastoid process

Opacified parotid gland

Mandibular ramus

Fig. 14-13 Tangential parotid gland showing opacification.

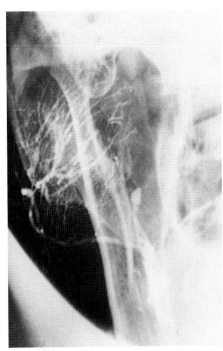

Fig. 14-14 Tangential parotid gland showing opacification.

LATERAL PROJECTION
R or L position

Image receptor: 8 × 10 inch (18 × 24 cm) lengthwise

Position of patient
• Place the patient in a semiprone or seated and upright position.

Position of part
Parotid gland
• With the affected side closest to the IR, extend the patient's neck so that the space between the cervical area of the spine and the mandibular rami is cleared.
• Center the IR to a point approximately 1 inch (2.5 cm) superior to the mandibular angle.
• Adjust the head so that the midsagittal plane is rotated approximately 15 degrees toward the IR from a true lateral position.

Submandibular gland
• Center the IR to the inferior margin of the angle of the mandible.
• Adjust the patient's head in a true lateral position (Fig. 14-15).
• An axiolateral or axiolateral oblique projection may also be performed. See Chapter 20 for positioning details.

• Iglauer[1] suggested depressing the floor of the mouth to displace the submandibular gland below the mandible. When the patient's throat is not too sensitive, accomplish this by having the patient place an index finger on the back of the tongue on the affected side.
• *Shield gonads.*
• *Respiration:* Suspend.

Central ray
• Perpendicular to the center of the IR and directed (1) at a point 1 inch (2.5 cm) superior to the mandibular angle to show the parotid gland or (2) at the inferior margin of the mandibular angle to show the submandibular gland

---

[1]Iglauer S: A simple maneuver to increase the visibility of a salivary calculus in the roentgenogram, *Radiology* 21:297, 1933.

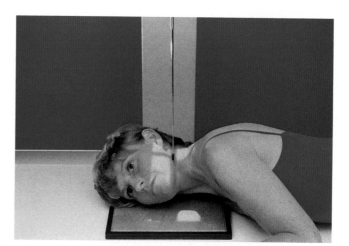

Fig. 14-15 Lateral submandibular gland.

Structures shown

A lateral image shows the bony structures and any calcific deposit or swelling in the unobscured areas of the parotid (Figs. 14-16 and 14-17) and submandibular glands (Fig. 14-18). The glands and their ducts are well outlined when an opaque medium is used.

EVALUATION CRITERIA

The following should be clearly shown:

- Mandibular rami free of overlap from the cervical vertebrae to show best the parotid gland superimposed over the ramus
- Superimposed mandibular rami and angles, if no tube angulation or head rotation is used for the submandibular gland
- Oblique position for the parotid gland
- Submandibular gland shown without superimposition of contralateral mandibular ramus, on axiolateral projections

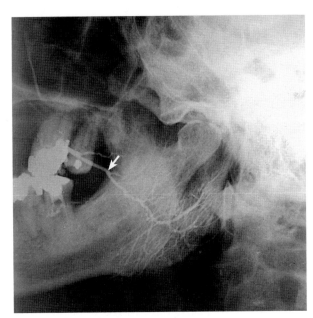

Fig. 14-16 Lateral parotid gland showing opacified gland and parotid duct (*arrow*).

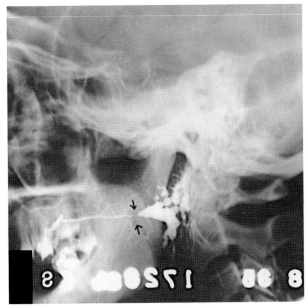

Fig. 14-17 Lateral parotid gland showing opacification and partial blockage of parotid duct (*arrows*).

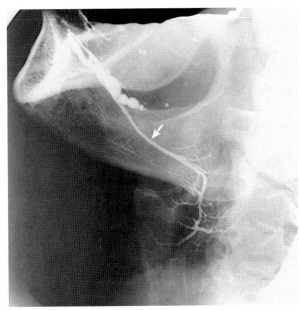

Fig. 14-18 Axiolateral submandibular gland showing opacification of submandibular duct (*arrow*).

15

ANTERIOR PART OF NECK

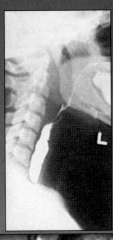

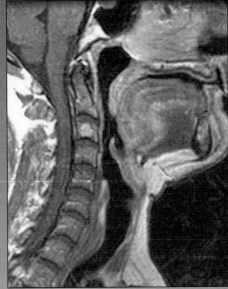

PROJECTIONS, POSITIONS, AND METHODS

Page	Essential	Anatomy	Projection	Position	Method
76		Pharynx and larynx	AP		
78		Soft palate, pharynx, and larynx	Lateral	R or L	

Neck

The *neck* occupies the region between the skull and the thorax (Figs. 15-1 and 15-2). For radiographic purposes, the neck is divided into posterior and anterior portions in accordance with tissue composition and function of the structures. The procedures that are required to show the osseous structures occupying the posterior division of the neck are described in the discussion of the cervical vertebrae in Chapter 8. The portions of the central nervous system and circulatory system that pass through the neck are described in Chapters 22 and 23.

The portion of the neck that lies in front of the vertebrae is composed largely of soft tissues. The upper parts of the respiratory and digestive systems are the principal structures. The thyroid and parathyroid glands and the larger part of the submandibular glands are also located in the anterior portion of the neck.

Thyroid Gland

The *thyroid gland* consists of two lateral lobes connected at their lower thirds by a narrow median portion called the *isthmus* (Fig. 15-3). The lobes are approximately 2 inches (5 cm) long, 1¼ inches (3.2 cm) wide, and ¾ inch (1.9 cm) thick. The isthmus lies at the front of the upper part of the trachea, and the lobes lie at the sides. The lobes reach from the lower third of the thyroid cartilage to the level of the first thoracic vertebra. Although the thyroid gland is normally suprasternal in position, it occasionally extends into the superior aperture of the thorax.

Parathyroid Glands

The *parathyroid glands* are small ovoid bodies, two on each side, *superior* and *inferior*. These glands are situated one above the other on the posterior aspect of the adjacent lobe of the thyroid gland.

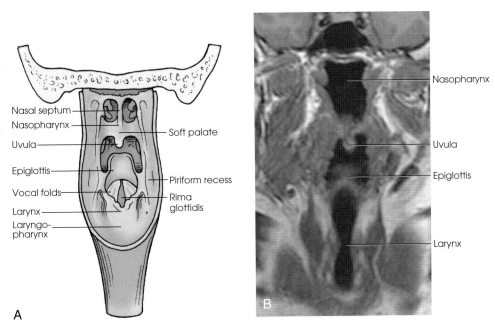

Fig. 15-1 A, Interior posterior view of neck. **B,** Coronal MRI of neck.

(**B,** Courtesy J. Louis Rankin, BS, RT(R)(MR).)

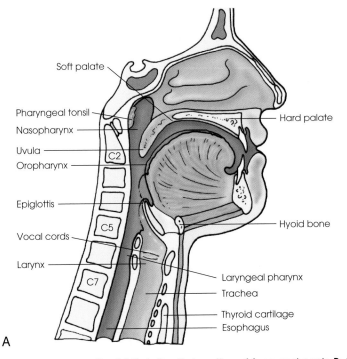

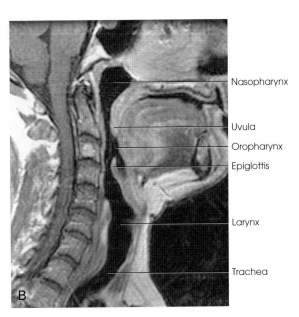

Fig. 15-2 A, Sagittal section of face and neck. **B,** Sagittal MRI of neck.

(**B,** Courtesy J. Louis Rankin, BS, RT(R)(MR).)

Pharynx

The *pharynx* serves as a passage for air and food and is common to the respiratory and digestive systems (see Fig. 15-2). The pharynx is a musculomembranous, tubular structure situated in front of the vertebrae and behind the nose, mouth, and larynx. Approximately 5 inches (13 cm) in length, the pharynx extends from the undersurface of the body of the sphenoid bone and the basilar part of the occipital bone inferiorly to the level of the disk between the sixth and seventh cervical vertebrae, where it becomes continuous with the esophagus. The pharyngeal cavity is subdivided into nasal, oral, and laryngeal portions.

The *nasopharynx* lies posteriorly above the *soft* and *hard* palates. (The upper part of the hard palate forms the floor of the nasopharynx.) Anteriorly, the nasopharynx communicates with the posterior apertures of the nose. Hanging from the posterior aspect of the soft palate is a small conical process, the *uvula*. On the roof and posterior wall of the nasopharynx, between the orifices of the auditory tubes, the mucosa contains a mass of lymphoid tissue known as the *pharyngeal tonsil* (or *adenoids* when enlarged). Hypertrophy of this tissue interferes with nasal breathing and is common in children. This condition is well shown in a lateral radiographic image of the nasopharynx.

The *oropharynx* is the portion extending from the soft palate to the level of the *hyoid bone*. The base, or root, of the tongue forms the anterior wall of the oropharynx. The *laryngeal pharynx* lies posterior to the larynx, its anterior wall being formed by the posterior surface of the larynx. The laryngeal pharynx extends inferiorly and is continuous with the esophagus.

The air-containing nasal and oral pharynges are well visualized in lateral images except during the act of phonation, when the soft palate contracts and tends to obscure the nasal pharynx. An opaque medium is required to show the lumen of the laryngeal pharynx, although it can be distended with air during the *Valsalva maneuver* (an increase in intrathoracic pressure produced by forcible expiration effort against the closed glottis).

Larynx

The larynx is the organ of voice (Figs. 15-4 and 15-5; see Figs. 15-1 through 15-3). Serving as the air passage between the pharynx and the trachea, the larynx is also one of the divisions of the respiratory system.

The larynx is a movable, tubular structure; is broader above than below; and is approximately $1\frac{1}{2}$ inches (3.8 cm) in length. Situated below the root of the tongue and in front of the laryngeal pharynx, the larynx is suspended from the hyoid bone and extends from the level of the superior margin of the fourth cervical vertebra to its junction with the trachea at the level of the inferior margin of the sixth cervical vertebra. The thin, leaf-shaped *epiglottis* is situated behind the root of the tongue and the hyoid bone and above the laryngeal entrance. It has been stated that the epiglottis serves as a trap to prevent leakage into the larynx between acts of swallowing. The *thyroid cartilage* forms the laryngeal prominence, or *Adam's apple*.

The inlet of the larynx is oblique, slanting posteriorly as it descends. A pouchlike fossa called the *piriform recess* is located on each side of the larynx and external to its orifice. The piriform recesses are well shown as triangular areas on frontal projections when insufflated with air (Valsalva maneuver) or when filled with an opaque medium.

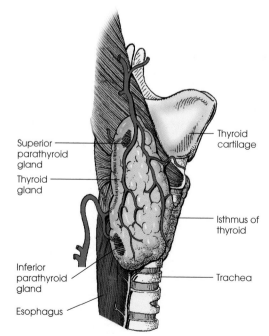

Superior parathyroid gland
Thyroid gland
Inferior parathyroid gland
Esophagus
Thyroid cartilage
Isthmus of thyroid
Trachea

Fig. 15-3 Lateral aspect of laryngeal area showing thyroid gland and isthmus that connects its two lobes.

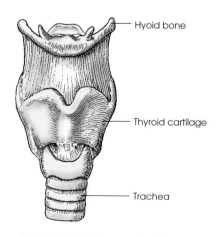

Hyoid bone
Thyroid cartilage
Trachea

Fig. 15-4 Anterior aspect of larynx.

The entrance of the larynx is guarded superiorly and anteriorly by the epiglottis and laterally and posteriorly by folds of mucous membrane. These folds, which extend around the margin of the laryngeal inlet from their junction with the epiglottis, function as a sphincter during swallowing. The *laryngeal cavity* is subdivided into three compartments by two pairs of mucosal folds that extend anteroposteriorly from its lateral walls. The superior pairs of folds are the *vestibular folds*, or false vocal cords. The space above them is called the *laryngeal vestibule*. The lower two folds are separated from each other by a median fissure called the *rima glottidis*. They are known as the *vocal folds*, or true vocal folds (see Fig. 15-5). The vocal cords are vocal ligaments that are covered by the vocal folds. The ligaments and the rima glottidis constitute the vocal apparatus of the larynx and are collectively referred to as the *glottis*.

SUMMARY OF ANATOMY

Thyroid gland	Pharynx	Larynx
Isthmus	Nasopharynx	Epiglottis
	Soft palate	Thyroid cartilage
Parathyroid glands	Hard palate	Piriform recess
Superior	Uvula	Laryngeal cavity
Inferior	Pharyngeal tonsil	Vestibular folds (false vocal cords)
	Oropharynx	Laryngeal vestibule
	Hyoid bone	Rima glottides
	Laryngeal pharynx	Vocal folds (true vocal cords)
		Glottis

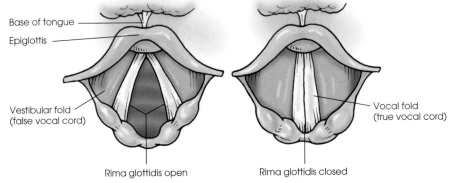

Base of tongue
Epiglottis
Vestibular fold (false vocal cord)
Vocal fold (true vocal cord)
Rima glottidis open
Rima glottidis closed

Fig. 15-5 Superior aspect of larynx (open and closed true vocal folds).

Anterior Part of Neck

Soft Palate, Pharynx, and Larynx: Methods of Examination

The throat structures may be examined with or without an opaque contrast medium. The technique employed depends on the abnormality being investigated. Computed tomography (CT) studies are often performed to show radiographically areas of the palate, pharynx, and larynx with little or no discomfort to the patient. Magnetic resonance imaging (MRI) is also used to evaluate the larynx. The radiologic modality selected is often determined by the institution and the physician. The only radiologic examination currently performed to evaluate structures of the anterior neck is positive-contrast pharyngography.

POSITIVE-CONTRAST PHARYNGOGRAPHY

Opaque studies of the pharynx are made with an ingestible contrast medium, usually a thick, creamy mixture of water and barium sulfate. This examination is frequently done using fluoroscopy with spot-film images only. These or conventional projections are made during deglutition (swallowing).

Deglutition

The act of swallowing is performed by the rapid and highly coordinated action of many muscles. The following points are important in radiography of the pharynx and upper esophagus:

1. The middle area of the tongue becomes depressed to collect the mass, or bolus, of material to be swallowed.
2. The base of the tongue forms a central groove to accommodate the bolus and then moves superiorly and inferiorly along the roof of the mouth to propel the bolus into the pharynx.

3. Simultaneously with the posterior thrust of the tongue, the larynx moves anteriorly and superiorly under the root of the tongue, the sphincteric folds nearly closing the laryngeal inlet (orifice).
4. The epiglottis divides the passing bolus and drains the two portions laterally into the piriform recesses as it lowers over the laryngeal entrance.

The bolus is projected into the pharynx at the height of the anterior movement of the larynx (Figs. 15-6 to 15-8). Synchronizing a rapid exposure with the peak of the act is necessary.

The shortest exposure time possible must be used for studies made during deglutition. The steps are as follows:

- Ask the patient to hold the barium sulfate bolus in the mouth until signaled and then to swallow the bolus in one movement.
- If a mucosal study is to be attempted, ask the patient to refrain from swallowing again.
- Take the mucosal study during the modified Valsalva maneuver for double-contrast delineation.

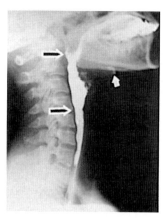

Fig. 15-6 Lateral projection with exposure made at peak of laryngeal elevation. Hyoid bone (*white arrow*) is almost at level of mandible. Pharynx (*between large arrows*) is completely distended with barium.

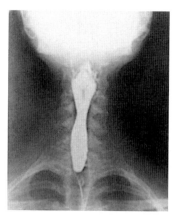

Fig. 15-7 AP projection of the same patient as in Fig. 15-6. Epiglottis divides bolus into two streams, filling the piriform recess below. Barium can also be seen entering upper esophagus.

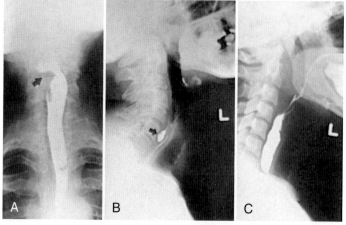

Fig. 15-8 AP projection of pharynx and upper esophagus with barium. **A,** Head was turned to right, with resultant asymmetric filling of pharynx. Bolus is passing through left piriform recess, leaving right side unfilled (*arrow*). **B,** Lateral projection after patient swallowed barium, showing diverticulum (*arrow*). **C,** Lateral projection made slightly later, showing only filling of upper esophagus.

Some fluoroscopic equipment can expose 12 frames per second using the 100-mm or 105-mm cut or roll film. Many institutions with such equipment use it to spot-image patients in rapid sequence during the act of swallowing. Another technique is to record the fluoroscopic image on videotape or cine film. The recorded image may be studied to identify abnormalities during the active progress of deglutition.

Gunson method

Gunson[1] offered a practical suggestion for synchronizing the exposure with the height of the swallowing act in deglutition studies of the pharynx and superior esophagus. Gunson's method consists of tying a dark-colored shoestring (metal tips removed) snugly around the patient's throat above the thyroid cartilage (Fig. 15-9). Anterior and superior movements of the larynx are shown by elevation of the shoestring as the thyroid cartilage moves anteriorly and immediately thereafter by displacement of the shoestring as the cartilage passes superiorly.

Having the exposure coincide with the peak of the anterior movement of the larynx—the instant at which the bolus of contrast material is projected into the pharynx—is desirable. As stated by Templeton and Kredel,[2] the action is so rapid that satisfactory filling is usually obtained if the exposure is made as soon as anterior movement is noted.

[1]Gunson EF: Radiography of the pharynx and upper esophagus: shoestring method, *Xray Tech* 33:1, 1961.
[2]Templeton FE, Kredel RA: The cricopharyngeal sphincter, *Laryngoscope* 53:1, 1943.

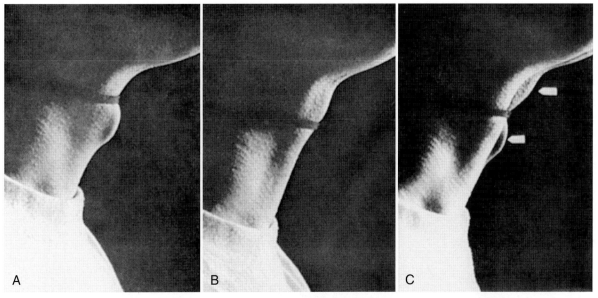

Fig. 15-9 A, An ordinary dark shoelace has been tied snugly around the patient's neck above the Adam's apple. **B,** Exposure was made at peak of superior and anterior movement of larynx during swallowing. Pharynx is completely filled with barium at this moment, which is the ideal instant for making an x-ray exposure. **C,** Double-exposure photograph emphasizing movement of Adam's apple during swallowing. Note extent of anterior and superior excursion (*arrows*).

AP PROJECTION

Radiographic studies of the pharyngo-laryngeal structures are made during breathing, phonation, stress maneuvers, and swallowing. To minimize the incidence of motion, the shortest possible exposure time must be used in the examinations. For the purpose of obtaining improved contrast on AP projections, use of a grid is recommended.

Image receptor: 8 × 10 inch (18 × 24 cm) or 10 × 12 inch (24 × 30 cm) lengthwise

Position of patient

• Except for tomographic studies, which require a recumbent body position (Fig. 15-10), place the patient in the upright position, seated or standing, whenever possible.

Position of part

• Center the midsagittal plane of the body to the midline of the vertical grid device.
• Ask the patient to sit or stand straight. If the standing position is used, have the patient distribute the weight of the body equally on the feet.
• Adjust the patient's shoulders to lie in the same horizontal plane to prevent rotation of the head and neck and resultant obliquity of the throat structures.
• Center the IR at the level of or just below the laryngeal prominence.
• Extend the patient's head only enough to prevent the mandibular shadow from obscuring the laryngeal area.
• *Shield gonads.*
• *Respiration:* Obtain preliminary images (AP and lateral) during the inspiratory phase of quiet nasal breathing to ensure that the throat passages are filled with air. To determine the optimal time for the exposure, watch the breathing movements of the chest. Make the exposure *just before* the chest comes to rest at the end of one of its inspiratory expansions (Fig. 15-11).

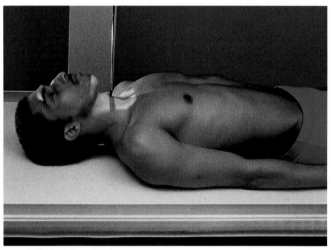

Fig. 15-10 AP pharynx and larynx with patient in supine position for tomography.

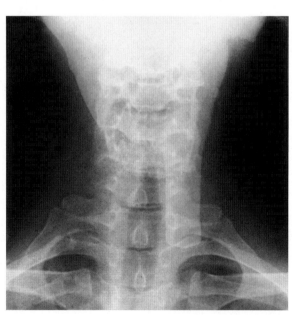

Fig. 15-11 AP pharynx and larynx during quiet breathing.

Central ray

- Perpendicular to the laryngeal prominence

Collimation

- Level of EAM to jugular notch and 1 inch (2.5 cm) beyond the skin edges on the sides

Additional studies

Additional necessary studies of the pharynx and larynx are usually determined fluoroscopically. These studies may be made at the following times:

1. During the Valsalva or modified Valsalva stress maneuver or both* (Fig. 15-12)
2. At the height of the act of swallowing a bolus of 1 tablespoon of creamy barium sulfate suspension. The patient holds the barium sulfate bolus in the mouth until signaled and then swallows it in one movement. The patient is asked to refrain from swallowing again if a double-contrast study is to be attempted.

---

*The Valsalva maneuver is performed by forcible exhalation against a closed airway, usually by closing the mouth and pinching the nose shut. The modified Valsalva maneuver is performed by forcible exhalation against a closed glottis.

3. During the modified Valsalva maneuver, immediately after the barium swallow for double-contrast delineation of the piriform recesses
4. During phonation and with the larynx in the rest position after its opacification with an iodinated contrast medium Tomographic studies of the larynx are made during phonation of a high-pitched *e-e-e*. After these studies, one or more sectional studies may be made at the selected level or levels with the larynx at rest (Fig. 15-13).

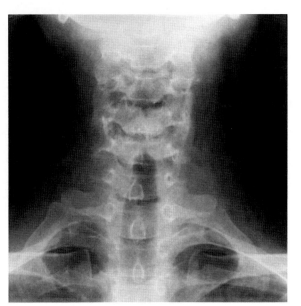

Fig. 15-12 AP pharynx and larynx showing Valsalva maneuver.

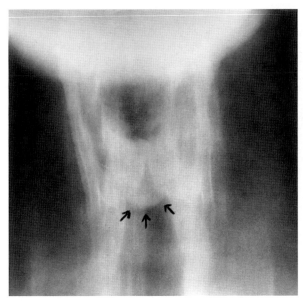

Fig. 15-13 AP pharynx and larynx with tomogram showing polypoid laryngeal mass (*arrows*).

LATERAL PROJECTION
R or L position

> **Image receptor:** 8 × 10 inch (18 × 24 cm) lengthwise

Position of patient
- Ask the patient to sit or stand laterally before the vertical grid device.
- Adjust the patient so that the coronal plane passing through or just anterior to the temporomandibular joints is centered to the midline of the IR.

Position of part
- Ask the patient to sit or stand straight, with the adjacent shoulder resting firmly against the stand for support.
- Adjust the body so that the midsagittal plane is parallel with the plane of the IR.
- Depress the shoulders as much as possible, and adjust them to lie in the same transverse plane. If necessary, have the patient clasp the hands in back to rotate the shoulders posteriorly.
- Extend the patient's head slightly.
- Immobilize the head by having the patient look at an object in line with the visual axis.

Central ray
- Perpendicular to the IR, center the IR (1) 1 inch (2.5 cm) below the level of the EAMs to show the nasopharynx and to perform cleft palate studies; (2) at the level of the mandibular angles to show the oropharynx; or (3) at the level of the laryngeal prominence to show the larynx, laryngeal pharynx, and upper end of the esophagus (Fig. 15-14).

Collimation
- Level of EAM to jugular notch; include all anterior oropharyngeal structures

Procedure
Preliminary studies of the pharyngolaryngeal structures are made during the inhalation phase of quiet nasal breathing to ensure filling of the passages with air (Fig. 15-15).

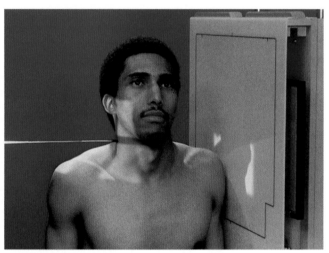

Fig. 15-14 Lateral pharynx and larynx.

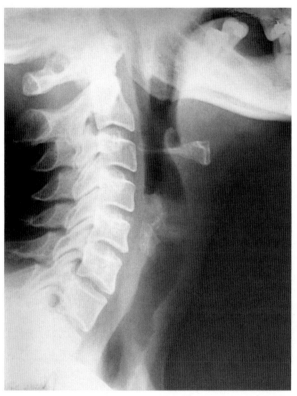

Fig. 15-15 Lateral pharynx and larynx during normal breathing.

According to the site and nature of the abnormality, further studies may be made. Each of the selected maneuvers must be explained to the patient and practiced just before actual use. The studies are obtained at one or more of the following:

1. During phonation of specified vowel sounds to show the vocal cords and to perform cleft palate studies (Fig. 15-16)
2. During Valsalva maneuver to distend the subglottic larynx and trachea with air (Fig. 15-17)
3. During modified Valsalva maneuver to distend the supraglottic larynx and the laryngeal pharynx with air
4. At the height of the act of swallowing a bolus of 1 tablespoon of creamy barium sulfate suspension to show the pharyngeal structures
5. With the larynx at rest or during phonation after opacification of the structure with an iodinated medium
6. During the act of swallowing a tuft or pledget of cotton (or food) saturated with a barium sulfate suspension to show nonopaque foreign bodies located in the pharynx or upper esophagus

EVALUATION CRITERIA

The following should be clearly shown:
- Evidence of proper collimation
- Exposure sufficient to demonstrate soft tissue pharyngolaryngeal structures
- Area from nasopharynx to the uppermost part of the lungs in preliminary studies
- Specific area of interest centered in detailed examinations
- No superimposition of the trachea by the shoulders
- Closely superimposed mandibular shadows
- Throat filled with air in preliminary studies

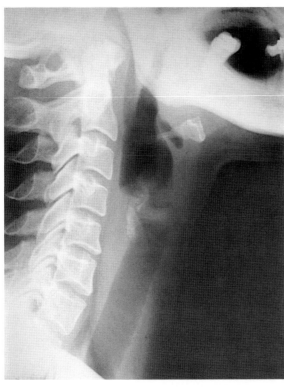

Fig. 15-16 Lateral pharynx and larynx during phonation of e-e-e.

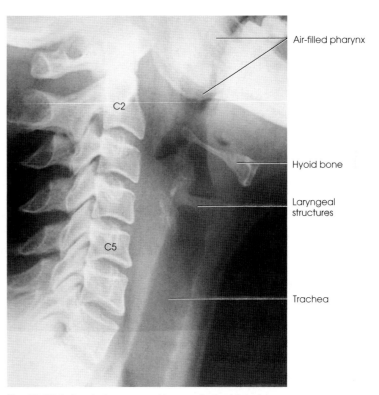

Fig. 15-17 Lateral pharynx and larynx during Valsalva maneuver.

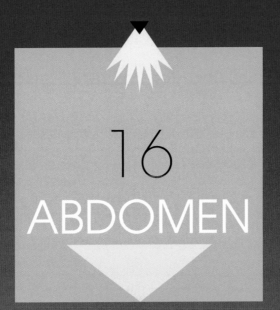

16

ABDOMEN

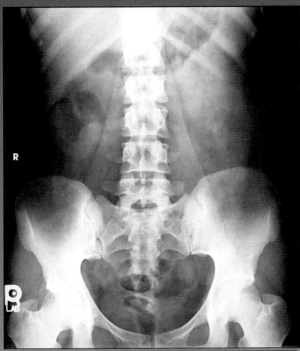

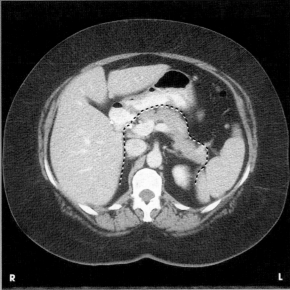

SUMMARY OF PROJECTIONS

PROJECTIONS, POSITIONS, AND METHODS

Page	Essential	Anatomy	Projection	Position	Method
89	🦃	Abdomen	AP	Supine; upright	
91	🦃	Abdomen	PA	Upright	
91	🦃	Abdomen	AP	L lateral decubitus	
93	🦃	Abdomen	Lateral	R or L	
94	🦃	Abdomen	Lateral	R or L dorsal decubitus	

Icons in the Essential column indicate projections frequently performed in the United States and Canada. Students should be competent in these projections.

Abdominopelvic Cavity

The *abdominopelvic* cavity consists of two parts: (1) a large superior portion, the abdominal cavity; and (2) a smaller inferior part, the pelvic cavity. The *abdominal cavity* extends from the diaphragm to the superior aspect of the bony pelvis. The abdominal cavity contains the stomach, small and large intestines, liver, gallbladder, spleen, pancreas, and kidneys. The *pelvic cavity* lies within the margins of the bony pelvis and contains the rectum and sigmoid of the large intestine, the urinary bladder, and the reproductive organs. Anatomists define the "true pelvis" as that portion of the abdominopelvic cavity inferior to a plane passing through the sacral promontory posteriorly and the superior surface of the pubic bones anteriorly.

The abdominopelvic cavity is enclosed in a double-walled seromembranous sac called the *peritoneum*. The outer portion of this sac, termed the *parietal peritoneum*, is in close contact with the abdominal wall, the greater (false) pelvic wall, and most of the undersurface of the diaphragm. The inner portion of the sac, known as the *visceral peritoneum*, is positioned over or around the contained organs. The peritoneum forms folds called the *mesentery* and *omenta*, which serve to support the viscera in position. The space between the two layers of the peritoneum is called the *peritoneal cavity* and contains serous fluid (Fig. 16-1). Because there are no mesenteric attachments of the intestines in the pelvic cavity, pelvic surgery can be performed without entry into the peritoneal cavity.

The *retroperitoneum* is the cavity behind the peritoneum. Organs such as the kidneys and pancreas lie in the retroperitoneum (Fig. 16-2).

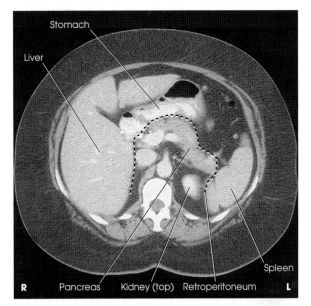

Fig. 16-2 Axial CT image of abdomen showing organs of upper abdomen. Retroperitoneum is posterior and medial to *dashed line*.

(From Kelley LL, Petersen CM: *Sectional anatomy for imaging professionals*, ed 2, St Louis, 2007, Mosby.)

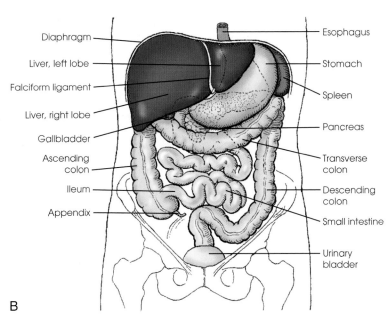

Fig. 16-1 A, Lateral aspect of abdomen showing peritoneal sac and its components.
B, Anterior aspect of abdominal viscera in relation to surrounding structures.

SUMMARY OF ANATOMY

Abdomen
Abdominopelvic cavity
Abdominal cavity
Pelvic cavity
Peritoneum
Parietal peritoneum
Mesentery
Omenta
Peritoneal cavity
Retroperitoneum
Visceral peritoneum

SUMMARY OF PATHOLOGY

Condition	Definition
Abdominal aortic aneurysm (AAA)	Localized dilation of abdominal aorta
Ascites	Fluid accumulation in the peritoneal cavity
Bowel obstruction	Blockage of bowel lumen
Ileus	Failure of bowel peristalsis
Metastasis	Transfer of a cancerous lesion from one area to another
Pneumoperitoneum	Presence of air in peritoneal cavity
Tumor	New tissue growth where cell proliferation is uncontrolled

SAMPLE EXPOSURE TECHNIQUE CHART ESSENTIAL PROJECTIONS

These techniques were accurate for the equipment used to produce each exposure. However, use caution when applying them in your department; generator output characteristics and IR energy sensitivities vary widely.[1]

This chart was created in collaboration with Dennis Bowman, AS, RT(R), Clinical Instructor, Community Hospital of the Monterey Peninsula, Monterey, CA. http://digitalradiographysolutions.com/.

ABDOMEN

Part	cm	kVp*	SID†	Collimation	CR‡ mAs	CR‡ Dose (mGy)‖	DR§ mAs	DR§ Dose (mGy)‖
AP¶	21	85	40"	14" × 17" (35 × 43 cm)	25**	3.700	10**	1.474
PA¶	21	85	40"	14" × 17" (35 × 43 cm)	22**	3.250	9**	1.321
AP/Lateral Decubitus¶	24	85	40"	17" × 14" (43 × 35 cm)	28**	4.480	11**	1.753
Lateral¶	30	90	40"	14" × 17" (35 × 43 cm)	50**	10.48	20**	4.170
Lateral/Dorsal Decubitus¶	30	90	40"	17" × 14" (43 × 35 cm)	65**	13.64	25**	5.230

[1]ACR-AAPM-SIMM Practice Guidelines for Digital Radiography, 2007.
*kVp values are for a high-frequency generator.
†40 inch minimum; 44 to 48 inches recommended to improve spatial resolution (mAs increase needed, but no increase in patient dose will result).
‡AGFA CR MD 4.0 General IP, CR 75.0 reader, 400 speed class, with 6:1 (178LPI) grid when needed.
§GE Definium 8000, with 13:1 grid when needed.
‖All doses are skin entrance for average adult (160 to 200 pound male, 150 to 190 pound female) at part thickness indicated.
¶Bucky/Grid.
**Large focal spot.

ABBREVIATIONS USED IN CHAPTER 16

AAA Abdominal aortic aneurysm
ERCP Endoscopic retrograde cholangiopancreatography
NPO Nil per os (nothing by mouth)
PTC Percutaneous transhepatic cholangiography
RUQ Right upper quadrant

See Addendum B for a summary of all abbreviations used in Volume 2.

Abdomen

Abdominal Radiographic Procedures

EXPOSURE TECHNIQUE

In examinations without a contrast medium, it is imperative to obtain maximal soft tissue differentiation throughout the different regions of the abdomen. Because of the wide range in the thickness of the abdomen and the delicate differences in physical density between the contained viscera, a proper balance of exposure factors is critical to show both solid organs, as well as adjacent structures, while delivering the lowest possible radiation dose. If the kilovolt peak (kVp) is too high, the possibility of not showing small or semiopaque gallstones increases (Fig. 16-3, A) particularly on film-screen radiographs.

The best criterion for assessing the quality of an abdominal radiographic image is the ability to visualize each of the following (Fig. 16-3, B):
- Sharply defined outlines of the psoas muscles
- Lower border of the liver
- Kidneys
- Ribs and transverse processes of the lumbar vertebrae

IMMOBILIZATION

A prime requisite in abdominal examinations is to prevent voluntary and involuntary movement. The following steps are observed:
- To prevent muscle contraction caused by tension, adjust the patient in a comfortable position so that he or she can relax.
- Explain the breathing procedure, and ensure that the patient understands exactly what is expected.

- If necessary, apply a compression band across the abdomen for *immobilization* but not for compression.
- Do not start the exposure for 1 to 2 seconds after suspension of respiration to allow the patient to come to rest and involuntary movement of the viscera to subside.

Voluntary motion produces a blurred outline of the structures that do not have involuntary movement, such as the liver, psoas muscles, and spine. Patient breathing during exposure results in blurring of bowel gas outlines in the upper abdomen as the diaphragm moves (Fig. 16-4). Involuntary motion caused by peristalsis may produce localized or generalized haziness of the image. Involuntary contraction of the abdominal wall or the muscles around the spine may cause movement of the entire abdominal area and may produce generalized image haziness.

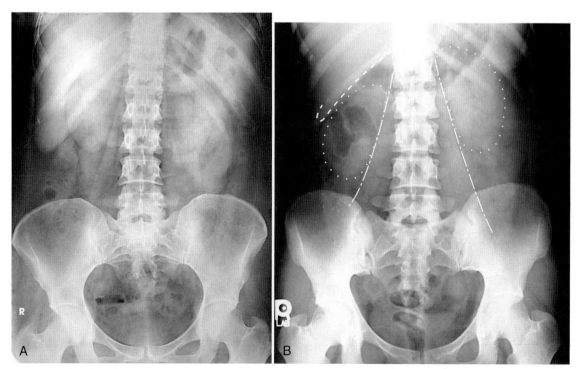

Fig. 16-3 A, AP abdomen showing proper positioning and collimation. **B,** AP abdomen showing kidney shadows (*dotted line*), margin of liver (*dashed line*), and psoas muscles (*dot-dash lines*).

RADIOGRAPHIC PROJECTIONS

Radiographic examination of the abdomen may include one or more projections. The most commonly performed is the supine AP projection, often called a *KUB* because it includes the *kidneys, ureters,* and *bladder.* Projections used to complement the supine AP include an upright AP abdomen or an AP projection in the lateral decubitus position (the left lateral decubitus is most often preferred), or both. Both images are useful in assessing the abdomen in patients with free air (pneumoperitoneum) and in determining the presence and location of air-fluid levels. Other abdominal projections include a lateral projection or a lateral projection in the supine (dorsal decubitus) body position. Many institutions also obtain a PA chest image to include the upper abdomen and diaphragm. The PA chest is indicated because any air escaping from the gastrointestinal tract into the peritoneal space rises to the highest level, usually just beneath the diaphragm.

POSITIONING PROTOCOLS

The required projections obtained to evaluate the patient's abdomen vary considerably depending on the institution and the physician. Some physicians consider the preliminary evaluation image (often termed a *scout* or *survey*) to consist of only the AP (supine) projection. Others obtain two projections: a supine and an upright AP abdomen (often called a *flat* and an *upright*). A three-way or acute abdomen series may be requested to rule out free air, bowel obstruction, and infection. The three projections usually include (1) AP with the patient supine, (2) AP with the patient upright, and (3) PA chest. If the patient cannot stand for the upright AP projection, the projection is performed using the left lateral decubitus position. The PA chest projection can be used to demonstrate free air that may accumulate under the diaphragm.

Positioning for radiographic examination of the abdomen is described in the following pages. (For a description of positioning for the PA chest, see Chapter 10.)

Abdominal Sequencing

To show small amounts of intraperitoneal gas in acute abdominal cases, Miller[1,2] recommended that the patient be kept in the left lateral position on a stretcher for 10 to 20 minutes before abdominal images are obtained. This position allows gas to rise into the area under the right hemidiaphragm, where the potential pathology would not be superimposed by the gastric gas bubble. If larger amounts of free air are present, many radiology departments suggest that the patient lie on the side for a minimum of 5 minutes before the exposure is made.

Projections of the abdomen are taken as follows:

- Perform an AP or PA projection of the chest and upper abdomen with the patient in the left lateral decubitus position.
- Use the chest exposure technique for this image (Fig. 16-5).
- Maintain the patient in the left lateral decubitus position while the patient is being moved onto a horizontally placed table. Tilt the table and the patient to the upright position.
- Turn the patient to obtain AP or PA projections of the chest and abdomen (Figs. 16-6 and 16-7).
- Return the table back to the horizontal position for a supine AP or PA projection of the abdomen (Fig. 16-8).

[1]Miller RE, Nelson SW: The roentgenologic demonstration of tiny amounts of free intraperitoneal gas: experimental and clinical studies, *AJR Am J Roentgenol* 112:574, 1971.
[2]Miller RE: The technical approach to the acute abdomen, *Semin Roentgenol* 8:267, 1973.

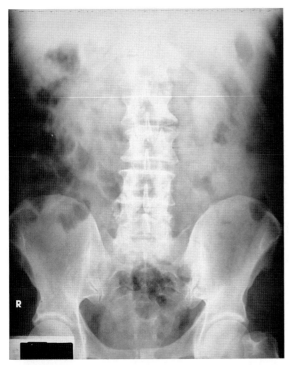

Fig. 16-4 AP abdomen showing blurred bowel gas in right upper quadrant (RUQ), caused by patient breathing during exposure.

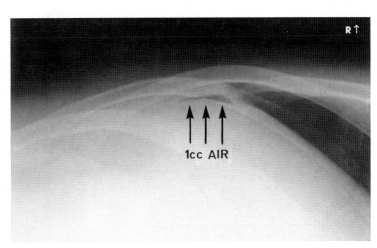

Fig. 16-5 Enlarged portion of AP abdomen, left lateral decubitus position in a patient injected with 1 mL of air into abdominal cavity.

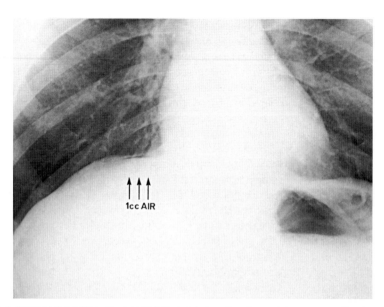

Fig. 16-6 Enlarged portion of upright AP chest showing free air in same patient as in Fig. 16-5.

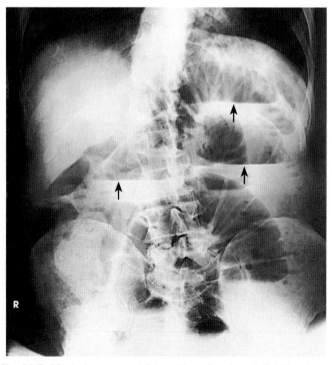

Fig. 16-7 AP abdomen, upright position, showing air-fluid levels (*arrows*) in intestine (same patient as in Fig. 16-8).

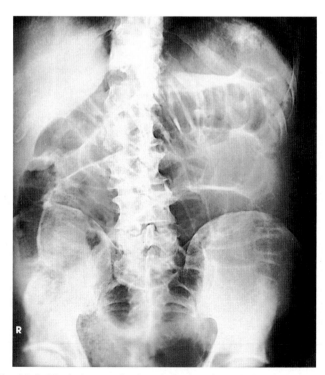

Fig. 16-8 AP abdomen. Supine study showing intestinal obstruction in same patient as in Fig. 16-7.

♠ AP PROJECTION
Supine; upright

Image receptor: 14 × 17 inch (35 × 43 cm) lengthwise

Position of patient
- For the AP abdomen, or KUB, projection, place the patient in either the supine or the upright position. The supine position is preferred for most initial examinations of the abdomen.

Position of part
- Center the midsagittal plane of the body to the midline of the grid device.
- If the patient is upright, distribute the weight of the body equally on the feet.

- Place the patient's arms where they do not cast shadows on the image.
- With the patient supine, place a support under the knees to relieve strain.
- For the *supine position,* center the IR/collimated field at the level of the iliac crests, and ensure that the pubic symphysis is included (Fig. 16-9).
- For the *upright position,* center the IR/collimated field 2 inches (5 cm) above the level of the iliac crests or high enough to include the diaphragm (Fig. 16-10).
- If the bladder is to be included on the upright image, center the IR/collimated field at the level of the iliac crests.
- If a patient is too tall to include the entire pelvic area, obtain a second

image to include the bladder, if necessary. The 10 × 12 inch (24 × 30 cm) IR or collimated field is oriented crosswise and is centered 2 to 3 inches (5 to 7.6 cm) above the upper border of the pubic symphysis.
- If necessary, apply a compression band across the abdomen with moderate pressure for immobilization.
- *Shield gonads:* Use local gonad shielding for examinations of male patients (not shown for illustrative purposes).
- *Respiration:* Suspend at the end of expiration so that the abdominal organs are not compressed.

Central ray
- Perpendicular to the IR at the level of the iliac crests for the supine position
- Horizontal and 2 inches (5 cm) above the level of the iliac crests to include the diaphragm for the upright position

Collimation
- Adjust to 14 × 17 inches (35 × 43 cm) on the collimator. For smaller patients, collimate to within 1 inch (2.5 cm) of shadow of the abdomen.

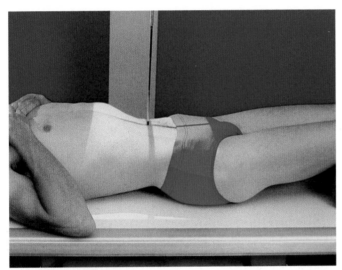

Fig. 16-9 AP abdomen, supine.

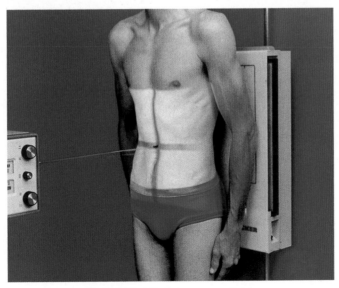

Fig. 16-10 AP abdomen, upright.

Abdomen

Structures shown

AP projection of the abdomen shows the size and shape of the liver, the spleen, and the kidneys and intra-abdominal calcifications or evidence of tumor masses (Fig. 16-11). Additional examples of supine and upright abdomen projections are shown in Figs. 16-7 and 16-8.

EVALUATION CRITERIA

The following should be clearly shown:
- Evidence of proper collimation
- Area from the pubic symphysis to the upper abdomen (two images may be necessary if the patient is tall or wide)
- Proper patient alignment, as ensured by the following:
  - ☐ Centered vertebral column
  - ☐ Ribs, pelvis, and hips equidistant to the edge of the image or collimated borders on both sides
- No rotation of the patient, as demonstrated by the following:
  - ☐ Spinous processes in the center of the lumbar vertebrae
  - ☐ Ischial spines of the pelvis symmetric, if visible
  - ☐ Alae or wings of the ilia symmetric

- Soft tissue brightness and contrast showing the following:
  - ☐ Lateral abdominal wall and properitoneal fat layer (flank stripe)
  - ☐ Psoas muscles, lower border of the liver, and kidneys
  - ☐ Inferior ribs
  - ☐ Transverse processes of the lumbar vertebrae
- Right or left marker visible but not lying over abdominal contents
- Diaphragm without motion on upright abdominal examinations (crosswise IR placement/collimated field is appropriate if the patient is large)
- Brightness and contrast on upright abdominal examination, similar to supine examination
- Upright abdomen identified with appropriate marker

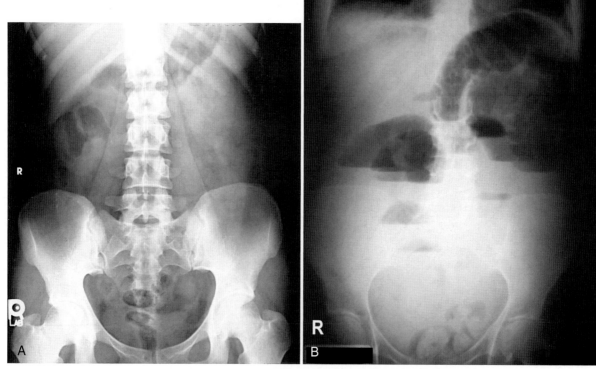

Fig. 16-11 A, AP abdomen, supine position. **B,** AP abdomen, upright position.

♠ PA PROJECTION
Upright

When the kidneys are not of primary interest, the upright PA projection should be considered. Compared with the AP projection, the PA projection of the abdomen greatly reduces patient gonadal dose.

> **Image receptor:** 14 × 17 inch (35 × 43 cm) lengthwise

Position of patient

- With the patient in the upright position, place the anterior abdominal surface in contact with the vertical grid device.
- Center the abdominal midline to the midline of the IR.
- Center the IR/collimated field 2 inches (5 cm) above the level of the iliac crests (Fig. 16-12), as previously described for the upright AP projection. The central ray, structures shown, and evaluation criteria are the same as for the upright AP projection.

♠ AP PROJECTION
L lateral decubitus position

> **Image receptor:** 14 × 17 inch (35 × 43 cm)

Position of patient

- If the patient is too ill to stand, place him or her in a lateral recumbent position lying on a radiolucent pad on a transportation cart. Use a left lateral decubitus position in most situations.
  - The radiolucent pad is particularly important to ensure inclusion of the entire dependent side when fluid demonstration is of primary concern.
- If possible, have the patient lie on the side for several minutes before the exposure to allow air to rise to its highest level within the abdomen.
- Place the patient's arms above the level of the diaphragm so that they are not projected over any abdominal contents.
- Flex the patient's knees slightly to provide stabilization.
- *Exercise care* to ensure that the patient does not fall off the cart; if a cart is used, *lock all wheels* securely in position.

Position of part

- Adjust the height of the vertical grid device so that the long axis of the IR is centered to the midsagittal plane.

- If the abdomen is too wide to include both flanks on one image, adjust patient and IR height to include side down when intraperitoneal fluid is suspected and to include side up when pneumoperitoneum is suspected.
- Position the patient so that the level of the iliac crests is centered to the IR. A slightly higher centering point, 2 inches (5 cm) above the iliac crests, may be necessary to ensure that the diaphragms are included in the image (Fig. 16-13).
- Adjust the patient to ensure that a true lateral position is attained.
- *Shield gonads.*
- *Respiration:* Suspend at the end of expiration.

▼ COMPENSATING FILTER

For patients with a large abdomen, a compensating filter improves image quality by preventing overexposure of the upper-side abdominal area.

Central ray

- Directed *horizontal* and perpendicular to the midpoint of the IR

Collimation

- Adjust to 14 × 17 inches (35 × 43 cm) on the collimator. For smaller patients, collimate to within 1 inch (2.5 cm) of shadow of the abdomen.

NOTE: A right lateral decubitus position is often requested or may be required when the patient cannot lie on the left side.

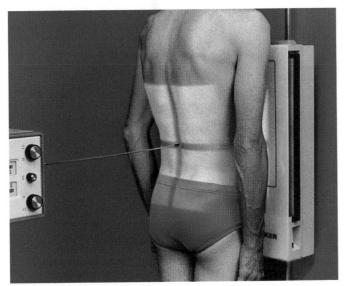

Fig. 16-12 PA abdomen, upright position. This projection is suggested for survey examination of the abdomen when the kidneys are not of primary interest.

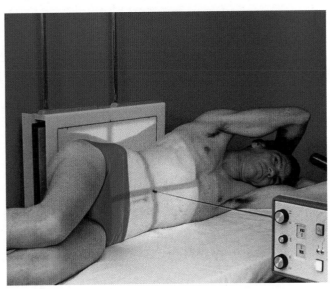

Fig. 16-13 AP abdomen, left lateral decubitus position.

Structures shown

In addition to showing the size and shape of the liver, spleen, and kidneys, the AP abdomen with the patient in the left decubitus position is most valuable for showing free air and air-fluid levels when an upright abdomen projection cannot be obtained (Fig. 16-14).

EVALUATION CRITERIA

The following should be clearly shown:
- Evidence of proper collimation
- Diaphragm without motion
- Both sides of the abdomen. If abdomen is too wide:
  □ Side down when fluid is suspected (ensure entire dependent side is included in the collimated field)
  □ Side up when free air is suspected
- Abdominal wall, flank structures, and diaphragm
- No rotation of patient, as demonstrated by the following:
  □ Spinous processes in the center of the lumbar vertebrae
  □ Ischial spines of the pelvis symmetric, if visible
  □ Alae or wings of the ilia symmetric
- Appropriate brightness and contrast to demonstrate abdominal contents
- Proper identification visible, including patient side and marking to indicate which side is up

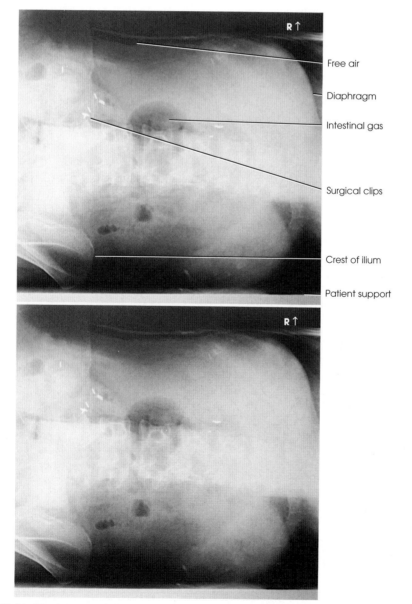

Free air

Diaphragm

Intestinal gas

Surgical clips

Crest of ilium

Patient support

Fig. 16-14 AP abdomen, left lateral decubitus position, showing free air collection along right flank. Note correct marker placement.

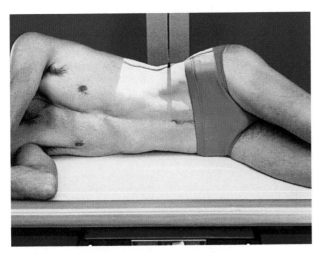

Fig. 16-15 Right lateral abdomen.

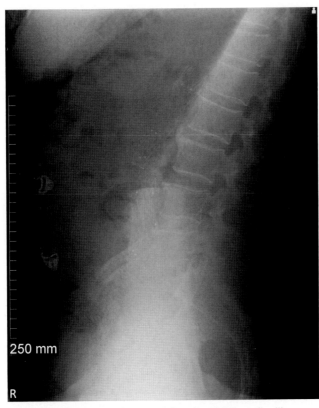

Fig. 16-16 Right lateral abdomen showing AAA graft with extensions into both common iliac arteries.

(Image courtesy of NEA Baptist Memorial Hospital, Jonesboro, AR.)

♠ LATERAL PROJECTION
R or L position

Image receptor: 14 × 17 inch (35 × 43 cm) lengthwise

Position of patient
- Turn the patient to a lateral recumbent position on the right or the left side.

Position of part
- Flex the patient's knees to a comfortable position, and adjust the body so that the midcoronal plane is centered to the midline of the grid.
- Place supports between the knees and the ankles.
- Flex the elbows, and place the hands under the patient's head (Fig. 16-15).
- Center the IR at the level of the iliac crests or 2 inches (5 cm) above the crests to include the diaphragm.
- Place a compression band across the pelvis for stability if necessary.
- *Shield gonads.*
- *Respiration:* Suspend at the end of expiration.

Central ray
- Perpendicular to the IR and entering the midcoronal plane at the level of the iliac crest or 2 inches (5 cm) above the iliac crest if the diaphragm is included

Collimation
- Adjust to 14 × 17 inches (35 × 43 cm) on the collimator. For smaller patients, collimate to within 1 inch (2.5 cm) of shadow of the abdomen.

Structures shown
A lateral projection of the abdomen shows the prevertebral space occupied by the abdominal aorta and any intra-abdominal calcifications or tumor masses. The lateral abdomen is also used to show proper placement of AAA grafts and other vascular interventional devices (Fig. 16-16).

EVALUATION CRITERIA
The following should be clearly shown:
- Evidence of proper collimation
- Appropriate brightness and contrast to demonstrate abdominal contents
- No rotation of patient, demonstrated by the following:
  - □ Superimposed ilia
  - □ Superimposed lumbar vertebrae pedicles and open intervertebral foramina
- As much of the remaining abdomen as possible when the diaphragm is included

93

♠ LATERAL PROJECTION
R or L dorsal decubitus position

Image receptor: 14 × 17 inch (35 × 43 cm)

Position of patient

- When the patient cannot stand or lie on the side, place the patient in the supine position on a transportation cart or other suitable support with the right or left side in contact with the vertical grid device.
- Place the patient's arms across the upper chest to ensure that they are not projected over any abdominal contents, or place them behind the patient's head.
- Flex the patient's knees slightly to relieve strain on the back.
- *Exercise care* to ensure that the patient does not fall from the cart or table; if a cart is used, *lock all wheels* securely in position.

Position of part

- Adjust the height of the vertical grid device so that the long axis of the IR is centered to the midcoronal plane.
- Position the patient so that a point approximately 2 inches (5 cm) above the level of the iliac crests is centered to the IR (Fig. 16-17).
- Adjust the patient to ensure that no rotation from the supine position occurs.
- *Shield gonads*.
- *Respiration:* Suspend at the end of expiration.

Central ray

- Directed *horizontal* and perpendicular to the center of the IR, entering the midcoronal plane 2 inches (5 cm) above the level of the iliac crests

Collimation

- Adjust to 14 × 17 inches (35 × 43 cm) on the collimator.

Structures shown

The lateral projection of the abdomen is valuable in showing the prevertebral space and is quite useful in determining air-fluid levels in the abdomen (Fig. 16-18).

EVALUATION CRITERIA

The following should be clearly shown:
- Evidence of proper collimation
- Diaphragm without motion
- Appropriate brightness and contrast to demonstrate abdominal contents
- Patient elevated so that entire abdomen is shown

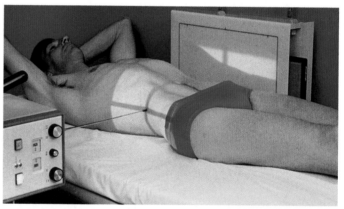

Fig. 16-17 Lateral abdomen, left dorsal decubitus position.

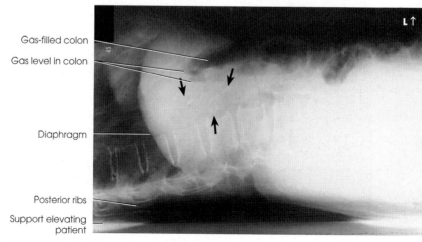

Gas-filled colon
Gas level in colon
Diaphragm
Posterior ribs
Support elevating patient

Fig. 16-18 Lateral abdomen, left dorsal decubitus position, showing calcified aorta (*arrows*). Note correct marker placement.

17

DIGESTIVE SYSTEM
Alimentary Canal

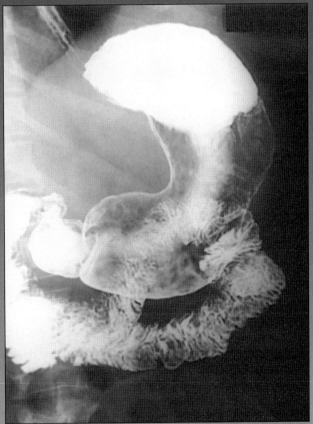

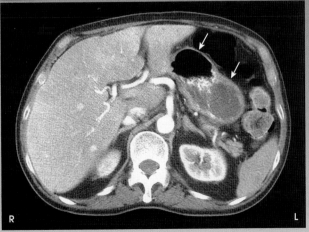

SUMMARY OF PROJECTIONS

PROJECTIONS, POSITIONS, AND METHODS

Page	Essential	Anatomy	Projection	Position	Method
118	♠	Esophagus	AP or PA		
118	♠	Esophagus	AP or PA oblique	RAO or LPO	
118	♠	Esophagus	Lateral	R or L	
124	♠	Stomach and duodenum	PA		
126		Stomach and duodenum	PA axial		
128	♠	Stomach and duodenum	PA oblique	RAO	
130	♠	Stomach and duodenum	AP oblique	LPO	
132	♠	Stomach and duodenum	Lateral	R only	
134	♠	Stomach and duodenum	AP		
136		Superior stomach and distal esophagus	PA oblique	RAO	WOLF
136		Stomach and duodenum serial and mucosal studies	PA oblique	RAO	
139	♠	Small intestine	PA or AP		
154	♠	Large intestine	PA		
156	♠	Large intestine	PA axial		
157	♠	Large intestine	PA oblique	RAO	
158	♠	Large intestine	PA oblique	LAO	
159	♠	Large intestine	Lateral	R or L	
160	♠	Large intestine	AP		
161	♠	Large intestine	AP axial		
162	♠	Large intestine	AP oblique	LPO	
163	♠	Large intestine	AP oblique	RPO	
165	♠	Large intestine	AP or PA	R lateral decubitus	
166	♠	Large intestine	PA or AP	L lateral decubitus	
167		Large intestine	Lateral	R or L ventral decubitus	
168	♠	Large intestine	AP, PA, oblique, lateral	Upright	
169		Large intestine	Axial		CHASSARD-LAPINÉ
174		Percutaneous transhepatic cholangiography	AP/AP oblique	Supine/RPO	
176		Postoperative (T-tube) cholangiography	AP/AP oblique	Supine/RPO	
178		Endoscopic retrograde cholangiopancreatography	AP/AP oblique	Supine/RPO	

Icons in the Essential column indicate projections frequently performed in the United States and Canada. Students should be competent in these projections.

Digestive System

The *digestive system* consists of two parts: the *accessory glands* and the *alimentary canal.* The accessory glands, which include the *salivary glands, liver, gallbladder,* and *pancreas,* secrete digestive enzymes into the alimentary canal. The alimentary canal is a musculomembranous tube that extends from the mouth to the anus. The regions of the alimentary canal vary in diameter according to functional requirements. The greater part of the canal, which is about 29 to 30 ft (8.6 to 8.9 m) long, lies in the abdominal cavity. The component parts of the alimentary canal (Fig. 17-1) are the *mouth,* in which food is masticated and converted into a bolus by insalivation; the *pharynx* and *esophagus,* which are the organs of swallowing; the *stomach,* in which the digestive process begins; the *small intestine,* in which the digestive process is completed; and the *large intestine,* which is an organ of egestion and water absorption that terminates at the *anus.*

Esophagus

The *esophagus* is a long, muscular tube that carries food and saliva from the laryngopharynx to the stomach (see Fig. 17-1). The adult esophagus is approximately 10 inches (24 cm) long and ¾ inch (1.9 cm) in diameter. Similar to the rest of the alimentary canal, the esophagus has a wall composed of four layers. Beginning with the outermost layer and moving in, the layers are as follows:

• Fibrous layer
• Muscular layer
• Submucosal layer
• Mucosal layer

The *esophagus* lies in the midsagittal plane. It originates at the level of the sixth cervical vertebra, or the upper margin of the thyroid cartilage. The esophagus enters the thorax from the superior portion of the neck. In the thorax, the esophagus passes through the mediastinum, anterior to the vertebral bodies and posterior to the trachea and heart (Fig. 17-1, *B*). In the lower thorax, the esophagus passes through the diaphragm at T10. Inferior to the diaphragm, the esophagus curves sharply left, increases in diameter, and joins the stomach at the *esophagogastric junction,* which is at the level of the xiphoid tip (T11). The expanded portion of the terminal esophagus, which lies in the abdomen, is called the *cardiac antrum.*

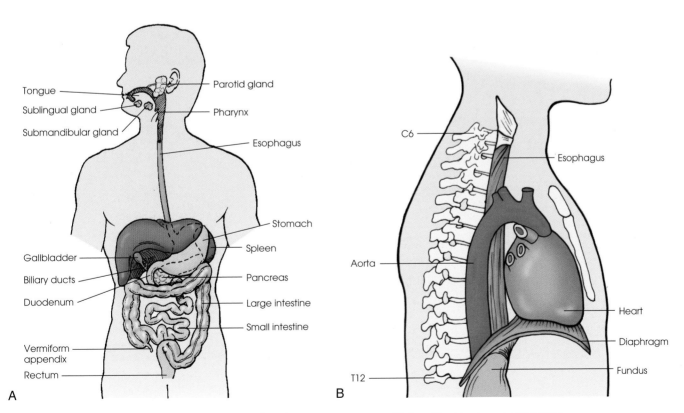

Fig. 17-1 A, Alimentary canal and accessory organs, with liver lifted to show gallbladder. **B,** Lateral view of thorax shows esophagus positioned anterior to vertebral bodies and posterior to trachea and heart.

Stomach

The *stomach* is the dilated, saclike portion of the digestive tract extending between the esophagus and the small intestine (Fig. 17-2). Its wall is composed of the same four layers as the esophagus.

The stomach is divided into the following four parts:
- Cardia
- Fundus
- Body
- Pyloric portion

The *cardia* of the stomach is the section immediately surrounding the esophageal opening. The *fundus* is the superior portion of the stomach that expands superiorly and fills the dome of the left hemidia-phragm. When the patient is in the upright position, the fundus is usually filled with gas; in radiography, this is referred to as the *gas bubble.* Descending from the fundus and beginning at the level of the cardiac notch is the *body* of the stomach. The inner mucosal layer of the body of the stomach contains numerous longitudinal folds called *rugae.* When the stomach is full, the rugae are smooth. The body of the stomach ends at a vertical plane passing through the *angular notch.* Distal to this plane is the *pyloric portion* of the stomach, which consists of the *pyloric antrum,* to the immediate right of the angular notch, and the narrow *pyloric canal,* which communicates with the duodenal bulb.

The stomach has anterior and posterior surfaces. The right border of the stomach is marked by the *lesser curvature.* The lesser curvature begins at the esophagogastric junction, is continuous with the right border of the esophagus, and is a concave curve ending at the pylorus. The left and inferior borders of the stomach are marked by the *greater curvature.* The greater curvature begins at the sharp angle at the esophagogastric junction, the *cardiac notch,* and follows the superior curvature of the fundus and then the convex curvature of the body down to the pylorus. The greater curvature is four to five times longer than the lesser curvature.

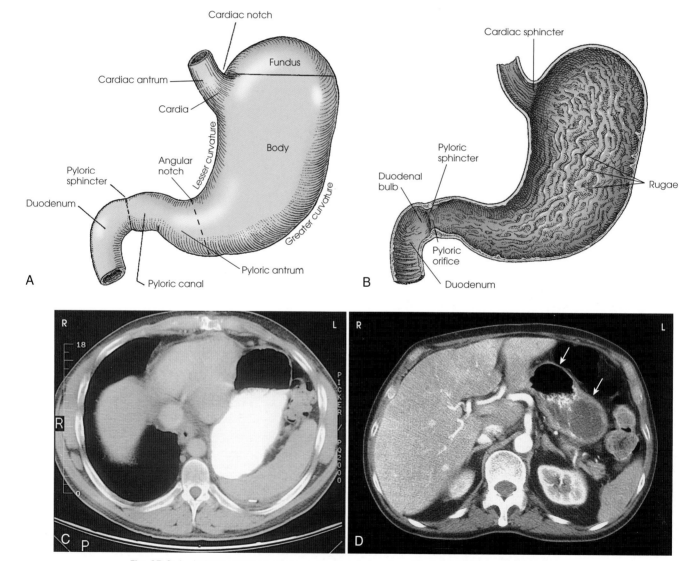

Fig. 17-2 A, Anterior surface of stomach. **B,** Interior view. **C,** Axial CT image of upper abdomen showing position of stomach in relation to surrounding organs. Note contrast media (*white*) and air (*black*) in stomach. **D,** Axial CT image showing stomach without contrast media. Note air (*upper arrow*) and empty stomach (*lower arrow*).

(**D,** Modified from Kelley LL, Petersen CM: *Sectional anatomy for imaging professionals,* ed 2, St Louis, 2007, Mosby.)

The entrance to and the exit from the stomach are controlled by a muscle sphincter. The esophagus joins the stomach at the esophagogastric junction through an opening termed the *cardiac orifice*. The muscle controlling the cardiac orifice is called the *cardiac sphincter*. The opening between the stomach and the small intestine is the *pyloric orifice,* and the muscle controlling the pyloric orifice is called the *pyloric sphincter.*

The size, shape, and position of the stomach depend on body habitus and vary with posture and the amount of stomach contents (Fig. 17-3). In persons with a hypersthenic habitus, the stomach is almost horizontal and is high, with its most dependent portion well above the umbilicus. In persons with an asthenic habitus, the stomach is vertical and occupies a low position, with its most dependent portion extending well below the transpyloric, or interspinous, line. Between these two extremes are the intermediate types of bodily habitus with corresponding variations in shape and position of the stomach. The habitus of 85% of the population is either sthenic or hyposthenic. Radiographers should become familiar with the various positions of the stomach in the different types of body habitus so that accurate positioning of the stomach is ensured.

The stomach has several functions in the digestive process. The stomach serves as a storage area for food until it can be digested further. It is also where food is broken down. Acids, enzymes, and other chemicals are secreted to break food down chemically. Food is also mechanically broken down through churning and peristalsis. Food that has been mechanically and chemically altered in the stomach is transported to the duodenum as a material called *chyme.*

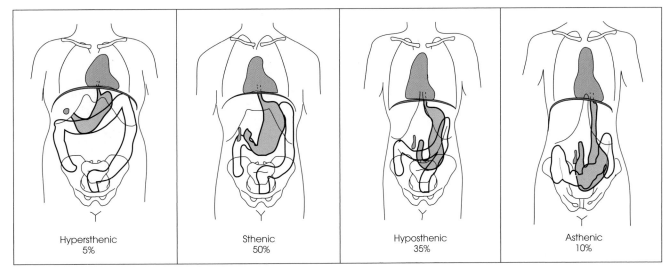

| Hypersthenic 5% | Sthenic 50% | Hyposthenic 35% | Asthenic 10% |

Fig. 17-3 Size, shape, and position of stomach and large intestine for the four different types of body habitus. Note extreme difference between hypersthenic and asthenic types.

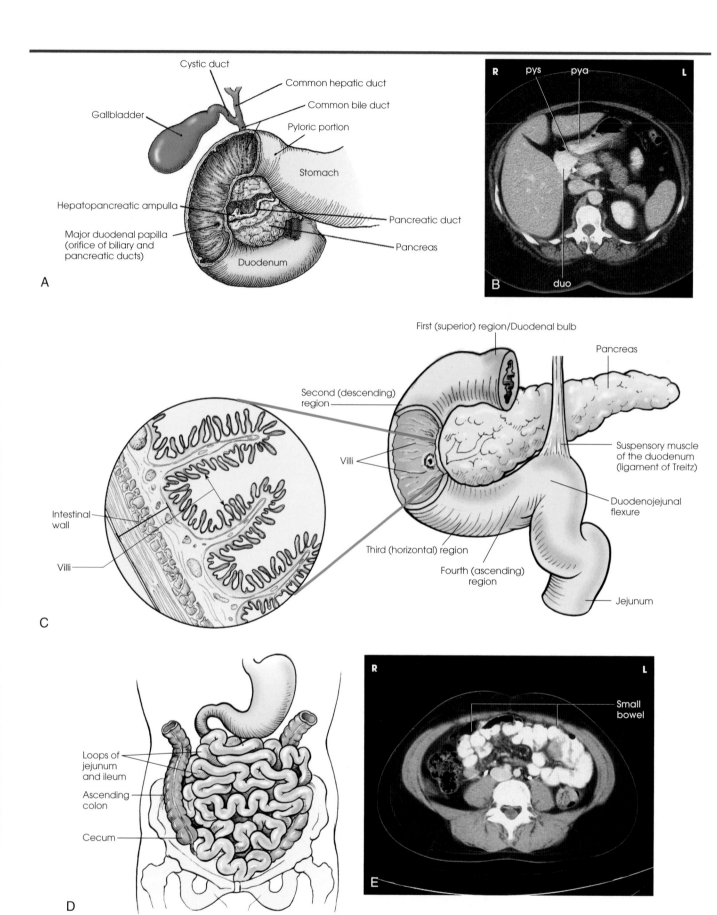

Fig. 17-4 A, Duodenal loop in relation to biliary and pancreatic ducts. **B,** CT axial image of pyloric antrum (*pya*), pyloric sphincter (*pys*), and duodenal bulb (*duo*). **C,** Anatomic areas of duodenum. *Inset:* Cross section of duodenum, showing villi. **D,** Loops of small intestine lying in central and lower abdominal cavity. **E,** CT axial image of small bowel loops with contrast media.

(**B** and **E,** Modified from Kelley LL, Petersen CM: *Sectional anatomy for imaging professionals,* ed 2, St Louis, 2007, Mosby.)

Small Intestine

The *small intestine* extends from the pyloric sphincter of the stomach to the ileocecal valve, where it joins the large intestine at a right angle. Digestion and absorption of food occur in this portion of the alimentary canal. The length of the adult small intestine averages about 22 ft (6.5 m), and its diameter gradually diminishes from approximately $1\frac{1}{2}$ inches (3.8 cm) in the proximal part to approximately 1 inch (2.5 cm) in the distal part. The wall of the small intestine contains the same four layers as the walls of the esophagus and stomach. The mucosa of the small intestine contains a series of fingerlike projections called *villi,* which assist the processes of digestion and absorption.

The small intestine is divided into the following three portions:
- Duodenum
- Jejunum
- Ileum

The *duodenum* is 8 to 10 inches (20 to 24 cm) long and is the widest portion of the small intestine (Fig. 17-4). It is retroperitoneal and is relatively fixed in position. Beginning at the pylorus, the duodenum follows a C-shaped course. Its four regions are described as the *first* (superior), *second* (descending), *third* (horizontal or inferior), and *fourth* (ascending) portions. The segment of the first portion is called the *duodenal bulb* because of its radiographic appearance when it is filled with an opaque contrast medium. The second portion is about 3 or 4 inches (7.6 to 10 cm) long. This segment passes inferiorly along the head of the pancreas and in close relation to the undersurface of the liver. The common bile duct and the pancreatic duct usually unite to form the *hepatopancreatic ampulla,* which opens on the summit of the *greater duodenal papilla* in the duodenum. The third portion passes toward the left at a slight superior inclination for a distance of about $2\frac{1}{2}$ inches (6 cm) and continues as the fourth portion on the left side of the vertebrae. This portion joins the jejunum at a sharp curve called the *duodenojejunal flexure* and is supported by the *suspensory muscle of the duodenum* (ligament of Treitz). The duodenal loop, which lies in the second portion, is the most fixed part of the small intestine and normally lies in the upper part of the umbilical region of the abdomen; however, its position varies with body habitus and with the amount of gastric and intestinal contents.

The remainder of the small intestine is arbitrarily divided into two portions, with the upper two fifths referred to as the *jejunum* and the lower three fifths referred to as the *ileum.* The jejunum and the ileum are gathered into freely movable loops, or gyri, and are attached to the posterior wall of the abdomen by the mesentery. The loops lie in the central and lower part of the abdominal cavity within the arch of the large intestine.

Large Intestine

The *large intestine* begins in the right iliac region, where it joins the ileum of the small intestine, forms an arch surrounding the loops of the small intestine, and ends at the anus (Fig. 17-5). The large intestine has four main parts, as follows:

- Cecum
- Colon
- Rectum
- Anal canal

The large intestine is about 5 ft (1.5 m) long and is greater in diameter than the small intestine. The wall of the large intestine contains the same four layers as the walls of the esophagus, stomach, and small intestine. The muscular portion of the intestinal wall contains an external band of longitudinal muscle that forms into three thickened bands called *taeniae coli*. One band is positioned anteriorly, and two are positioned posteriorly. These bands create a pulling muscle tone that forms a series of pouches called the *haustra*. The main functions of the large intestine are reabsorption of fluids and elimination of waste products.

The *cecum* is the pouchlike portion of the large intestine that is below the junction of the ileum and the colon. The cecum is approximately $2\frac{1}{2}$ inches (6 cm) long and 3 inches (7.6 cm) in diameter. The *vermiform appendix* is attached to the posteromedial side of the cecum. The appendix is a narrow, wormlike tube that is about 3 inches (7.6 cm) long. The *ileocecal valve* is just below the junction of the ascending colon and the cecum. The valve projects into the lumen of the cecum and guards the opening between the ileum and the cecum.

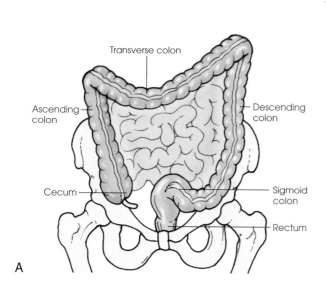

A

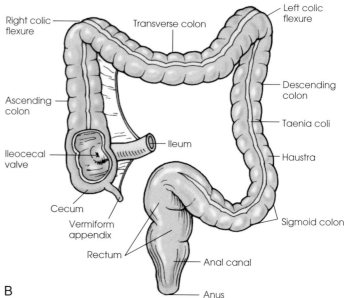

B

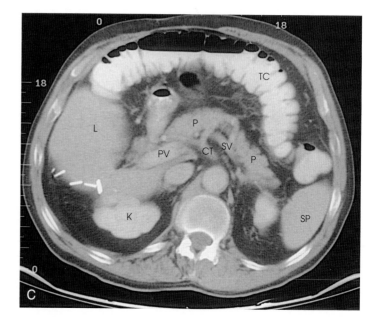

C

Fig. 17-5 A, Anterior aspect of large intestine positioned in abdomen. **B,** Anterior aspect of large intestine. **C,** Axial CT image of upper abdomen showing actual image of transverse colon positioned in anterior abdomen.

The *colon* is subdivided into ascending, transverse, descending, and sigmoid portions. The *ascending colon* passes superiorly from its junction with the cecum to the undersurface of the liver, where it joins the transverse portion at an angle called the *right colic flexure* (formerly hepatic flexure). The *transverse colon,* which is the longest and most movable part of the colon, crosses the abdomen to the undersurface of the spleen. The transverse portion makes a sharp curve, called the *left colic flexure* (formerly splenic flexure), and ends in the descending portion. The *descending colon* passes inferiorly and medially to its junction with the *sigmoid portion* at the superior aperture of the lesser pelvis. The sigmoid colon curves to form an S-shaped loop and ends in the rectum at the level of the third sacral segment.

The *rectum* extends from the sigmoid colon to the anal canal. The *anal canal* terminates at the *anus,* which is the external aperture of the large intestine (Fig. 17-6). The rectum is approximately 6 inches (15 cm) long. The distal portion, which is about 1 inch (2.5 cm) long, is constricted to form the anal canal. Just above the anal canal is a dilatation called the *rectal ampulla.* Following the sacrococcygeal curve, the rectum passes inferiorly and posteriorly to the level of the pelvic floor and bends sharply anteriorly and inferiorly into the anal canal, which extends to the anus. The rectum and anal canal have two AP curves; this fact must be remembered when an enema tube is inserted.

The size, shape, and position of the large intestine vary greatly, depending on body habitus (see Fig. 17-3). In hypersthenic patients, the large intestine is positioned around the periphery of the abdomen and may require more images to show its entire length. The large intestine of asthenic patients, which is bunched together and positioned low in the abdomen, is at the other extreme.

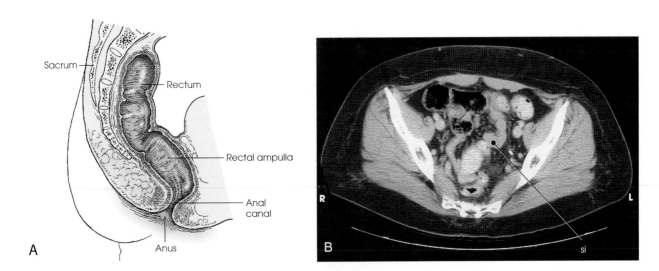

Fig. 17-6 A, Sagittal section showing direction of anal canal and rectum. **B,** Axial CT image of lower pelvis showing rectum and sigmoid colon (*si*) in relation to surrounding organs.

(**B,** From Kelley LL, Petersen CM: *Sectional anatomy for imaging professionals,* ed 2, St Louis, 2007, Mosby.)

Liver and Biliary System

The *liver,* the largest gland in the body, is an irregularly wedge-shaped gland. It is situated with its base on the right and its apex directed anteriorly and to the left (Fig. 17-7). The deepest point of the liver is the inferior aspect just above the right kidney. The diaphragmatic surface of the liver is convex and conforms to the under-surface of the diaphragm. The visceral surface is concave and is molded over the viscera on which it rests. Almost all of the right hypochondrium and a large part of the epigastrium are occupied by the liver. The right portion extends inferiorly into the right lateral region as far as the fourth lumbar vertebra, and the left extremity extends across the left hypochondrium.

At the *falciform ligament,* the liver is divided into a large *right lobe* and a much smaller *left lobe*. Two minor lobes are located on the medial side of the right lobe: the *caudate lobe* on the posterior surface and the *quadrate lobe* on the inferior surface (Fig. 17-8, *A*). The hilum of the liver, called the *porta hepatis,* is situated transversely between the two minor lobes.

The *portal vein* and the *hepatic artery,* both of which convey blood to the liver, enter the porta hepatis and branch out through the liver substance (Fig. 17-8, *C*). The portal vein ends in the sinusoids, and the hepatic artery ends in capillaries that communicate with sinusoids. In addition to the usual arterial blood supply, the liver receives blood from the portal system.

The portal system, of which the portal vein is the main trunk, consists of the veins arising from the walls of the stomach, from the greater part of the intestinal tract and the gallbladder, and from the pancreas and the spleen. The blood circulating through these organs is rich in nutrients and is carried to the liver for modification before it is returned to the heart. The *hepatic veins* convey the blood from the liver sinusoids to the inferior vena cava.

The liver has numerous physiologic functions. The primary consideration from the radiographic standpoint is the formation of *bile*. The gland secretes bile at the rate of 1 to 3 pints ($\frac{1}{2}$ to $1\frac{1}{2}$ L) each day. Bile, the channel of elimination for the waste products of red blood cell destruction, is an excretion and a secretion. As a secretion, it is an important aid in the emulsification and assimilation of fats. The bile is collected from the liver cells by the ducts and is carried to the gallbladder for temporary storage or is poured directly into the duodenum through the common bile duct.

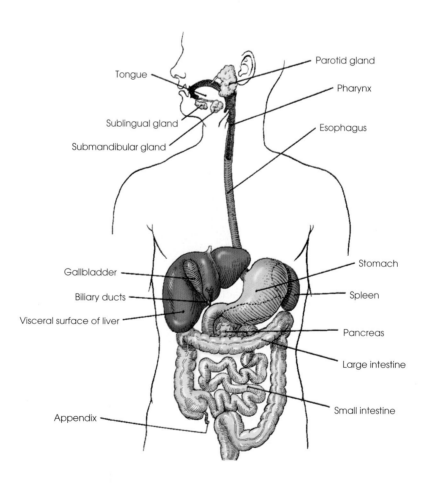

Fig. 17-7 Alimentary tract and accessory organs. To show position of gallbladder in relation to liver, the liver is shown with inferior portion pulled anteriorly and superiorly, placing the liver in an atypical position.

The biliary, or excretory, system of the liver consists of the bile ducts and gallbladder (see Fig. 17-8). Beginning within the lobules as bile capillaries, the ducts unite to form larger and larger passages as they converge, finally forming two main ducts, one leading from each major lobe. The two main *hepatic ducts* emerge at the porta hepatis and join to form the *common hepatic duct,* which unites with the *cystic duct* to form the *common bile duct.* The hepatic and cystic ducts are each about 1½ inches (3.8 cm) long. The common bile duct passes inferiorly for a distance of approximately 3 inches (7.6 cm). The common bile duct joins the pancreatic duct, and they enter together or side by side into an enlarged chamber known as the *hepatopancreatic ampulla,* or *ampulla of Vater.* The ampulla opens into the descending portion of the duodenum. The distal end of the common bile duct is controlled by the *choledochal sphincter* as it enters the duodenum. The hepatopancreatic ampulla is controlled by a circular muscle known as the *sphincter of the hepatopancreatic ampulla,* or *sphincter of Oddi.* During interdigestive periods, the sphincter remains in a contracted state, routing most of the bile into the gallbladder for concentration and temporary storage; during digestion, it relaxes to permit the bile to flow from the liver and gallbladder into the duodenum. The hepatopancreatic ampulla opens on an elevation on the duodenal mucosa known as the *major duodenal papilla.*

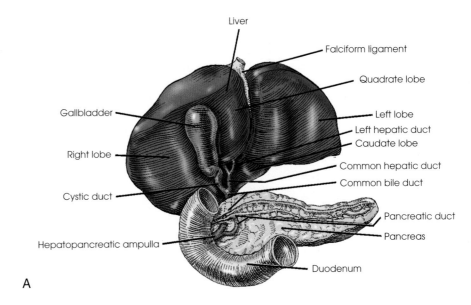

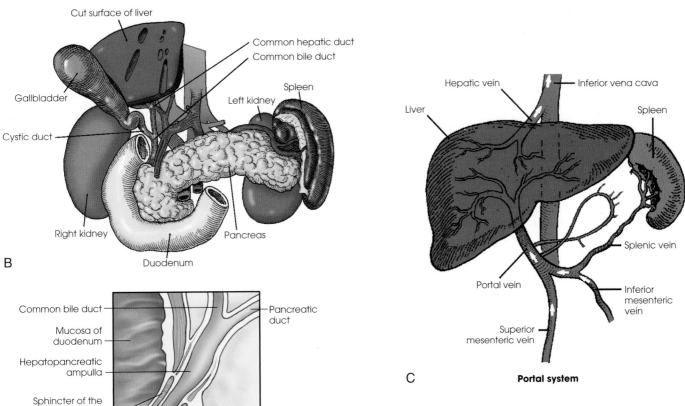

Fig. 17-8 A, Visceral surface (inferoposterior aspect) of liver and gallbladder. **B,** Visceral (inferoposterior) surface of gallbladder and bile ducts. **C,** Portal system showing hepatic artery and vein and other surrounding vessels. **D,** Detail of drainage system into duodenum.

The *gallbladder* is a thin-walled, more or less pear-shaped, musculomembranous sac with a capacity of approximately 2 oz. The gallbladder concentrates bile through absorption of the water content; stores bile during interdigestive periods; and, by contraction of its musculature, evacuates the bile during digestion. The muscular contraction of the gallbladder is activated by a hormone called *cholecystokinin*. This hormone is secreted by the duodenal mucosa and is released into the blood when fatty or acid chyme passes into the intestine. The gallbladder consists of a narrow neck that is continuous with the *cystic duct;* a body or main portion; and a fundus, which is its broad lower portion. The gallbladder is usually lodged in a fossa on the visceral (inferior) surface of the right lobe of the liver, where it lies in an oblique plane inferiorly and anteriorly. Measuring about 1 inch (2.5 cm) in width at its widest part and 3 to 4 inches (7.5 to 10 cm) long, the gallbladder extends from the lower right margin of the porta hepatis to a variable distance below the anterior border of the liver. The position of the gallbladder varies with body habitus; it is high and well away from the midline in hypersthenic persons and low and near the spine in asthenic persons (Fig. 17-9). The gallbladder is sometimes embedded in the liver and frequently hangs free below the inferior margin of the liver.

Pancreas and Spleen

The *pancreas* is an elongated gland situated across the posterior abdominal wall. Extending from the duodenum to the spleen (Fig. 17-10; see Fig. 17-8), the pancreas is about 5½ inches (14 cm) long and consists of a head, neck, body, and tail. The *head,* which is the broadest portion of the organ, extends inferiorly and is enclosed within the curve of the duodenum at the level of the second or third lumbar vertebra. The *body* and *tail* of the pancreas pass transversely behind the stomach and in front of the left kidney, with the narrow tail terminating near the spleen. The pancreas cannot be seen on plain radiographic studies.

The pancreas is an *exocrine* and an *endocrine* gland. The exocrine cells of the pancreas are arranged in lobules with a highly ramified duct system. This exocrine portion of the gland produces *pancreatic juice,* which acts on proteins, fats, and carbohydrates. The endocrine portion of the gland consists of clusters of islet cells, or islets of Langerhans, which are randomly distributed throughout the pancreas. Each islet comprises clusters of cells surrounding small groups of capillaries. These cells produce the hormones *insulin* and *glucagon,* which are respon-sible for glucose metabolism. The islet cells do not communicate directly with the ducts but release their secretions directly into the blood through a rich capillary network.

The digestive juice secreted by the exocrine cells of the pancreas is conveyed into the *pancreatic duct* and from there into the duodenum. The pancreatic duct often unites with the common bile duct to form a single passage via the hepatopancreatic ampulla, which opens directly into the descending duodenum.

The *spleen* is included in this section only because of its location; it belongs to the lymphatic system. The spleen is a glandlike but ductless organ that produces lymphocytes and stores and removes dead or dying red blood cells. The spleen is more or less bean-shaped and measures about 5 inches (13 cm) long, 3 inches (7.6 cm) wide, and 1½ inches (3.8 cm) thick. Situated obliquely in the left upper quadrant, the spleen is just below the diaphragm and behind the stomach. It is in contact with the abdominal wall laterally, with the left suprarenal gland and left kidney medially, and with the left colic flexure of the colon inferiorly. The spleen is visualized with and without contrast media.

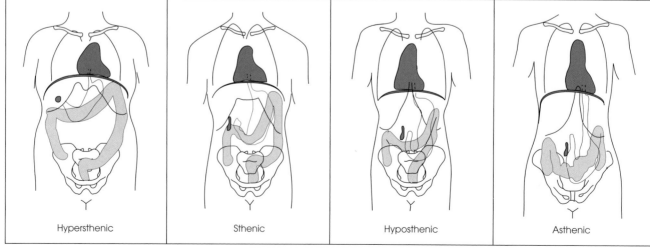

| Hypersthenic | Sthenic | Hyposthenic | Asthenic |

Fig. 17-9 Gallbladder (*green*) position varies with body habitus. Note extreme difference in position of gallbladder between hypersthenic and asthenic habitus.

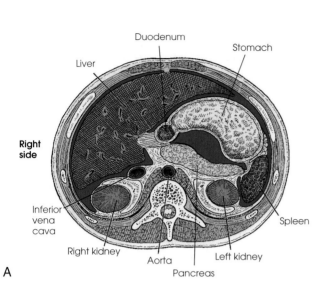

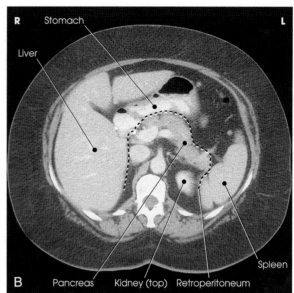

Fig. 17-10 A, Sectional image of upper abdomen (viewed from the patient's feet upward), showing relationship of digestive system components. **B,** Axial CT image of same area of abdomen as in **A.**

(**B,** From Kelley LL, Petersen CM: *Sectional anatomy for imaging professionals,* ed 2, St Louis, 2007, Mosby.)

ABBREVIATIONS USED IN CHAPTER 17	
BE	Barium enema
CTC	CT colonography
MPR	Multiplanar reconstruction
UGI	Upper gastrointestinal
VC	Virtual colonoscopy

See Addendum B for a summary of all abbreviations used in Volume 2.

These techniques were accurate for the equipment used to produce each exposure. However, use caution when applying them in your department because generator output characteristics and IR energy sensitivities vary widely.[1]

This chart was created in collaboration with Dennis Bowman, AS, RT(R), Clinical Instructor, Community Hospital of the Monterey Peninsula, Monterey, CA.

http://digitalradiographysolutions.com/

DIGESTIVE SYSTEM, ALIMENTARY CANAL

Part	cm	kVp*	SID[†]	Collimation	CR[‡] mAs	CR Dose (mGy)[‖]	DR[§] mAs	DR Dose (mGy)[‖]
Esophagus								
AP and PA[¶]	16	120	40″	10″ × 17″ (24 × 43 cm)	8**	1.832	4**	0.904
Obliques[¶]	21	120	40″	10″ × 17″ (24 × 43 cm)	12**	3.230	6**	1.621
Lateral[¶]	30	120	40″	10″ × 17″ (24 × 43 cm)	24**	8.230	12**	4.085
Stomach and duodenum								
PA and AP[¶]	21	120	40″	10″ × 12″ (24 × 30 cm)	10**	2.610	5**	1.291
PA and AP oblique[¶]	24	120	40″	10″ × 12″ (24 × 30 cm)	15**	4.495	7.5**	2.245
Lateral[¶]	27	120	40″	10″ × 12″ (24 × 30 cm)	30**	9.770	15**	4.860
Small intestine								
PA and AP[¶]	21	120	40″	14″ × 17″ (35 × 43 cm)	16**	4.320	8**	2.160
Large intestine								
PA and AP[¶]	21	120	40″	14″ × 17″ (35 × 43 cm)	20**	5.420	10**	2.700
PA and AP[¶] axial	24	120	40″	14″ × 17″ (35 × 43 cm)	32**	9.365	16**	4.650
PA and AP oblique[¶]	24	120	40″	14″ × 17″ (35 × 43 cm)	25**	7.310	12.5**	3.635
Lower lateral (rectum)[¶]	31	120	40″	10″ × 12″ (24 × 30 cm)	60**	22.21	30**	10.89
AP and PA decubitus (air contrast)[¶]	24	120	40″	17″ × 14″ (43 × 35 cm)	25**	7.320	12.5**	3.640

[1]ACR-AAPM-SIMM Practice Guidelines for Digital Radiography, 2007.
*kVp values are for a high-frequency generator.
[†]40 inch *minimum*; 44 to 48 inches recommended to improve spatial resolution (mAs increase needed, but no increase in patient dose will result).
[‡]AGFA CR MD 4.0 General IP, CR 75.0 reader, 400 speed class, with 6:1 (178LPI) grid when needed.
[§]GE Definium 8000, with 13:1 grid when needed.
[‖]All doses are skin entrance for average adult (160 to 200 pound male, 150 to 190 pound female) at part thickness indicated.
[¶]Bucky/Grid.
**Large focal spot.

SUMMARY OF ANATOMY

Digestive system
Alimentary canal
Mouth
Pharynx
Esophagus
Stomach
Small intestine
Large intestine (colon)
Anus

Accessory glands
Salivary glands
Liver
Gallbladder
Pancreas

Esophagus
Fibrous layer
Muscular layer
Submucosal layer
Esophagogastric junction
Cardiac antrum
Cardiac notch

Stomach
Cardia
Fundus

Body
  Rugae
Angular notch
Pyloric portion
  Pyloric antrum
  Pyloric canal
Lesser curvature
Cardiac notch
Greater curvature
Cardiac orifice
Cardiac sphincter
Pyloric orifice
Pyloric sphincter
Chyme

Small intestine
Villi
Duodenum (four regions)
  First (superior)—duodenal bulb
  Second (descending)—major duodenal papilla
  Third (horizontal)
  Fourth (ascending)—duodenojejunal flexure; suspensory muscle of duodenum

Jejunum
Ileum

Large intestine
Taeniae coli
Haustra
Cecum
Vermiform appendix
Ileocecal valve
Colon
  Ascending colon
  Right colic flexure
  Transverse colon
  Left colic flexure
  Descending colon
  Sigmoid colon
Rectum
  Rectal ampulla
  Anal canal
  Anus

Liver and biliary system
Falciform ligament
Right lobe
Left lobe
Caudate lobe
Quadrate lobe

Porta hepatis
Hepatic artery
Portal vein
Hepatic veins
Hepatic ducts
Common hepatic duct
Cystic duct
Common bile duct
Hepatopancreatic ampulla
Sphincter of hepatopancreatic ampulla
Major duodenal papilla
Gallbladder

Pancreas and spleen
Pancreas
  Head
  Body
  Tail
Exocrine gland
  Pancreatic juice
Endocrine gland
  Islet cells
Pancreatic duct
Spleen

Digestive System

SUMMARY OF PATHOLOGY

Condition	Definition
Achalasia	Failure of smooth muscle of alimentary canal to relax
Appendicitis	Inflammation of the appendix
Barrett esophagus	Peptic ulcer of lower esophagus, often with stricture
Bezoar	Mass in the stomach formed by material that does not pass into the intestine
Biliary stenosis	Narrowing of bile ducts
Carcinoma	Malignant new growth composed of epithelial cells
Celiac disease or sprue	Malabsorption disease caused by mucosal defect in the jejunum
Cholecystitis	Acute or chronic inflammation of gallbladder
Choledocholithiasis	Calculus in common bile duct
Cholelithiasis	Presence of gallstones
Colitis	Inflammation of the colon
Diverticulitis	Inflammation of diverticula in the alimentary canal
Diverticulosis	Diverticula in the colon without inflammation or symptoms
Diverticulum	Pouch created by herniation of the mucous membrane through the muscular coat
Esophageal varices	Enlarged tortuous veins of lower esophagus, resulting from portal hypertension
Gastritis	Inflammation of lining of stomach
Gastroesophageal reflux	Backward flow of stomach contents into the esophagus
Hiatal hernia	Protrusion of the stomach through the esophageal hiatus of the diaphragm
Hirschsprung disease or congenital aganglionic megacolon	Absence of parasympathetic ganglia, usually in the distal colon, resulting in the absence of peristalsis
Ileus	Failure of bowel peristalsis
Inguinal hernia	Protrusion of the bowel into the groin
Intussusception	Prolapse of a portion of the bowel into the lumen of an adjacent part
Malabsorption syndrome	Disorder in which subnormal absorption of dietary constituents occurs
Meckel diverticulum	Diverticulum of the distal ileum, similar to the appendix
Pancreatic pseudocyst	Collection of debris, fluid, pancreatic enzymes, and blood as a complication of acute pancreatitis
Pancreatitis	Acute or chronic inflammation of the pancreas
Polyp	Growth or mass protruding from a mucous membrane
Pyloric stenosis	Narrowing of pyloric canal causing obstruction
Regional enteritis or Crohn disease	Inflammatory bowel disease, most commonly involving the distal ileum
Ulcer	Depressed lesion on the surface of the alimentary canal
Ulcerative colitis	Recurrent disorder causing inflammatory ulceration in the colon
Volvulus	Twisting of a bowel loop on itself
Zenker diverticulum	Diverticulum located just above the cardiac portion of the stomach

Technical Considerations

GASTROINTESTINAL TRANSIT

Peristalsis is the term applied to the contraction waves by which the digestive tube propels its contents toward the rectum. Normally three or four waves per minute occur in the filled stomach. The waves begin in the upper part of the organ and travel toward the pylorus. The average emptying time of a normal stomach is 2 to 3 hours.

Peristaltic action in the intestines is greatest in the upper part of the canal and gradually decreases toward the lower portion. In addition to peristaltic waves, localized contractions occur in the duodenum and the jejunum. These contractions usually occur at intervals of 3 to 4 seconds during digestion. The first part of a "barium meal" normally reaches the ileocecal valve in 2 to 3 hours, and the last portion reaches the ileocecal valve in 4 to 5 hours. The barium usually reaches the rectum within 24 hours.

The specialized procedures commonly used in radiologic examinations of the esophagus, stomach, and intestines are discussed in this section. The esophagus extends between the pharynx and the cardiac end of the stomach and occupies a constant position in the posterior part of the mediastinum; it is easy to show the esophagus on radiographic images when a contrast medium is used. The stomach and intestines vary in size, shape, position, and muscular tonus according to the body habitus (see Fig. 17-3). In addition to normal structural and functional differences, various gastrointestinal abnormalities can cause further changes in location and motility. These variations make the gastrointestinal investigation of every patient an individual study, and meticulous attention must be given to each detail of the examination procedure.

EXAMINATION PROCEDURE

The alimentary canal may be imaged using only fluoroscopy or using a combination of fluoroscopy and radiography. Fluoroscopy makes it possible to observe the canal in motion, perform special mucosal studies, and determine the subsequent procedure required for a complete examination. Depending on the radiologist's preference, all images may be obtained during fluoroscopy, thus the radiographer's role is to communicate with and assist the patient before and after contrast administration while assisting the fluoroscopist during the procedure. Some facilities still obtain radiographic images after the fluoroscopy examination, and these images are the responsibility of the radiographer. In both types of examinations, the essential projections described in this chapter are obtained to provide a permanent record of the findings. Radiographers must be proficient in recognizing the pertinent anatomy shown in each position and projection to provide proper patient assistance in fluoroscopy-only procedures and to obtain accurate radiographic images in the combination examinations.

Contrast media

Because the thin-walled alimentary canal does not have sufficient density to be shown through the surrounding structures, demonstration of it on radiographic images requires the use of an artificial contrast medium. *Barium sulfate,* which is a water-insoluble salt of the metallic element barium, is the contrast medium universally used in examinations of the alimentary canal (Fig. 17-11). The barium sulfate used for this purpose is a specially prepared, chemically pure product to which various chemical substances have been added. Barium sulfate is available as a dry powder or as a liquid. The powdered barium has different concentrations and is mixed with plain water. The concentration depends on the part to be examined and the preference of the physician.

Many special barium sulfate products are also available. Products with finely divided barium sulfate particles tend to resist precipitation and remain in suspension longer than regular barium preparations. Some barium preparations contain gums or other suspending or dispersing agents and are referred to as *suspended* or *flocculation-resistant* preparations. The speed with which the barium mixture passes through the alimentary canal depends on the suspending medium, the temperature of the medium, the consistency of the preparation, and the motile function of the alimentary canal.

In addition to barium sulfate, *water-soluble, iodinated contrast media* suitable for opacification of the alimentary canal are available (Fig. 17-12). These preparations are modifications of basic IV urographic media, such as diatrizoate sodium and diatrizoate meglumine.

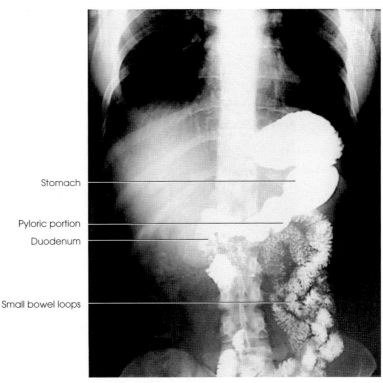

Fig. 17-11 Barium sulfate suspension in stomach, sthenic body habitus.

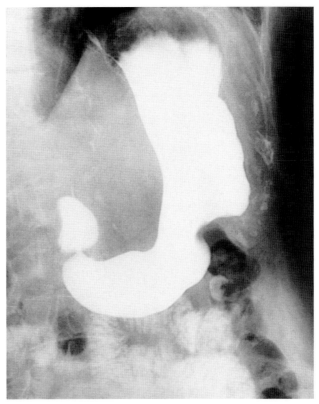

Fig. 17-12 Water-soluble, iodinated solution in stomach.

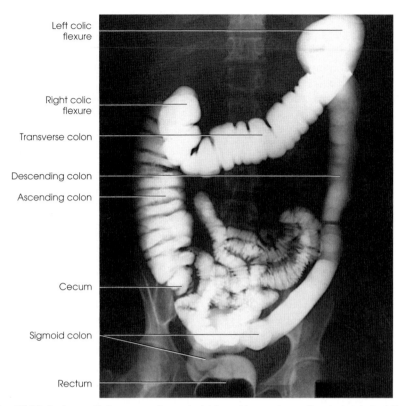

Left colic
flexure

Right colic
flexure

Transverse colon

Descending colon

Ascending colon

Cecum

Sigmoid colon

Rectum

Fig. 17-13 Barium sulfate suspension administered by rectum, sthenic body habitus.

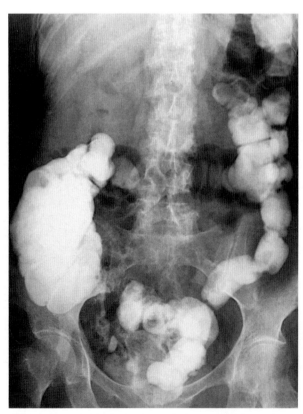

Fig. 17-14 Water-soluble, iodinated solution administered by mouth.

Iodinated solutions move through the gastrointestinal tract quicker than barium sulfate suspensions (Figs. 17-13 and 17-14). An iodinated solution normally clears the stomach in 1 to 2 hours, and the entire iodinated contrast column reaches and outlines the colon in about 4 hours. An orally administered iodinated medium differs from barium sulfate in the following ways:

1. It outlines the esophagus, but it does not adhere to the mucosa as well as a barium sulfate suspension does.

2. It affords an entirely satisfactory examination of the stomach and duodenum including mucosal delineation.

3. It permits a rapid survey of the entire small intestine but fails to provide clear anatomic detail of this portion of the alimentary canal. This failure results from dilution of the contrast medium and the resultant decrease in opacification.

4. Because of the normal rapid absorption of water through the colonic mucosa, the medium again becomes densely concentrated in the large intestine. Consequently, the entire large intestine is opacified with retrograde filling using a barium sulfate suspension. As a result of its increased concentration and accelerated transit time, rapid investigation of the large intestine can be performed by the oral route when a patient cannot cooperate for a satisfactory enema study.

A great advantage of water-soluble media is that they are easily removed by aspiration before or during surgery. If a water-soluble, iodinated medium escapes into the peritoneum through a preexisting perforation of the stomach or intestine, no ill effects result. The medium is readily absorbed from the peritoneal cavity and excreted by the kidneys. This provides a definite advantage when perforated ulcers are being investigated.

A disadvantage of iodinated preparations is their strongly bitter taste, which can be masked only to a limited extent. Patients should be forewarned so that they can more easily tolerate ingestion of these agents. In addition, these iodinated contrast media are hyperosmolar, encouraging movement of excess fluid into the gastrointestinal tract lumen.

Radiologic apparatus

The fluoroscopic equipment used today contains highly sophisticated image intensification systems (Fig. 17-15). These systems can be connected to accessory units, such as cine film recorders, television systems, spot-film cameras, digital-image cameras, and video recorders. Remote control fluoroscopic rooms are also available and are used by the fluoroscopist in an adjacent control area (Fig. 17-16). Although conventional IR-loaded spot-image devices are still used with image intensification, digital fluoroscopic units that permit the recording of multiple fluoroscopic images are increasingly more common.

Compression and palpation of the abdomen are often performed during an examination of the alimentary canal. Many types of compression devices are available. The fluoroscopic unit shown in Fig. 17-15 shows a compression cone in contact with the patient's abdomen. This device is often used during general fluoroscopic examinations.

Other types of commercial compression devices include the pneumatic compression paddle shown in Fig. 17-17. This device is often placed under the duodenal bulb and inflated to place pressure on the abdomen. The air is slowly released, and the compression on the body part is eliminated.

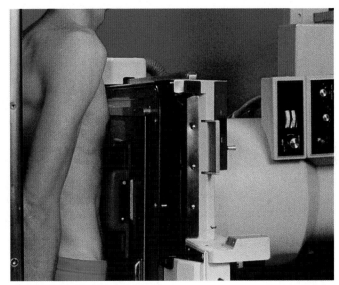

Fig. 17-15 Image intensification system, with compression cone in contact with abdomen.

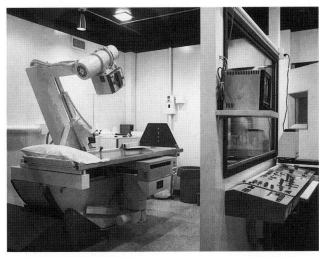

Fig. 17-16 Remote control fluoroscopic room, showing patient fluoroscopic table (*left*) and fluoroscopist's control console (*right*). The fluoroscopist views the patient through the large window.

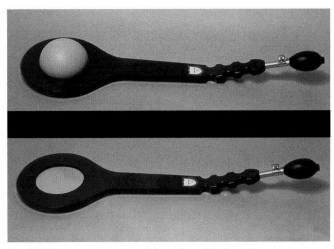

Fig. 17-17 Compression paddle: inflated (*above*) and noninflated (*below*).

Preparation of examining room

The examining room should be completely prepared before the patient enters. In preparing the room, the radiographer should do the following:

- Adjust equipment controls to the appropriate settings.
- Have the footboard and shoulder support available.
- Check for proper operation of the imaging and recording devices.
- Prepare the required type and amount of contrast medium.

Before beginning the examination, the radiographer must communicate with the patient in the following ways:

- Explain the type and administration route of the contrast media.
  - Use lay terminology, such as "drinking" for orally administered agents.
  - Explain the taste and texture of the contrast agent, such as "chalky and thick" for barium and "bitter" for iodinated agents.
  - For an enema examination, show the tube tip and explain insertion and the potential abdominal sensations that often accompany the flow of contrast into the colon.
- Point out that the lights are dimmed in the room during fluoroscopy, and explain the need for a darkened room during the procedure.
- The fluoroscopist will instruct the patient to move into certain positions and will provide breathing instructions. Assure the patient that you will assist, as needed.
  - If radiographic images are obtained post fluoroscopy, inform the patient of the approximate number of images you will be obtaining when the fluoroscopist leaves the room.
- After you have verified that the patient understands the overall procedure, introduce the patient and the fluoroscopist to each other when the fluoroscopist enters the examining room.

Exposure time

One of the most important considerations in gastrointestinal radiography is the elimination of motion. The highest degree of motor activity is normally found in the stomach and proximal part of the small intestine. Activity gradually decreases along the intestinal tract until it becomes fairly slow in the distal part of the large bowel. Peristaltic speed also depends on the individual patient's body habitus and is influenced by pathologic changes, use of narcotic pain medication, body position, and respiration. The amount of exposure time for each region must be based on these factors.

In esophageal examinations, the radiographer should observe the following guidelines, if obtaining radiographic images post fluoroscopy:

- Use an exposure time of 0.1 second or less for upright images. The time may be slightly longer for recumbent images because the barium descends more slowly when patients are in a recumbent position.
- Barium passes through the esophagus fairly slowly if it is swallowed at the end of full inspiration. The rate of passage is increased if the barium is swallowed at the end of moderate inspiration. The barium is delayed in the lower part for several seconds, however, if it is swallowed at the end of full expiration.
- Respiration is inhibited for several seconds after the beginning of deglutition, which allows sufficient time for the exposure to be made without the need to instruct the patient to hold his or her breath after swallowing.

In examinations of the stomach and small intestine, the radiographer should observe the following guidelines:

- Use an exposure time no longer than 0.2 second for patients with normal peristaltic activity and never longer than 0.5 second; exposure time should be 0.1 second or less for patients with hypermotility.
- Make exposures of the stomach and intestines at the end of expiration in the routine procedure.

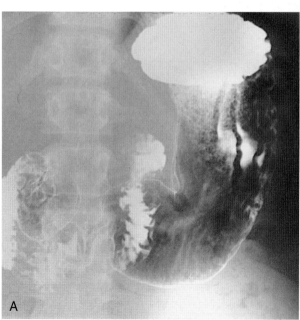

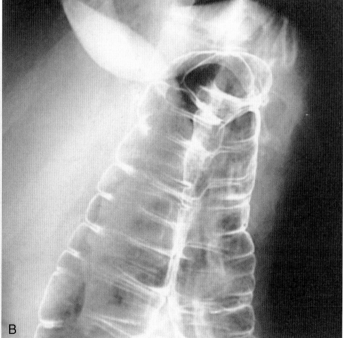

Fig. 17-18 A, AP spot image of barium-filled fundus of stomach. **B,** Spot image of air-contrast colon, showing left colic flexure.

Radiation Protection

The patient receives radiation during fluoroscopy, while the procedure is recorded and images obtained (Fig. 17-18). When radiographic images are a required part of a partial or complete gastrointestinal examination, even more radiation is delivered to the patient. It is taken for granted that properly added filtration is in place at all times in each x-ray tube in the radiology department. It is further assumed that based on the capacity of the machines and the best available accessory equipment, exposure factors are adjusted to deliver the least possible radiation to the patient.

Protection of the patient from unnecessary radiation is a professional responsibility of the radiographer. (See Chapter 1 in Volume 1 of this atlas for specific guidelines.) In this chapter, the *Shield gonads* statement at the end of the *Position of part* section indicates that the patient is to be protected from unnecessary radiation by *restricting the radiation beam using proper collimation to include only the primary anatomy of interest*. Placing lead shielding between the gonads and the radiation source when the clinical objectives of the examination are not compromised is also appropriate.

Esophagus
CONTRAST MEDIA STUDIES

The esophagus may be examined by performing a *full-column, single-contrast* study in which only barium or water-soluble, iodinated contrast agent is used to fill the esophageal lumen. A *double-contrast* procedure also may be used. For this study, high-density barium and carbon dioxide crystals (which liberate carbon dioxide when exposed to water) are the two contrast agents. No preliminary preparation of the patient is necessary. These contrast media procedures show intrinsic lesions and extrinsic pathology impressing on the esophagus. Anatomic structures normally indenting the esophagus must be appreciated to identify pathology. Normally indenting structures include the aortic arch, left main stem bronchus, and left atrium (Fig. 17-19).

Barium sulfate mixture

A 30% to 50% weight/volume suspension[1] is useful for the full-column, single-contrast technique. A low-viscosity, high-density barium developed for double-contrast gastric examinations may be used for a double-contrast examination. Whatever the weight/volume concentration of the barium, the most important criterion is that the barium flows sufficiently to coat the walls of the esophagus. The mixing instructions of the barium manufacturer must be followed closely to attain optimal performance of the contrast medium.

[1]Scukas J: Contrast media. In Margulis AR, Burhenne HJ, editors: *Alimentary tract radiology,* vol 1, ed 4, St Louis, 1989, Mosby.

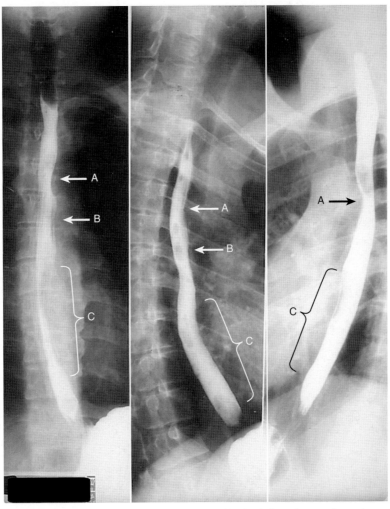

Fig. 17-19 Esophagogram images showing luminal indentations from adjacent anatomy. Normally indented structures include aortic arch (*A*), left main stem bronchus (*B*), and left atrium (*C*).

Examination procedures

For a single-contrast examination (Figs. 17-20 to 17-22), the following steps are taken:

- Start the fluoroscopic and spot-image examinations with the patient in the upright position when possible.

- Use the horizontal and Trendelenburg positions as indicated.
- After the fluoroscopic examination of the heart and lungs and when the patient is upright, instruct the patient to take the cup containing the barium suspension into the left hand and to drink it on request.

The radiologist asks the patient to swallow several mouthfuls of the barium so that the act of deglutition can be observed to determine whether any abnormality is present. The radiologist instructs the patient to perform various breathing maneuvers under fluoroscopic observation so that spot images of areas or lesions not otherwise shown can be obtained.

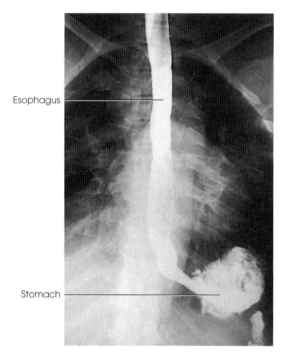

Fig. 17-20 AP esophagus, single-contrast study.

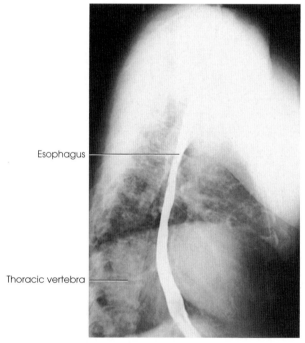

Fig. 17-21 Lateral esophagus, single-contrast study.

Performance of a *double-contrast* esophageal examination (Fig. 17-23) is similar to that of a single-contrast examination. For a double-contrast examination, free-flowing, high-density barium must be used. A gas-producing substance, usually carbon dioxide crystals, can be added to the barium mixture or given by mouth immediately *before* the barium suspension is ingested. Spot images are taken during the examination, and delayed images may be obtained on request.

OPAQUE FOREIGN BODIES

Opaque foreign bodies lodged in the pharynx or in the upper part of the esophagus can usually be shown without the use of a contrast medium. A soft tissue neck or lateral projection of the retrosternal area may be taken for this purpose. A lateral neck image should be obtained at the height of swallowing for the delineation of opaque foreign bodies in the upper end of the intrathoracic esophagus. Swallowing elevates the intrathoracic esophagus a distance of two cervical segments, placing it above the level of the clavicles.

Tufts or pledgets of cotton saturated with a thin barium suspension are sometimes used to show an obstruction or to detect *nonopaque foreign bodies* in the pharynx and upper esophagus (Fig. 17-24).

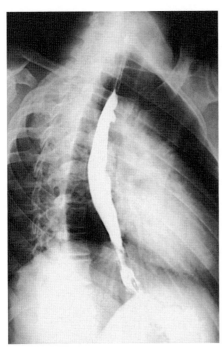

Fig. 17-22 PA oblique esophagus, RAO position, single-contrast study.

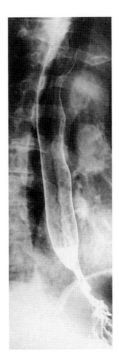

Fig. 17-23 PA oblique distal esophagus, RAO position, double-contrast spot image.

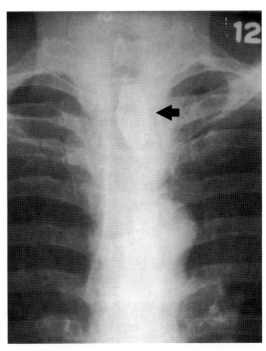

Fig. 17-24 Barium-soaked cotton ball showing nonopaque foreign body in upper esophagus (*arrow*).

✦ AP, PA, OBLIQUE, AND LATERAL PROJECTIONS

Image receptor: 14 × 17 inch (35 × 43 cm) lengthwise and centered so that the top of the IR is positioned at the level of the mouth for inclusion of the entire esophagus

Position of patient

- Position the patient as for chest images (AP, PA, oblique, and lateral; see Chapter 10, Volume 1). Because the RAO position of 35 to 40 degrees (Fig. 17-25) makes it possible to obtain a wider space for an unobstructed image of the esophagus between the vertebrae and the heart, it is usually used in preference to the LAO position. The LPO position has also been recommended.[1]
- Unless the upright position is specified, place the patient in the recumbent position for esophageal studies. The recumbent position is used to obtain more complete contrast filling of the esophagus (especially filling of the proximal part) by having the barium column flow against gravity. The recumbent position is routinely used to show variceal distentions of the esophageal veins because varices are best filled by having the blood flow against gravity. Variceal filling is more complete during increased venous pressure, which may be applied by full expiration or by the Valsalva maneuver (see Chapter 15, p. 77).

[1]Cockerill EM et al: Optimal visualization of esophageal varices, *AJR Am J Roentgenol* 126:512, 1976.

✦ AP OR PA PROJECTION

The following steps are taken:
- Place the patient in the supine or prone position with the arms above the head in a comfortable position.
- Center the midsagittal plane to the grid.
- Turn the head slightly, if necessary, to assist drinking of the barium mixture.
- *Shield gonads.*

✦ AP OR PA OBLIQUE PROJECTION
RAO OR LPO POSITION

The steps are as follows:
- Position the patient in the RAO or LPO position with the midsagittal plane forming an angle of 35 to 40 degrees from the grid device.
- For the RAO position, adjust the patient's side-down arm at the side and the side-up arm on the pillow by the head. For the LPO position, do the same, with the side-down arm at the side and the side-up arm on the pillow.
- Center the elevated side to the grid through a plane approximately 2 inches (5 cm) lateral to the midsagittal plane (Fig. 17-26).
- *Shield gonads.*

✦ LATERAL PROJECTION
R OR L POSITION

The steps are as follows:
- Place the patient's arms forward, with the forearm on the pillow near the head.

- Center the midcoronal plane to the grid.
- *Shield gonads.*

Central ray

- Perpendicular to the midpoint of the IR (the central ray is at the level of T5-6)

Collimation

- Adjust to 12 × 17 inches (30 × 43 cm) on the collimator.

Structures shown

The contrast medium–filled esophagus should be shown from the lower part of the neck to the esophagogastric junction, where the esophagus joins the stomach.

EVALUATION CRITERIA

The following should be clearly shown:

General

- Evidence of proper collimation
- Esophagus from the lower part of the neck to its entrance into the stomach
- Esophagus filled with barium
- Penetration of the barium

AP or PA projection (see Fig. 17-20)

- Brightness and contrast sufficient to visualize the esophagus through the superimposed thoracic vertebrae
- No rotation of the patient

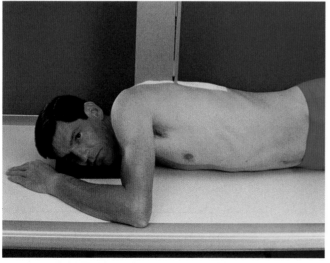

Fig. 17-25 PA oblique esophagus, RAO position.

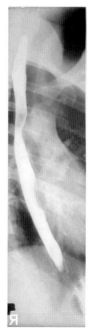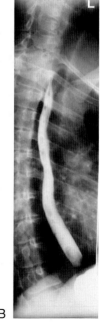

Fig. 17-26 A, PA oblique esophagus, RAO position. **B,** AP oblique esophagus, LPO position.

Oblique projection (see Fig. 17-26)

■ Esophagus between the vertebrae and the heart

Lateral projection (see Fig. 17-21)

■ Patient's arm not interfering with visualization of the proximal esophagus
■ Ribs posterior to the vertebrae superimposed to show that the patient was not rotated

NOTE: The general criteria apply to all projections: AP or PA, oblique, and lateral.

Barium administration and respiration

• Feed the barium sulfate suspension to the patient by spoon, by cup, or through a drinking straw, depending on its consistency.
• Ask the patient to swallow several mouthfuls of barium in rapid succession and then to hold a mouthful until immediately before the exposure.

• To show esophageal varices, instruct the patient (1) to exhale fully and then swallow the barium bolus and avoid inspiration until the exposure has been made, or (2) to take a deep breath and, while holding the breath, swallow the bolus and then perform the Valsalva maneuver (Fig. 17-27, A).
• For other conditions, instruct the patient simply to swallow the barium bolus, which is normally done during moderate inspiration (Fig. 17-27, B). Because respiration is inhibited for about 2 seconds after swallowing, the patient does not have to hold his or her breath for the exposure. If the contrast medium is swallowed at the end of full inspiration, make two or three exposures in rapid succession before the contrast medium passes into the stomach. To show the entire esophagus, it is sometimes necessary to make the exposure while the patient is drinking the barium suspension through a straw in rapid and continuous swallows.
• Ask the patient to swallow a barium tablet to evaluate the degree of lumen narrowing with esophageal stricture (Fig. 17-28).

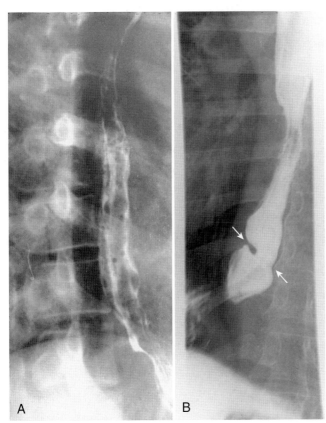

Fig. 17-27 A, Spot-film studies showing esophageal varices. **B,** Barium bolus clearly shows Schatzki ring (*arrows*).

(Courtesy Michael J. Kudlas, MEd, RT(R)(QM).)

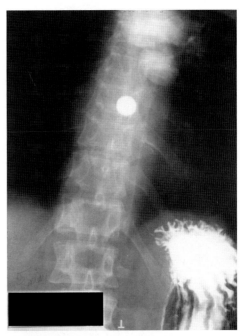

Fig. 17-28 AP projection showing barium pill in distal esophagus, at the site of luminal stricture.

Stomach: Gastrointestinal Series

Upper gastrointestinal (UGI) tract images are used to evaluate the distal esophagus, the stomach, and some or all of the small intestine. A UGI examination (Fig. 17-29), usually called a *gastrointestinal* or *UGI series,* may include the following:

1. A preliminary image of the abdomen to delineate the liver, spleen, kidneys, psoas muscles, and bony structures and to detect any abdominal or pelvic calcifications or tumor masses. Detection of calcifications and tumor masses requires that the survey image of the abdomen be taken after preliminary cleansing of the intestinal tract but before administration of the contrast medium.
2. Fluoroscopic recorded images only or a combination of fluoroscopic and radiographic images after contrast administration. Images will include the esophagus, stomach, and duodenum using an ingested opaque mixture, usually barium sulfate.
3. When requested, a small intestine study consisting of images obtained at frequent intervals during passage of the contrast column through the small intestine, at which time the vermiform appendix and the ileocecal region may be examined.

Nonambulatory outpatients or acutely ill patients, such as patients with a bleeding ulcer, are usually examined in the supine position using a fluoroscopic and spot-imaging procedure. Everything possible should be done to expedite the procedure. Any contrast preparation must be ready, and the examination room must be fully prepared before the patient is brought into the radiology department.

PRELIMINARY PREPARATION
Preparation of patient

Because a gastrointestinal series is time-consuming, the patient should be told the approximate time required for the procedure before being assigned an appointment for an examination. The patient also needs to understand the reason for preliminary preparation so that full cooperation can be given.

The stomach must be empty for an examination of the UGI tract (the stomach and small intestine). It is also desirable to have the colon free of gas and fecal material. When the patient is constipated, a non–gas-forming laxative may be administered 1 day before the examination.

An empty stomach is ensured by withholding food and water after midnight for 8 to 9 hours before the examination. When a small intestine study is to be made, food and fluid are withheld after the evening meal.

Because some research suggests that nicotine and chewing gum stimulate gastric secretion and salivation, some physicians tell patients not to smoke or chew gum after midnight on the night before the examination. This restriction is intended to prevent excessive fluid from accumulating in the stomach and diluting the barium suspension enough to interfere with its coating property. Radiographers should verify patient compliance with the preliminary preparation before obtaining the scout abdominal image, and should inform the fluoroscopist of the patient's answer when the scout image is provided for preliminary inspection.

Barium sulfate suspension

The contrast medium generally used in routine gastrointestinal examinations is barium sulfate mixed with water. The preparation must be thoroughly mixed according to the manufacturer's instructions. Specially formulated high-density barium is also available. Advances in the production of barium have all but eliminated the use of a single barium formula for most gastrointestinal examinations performed in the radiology department.

Most physicians use one of the many commercially prepared barium suspensions. These products are available in several flavors, and some are conveniently packaged in individual cups containing the dry ingredients. To these products, the radiographer merely has to add water, recap the cup, and shake it to obtain a smooth suspension. Other barium suspensions are completely mixed and ready to use.

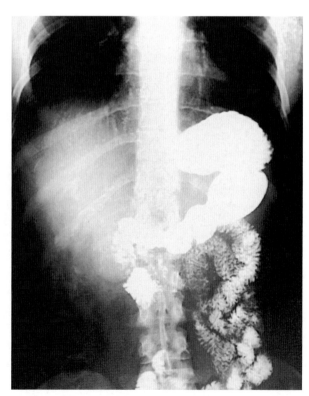

Fig. 17-29 Barium-filled AP stomach and small bowel.

Contrast Studies

Two general procedures are routinely used to examine the stomach: the *single-contrast* method and the *double-contrast* method. A *biphasic* examination is a combination of the single-contrast and double-contrast methods during the same procedure. *Hypotonic duodenography* is another, less commonly used examination.

SINGLE-CONTRAST EXAMINATION

In the single-contrast method (Fig. 17-30), a barium sulfate suspension is administered during the initial fluoroscopic examination. The barium suspension used for this study is usually in the 30% to 50% weight/volume range.[1] The procedure is as follows:

- Whenever possible, begin the examination with the patient in the upright position.
- The radiologist may first examine the heart and lungs fluoroscopically and observe the abdomen to determine whether food or fluid is in the stomach.
- Give the patient a glass of barium and instruct the patient to drink it as requested by the radiologist. If the patient is in the recumbent position, administer the suspension through a drinking straw.
- The radiologist asks the patient to swallow two or three mouthfuls of barium. During this time, the radiologist examines and exposes any indicated spot images of the esophagus. By manual manipulation of the stomach through the abdominal wall, the radiologist then coats the gastric mucosa.
- Images are obtained with the spot-imaging device or another compression device to show a mucosal lesion of the stomach or duodenum.
- After studying the rugae and as the patient drinks the remainder of the barium suspension, the radiologist observes filling of the stomach and examines the duodenum further. Based on this examination, the following can be accomplished:
  1. Determine the size, shape, and position of the stomach.
  2. Examine the changing contour of the stomach during peristalsis.
  3. Observe the filling and emptying of the duodenal bulb.

4. Detect any abnormal alteration in the function or contour of the esophagus, stomach, and duodenum.
5. Record spot images as indicated.

The contrast medium normally begins to pass into the duodenum almost immediately. Nervous tension of the patient may delay transit of the contrast material, however.

Fluoroscopy is performed with the patient in the upright and recumbent positions while the body is rotated and the table is angled, so that all aspects of the esophagus, stomach, and duodenum are shown. Spot images are exposed as indicated. If esophageal involvement is suspected, a study is usually made with a thick barium suspension. In facilities in which subsequent radiographic images of the stomach and duodenum are required, the required projections should be obtained immediately after fluoroscopy before any considerable amount of the barium suspension passes into the jejunum.

Position of patient

The stomach and the duodenum may be examined using PA, AP, oblique, and lateral projections with the patient in the upright and recumbent positions, as indicated by the fluoroscopic findings.

One variation of the supine position is the LPO position. In another variation, the head end of the table is lowered 25 to 30 degrees to show a hiatal hernia. Finally, to show esophageal regurgitation and hiatal hernias, the head end of the table is lowered 10 to 15 degrees and the patient is rotated slightly toward the right side to place the esophagogastric (gastroesophageal) junction in profile to the right of the spine. The medical significance of diagnosing hiatal hernia is a topic that has received much attention in recent years. Some authors report little correlation between the presence of a hiatal hernia and gastrointestinal symptoms. If little correlation exists, radiographic evaluation is of little value in most hiatal hernias.

[1]Skucas J: Contrast media. In Margulis AR, Burhenne HJ, editors: *Alimentary tract radiology,* vol 1, ed 4, St Louis, 1989, Mosby.

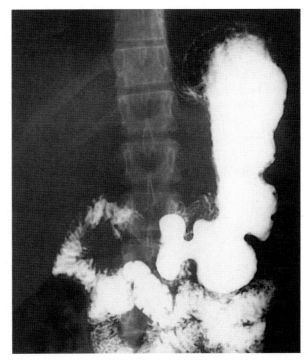

Fig. 17-30 Barium-filled PA stomach, single-contrast study.

DOUBLE-CONTRAST EXAMINATION

A second approach to examination of the gastrointestinal tract is the *double-contrast* technique (Fig. 17-31). The principal advantages of this method over the single-contrast method are that small lesions are less easily obscured and the mucosal lining of the stomach can be more clearly visualized. For successful results, the patient must be able to move with relative ease throughout the examination.

For double-contrast studies, the procedure is as follows:

- To begin the examination, place the patient on the fluoroscopic table in the upright position.
- Give the patient a gas-producing substance in the form of a powder, crystals, pills, or a carbonated beverage. (An older technique involved placing pinholes in the sides of a drinking straw so that the patient ingested air while drinking the barium suspension during the examination.)
- Give the patient a small amount of commercially available, high-density barium suspension. For even coating of the stomach walls, the barium must flow freely and have low viscosity. Many high-density barium products are available; these suspensions have weight/volume ratios of up to 250%.
- Place the patient in the recumbent position, and instruct him or her to turn from side to side or to roll over a few times. This movement serves to coat the mucosal lining of the stomach as the carbon dioxide continues to expand. The patient may feel the need to belch but should refrain from doing so until the examination is finished to ensure that an optimal amount of contrast material (gas) remains for the duration of the examination.

- Just before the examination, the patient may be given glucagon or other anticholinergic medications intravenously or intramuscularly to relax the gastrointestinal tract. These medications improve visualization by inducing greater distention of the stomach and intestines. Before administering these agents, the radiologist must consider numerous factors, including side effects, contraindications, availability, and cost.

Radiographic imaging procedure

The conventional images obtained after the fluoroscopic examination may be the same as images obtained for the single-contrast examination. Often the images with the greatest amount of diagnostic information are the spot images taken during fluoroscopy. In most cases, the radiologist will have already obtained most of the necessary diagnostic images. Nonfluoroscopic images may be unnecessary.

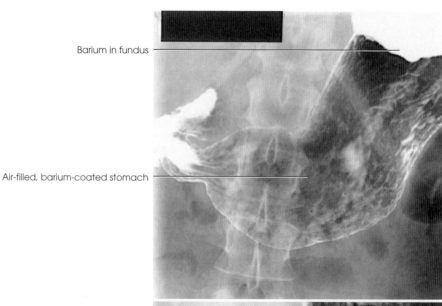

Barium in fundus

Air-filled, barium-coated stomach

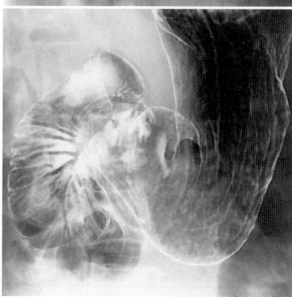

Fig. 17-31 Double-contrast stomach spot images.

BIPHASIC EXAMINATION

The *biphasic* gastrointestinal examination incorporates the advantages of single-contrast and double-contrast UGI examinations, with both examinations performed during the same procedure. The patient first undergoes a double-contrast examination of the UGI tract. When this study is completed, the patient is given an approximately 15% weight/volume barium suspension, and a single-contrast examination is performed. This biphasic approach increases the accuracy of diagnosis without significantly increasing the cost of the examination.

HYPOTONIC DUODENOGRAPHY

The use of *hypotonic duodenography* as a primary diagnostic tool has decreased in recent years. When lesions beyond the duodenum are suspected, the double-contrast gastrointestinal examination described can aid in the diagnosis. When pancreatic disease is suspected, computed tomography (CT) or needle biopsy can also be used. Hypotonic duodenography is less frequently necessary.

First described by Liotta,[1] hypotonic duodenography requires intubation (Figs. 17-32 and 17-33) and is used to evaluate postbulbar duodenal lesions and to detect pancreatic disease. A newer tubeless technique requires temporary drug-induced duodenal paralysis so that a double-contrast examination can be performed without interference from peristaltic activity. During the atonic state, when the duodenum is distended with contrast medium to two or three times its normal size, it presses against and outlines any abnormality in the contour of the head of the pancreas.

---

[1]Liotta D: Pour le diagnostic des tumeus du pancréas: la duodénographic hypotonique, *Lyon Chir* 50:445, 1955.

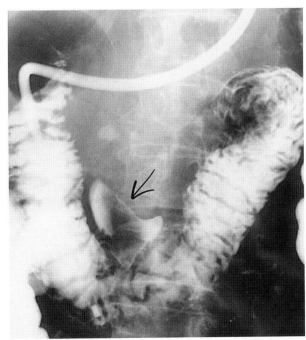

Fig. 17-32 Hypotonic duodenogram showing deformity of duodenal diverticulum by small carcinoma of head of pancreas (*arrow*).

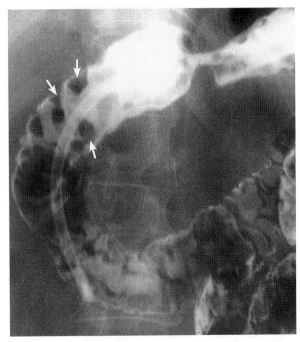

Fig. 17-33 Hypotonic duodenogram showing multiple defects (*arrows*) in duodenal bulb and proximal duodenum, caused by hypertrophy of Brunner glands.

✷ PA PROJECTION

Image receptor: 10 × 12 inch (24 × 30 cm), 11 × 14 inch (30 × 35 cm), or 14 × 17 inch (35 × 43 cm) lengthwise, depending on availability and radiologist preference

Position of patient
- For radiographic studies of the stomach and duodenum, place the patient in the recumbent position. The upright position is sometimes used to show the relative position of the stomach.
- When adjusting thin patients in the prone position, support the weight of the body on pillows or other suitable pads positioned under the thorax and pelvis. This adjustment keeps the stomach or duodenum from pressing against the vertebrae, with resultant pressure-filling defects.

Position of part
- Adjust the patient's position recumbent or upright so that the midline of the grid coincides with a sagittal plane passing halfway between the vertebral column and the left lateral border of the abdomen (Fig. 17-34).
- Center the IR about 1 to 2 inches (2.5 to 5 cm) above the lower rib margin at the level of L1-2 when the patient is prone (Figs. 17-35 and 17-36).
- For upright images, center the IR 3 to 6 inches (7.6 to 15 cm) lower than L1-2. The greatest visceral movement between prone and upright positions occurs in asthenic patients.
- Do not apply an immobilization band for standard radiographic projections of the stomach and intestines because the pressure is likely to cause filling defects and to interfere with emptying and filling of the duodenal bulb—factors that are important in serial studies.
- *Shield gonads.*
- *Respiration:* Suspend at the end of expiration unless otherwise requested.

Central ray
- Perpendicular to the center of the IR

Collimation
- Adjust to 10 × 12 inches (24 × 30 cm) on the collimator. If a 14 × 17-inch (35 × 43 cm) IR is used for larger patients, collimate to 11 × 14 inches (28 × 35 cm).

Structures shown
A PA projection of the contour of the barium-filled stomach and duodenal bulb is shown. The upright projection shows the size, shape, and relative position of the filled stomach, but it does not adequately show the unfilled fundic portion of the organ. In the prone position, the stomach moves superiorly 1½ to 4 inches (3.8 to 10 cm) according to the patient's body habitus (Figs. 17-37 to 17-40). At the same time, the stomach spreads horizontally, with a comparable decrease in its length. (Note that the fundus usually fills in asthenic patients.)

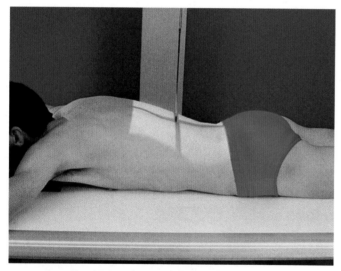

Fig. 17-34 PA stomach and duodenum.

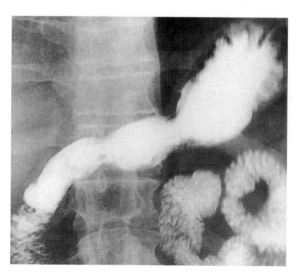

Fig. 17-35 Single-contrast PA stomach and duodenum.

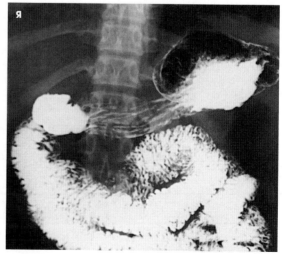

Fig. 17-36 Double-contrast PA stomach and duodenum.

The pyloric canal and the duodenal bulb are well shown in patients with an asthenic or hyposthenic habitus. These structures are often partially obscured in patients with a sthenic habitus and, except in the PA axial projection, are completely obscured by the prepyloric portion of the stomach in patients with a hypersthenic habitus.

EVALUATION CRITERIA

The following should be clearly shown:
- Evidence of proper collimation
- Entire stomach and duodenal loop
- Stomach centered at the level of the pylorus

- No rotation of the patient
- Exposure technique that shows the anatomy

NOTE: A 14 × 17-inch (35 × 43-cm) IR is often used when the distal esophagus or the small bowel is to be visualized along with the stomach.

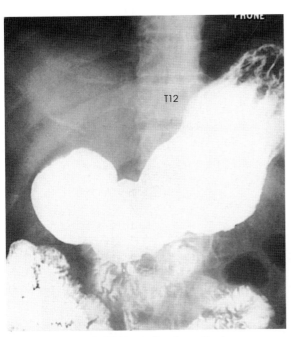

Fig. 17-37 Hypersthenic patient.

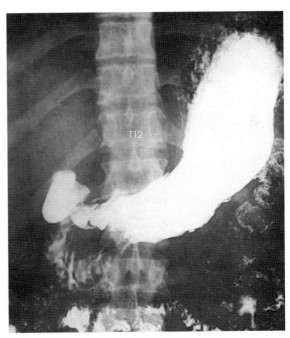

Fig. 17-38 Sthenic patient.

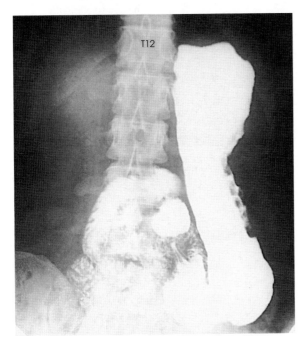

Fig. 17-39 Hyposthenic patient.

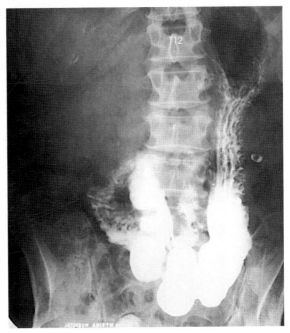

Fig. 17-40 Asthenic patient.

PA AXIAL PROJECTION

Image receptor: 14 × 17 inch (35 × 43 cm) lengthwise

Position of patient
- Place the patient in the prone position.

Position of part
- Adjust the patient's body so that the midsagittal plane is centered to the grid.

- For a sthenic patient, center the IR at the level of L2 (Fig. 17-41); center it higher for a hypersthenic patient and lower for an asthenic patient. L2 lies about 1 to 2 inches (2.5 to 5 cm) above the lower rib margin.
- *Shield gonads.*
- *Respiration:* Suspend respiration at the end of expiration unless otherwise requested.

Central ray
- Directed to the midpoint of the IR at an angle of 35 to 45 degrees cephalad. Gugliantini[1] recommended cephalic angulation of 20 to 25 degrees to show the stomach in infants.

Collimation
- Adjust to 14 × 17 inches (35 × 43 cm) on the collimator.

---

[1]Gugliantini P: Utilitá delle incidenze oblique caudocraniali nello studio radiologico della stenosi congenita ipertrofica del piloro, *Ann Radiol [Diagn]* 34:56, 1961. Abstract, *AJR Am J Roentgenol* 87:623, 1962.

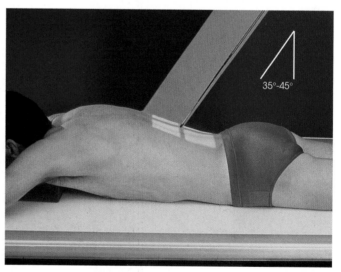

Fig. 17-41 PA axial stomach.

Structures shown

Gordon[1] developed the PA axial projection to "open up" the high, horizontal (hypersthenic-type) stomach to show the greater and lesser curvatures, the antral portion of the stomach, the pyloric canal, and the duodenal bulb. The resultant image gives a hypersthenic stomach much the same configuration as the average sthenic type of stomach (Fig. 17-42).

[1]Gordon SS: The angled posteroanterior projection of the stomach: an attempt at better visualization of the high transverse stomach, *Radiology* 69:393, 1957.

EVALUATION CRITERIA

The following should clearly be shown:
- Evidence of proper collimation
- Entire stomach and proximal duodenum
- Stomach centered at the level of the pylorus
- Exposure technique that shows the anatomy

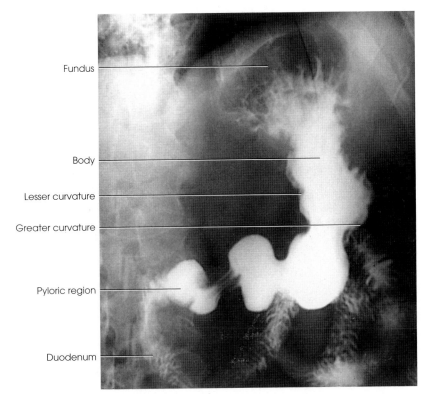

Fundus
Body
Lesser curvature
Greater curvature
Pyloric region
Duodenum

Fig. 17-42 PA axial stomach, sthenic habitus.

♠ PA OBLIQUE PROJECTION
RAO position

Image receptor: 10 × 12 inch (24 × 30 cm), 11 × 14 inch (30 × 35 cm), or 14 × 17 inch (35 × 43 cm) lengthwise, depending on availability

Position of patient
- Place the patient in the recumbent position.

Position of part
- After the PA projection, instruct the patient to rest the head on the right cheek and to place the right arm along the side of the body.
- Have the patient raise his or her left side and support the body on the left forearm and flexed left knee.
- Adjust the patient's position so that a sagittal plane passing midway between the vertebrae and the lateral border of the elevated side coincides with the midline of the grid (Fig. 17-43).
- Center the IR about 1 to 2 inches (2.5 to 5 cm) above the lower rib margin, at the level of L1-2, when the patient is prone.

- Make the final adjustment in body rotation. The approximately 40 to 70 degrees of rotation required to give the best image of the pyloric canal and duodenum depends on the size, shape, and position of the stomach. Generally, hypersthenic patients require a greater degree of rotation than sthenic and asthenic patients.
- The RAO position is used for serial studies of the pyloric canal and the duodenal bulb because gastric peristalsis is usually more active when the patient is in this position.
- *Shield gonads.*
- *Respiration:* Suspend at the end of expiration unless otherwise requested.

Central ray
- Perpendicular to the center of the IR

Collimation
- Adjust to 10 × 12 inches (24 × 30 cm) on the collimator. If the 14 × 17-inch (35 × 43-cm) IR is used for larger patients, collimate to 11 × 14 inches (28 × 35 cm).

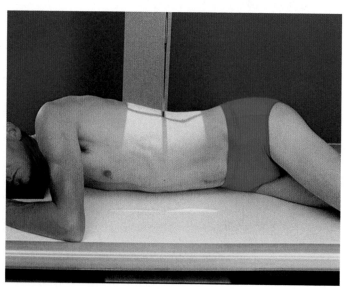

Fig. 17-43 PA oblique stomach and duodenum, RAO position.

Structures shown

A PA oblique projection of the stomach and entire duodenal loop is presented. This projection gives the best image of the pyloric canal and the duodenal bulb in patients whose habitus approximates the sthenic type (Figs. 17-44 and 17-45).

Because gastric peristalsis is generally more active with the patient in the RAO position, a serial study of several exposures is sometimes obtained at intervals of 30 to 40 seconds to delineate the pyloric canal and duodenal bulb.

EVALUATION CRITERIA

The following should be clearly shown:

- Evidence of proper collimation
- Entire stomach and duodenal loop
- No superimposition of the pylorus and duodenal bulb
- Duodenal bulb and loop in profile
- Stomach centered at the level of the pylorus
- Exposure technique that shows the anatomy

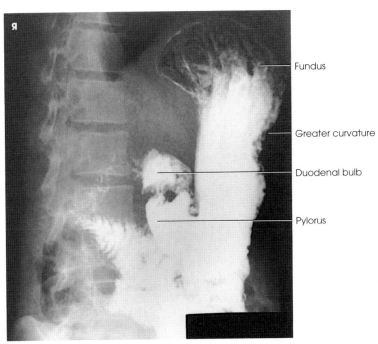

Fundus

Greater curvature

Duodenal bulb

Pylorus

Fig. 17-44 Single-contrast PA oblique stomach and duodenum, RAO position.

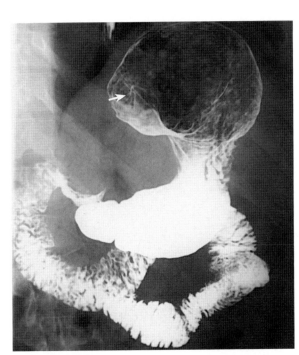

Fig. 17-45 Double-contrast PA oblique stomach and duodenum. Note esophagus entering stomach (*arrow*).

☀ AP OBLIQUE PROJECTION
LPO position

Image receptor: 10×12 inch (24×30 cm), 11×14 inch (30×35 cm), or 14×17 inch (35×43 cm) lengthwise, depending on availability

Position of patient
- Place the patient in the supine position.

Position of part
- Have the patient abduct the left arm and place the hand near the head, or place the extended arm alongside the body.
- Place the right arm alongside the body or across the upper chest, as preferred.
- Have the patient turn toward the left, resting on the left posterior body surface.
- Flex the patient's right knee, and rotate the knee toward the left for support.
- Place a positioning sponge against the patient's elevated back for immobilization.
- Adjust the patient's position so that a sagittal plane passing approximately midway between the vertebrae and the left lateral margin of the abdomen is centered to the IR.

- Adjust the center of the IR at the level of the body of the stomach. Centering would be adjusted at a point midway between the xiphoid process and the lower margin of the ribs (Fig. 17-46).
- The degree of rotation required to show the stomach best depends on the patient's body habitus. An average angle of 45 degrees should be sufficient for a sthenic patient, but the degree of angulation can vary from 30 to 60 degrees.
- *Shield gonads.*
- *Respiration:* Suspend at the end of expiration unless otherwise instructed.

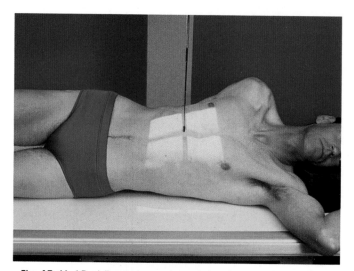

Fig. 17-46 AP oblique stomach and duodenum, LPO position.

Central ray

- Perpendicular to the center of the IR

Collimation

- Adjust to 10 × 12 inches (24 × 30 cm) on the collimator. If the 14 × 17-inch (35 × 43-cm) IR is used for larger patients, collimate to 11 × 14 inches (28 × 35 cm).

Structures shown

The AP oblique projection shows the fundic portion of the stomach (Fig. 17-47). Because of the effect of gravity, the pyloric canal and the duodenal bulb are not as filled with barium as they are in the opposite and complementary position (the RAO position; see Figs. 17-43 to 17-45).

The following should be clearly shown:
- Evidence of proper collimation
- Entire stomach and duodenal loop
- Fundic portion of stomach
- No superimposition of pylorus and duodenal bulb
- Body of the stomach centered to the image
- Exposure technique that shows the anatomy
- Body and pyloric antrum with double-contrast visualization

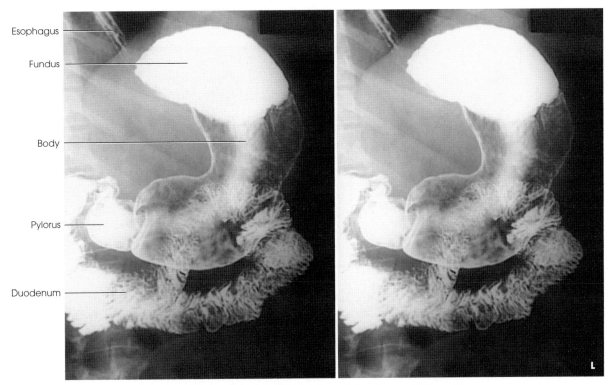

Fig. 17-47 Double-contrast AP oblique stomach and duodenum, LPO position.

Esophagus

Fundus

Body

Pylorus

Duodenum

Stomach and Duodenum

131

⚘ LATERAL PROJECTION
R position

Image receptor: 10 × 12 inch (24 × 30 cm), 11 × 14 (30 × 35 cm), or 14 × 17 inch (35 × 43 cm) lengthwise, depending on availability

Position of patient

- Place the patient in the *upright left lateral position* to show the left retrogastric space and in the *recumbent right lateral position* to show the right retrogastric space, duodenal loop, and duodenojejunal junction.

Position of part

- With the patient in the upright or recumbent position, adjust the body so that a plane passing midway between the midcoronal plane and the anterior surface of the abdomen coincides with the midline of the grid.
- Center the IR at the level of L1-2 for the recumbent position (about 1 to 2 inches [2.5 to 5 cm] above the lower rib margin) and at L3 for the upright position.
- Adjust the body in a true lateral position (Fig. 17-48).
- *Shield gonads.*
- *Respiration:* Suspend at the end of expiration unless otherwise requested.

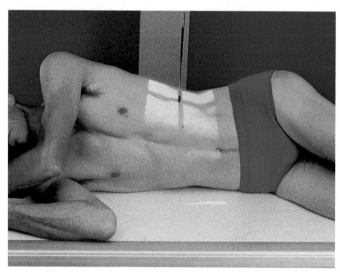

Fig. 17-48 Right lateral stomach and duodenum.

Central ray

- Perpendicular to the center of the IR

Collimation

- Adjust to 10 × 12 inches (24 × 30 cm) on the collimator. If the 14 × 17-inch (35 × 43-cm) IR is used for larger patients, collimate to 11 × 14 inches (28 × 35 cm).

Structures shown

A lateral projection shows the anterior and posterior aspects of the stomach, the pyloric canal, and the duodenal bulb (Figs. 17-49 and 17-50). The right lateral projection commonly affords the best image of the pyloric canal and the duodenal bulb in patients with a hypersthenic habitus.

The following should be clearly shown:
- Evidence of proper collimation
- Entire stomach and duodenal loop
- No rotation of the patient, as shown by the vertebrae
- Stomach centered at the level of the pylorus
- Exposure technique that shows the anatomy

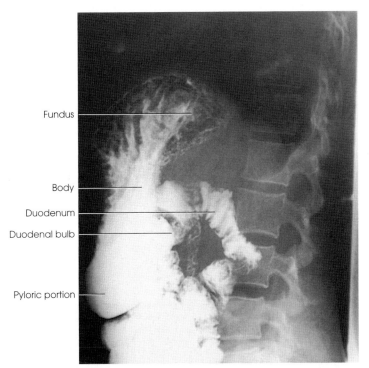

Fundus

Body

Duodenum

Duodenal bulb

Pyloric portion

Fig. 17-49 Single-contrast right lateral stomach and duodenum.

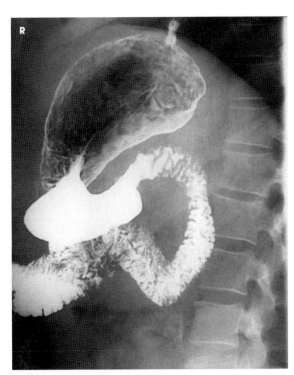

R

Fig. 17-50 Double-contrast right lateral stomach and duodenum.

♠ AP PROJECTION

Image receptor: 10 × 12 inch (24 × 30 cm) lengthwise for small hiatal hernias; 14 × 17 inch (35 × 43 cm) lengthwise for large diaphragmatic herniations or for the stomach and small bowel

Position of patient

- Place the patient in the supine position. The stomach moves superiorly and to the left in this position, and, except in thin patients, its pyloric end is elevated so that the barium flows into and fills its cardiac or fundic portions or both. Filling of the fundus displaces the gas bubble into the pyloric end of the stomach, where it allows double-contrast delineation of posterior wall lesions when a single-contrast examination is performed. If the patient is thin, the intestinal loops do not move superior enough to tilt the stomach for fundic filling. Rotating the patient's body toward the left or angling the head end of the table downward is necessary.
- Tilt the table to full or partial Trendelenburg angulation to show diaphragmatic herniations (Fig. 17-51). In the Trendelenburg position, the involved organ or organs, which may appear to be normally located in all other body positions, shift upward and protrude through the hernial orifice (most commonly through the esophageal hiatus).

NOTE: Valsalva maneuver may be used in conjunction with or as an alternative to the Trendelenburg position.

Position of part

- Adjust the position of the patient so that the midline of the grid coincides (1) with the midline of the body when a 14 × 17-inch (35 × 43-cm) IR is used (see Fig. 17-51) or (2) with a sagittal plane passing midway between the midline and the left lateral margin of the abdomen when a 10 × 12-inch (24 × 30-cm) IR is used (Fig. 17-52). Longitudinal centering of the large IR depends on the extent of hernial protrusion into the thorax and is determined during fluoroscopy.
- For the stomach and duodenum, center the 10 × 12-inch (24 × 30-cm) IR at a level midway between the xiphoid process and the lower rib margin (approximately L1-2). For the 14 × 17-inch (35 × 43-cm) IR, center it at the same level and adjust up or down slightly, depending on whether the diaphragm or the small bowel needs to be seen.
- *Shield gonads.*
- *Respiration:* Suspend at the end of expiration unless otherwise requested.

Central ray

- Perpendicular to the center of the IR

Collimation

- Adjust to 10 × 12 inches (24 × 30 cm) (for stomach) or 14 × 17 inches (35 × 43 cm) (for stomach and small bowel) on the collimator.

Structures shown

Stomach. An AP projection of the stomach shows a well-filled fundic portion and usually a double-contrast delineation of the body, pyloric portion, and duodenum (Fig. 17-53). Because of the elevation and superior displacement of the stomach, this projection affords the best AP projection of the retrogastric portion of the duodenum and jejunum.

Diaphragm. An AP projection of the abdominothoracic region shows the organ or organs involved in, and the location and extent of, any gross hernial protrusion through the diaphragm (Figs. 17-54 and 17-55).

EVALUATION CRITERIA

The following should be clearly shown:
- Evidence of proper collimation
- Entire stomach and duodenal loop
- Double-contrast visualization of the gastric body, pylorus, and duodenal bulb
- Retrogastric portion of the duodenum and jejunum
- Lower lung fields on 14 × 17-inch (35 × 43-cm) images to show diaphragmatic hernias
- Stomach centered at the level of the pylorus on 10 × 12-inch (24 × 30-cm) and 11 × 14- inch (28 × 35-cm) images
- No rotation of the patient
- Exposure technique that shows the anatomy

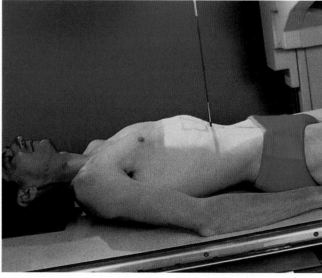

Fig. 17-51 AP stomach and duodenum with table in partial Trendelenburg position.

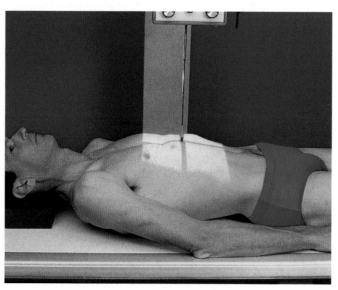

Fig. 17-52 AP stomach and duodenum.

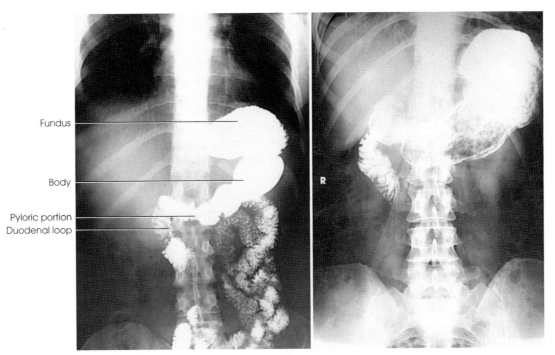

Fundus

Body

Pyloric portion
Duodenal loop

Fig. 17-53 AP stomach and duodenum, sthenic habitus.

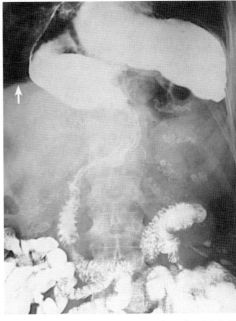

Fig. 17-54 AP stomach and duodenum, showing hiatal hernia above level of diaphragm (*arrow*).

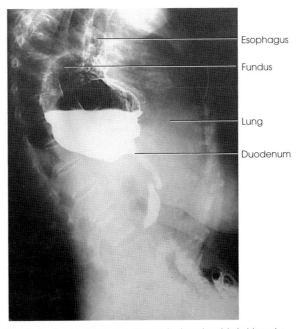

Esophagus

Fundus

Lung

Duodenum

Fig. 17-55 Upright left lateral stomach showing hiatal hernia. (Comparison lateral images are shown in Figs. 17-49 and 17-50.)

PA OBLIQUE PROJECTION
WOLF METHOD (FOR HIATAL HERNIA)
RAO position

Image receptor: 14 × 17 inch (35 × 43 cm) lengthwise

The Wolf method[1] is a modification of the Trendelenburg position. The technique was developed for the purpose of applying greater intra-abdominal pressure than is provided by body angulation alone and ensuring more consistent results in the radiographic demonstration of small, sliding gastroesophageal herniations through the esophageal hiatus.

The Wolf method requires the use of a semicylindric radiolucent compression device measuring 22 inches (55 cm) in length, 10 inches (24 cm) in width, and 8 inches (20 cm) in height. (The compression sponge depicted in Fig. 17-56 is slightly smaller than the one described by Wolf.)

---

[1]Wolf BS, Guglielmo J: Method for the roentgen demonstration of minimal hiatal herniation, *J Mt Sinai Hosp NY* 23:738, 741, 1956.

Wolf and Guglielmo[1] stated that this compression device not only provides Trendelenburg angulation of the patient's trunk, it also increases intra-abdominal pressure enough to permit adequate contrast filling and maximal distention of the entire esophagus. A further advantage of the device is that it does not require angulation of the table; the patient can hold the barium container and ingest the barium suspension through a straw with comparative ease.

NOTE: Valsalva maneuver also increases intra-abdominal pressure and may be used instead of the Wolf method.

---

[1]Wolf BS, Guglielmo J: The roentgen demonstration of minimal hiatus hernia, *Med Radiogr Photogr* 33:90, 1957.

Position of patient
- Place the patient in the prone position on the radiographic table.

Position of part
- Instruct the patient to assume a modified knee-chest position during placement of the compression device.
- Place the compression device horizontally under the abdomen and just below the costal margin.
- Adjust the patient in a 40- to 45-degree RAO position, with the thorax centered to the midline of the grid.
- Instruct the patient to ingest the barium suspension in rapid, continuous swallows.
- To allow for complete filling of the esophagus, make the exposure during the third or fourth swallow (see Fig. 17-56).
- *Shield gonads.*
- *Respiration:* Suspend at the end of expiration.

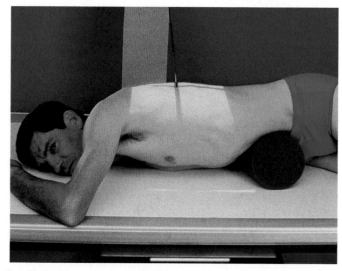

Fig. 17-56 PA oblique stomach with compression sponge, RAO position.

Central ray

• Perpendicular to the long axis of the patient's back and centered at the level of T6 or T7. This position usually results in 10- to 20-degree caudad angulation of the central ray.

Collimation

• Adjust to 14 × 17 inches (35 × 43 cm) on the collimator.

Structures shown

The Wolf method shows the relationship of the stomach to the diaphragm and is useful in diagnosing a hiatal hernia (Fig. 17-57).

EVALUATION CRITERIA

The following should be clearly shown:
■ Evidence of proper collimation
■ Middle or distal aspects of the esophagus and the upper aspect of the stomach
■ Esophagus visible between the vertebral column and the heart
■ Exposure technique that shows the anatomy

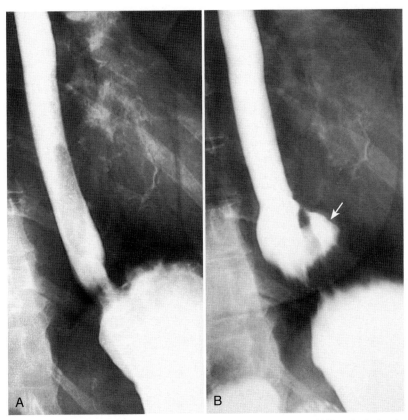

Fig. 17-57 Comparison PA axial oblique images in one patient. **A,** Without abdominal compression: no evidence of hernia. **B,** With abdominal compression: obvious large sliding hernia (*arrow*).

Small Intestine

Radiologic examinations of the small intestine are performed by administering a barium sulfate preparation (1) by *mouth;* (2) by complete *reflux filling* with a large-volume barium enema (BE); or (3) by direct injection into the bowel through an intestinal tube—a technique that is called *enteroclysis,* or small intestine enema. The latter two methods are used when the oral method fails to provide conclusive information.[1] Enteroclysis is technically difficult, so its use is usually limited to larger medical facilities.

PREPARATION FOR EXAMINATION

Preferably, the patient has a soft or low-residue diet for 2 days before the small intestine study. Because of economics, however, it often is impossible to delay the examination for 2 days. Food and fluid are usually withheld after the evening meal of the day before the examination, and breakfast is withheld on the day of the study. A cleansing enema may be administered to clear the colon; however, an enema is not always recommended for enteroclysis because enema fluid may be retained in the small intestine. The barium formula varies depending on the method of examination. The patient's bladder should be empty before and during the procedure to avoid displacing or compressing the ileum.

[1]Fitch D: The small-bowel see-through: an improved method of radiographic small bowel visualization, *Can J Med Radiat Technol* 26:167, 1995.

ORAL METHOD OF EXAMINATION

The radiographic examination of the small intestine is usually termed a *small bowel series* because several identical images are done at timed intervals. The oral examination, or ingestion of barium through the mouth, is usually preceded by a preliminary image of the abdomen. Each image of the small intestine is identified with a time marker indicating the interval between its exposure and ingestion of barium. Studies are made with the patient in the supine or the prone position. The supine position is used (1) to take advantage of the superior and lateral shift of the barium-filled stomach for visualization of retrogastric portions of the duodenum and jejunum and (2) to prevent possible compression overlapping of loops of the intestine. The prone position is used to compress the abdominal contents; this enhances radiographic image quality. For the final images in thin patients, it may be necessary to angle the table into the Trendelenburg position to "unfold" low-lying and superimposed loops of the ileum.

The first exposure of the small intestine is usually taken 15 minutes after the patient drinks the barium. The interval to the next exposure varies from 15 to 30 minutes depending on the average transit time of the barium sulfate preparation used. Regardless of the barium preparation used, the radiologist inspects the images as they are processed and varies the procedure according to requirements for the individual patient. Fluoroscopic and radiographic studies (spot or conventional) may be made of any segment of the bowel as the loops become opacified.

Some radiologists request that a glass of ice water (or another routinely used food stimulant) be given to a patient with hypomotility after 3 or 4 hours of administrating barium sulfate to accelerate peristalsis. Others give patients a water-soluble gastrointestinal contrast medium, tea, or coffee to stimulate peristalsis. Other radiologists administer peristaltic stimulants every 15 minutes through the transit time. With these methods, transit of the medium is shown fluoroscopically, spot and conventional radiographic images are exposed as indicated, and the examination is usually completed in 30 to 60 minutes.

🦅 PA OR AP PROJECTION

Image receptor: 14 × 17 inch (35 × 43 cm) lengthwise

Position of patient
• Place the patient in the prone or supine position.

Position of part
• Adjust the patient so that the midsagittal plane is centered to the grid.
• For a sthenic patient, center the IR at the level of L2 for images taken within 30 minutes after the contrast medium is administered (Fig. 17-58).
• For delayed images, center the IR at the level of the iliac crests.
• *Shield gonads.*
• *Respiration:* Suspend at the end of expiration unless otherwise requested.

Central ray
• Perpendicular to the midpoint of the IR (L2) for early images or at the level of the iliac crests for delayed sequence exposures

Collimation
• Adjust to 14 × 17 inches (35 × 43 cm) on the collimator.

Structures shown
The PA or AP projection shows the small intestine progressively filling until barium reaches the ileocecal valve (Figs. 17-59 to 17-62). When barium has reached the ileocecal region, fluoroscopy may be performed, and compression radiographic images may be obtained (Fig. 17-63). The examination is usually completed when the barium is visualized in the cecum, typically within about 2 hours for a patient with normal intestinal motility.

The following should be clearly shown:
■ Evidence of proper collimation
■ Entire small intestine on each image
■ Stomach on initial images
■ Time marker
■ Vertebral column centered on the image
■ No rotation of the patient
■ Exposure technique that shows the anatomy
■ Complete examination when barium reaches the cecum

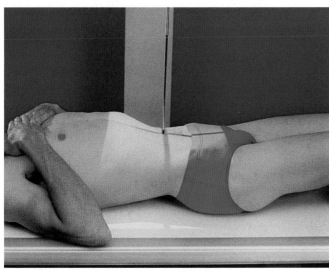

Fig. 17-58 AP small intestine.

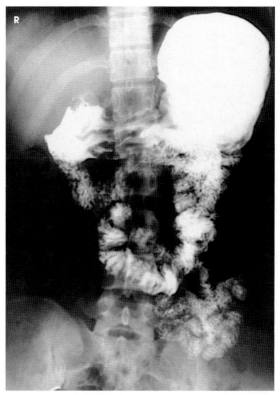

Fig. 17-59 Immediate AP small intestine.

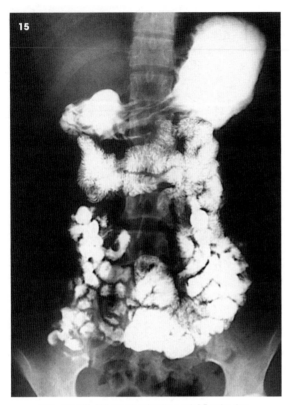

Fig. 17-60 AP small intestine at 15 minutes.

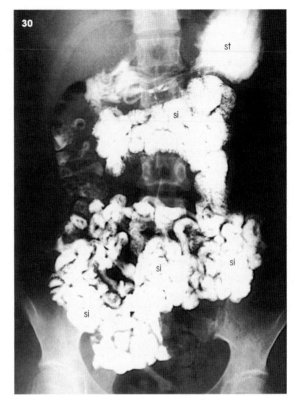

Fig. 17-61 AP small intestine at 30 minutes, showing stomach (*st*) and small intestine (*si*).

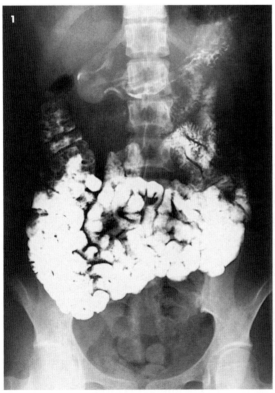

Fig. 17-62 AP small intestine at 1 hour, showing barium-filled cecum.

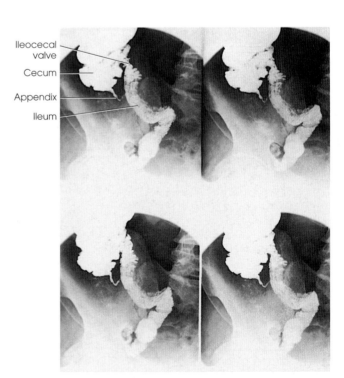

Fig. 17-63 Ileocecal studies.

Digestive System

COMPLETE REFLUX EXAMINATION

For a complete reflux examination of the small intestine,[1,2] the patient's colon and small intestine are filled by a BE administered to show the colon and small bowel. Before the examination, glucagon may be administered to relax the intestine. Diazepam (Valium) may also be given to diminish patient discomfort during initial filling of the bowel. A 15% ± 5% weight/volume barium suspension is often used, and a large amount of the suspension (about 4500 mL) is required to fill the colon and small intestine.

A retention enema tip is used, and the patient is placed in the supine position for the examination. The barium suspension is allowed to flow until it is observed in the duodenal bulb. The enema bag is lowered to the floor to drain the colon before images of the small intestine are obtained (Fig. 17-64).

[1]Miller RE: Complete reflux small bowel examination, *Radiology* 84:457, 1965.

[2]Miller RE: Localization of the small bowel hemorrhage: complete reflux small bowel examination, *Am J Dig Dis* 17:1019, 1972.

ENTEROCLYSIS PROCEDURE

Enteroclysis (the injection of nutrient or medicinal liquid into the bowel) is a radiographic procedure in which contrast medium is injected into the duodenum under fluoroscopic control for examination of the small intestine. Contrast medium is injected through a specially designed enteroclysis catheter, historically a Bilbao or Sellink tube.

Before the procedure is begun, the patient's colon must be thoroughly cleansed. Enemas are not recommended as preparation for enteroclysis because some enema fluid may be retained in the small intestine. Under fluoroscopic control, the enteroclysis catheter with a stiff guidewire is advanced to the end of the duodenum at the duodenojejunal flexure, near the ligament of Treitz. The retention balloon, if present, is filled with sterile water or saline. Barium is instilled through the tube at a rate of approximately 100 mL/min (Fig. 17-65). Spot images, with and without compression, are taken as required. In some patients, air is injected after contrast fluid has reached the distal small intestine (Fig. 17-66). When CT is to be performed, an iodinated contrast medium (Figs. 17-67 and 17-68) or tap water (Figs. 17-69 and 17-70) may be used.

After fluoroscopic examination of the patient's small intestine, images of the small intestine may be requested. The projections most often requested include AP, PA, oblique, and lateral. Recumbent and upright images may be requested. (Positioning descriptions involving the abdomen are presented in Chapter 16.)

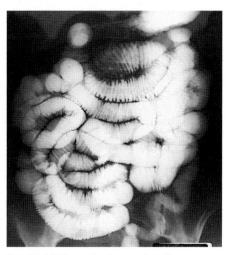

Fig. 17-64 Normal retrograde reflux examination of small intestine.

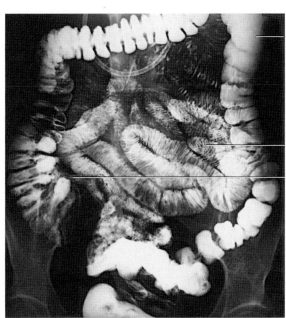

Barium in colon

Small intestine

Terminal ileum

Fig. 17-65 Enteroclysis procedure with barium visualized in colon.

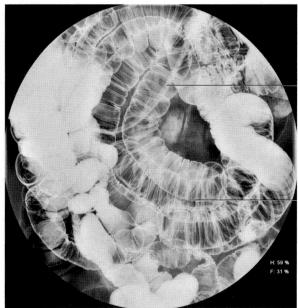

Enteroclysis catheter

Barium air in small intestine

Fig. 17-66 Air-contrast enteroclysis.

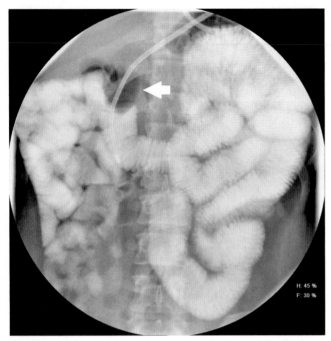

Fig. 17-67 Enteroclysis with iodinated contrast medium. Filled retention balloon is seen in duodenum (*arrow*). (Courtesy Michelle Alting, AS, RT(R).)

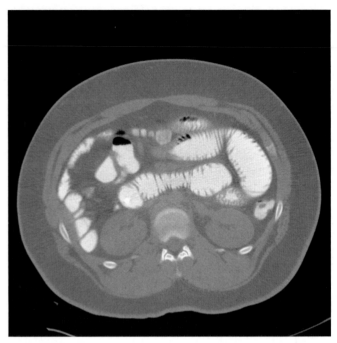

Fig. 17-68 Axial CT enteroclysis of the patient in Fig. 17-67.

Colon   Small intestine

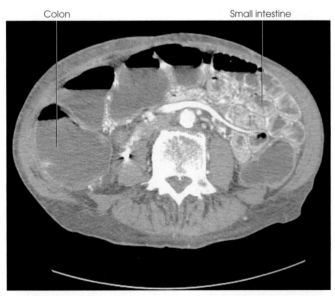

Fig. 17-69 Axial CT enteroclysis with tap water and intravenous iodinated contrast medium. Intraluminal water (*dark gray*) is clearly delineated from bowel wall (*light gray*).

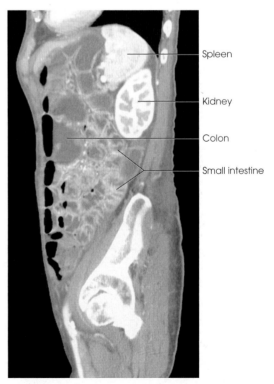

Spleen

Kidney

Colon

Small intestine

Fig. 17-70 Sagittal reconstruction of CT enteroclysis from Fig. 17-69.

INTUBATION EXAMINATION PROCEDURES

Gastrointestinal intubation is a procedure in which a long, specially designed tube is inserted through the nose and passed into the stomach. From there, the tube is carried inferiorly by peristaltic action. Gastrointestinal intubation is used for therapeutic and diagnostic purposes.

When gastrointestinal intubation is used therapeutically, the tube is connected to a suction system for continuous siphoning of gas and fluid contents of the gastrointestinal tract. The purpose of the maneuver is to prevent or relieve postoperative distention or to deflate or decompress an obstructed small intestine.

Although used much less frequently than in the past, a *Miller-Abbott* double-lumen, single-balloon tube (or other similar tubing) can be used to intubate the small intestine. Just above the tip of the Miller-Abbott tube is a small, thin rubber balloon. Marks on the tube, beginning at the distal end, indicate the extent of the tube's passage and are read from the edge of the nostril. The marks are graduated in centimeters up to 85 cm and are given in feet thereafter. The lumen of the tube is asymmetrically divided into (1) a small balloon lumen that communicates with the balloon only and is used for inflation and deflation of the balloon and for injection of mercury to weight the balloon and (2) a large aspiration lumen that communicates with the gastrointestinal tract through perforations near and at the distal end of the tube. Gas and fluids are withdrawn through the aspiration lumen, and liquids are injected through it.

The introduction of an intestinal tube is an unpleasant experience for a patient, especially one who is acutely ill. Depending on the condition of the patient, the tube is more readily passed if the patient can sit erect and lean slightly forward, or if the patient can be elevated almost to a sitting position.

With the intestinal tube in place, the patient is turned to an RAO position, a syringe is connected to the balloon lumen, and mercury is poured into the syringe and allowed to flow into the balloon. Air is slowly withdrawn from the balloon. The tube is secured with an adhesive strip beside the nostril to prevent regurgitation or advancement of the tube. The stomach is aspirated by using a syringe or by attaching the large position of the lumen to the suction apparatus.

With the tip of the tube situated close to the pyloric sphincter and the patient in the RAO position (a position in which gastric peristalsis is usually more active), the tube should pass into the duodenum in a reasonably short time. Without intervention, this process sometimes takes many hours. Having the patient drink ice water to stimulate peristalsis is often successful. When this measure fails, the examiner guides the tube into the duodenum by manual manipulation under fluoroscopic observation. After the tube enters the duodenum, it is inflated again to provide a bolus that peristaltic waves can more readily move along the intestine.

When the tube is inserted for decompression of an intestinal obstruction and possible later radiologic investigation, the adhesive strip is removed and replaced with an adhesive loop attached to the forehead. The tube can slide through the loop without tension as it advances toward the obstructed site. The patient is then returned to the hospital room. Radiographic images of the abdomen may be taken to check the progress of the tube and the effectiveness of decompression. Simple obstructions are sometimes relieved by suction; others require surgical intervention.

If passage of the intestinal tube is arrested, suction is discontinued, and the patient is returned to the radiology department for a Miller-Abbott tube study. The contrast medium used for studies of a localized segment of the small intestine may be a water-soluble, iodinated solution (Fig. 17-71, *A*) or a thin barium sulfate suspension. Under fluoroscopic observation, the contrast agent is injected through the large lumen of the tube with a syringe. Spot and conventional images are obtained as indicated.

When the intestinal tube is introduced for the purpose of performing a small intestine enema, the tube is advanced into the proximal loop of the jejunum and is secured at this level with an adhesive strip taped beside the nose. Medical opinion varies regarding the quantity of barium suspension required for this examination (Fig. 17-71, *B*). The medium is injected through the aspiration lumen of the tube in a continuous, low-pressure flow. Spot and conventional images are exposed as indicated. Except for the presence of the tube in the upper jejunum, resultant images resemble those obtained by the oral method.

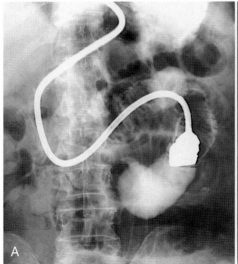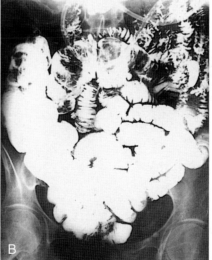

Fig. 17-71 A, Miller-Abbott tube study with water-soluble medium. **B,** Small bowel examination by Miller-Abbott tube with injection of barium sulfate.

CONTRAST MEDIA STUDIES

The two basic radiologic methods of examining the large intestine by means of contrast media enemas are (1) the *single-contrast* method (Fig. 17-72), in which the colon is examined with a barium sulfate suspension or water-soluble iodide only, and (2) the *double-contrast* method (Fig. 17-73), which may be performed as a two-stage or single-stage procedure. In the *two-stage, double-contrast procedure,* the colon is examined with a barium sulfate suspension and then, immediately after evacuation of the barium suspension, with an air enema or another gaseous enema. In the *single-stage, double-contrast procedure,* the fluoroscopist selectively injects the barium suspension and the gas.

Positive contrast medium shows the anatomy and tonus of the colon and most of the abnormalities to which it is subject. The gaseous medium serves to distend the lumen of the bowel and to render visible, through the transparency of its shadow, all parts of the barium-coated mucosal lining of the colon and any small intraluminal lesions, such as polypoid tumors.

A more recent development in radiographic examination of the large intestine is *computed tomography colonography* (CTC), also called *virtual colonoscopy* (VC)—a procedure used as a primary screening tool for colorectal cancer or after a failed conventional colonoscopy. This software-driven technique combines helical CT and virtual reality software to create three-dimensional and multiplanar images of the colonic mucosa. Examples of currently available CTC techniques include the perspective-filet or virtual dissection view, the three-dimensional topographic view, the multiplanar reformatted (MPR) view, and the colonoscopic-like endoluminal view (Figs. 17-74 to 17-76).

Contrast media

Commercially prepared barium sulfate products are generally used for routine retrograde examinations of the large intestine. Some of these products are referred to as *colloidal preparations* because they have finely divided barium particles that resist precipitation, whereas others are referred to as suspended or *flocculation-resistant preparations* because they contain some form of suspending or dispersing agent.

The newest barium products available are referred to as *high-density barium sulfate*. These products absorb a greater percentage of radiation, similar to older "thick" barium products. High-density barium is particularly useful for double-contrast studies of the alimentary canal in which uniform coating of the lumen is required.

Air is the gaseous medium usually used in the double-contrast enema study. The procedure is generally called an *air-contrast study*. Carbon dioxide may also be used because it is more rapidly absorbed than the nitrogen in air when evacuation of the gaseous medium is incomplete. Use of air as a contrast medium for radiographic evaluation of the colon is not limited to the double-contrast enema procedure. Air or carbon dioxide insufflation of the colon is used to perform CTC or VC.

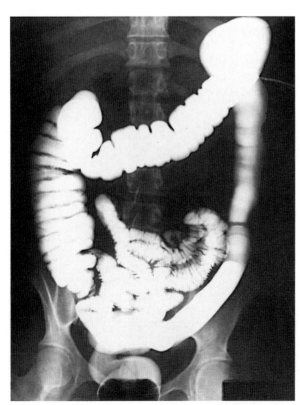

Fig. 17-72 Large intestine, single-contrast study.

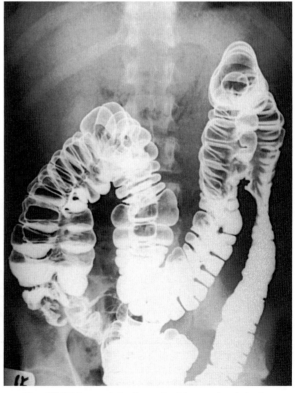

Fig. 17-73 Large intestine, double-contrast study.

Water-soluble, iodinated contrast media enemas are performed when colon perforation or leak is suspected. These iodinated contrast agents are administered orally to selected patients when retrograde filling of the colon with barium is impossible or is contraindicated. A disadvantage of iodinated solutions is that evacuation often is insufficient for satisfactory double-contrast visualization of the mucosal pattern. When a patient is unable to cooperate for a successful enema study, orally administered iodinated medium allows satisfactory examination of the colon. With these oral agents, transit time from ingestion to colonic filling is fast, averaging 3 to 4 hours. Iodinated solutions are practically nonabsorbable from the gastrointestinal mucosa. As a result, the oral dose reaches and outlines the entire large bowel. In contrast to an ingested barium sulfate suspension, this medium is not subject to drying, flaking, and unequal distribution in the colon. It frequently delineates the intestine almost as well as the BE does.

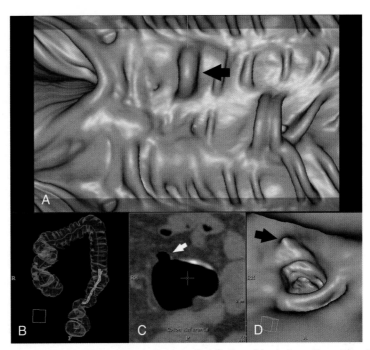

Fig. 17-74 Examples of CTC or VC. **A,** Perspective-filet or virtual dissection view, showing diverticulum (*arrow*). **B,** Three-dimensional topographic view: *Purple line* in the sigmoid shows length of filet in **A. C,** Axial MPR, showing same diverticulum as in **A** (*arrow*). **D,** Endoluminal view showing opening (*arrow*) of diverticulum from **A.**

(**D,** Courtesy J. Louis Rankin, BS, RT(R)(MR).)

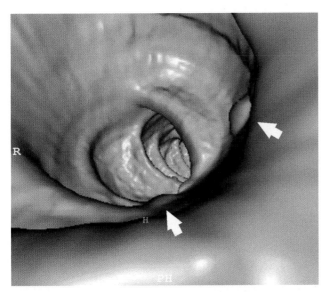

Fig. 17-75 Endoluminal CTC image, showing two tubular adenomas (*arrows*).

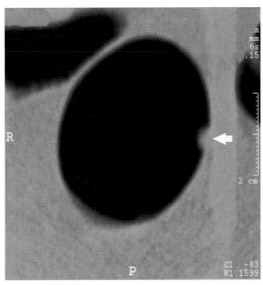

Fig. 17-76 Axial MPR image of upper tubular adenoma (*arrow*) from Fig. 17-75.

Preparation of intestinal tract

Medical opinion about preparation measures varies. Members of the medical profession usually agree, however, that the large intestine must be completely emptied of its contents to render all portions of its inner wall visible for inspection. When coated with a barium sulfate suspension, retained fecal masses are likely to simulate the appearance of polypoid or other small tumor masses (Fig. 17-77); this makes thorough cleansing of the entire colon a matter of prime importance. Preliminary preparation of the intestinal tract of patients who have a condition such as severe diarrhea, gross bleeding, or symptoms of obstruction is limited. Other patients are prepared, with modification as indicated, according to specifications established by the examining physician. The preliminary preparation usually includes dietary restrictions ("clear" liquids only) and a bowel cleansing regimen. Methods of bowel cleansing include the following:

- Complete intestinal tract cleansing kits
- Gastrointestinal lavage preparations
- Cleansing enema

Standard barium enema apparatus

Disposable soft plastic enema tips and enema bags are commercially available in different sizes. A soft rubber rectal catheter of small caliber should be used in patients who have inflamed hemorrhoids, fissures, a stricture, or other abnormalities of the anus.

Disposable rectal *retention tips* (Fig. 17-78) have replaced the older retention catheters, such as the Bardex or Foley catheter. The retention tip is a double-lumen tube with a thin balloon at its distal end. Because of the danger of intestinal wall damage, the retention tip must be inserted with extreme care. The enema retention tip is used in a patient who has a relaxed anal sphincter or another condition that makes it difficult or impossible to retain an enema. Some radiologists routinely use retention enema tips and inflate them if necessary.

The disposable rectal retention tip has a balloon cuff that fits snugly against the enema nozzle before inflation and after deflation so that it can be inserted and removed with little discomfort to the patient. A reusable squeeze inflator is rec-ommended to limit air capacity to approximately 90 mL. One complete squeeze of the inflator provides adequate distention of the retention balloon without danger of overinflation. Disposable retention tips are available for double-contrast and single-contrast enemas. For the safety of the patient, any retention balloon must be inflated with caution, using fluoroscopy, just before the examination.

For performance of a double-contrast BE examination, a special rectal tip is necessary to instill air in the colon (Fig. 17-79). Alternatively, air can simply be pumped into the colon using a sphygmomanometer bulb. Double-contrast retention tips are also available.

Most enema bags have a capacity of 3 qt (3000 mL) when completely filled and have graduated quantity markings on the side. A filter may be incorporated within the bag to prevent passage of any unmixed lumps of barium. The tubing is approximately 6 ft (1.8 m) long. Smaller enema bags (500 mL) with short, large-diameter tubing have been developed for double-contrast BE procedures.

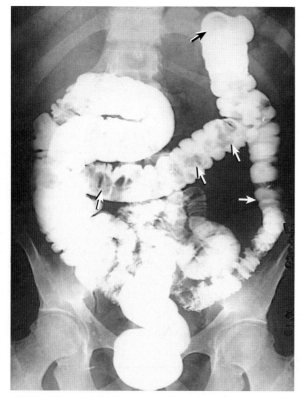

Fig. 17-77 Single-contrast, barium-filled colon, showing fecal material that simulates or masks pathologic condition (*arrows*).

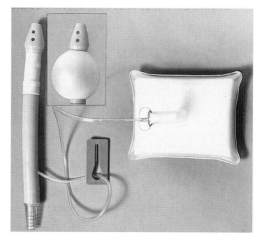

Fig. 17-78 Disposable retention enema tip. Uninflated balloon fits snugly. *Inset:* Balloon cuff inflated with 90 mL of air (one complete squeeze of inflator).

Preparation of barium suspensions

The concentration of barium sulfate suspensions used for single-contrast colonic enemas varies considerably. The often recommended range is 12% to 25% for weight/volume. For double-contrast examinations, a relatively high-density barium product is used. A 75% to 95% weight/volume ratio is common.

Commercial BE preparations are available as premixed liquids that can be poured into the disposable enema kit bag. Powdered barium is also available in single-contrast disposable kit bags. Water is added, and the solution is mixed by shaking the bag. Instructions for mixing a barium preparation vary according to the manufacturer and the type of barium used. The best recommendation is to follow the manufacturer's instructions precisely.

If warm BEs are administered, the temperature should be below body temperature—about 85° F to 90° F (29° C to 30° C). In addition to being unpleasant and debilitating, an enema that is too warm is injurious to intestinal tissues and produces so much irritation that it is difficult, if not impossible, for the patient to retain the enema long enough to permit a satisfactory examination.

Preparation and care of patient

In no radiologic examination is the full cooperation of the patient more essential to success than in the retrograde examination of the colon. Few patients who are physically able to retain the enema fail to do so when they understand the procedure and realize that in large measure the success of the examination depends on them. The radiographer should observe the following guidelines in preparing a patient for retrograde examination of the colon:

- Take time to explain the procedural differences between an ordinary cleansing enema and a diagnostic enema: (1) With the diagnostic enema, the fluoroscopist examines all portions of the bowel as it is being filled with contrast medium under fluoroscopic observation; (2) this part of the examination involves palpation of the abdomen, rotation of the body as required to visualize different segments of the colon, and taking of spot images without and, when indicated, with compression; (3) a series of large radiographic images are taken before the colon can be evacuated.
- Assure the patient that retention of the diagnostic enema preparation is comparatively easy because its flow is controlled under fluoroscopic observation.
- Instruct the patient to (1) keep the anal sphincter tightly contracted against the tubing to hold it in position and prevent leakage; (2) relax the abdominal muscles to prevent intra-abdominal pressure; and (3) concentrate on deep oral breathing to reduce the incidence of colonic spasm and resultant cramps.
- Assure the patient that the flow of the enema would be stopped for the duration of any cramping.

A patient who has not had a previous colonic examination is usually fearful of being embarrassed by inadequate draping and failure to retain the enema for the required time. The radiographer can dispel or greatly relieve the patient's anxiety by taking the following steps:

- Assure the patient that he or she will be properly covered.
- Assure the patient that although there is little chance of "mishap," he or she will be well protected, and there is no need to feel embarrassed should one occur.
- Keep a bedpan in the examining room for a patient who cannot or may not be able to make the trip to the toilet.

The preliminary preparation required for a retrograde study of the colon is strenuous for the patient. The examination itself further depletes the patient's strength. Feeble patients, particularly elderly patients, are likely to become weak and faint from the exertion of the preparation, the examination, and the effort made to expel the enema. The strenuous nature of these procedures presents an increased risk for patients with a history of heart disease. An emergency call button should be available in the lavatory so that the patient can summon help if necessary. Although the patient's privacy must be respected, the radiographer or an aide should frequently inquire to ensure that the patient is all right.

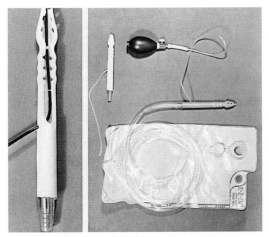

Fig. 17-79 Air-contrast enema tip shown with air tube filled with ink to show position.

Insertion of enema tip

In preparation for insertion of the enema tip, the following steps are taken:

- Instruct the patient to turn onto the left side, roll forward about 35 to 40 degrees, and rest the flexed right knee on the table, above and in front of the slightly flexed left knee (Sims position). This position relaxes the abdominal muscles, which decreases intra-abdominal pressure on the rectum and makes relaxation of the anal sphincter less difficult.
- Adjust the IV pole so that the enema contents are no higher than 24 inches (61 cm) above the level of the anus.
- Adjust the overlapping back of the gown or other draping to expose the anal region only, but keep the patient otherwise well covered. The anal orifice is commonly partially obscured by distended hemorrhoids or a fringe of undistended hemorrhoids. Sometimes there is a contraction or other abnormality of the orifice. It is necessary for the anus to be exposed and sufficiently well lighted for the orifice to be clearly visible, so that the enema tip can be inserted without injury or discomfort.

- Run a little of the barium mixture into a waste basin to free the tubing of air, and then lubricate the rectal tube well with a water-soluble lubricant.
- Advise the patient to relax and take deep breaths so that no discomfort is felt when the tube is inserted.
- Elevate the right buttock laterally to open the gluteal fold.
- As the abdominal muscles and anal sphincter are relaxed during the expiration phase of a deep breath, insert the rectal tube gently and slowly into the anal orifice. Following the angle of the anal canal, direct the tube anteriorly 1 to 1½ inches (2.5 to 3.8 cm). Then, while following the curve of the rectum, direct the tube slightly superiorly.
- Insert the tube for a total distance of no more than 4 inches (10 cm). Insertion for a greater distance not only is unnecessary but also may injure the rectum.
- If the tube cannot be entered easily, ask the patient to assist if he or she is capable.
- *Never* forcibly insert a rectal tube because the patient may have distended internal hemorrhoids or another condition that makes forced insertion of the tube dangerous.

- After the enema tip is inserted, hold it in position to prevent slipping while the patient turns to the supine or prone position for fluoroscopy, according to the preference of the fluoroscopist. The retention cuff may be inflated at this time.
- Adjust the protective underpadding and relieve any pressure on the tubing, so that the enema mixture flows freely.

SINGLE-CONTRAST BARIUM ENEMA

Administration of contrast medium

After preparing the patient for the examination, the radiographer observes the following steps:

- Notify the radiologist as soon as everything is ready for the examination.
- If the patient has not been introduced to the radiologist, make the introduction at this time.
- At the radiologist's request, release the control clip and ensure the enema flow.
- When occlusion of the enema tip occurs, displace soft fecal material by withdrawing the rectal tube about 1 inch (2.5 cm). Before reinserting the tip, temporarily elevate the enema bag to increase fluid pressure.

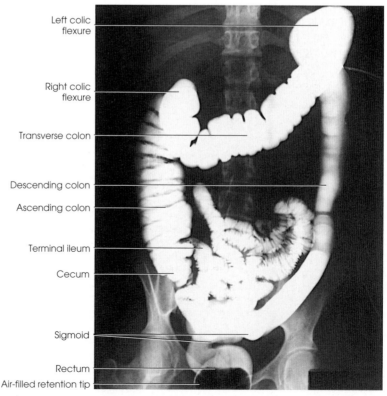

Left colic flexure
Right colic flexure
Transverse colon
Descending colon
Ascending colon
Terminal ileum
Cecum
Sigmoid
Rectum
Air-filled retention tip

Fig. 17-80 Single-contrast BE image, sthenic habitus.

The rectal ampulla fills slowly. Unless the barium flow is stopped for a few seconds after the rectal ampulla is full, the suspension flows through the sigmoid and descending portions of the colon at a fairly rapid rate, frequently causing a severe cramp and acute stimulation of the defecation impulse. The flow of the barium suspension is usually stopped for several seconds at frequent intervals during fluoroscopically controlled filling of the colon.

During the fluoroscopic procedure, the radiologist rotates the patient to inspect all segments of the bowel. The radiologist takes spot images as indicated and determines the positions to be used for subsequent radiographic studies. On completion of the fluoroscopic examination, the enema tip is usually removed so the patient can be maneuvered more easily, and so the tip is not accidentally displaced during the imaging procedure. A retention tube is not removed until the patient is placed on a bedpan or the toilet.

After the IRs have been exposed (Fig. 17-80), the patient is escorted to a toilet or placed on a bedpan and is instructed to expel as much of the barium suspension as possible. A postevacuation image is then taken (Fig. 17-81). If this image shows evacuation to be inadequate for satisfactory delineation of the mucosa, the patient may be given a hot beverage (tea or coffee) to stimulate further evacuation.

Positioning of opacified colon

The most commonly obtained projections for single-contrast BE are PA or AP and PA obliques, axial for the sigmoid, and lateral to show the rectum.

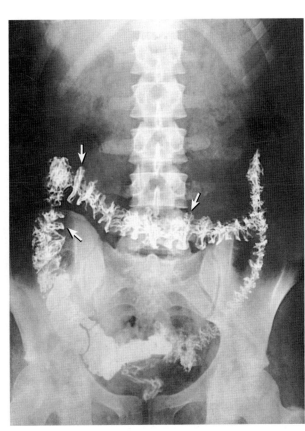

Fig. 17-81 Postevacuation image showing mucosal pattern (*arrows*). Hyposthenic habitus.

DOUBLE-CONTRAST BARIUM ENEMA

Two approaches to administering double-contrast BEs are currently in use. The first technique is a *two-stage procedure,* described by Welin,[1] in which the entire colon is filled with a barium suspension. After administration of the enema, the patient evacuates the barium and immediately returns to the fluoroscopic table, where air or another gaseous medium is injected into the colon. The second approach is the *single-stage, double-contrast examination.* The popularity of this approach can be attributed primarily to more recent advancements in the manufacture of high-density barium sulfate.

Single-stage procedure

In performing the single-stage, double-contrast enema, certain requirements must be met to ensure an adequate examination. The most important requirement is that the patient's colon must be exceptionally clean. Residual fecal material can obscure

small polyps or tumor masses. A second requirement is that a suitable barium suspension must be used. A barium mixture that clumps or flakes neither clearly shows the lumen nor properly drains from the colon.

Currently available, premixed liquid barium products are generally more uniform for radiographic use than most barium suspensions mixed in the health care institution. A barium product with a density of 200% weight/volume may be used for a single-stage, double-contrast examination of the colon. The most important criterion is that the barium flows sufficiently to coat the walls of the colon.

With advances in the manufacture of high-density barium, high-quality double-contrast colon images can be consistently obtained during one filling of the colon. In the single-stage procedure, barium and air are instilled in a single procedure. Miller[1] described a *7-pump* method for performing single-stage, double-contrast examinations. This method reduces cost, saves

time, and reduces radiation exposure to the patient. (A more complete description of the 7-pump method is provided in the seventh edition or earlier editions of this atlas.)

Fluoroscopy is performed to check the location of the barium, and additional air is instilled under fluoroscopic control. The patient is slowly rotated 360 degrees and is placed in the supine position. Spot images and overhead radiographic images are then taken (Figs. 17-82 and 17-83).

In addition to the 7-pump method, a single-stage, double-contrast examination can be performed using a technique that does not employ a special air-contrast enema tip. With this technique, barium and air are instilled through the closed enema bag system (Fig. 17-84).

[1]Welin S: Modern trends in diagnostic roentgenology of the colon, *Br J Radiol* 31:453, 1958.

[1]Miller RE: Barium pneumocolon: technologist-performed "7-pump" method, *AJR Am J Roentgenol* 139:1230, 1982.

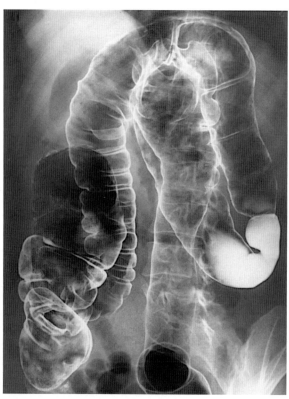

Fig. 17-82 AP oblique colon, RPO position, double-contrast study.

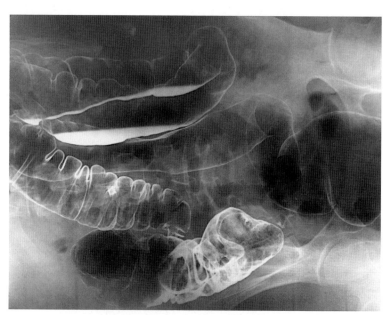

Fig. 17-83 AP colon, right lateral decubitus position.

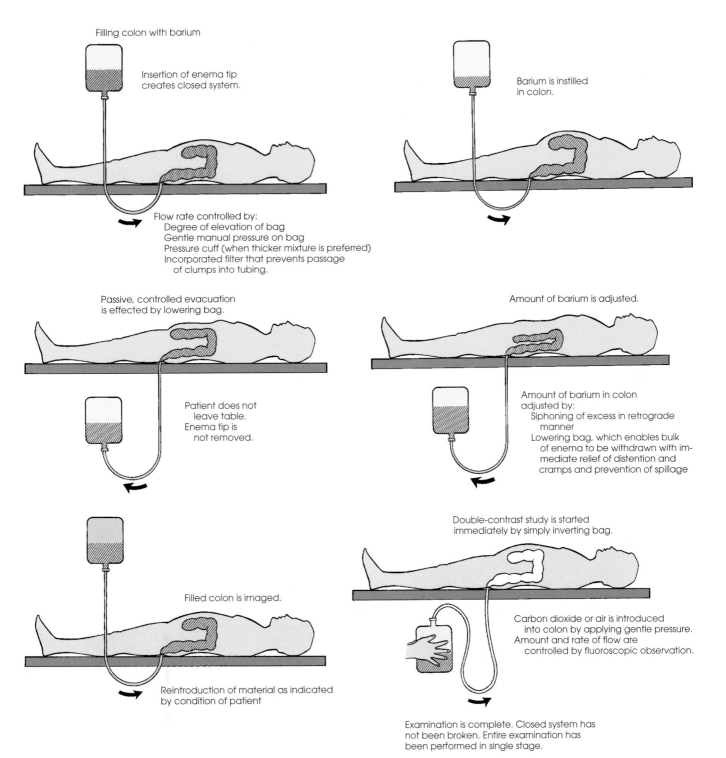

Filling colon with barium

Insertion of enema tip creates closed system.

Flow rate controlled by:
  Degree of elevation of bag
  Gentle manual pressure on bag
  Pressure cuff (when thicker mixture is preferred)
  Incorporated filter that prevents passage
    of clumps into tubing.

Passive, controlled evacuation is effected by lowering bag.

Patient does not leave table. Enema tip is not removed.

Filled colon is imaged.

Reintroduction of material as indicated by condition of patient

Barium is instilled in colon.

Amount of barium is adjusted.

Amount of barium in colon adjusted by:
  Siphoning of excess in retrograde manner
  Lowering bag, which enables bulk of enema to be withdrawn with immediate relief of distention and cramps and prevention of spillage

Double-contrast study is started immediately by simply inverting bag.

Carbon dioxide or air is introduced into colon by applying gentle pressure. Amount and rate of flow are controlled by fluoroscopic observation.

Examination is complete. Closed system has not been broken. Entire examination has been performed in single stage.

Fig. 17-84 Conduction of single-stage, closed-system, double-contrast examination.

(From Pochaczevsky R, Sherman RS: A new technique for roentgenologic examination of the colon, *AJR Am J Roentgenol* 89:787, 1963.)

Welin method

Welin[1,2] developed a technique for double-contrast enema that reveals even the smallest intraluminal lesions (Figs. 17-85 and 17-86). He stated that this method of examination is extremely valuable in the early diagnosis of conditions such as ulcerative colitis, regional colitis, and polyps.

Welin stressed the importance of preparing the intestine for the examination, stating that (1) the colon must be cleansed as thoroughly as possible, and (2) the colonic mucosa must be prepared in such a way that an extremely thin, even coating of barium can adhere to the colonic wall. He recommended regulation of evacuation so that the two stages of the examination can be carried out at short intervals to avoid unnecessary waiting time, and the patient does not have to be in the examining room for longer than 20 to 25 minutes.

[1]Welin S: Modern trends in diagnostic roentgenology of the colon, *Br J Radiol* 31:453, 1958.
[2]Welin S: Results of the Malmo technique of colon examination, *JAMA* 199:369, 1967.

Stage 1. With the patient in the prone position to prevent possible ileal leak, the colon is filled to the left colic flexure, after which a conventional radiographic image is taken (i.e., a right lateral projection of the barium-filled rectum). The patient is sent to the lavatory to evacuate the barium. Afterward, if the patient feels the need to do so, he or she is allowed to lie down and rest.

Stage 2. When the patient returns to the examining table, the enema tip is inserted, and the patient is again turned to the prone position. The prone position not only prevents ileal leakage with resultant opacification and overlap of the small intestine on the rectosigmoid area, it also aids in providing adequate drainage of excess barium from the rectum.

The radiologist allows the barium mixture to run up to the middle of the sigmoid colon (slightly farther if the sigmoid is long). The patient is turned onto the right side, and air is instilled through the enema tip. The air forces the barium along, distributing it throughout the colon, and the patient is turned as required for even coating of the entire colon. Spot images are made as indicated. If barium flows back into the rectum, it is drained out through the enema tip. More air is then instilled. Welin stressed the importance of instilling enough air ($\approx$1800 to 2000 cc) to obtain proper distention of the colon.

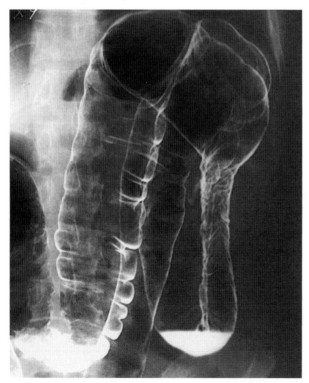

Fig. 17-85 Upright oblique position of flexure after implementation of Welin method.

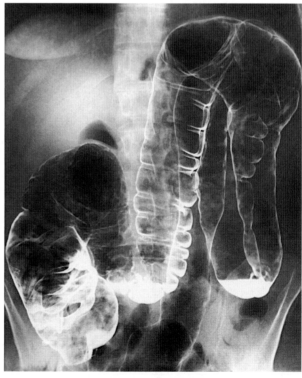

Fig. 17-86 Upright PA colon after implementation of Welin method.

When sufficient distention of the colon has been obtained, 14 × 17-inch (35 × 43-cm) images are obtained (Fig. 17-87) to include the rectum, using the following sequence: PA projection, PA oblique (LAO and RAO) projections, and right lateral projection 10 × 12 inches (24 × 30 cm). The patient is then turned to the supine position for an AP projection and two AP oblique (LPO and RPO) projec- tions, all to include the transverse colon and its flexures. These studies are fol- lowed by AP projections in the right and left lateral decubitus positions to include the rectum. Finally, the patient is placed in the erect position for PA and PA oblique (RAO and LAO) projections of the hori- zontal colon and the left and right colic flexures.

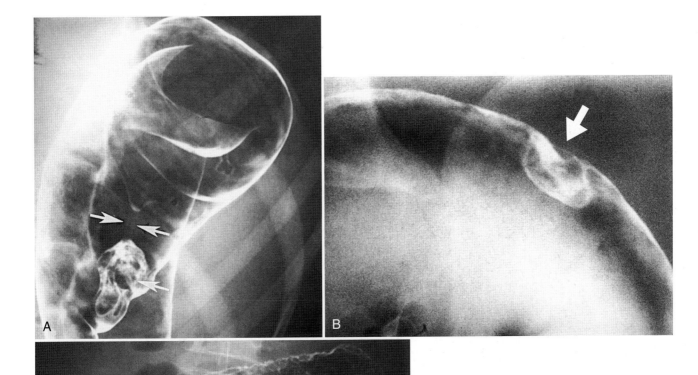

Fig. 17-87 A, Pedunculated polyps (*arrows*) during stage 2 of Welin method. **B,** Small carcinoma with intubation (*arrow*) during stage 2 of Welin method. **C,** Cobblestone appearance of granulomatous colitis in image obtained during stage 2 of Welin method.

OPACIFIED COLON

Radiographic studies of the adult colon are made on 14 × 17-inch (35 × 43-cm) IRs. Except for axial projections, these IRs may be centered at the level of the iliac crests on patients of sthenic build—higher for hypersthenic patients and lower for asthenic patients. AP and PA projections of the colon and abdomen may require two exposures, with the IRs placed crosswise: The first is centered high enough to include the diaphragm, and the second is centered low enough to include the rectum. Localized studies of the rectum and rectosigmoid junction are often exposed on 10 × 12-inch (24 × 30-cm) IRs centered at or slightly above the level of the pubic symphysis. Preevacuation images of the colon include one or more images to show otherwise obscured flexed and curved areas of the large intestine.

Depending on the preference of the radiologist, the radiographic projections taken after fluoroscopy vary considerably. Any combination of the following images may be taken to complete the examination.

⚹ PA PROJECTION

Image receptor: 14 × 17 inch (35 × 43 cm) lengthwise

Position of patient
- Place the patient in the prone position.

Position of part
- Center the midsagittal plane to the grid.
- Adjust the center of the IR at the level of the iliac crests (Fig. 17-88).
- In addition to positioning for the PA projection, place the fluoroscopic table in a slight Trendelenburg position if necessary. This table position helps separate redundant and overlapping loops of the bowel by "spilling" them out of the pelvis.
- *Shield gonads.*
- *Respiration:* Suspend.

Central ray
- Perpendicular to the IR to enter the midline of the body at the level of the iliac crests

Collimation
- Adjust to 14 × 17 inches (35 × 43 cm) on the collimator.

Structures shown
The PA projection shows the entire colon with the patient prone (Figs. 17-89 to 17-91).

EVALUATION CRITERIA
The following should be clearly shown:
- ■ Evidence of proper collimation
- ■ Entire colon including the flexures and the rectum (two IRs may be necessary for hypersthenic patients)
- ■ Vertebral column centered so that ascending and descending portions of the colon are included
- ■ Exposure technique that shows the anatomy

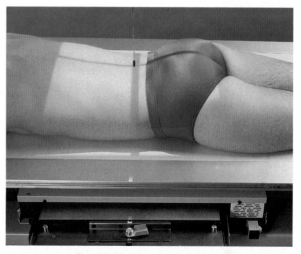

Fig. 17-88 PA large intestine.

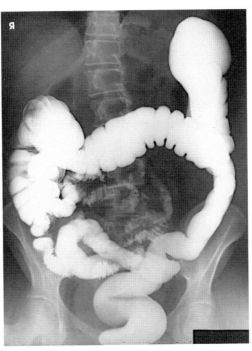

Fig. 17-89 Single-contrast PA large intestine.

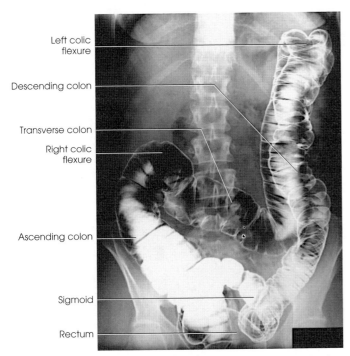

Left colic flexure

Descending colon

Transverse colon

Right colic flexure

Ascending colon

Sigmoid

Rectum

Fig. 17-90 Double-contrast PA large intestine, hyposthenic body habitus.

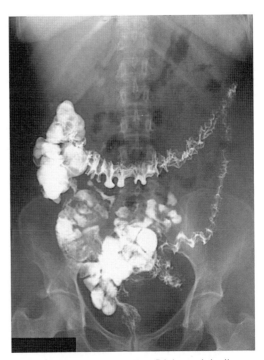

Fig. 17-91 Postevacuation PA large intestine.

🔥 PA AXIAL PROJECTION

Image receptor: 14 × 17 inch (35 × 43 cm) or 10 × 12 inch (24 × 30 cm) lengthwise

Position of patient

- Place the patient in the prone position.

Position of part

- Center the midsagittal plane to the grid.
- Adjust the center of the IR at the level of the iliac crests (Fig. 17-92).
- *Shield gonads.*
- *Respiration:* Suspend.

Central ray

- Directed 30 to 40 degrees caudad to enter the midline of the body at the level of the anterior superior iliac spine (ASIS)

Collimation

- Adjust to 14 × 17 inches (35 × 43 cm) or 10 × 12 inches (24 × 30) on the collimator.

Structures shown

The PA axial projection best shows the rectosigmoid area of the colon (Figs. 17-93 and 17-94).

NOTE: This axial projection is sometimes performed with the patient in the RAO position, to further reduce superimposition in the rectosigmoid area.

The following should be clearly shown:

- Evidence of proper collimation
- Rectosigmoid area centered to image when a 10 × 12-inch (24 × 30-cm) IR is used
- Rectosigmoid area with less superimposition than in PA projection because of angulation of the central ray
- Transverse colon and both flexures not always included
- Exposure technique that shows the anatomy

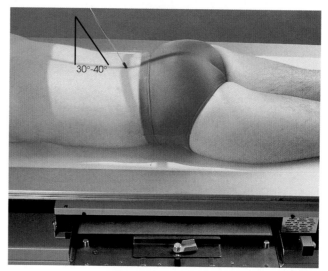

Fig. 17-92 PA axial large intestine.

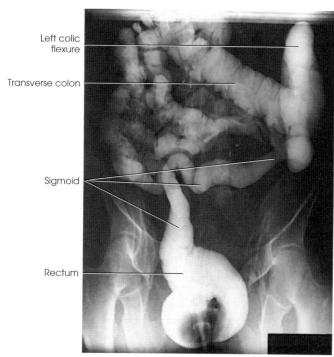

Left colic flexure

Transverse colon

Sigmoid

Rectum

Fig. 17-93 Single-contrast PA axial (30-degree angulation) large intestine.

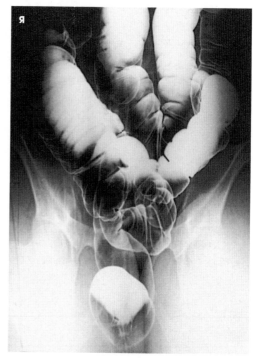

Fig. 17-94 Double-contrast PA axial (40-degree angulation) large intestine.

Digestive System

⚓ PA OBLIQUE PROJECTION
RAO position

Image receptor: 14 × 17 inch (35 × 43 cm) lengthwise

Position of patient
- Place the patient in the prone position.

Position of part
- With the patient's right arm by the side of the body and the left hand by the head, have the patient roll onto the right hip to obtain a 35- to 45-degree rotation from the radiographic table.
- Flex the patient's left knee to provide stability.
- Center the patient's body to the midline of the grid.
- Adjust the center of the IR at the level of the iliac crests (Fig. 17-95).
- *Shield gonads.*
- *Respiration:* Suspend.

Central ray
- Perpendicular to the IR and entering approximately 1 to 2 inches (2.5 to 5 cm) lateral to the midline of the body on the elevated side at the level of the iliac crest

Collimation
- Adjust to 14 × 17 inches (35 × 43 cm) on the collimator.

Structures shown
The RAO position best shows the right colic flexure, the ascending portion of the colon, and the sigmoid portion of the colon (Figs. 17-96 and 17-97).

The following should be clearly shown:
- Evidence of proper collimation
- Entire colon
- Right colic flexure less superimposed or open compared with the PA projection
- Ascending colon, cecum, and sigmoid colon
- Exposure technique that shows the anatomy

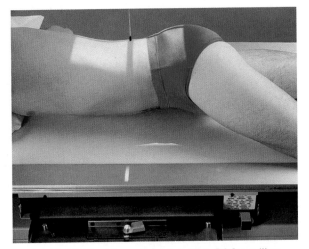

Fig. 17-95 PA oblique large intestine, RAO position.

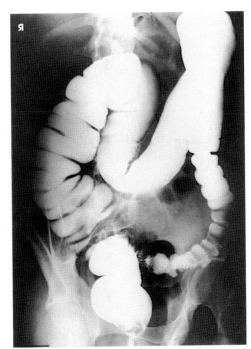

Fig. 17-96 Single-contrast PA oblique large intestine, RAO position.

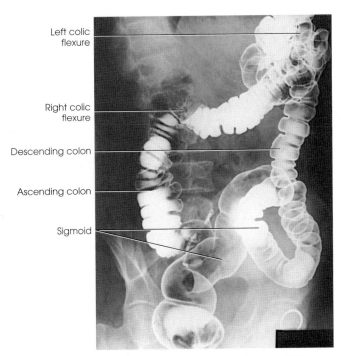

Left colic flexure

Right colic flexure

Descending colon

Ascending colon

Sigmoid

Fig. 17-97 Double-contrast PA oblique large intestine, RAO position.

♠ PA OBLIQUE PROJECTION
LAO position

Image receptor: 14 × 17 inch (35 × 43 cm) lengthwise

Position of patient
- Place the patient in the prone position.

Position of part
- With the patient's left arm by the side of the body and the right hand by the head, have the patient roll onto the left hip to obtain a 35- to 45-degree rotation from the radiographic table.
- Flex the patient's right knee to provide stability.
- Center the patient's body to the midline of the grid.
- Adjust the center of the IR at the level of the iliac crest (Fig. 17-98).
- *Shield gonads.*
- *Respiration:* Suspend.

Central ray
- Perpendicular to the IR and entering approximately 1 to 2 inches (2.5 to 5 cm) lateral to the midline of the body on the elevated side at the level of the iliac crest

Collimation
- Adjust to 14 × 17 inches (35 × 43 cm) on the collimator.

Structures shown
The LAO position best shows the left colic flexure and the descending portion of the colon (Figs. 17-99 and 17-100).

The following should be clearly shown:
- ■ Evidence of proper collimation
- ■ Entire colon
- ■ Left colic flexure less superimposed or open compared with the PA projection
- ■ Descending colon
- ■ Exposure technique that shows the anatomy

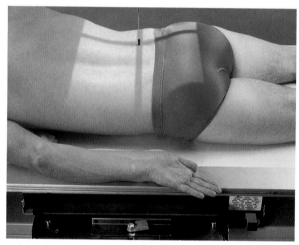

Fig. 17-98 PA oblique large intestine, LAO position.

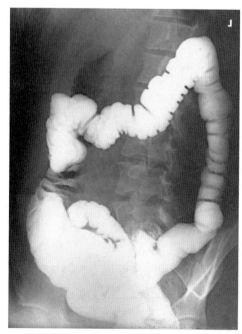

Fig. 17-99 Single-contrast PA oblique large intestine, LAO position.

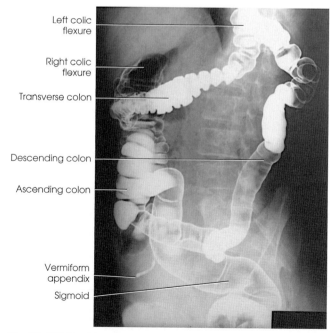

Left colic flexure

Right colic flexure

Transverse colon

Descending colon

Ascending colon

Vermiform appendix

Sigmoid

Fig. 17-100 Double-contrast PA oblique large intestine, LAO position.

Digestive System

♠ LATERAL PROJECTION
R or L position

Image receptor: 10 × 12 inch (24 × 30 cm) lengthwise

Position of patient
- Place the patient in the lateral recumbent position on the left or the right side.

Position of part
- Center the midcoronal plane to the center of the grid.
- Flex the patient's knees slightly for stability, and place a support between the knees to keep the pelvis lateral.
- Adjust the patient's shoulders and hips to be perpendicular (Fig. 17-101).
- Adjust the center of the IR to the ASIS.
- *Shield gonads.*
- *Respiration:* Suspend.

Central ray
- Perpendicular to the IR to enter the midcoronal plane at the level of the ASIS

Collimation
- Adjust to 10 × 12 inches (24 × 30 cm) on the collimator.

Structures shown
The lateral projection best shows the rectum and the distal sigmoid portion of the colon (Figs. 17-102 and 17-103).

The following should be clearly shown:
- Evidence of proper collimation
- Rectosigmoid area in the center of the image
- No rotation of the patient
- Superimposed hips and femora
- Superior portion of colon not included when the rectosigmoid region is the area of interest
- Exposure technique that shows the anatomy

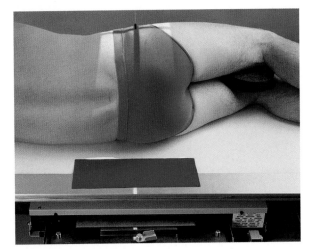

Fig. 17-101 Left lateral rectum.

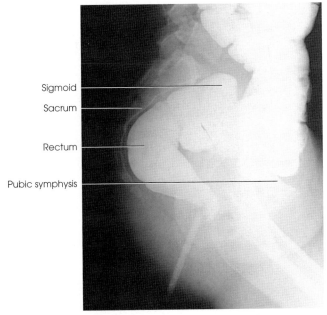

Sigmoid

Sacrum

Rectum

Pubic symphysis

Fig. 17-102 Single-contrast left lateral rectum.

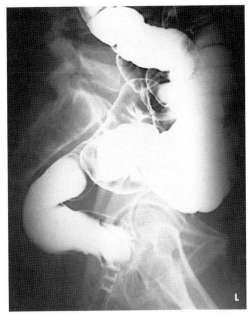

Fig. 17-103 Double-contrast left lateral rectum.

Large Intestine

🔥 AP PROJECTION

Image receptor: 14 × 17 inch (35 × 43 cm) lengthwise

Position of patient
- Place the patient in the supine position.

Position of part
- Center the midsagittal plane to the grid.
- Adjust the center of the IR at the level of the iliac crests (Fig. 17-104).
- *Shield gonads.*
- *Respiration:* Suspend.

Central ray
- Perpendicular to the IR to enter the midline of the body at the level of the iliac crests

Collimation
- Adjust to 14 × 17 inches (35 × 43 cm) on the collimator

Structures shown
AP projection shows the entire colon with the patient supine (Figs. 17-105 and 17-106).

The following should be clearly shown:
- Evidence of proper collimation
- Entire colon including the splenic flexure and the rectum (two IRs may be necessary for hypersthenic patients)
- Vertebral column centered so that the ascending colon and the descending colon are completely included
- Exposure technique that shows the anatomy

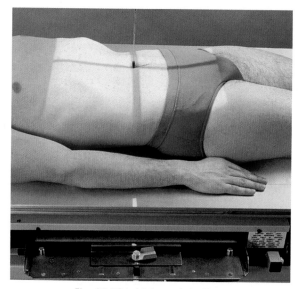

Fig. 17-104 AP large intestine.

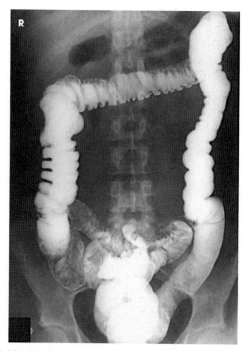

Fig. 17-105 Single-contrast AP large intestine, sthenic habitus.

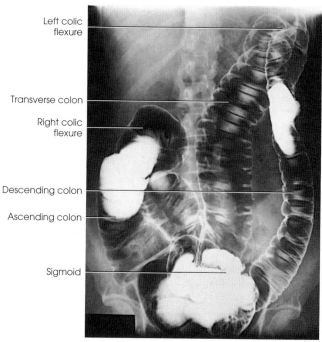

Left colic flexure

Transverse colon

Right colic flexure

Descending colon

Ascending colon

Sigmoid

Fig. 17-106 Double-contrast AP large intestine, asthenic habitus.

Digestive System

✸ AP AXIAL PROJECTION

Image receptor: 14 × 17 inch (35 × 43 cm) or 10 × 12 inch (24 × 30 cm) lengthwise

Position of patient
• Place the patient in the supine position.

Position of part
• Center the midsagittal plane to the grid.
• Adjust the center of the IR at a level approximately 2 inches (5 cm) above the level of the iliac crests (Fig. 17-107).
• *Shield gonads.*
• *Respiration:* Suspend.

Central ray
• Directed 30 to 40 degrees cephalad to enter the midline of the body approximately 2 inches (5 cm) below the level of the ASIS
• Directed to enter the inferior margin of the pubic symphysis when a collimated image is desired to show the rectosigmoid region

Collimation
• Adjust to 14 × 17 inches (35 × 43 cm) or 10 × 12 inches (24 × 30 cm) on the collimator

Structures shown
The AP axial projection best shows the rectosigmoid area of the colon (Figs. 17-108 and 17-109). A similar image is obtained when the patient is prone (see Fig. 17-92).

NOTE: This axial projection is sometimes performed with the patient in the LPO position, to further reduce superimposition in the rectosigmoid area.

The following should be clearly shown:
■ Evidence of proper collimation
■ Rectosigmoid area centered when a 10 × 12-inch (24 × 30-cm) IR is used
■ Rectosigmoid area with less superimposition than in the AP projection because of the angulation of the central ray
■ Transverse colon and flexures not included
■ Exposure technique that shows the anatomy

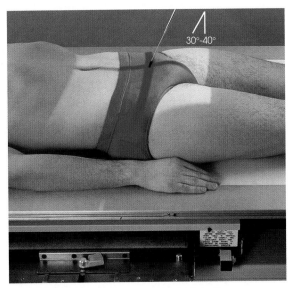

Fig. 17-107 AP axial large intestine.

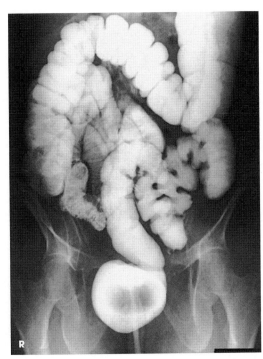

Fig. 17-108 Single-contrast AP axial large intestine.

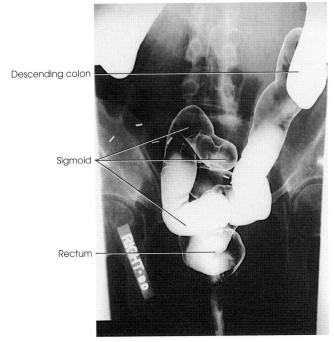

Descending colon

Sigmoid

Rectum

Fig. 17-109 Double-contrast AP axial large intestine.

♠ AP OBLIQUE PROJECTION
LPO position

Image receptor: 14 × 17 inch (35 × 43 cm) lengthwise

Position of patient
- Place the patient in the supine position.

Position of part
- With the patient's left arm by the side of the body and the right arm across the superior chest, have the patient roll onto the left hip to obtain a 35- to 45-degree rotation from the table.
- Use a positioning sponge and flex the patient's right knee for stability, if necessary.
- Center the patient's body to the midline of the grid.
- Adjust the center of the IR at the level of the iliac crests (Fig. 17-110).
- *Shield gonads.*
- *Respiration:* Suspend.

Central ray
- Perpendicular to the IR to enter approximately 1 to 2 inches (2.5 to 5 cm) lateral to the midline of the body on the elevated side at the level of the iliac crest

Collimation
- Adjust to 14 × 17 inches (35 × 43 cm) on the collimator

Structures shown
The LPO position best shows the right colic flexure and the ascending and sigmoid portions of the colon (Figs. 17-111 and 17-112).

The following should be clearly shown:
- Evidence of proper collimation
- Entire colon
- Right colic flexure less superimposed or open compared with the AP projection
- Ascending colon, cecum, and sigmoid colon
- Exposure technique that shows the anatomy

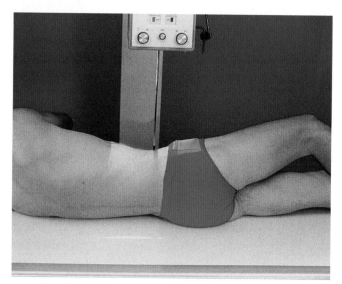

Fig. 17-110 AP oblique large intestine, LPO position.

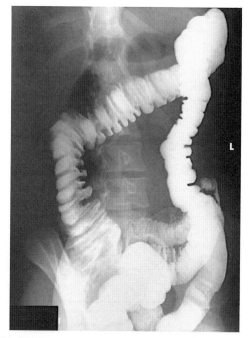

Fig. 17-111 Single-contrast AP oblique large intestine, LPO position.

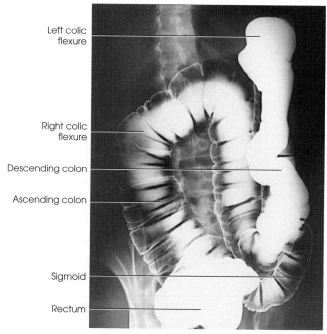

Left colic flexure
Right colic flexure
Descending colon
Ascending colon
Sigmoid
Rectum

Fig. 17-112 Double-contrast AP oblique large intestine, LPO position.

▲ AP OBLIQUE PROJECTION
RPO position

Image receptor: 14 × 17 inch (35 × 43 cm) lengthwise

Position of patient
• Place the patient in the supine position.

Position of part
• With the patient's right arm by the side of the body and the left arm across the superior chest, have the patient roll onto the right hip to obtain a 35- to 45-degree rotation from the radiographic table.
• Use a positioning sponge and flex the patient's right knee for stability, if needed.
• Center the patient's body to the midline of the grid.
• Adjust the center of the IR at the level of the iliac crests (Fig. 17-113).
• *Shield gonads.*
• *Respiration:* Suspend.

Central ray
• Perpendicular to the IR to enter approximately 1 to 2 inches (2.5 to 5 cm) lateral to the midline of the body on the elevated side at the level of the iliac crest

Collimation
• Adjust to 14 × 17 inches (35 × 43 cm) on the collimator

Structures shown
RPO position best shows the left colic flexure and the descending colon (Figs. 17-114 and 17-115).

The following should be clearly shown:
■ Evidence of proper collimation
■ Entire colon
■ Left colic flexure and descending colon
■ Exposure technique that shows the anatomy

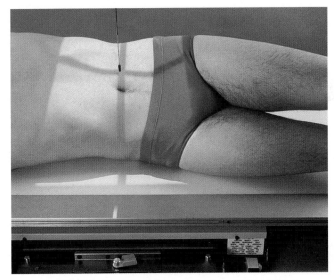

Fig. 17-113 AP oblique large intestine, RPO position.

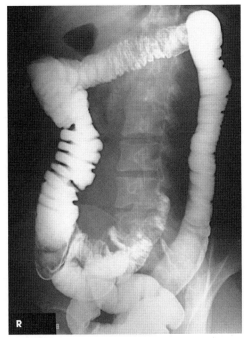

Fig. 17-114 Single-contrast AP oblique large intestine, RPO position.

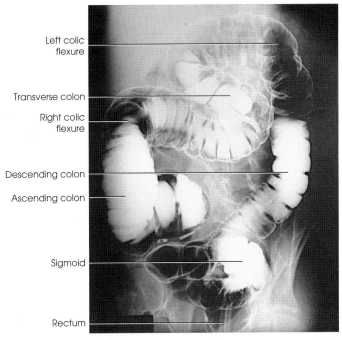

Left colic flexure
Transverse colon
Right colic flexure
Descending colon
Ascending colon
Sigmoid
Rectum

Fig. 17-115 Double-contrast AP oblique large intestine, RPO position.

Decubitus Positions

When a patient is being prepared for an examination in a decubitus position, the following general guidelines are observed:

- Take all decubitus images (1) with the patient lying on the fluoroscopic table and a grid IR firmly supported behind the patient's body; (2) with the patient lying on a patient cart with the body against an upright table or chest device; or (3) with the patient lying on a table or cart and a specially designed vertical grid device behind the patient.

- To ensure that the side on which the patient is lying is shown, elevate the patient on a suitable radiolucent support. If this is not done, the image records artifacts from the mattress or from the table edge and superimposes these images over the portion of the patient's colon on the "down" side.

- For all decubitus procedures, *exercise extreme caution* to ensure that the *wheels of the cart are securely locked* so that the patient will not fall.

- For lateral decubitus images, have the patient put the back or abdomen against the vertical grid device. Most patients find it more comfortable to have their back against the vertical grid device than to have their abdomen against the same device.

- If both lateral decubitus images are requested (which is often the case with air-contrast examinations), take one image with the patient's anterior body surface against the vertical grid device and the second image with the posterior body surface against the vertical grid device.

⚘ AP OR PA PROJECTION
Right lateral decubitus position

Image receptor: 14 × 17 inch (35 × 43 cm) lengthwise

Position of patient
- Place the patient on the right side with the back or abdomen in contact with the vertical grid device.
- *Exercise care* to ensure that the patient does not fall from the cart or table; if a cart is used, *lock all wheels* securely.

Position of part
- With the patient lying on an elevated radiolucent support, center the midsagittal plane to the grid.
- Adjust the center of the IR to the level of the iliac crests (Fig. 17-116).
- *Shield gonads.*
- *Respiration:* Suspend.

Central ray
- *Horizontal* and perpendicular to the IR to enter the midline of the body at the level of the iliac crests

Collimation
- Adjust to 14 × 17 inches (35 × 43 cm) on the collimator.

Structures shown
The right lateral decubitus position shows an AP or PA projection of the contrast-filled colon. This position best shows the "up" medial side of the ascending colon and the lateral side of the descending colon when the colon is inflated with air (Figs. 17-117 and 17-118).

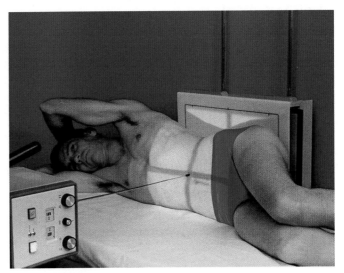

Fig. 17-116 AP large intestine, right lateral decubitus position.

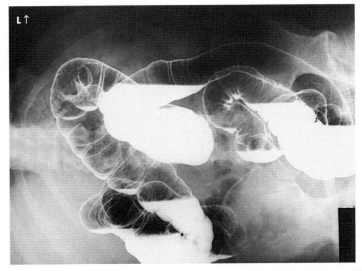

Fig. 17-117 Double-contrast AP large intestine, right lateral decubitus position.

EVALUATION CRITERIA
The following should be clearly shown:
- Evidence of proper collimation
- Area from the left colic flexure to the rectum
- No rotation of the patient, as demonstrated by symmetry of the ribs and pelvis
- For single-contrast examinations, adequate penetration of the barium; for double-contrast examinations, the air-inflated portion of the colon is of primary importance and should not be overpenetrated

◥ COMPENSATING FILTER
Image quality can be improved on larger patients with the use of a special decubitus filter.

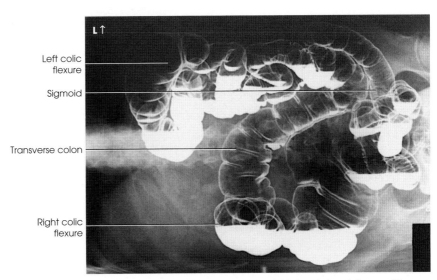

Fig. 17-118 Double-contrast AP large intestine, right lateral decubitus position.

Left colic flexure
Sigmoid
Transverse colon
Right colic flexure

⚹ PA OR AP PROJECTION
Left lateral decubitus position

Image receptor: 14 × 17 inch (35 × 43 cm) lengthwise

Position of patient
- Place the patient on the left side with the abdomen or back in contact with the vertical grid device.
- *Exercise care* to ensure that the patient does not fall from the cart or table; if a cart is used, *lock all wheels* securely in position.

Position of part
- With the patient lying on an elevated radiolucent support, center the midsagittal plane to the grid.
- Adjust the center of the IR at the level of the iliac crests (Fig. 17-119).
- *Shield gonads.*
- *Respiration:* Suspend.

Central ray
- *Horizontal* and perpendicular to the IR to enter the midline of the body at the level of the iliac crests

Collimation
- Adjust to 14 × 17 inches (35 × 43 cm) on the collimator.

Structures shown
The left lateral decubitus position shows a PA or AP projection of the contrast-filled colon. This position best shows the "up" lateral side of the ascending colon and the medial side of the descending colon when the colon is inflated with air (Figs. 17-120 and 17-121).

EVALUATION CRITERIA
The following should be clearly shown:
- Evidence of proper collimation
- Area from the left colic flexure to the rectum
- No rotation of the patient, as demonstrated by symmetry of the ribs and pelvis
- For single-contrast examinations, adequate penetration of the barium; for double-contrast examinations, the air-inflated portion of the colon is of primary importance and should not be overpenetrated

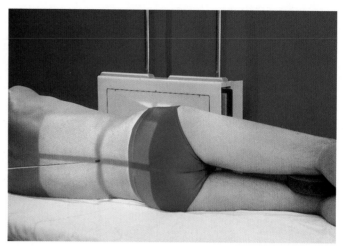

Fig. 17-119 PA large intestine, left lateral decubitus position.

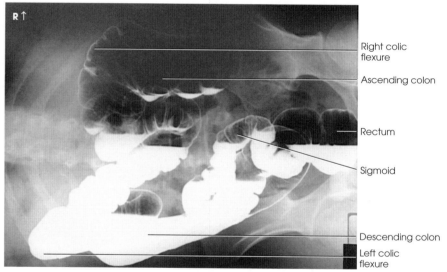

Right colic flexure

Ascending colon

Rectum

Sigmoid

Descending colon

Left colic flexure

Fig. 17-120 Double-contrast PA large intestine, left lateral decubitus position.

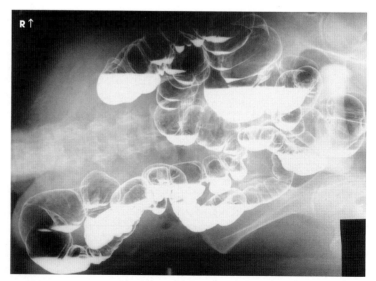

Fig. 17-121 Double-contrast PA large intestine, left lateral decubitus position.

LATERAL PROJECTION
R or L ventral decubitus position

Image receptor: 14 × 17 inch (35 × 43 cm) lengthwise

Position of patient
- Place the patient in the prone position with the right side or the left side against the vertical grid device.

Position of part
- Elevate the patient on a radiolucent support, and center the midcoronal plane to the grid.
- Adjust the center of the IR at the level of the iliac crests.
- *Shield gonads.*
- *Respiration:* Suspend.

Central ray
- *Horizontal* and perpendicular to the IR to enter the midcoronal plane of the body at the level of the iliac crests

Collimation
- Adjust to 14 × 17 inches (35 × 43 cm) on the collimator.

Structures shown
The ventral decubitus position shows a lateral projection of the contrast-filled colon. This position best shows the "up" posterior portions of the colon and is most valuable in double-contrast examinations (Fig. 17-122).

The following should be clearly shown:
- Evidence of proper collimation
- Area from the flexures to the rectum
- No rotation of the patient
- For single-contrast examinations, adequate penetration of the barium; for double-contrast examinations, the air-inflated portion of the colon is of primary importance and should not be overpenetrated
- Enema tip removed for an unobstructed image of the rectum

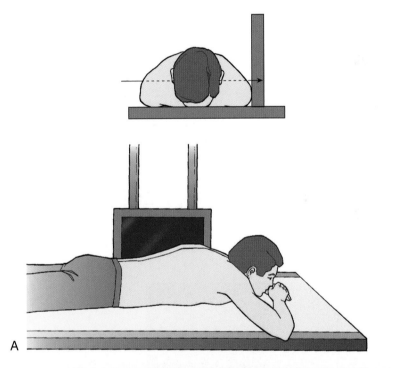

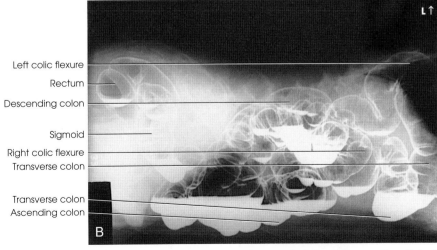

Fig. 17-122 A, Patient in position for lateral projection, ventral decubitus position. **B,** Left lateral large intestine, ventral decubitus position.

✦ AP, PA, OBLIQUE, AND LATERAL PROJECTIONS
Upright position

Upright AP, PA, oblique, and lateral projections may be taken as requested. The positioning and evaluation criteria for upright images are identical to criteria required for the recumbent positions. The IR is placed at a lower level, however, to compensate for the drop of the bowel caused by the effect of gravity (Figs. 17-123 to 17-125).

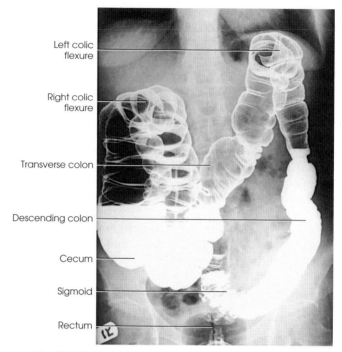

Left colic flexure

Right colic flexure

Transverse colon

Descending colon

Cecum

Sigmoid

Rectum

Fig. 17-123 Upright double-contrast AP large intestine.

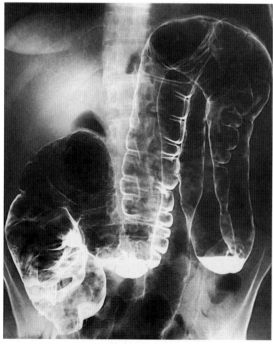

Fig. 17-124 Upright double-contrast PA large intestine.

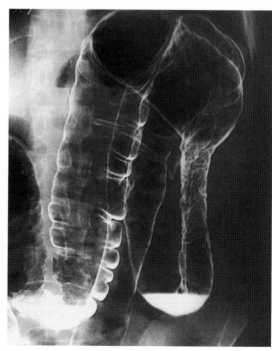

Fig. 17-125 Upright double-contrast AP oblique large intestine, RPO position.

AXIAL PROJECTION

CHASSARD-LAPINÉ METHOD

The Chassard-Lapiné method is used to show the rectum, rectosigmoid junction, and sigmoid. This projection, which is made at almost a right angle to the AP projection, shows the anterior and posterior surfaces of the lower portion of the bowel and permits the coils of the sigmoid to be projected free from overlapping.[1-3] The projection may be exposed after evacuation of the large intestine, although a preevacuation image can be exposed when the patient has reasonable sphincteric control.[1]

Image receptor: 11 × 14 inch (30 × 35 cm) or 14 × 17 inch (35 × 43 cm) lengthwise, depending on availability

Position of patient

- Seat the patient on the radiographic table.

Position of part

- Instruct the patient to sit well back on the side of the table so that the midcoronal plane of the body is as close as possible to the midline of the table.
- If necessary, shift the transversely placed IR forward in the Bucky tray so that its transverse axis coincides as nearly as possible with the midcoronal plane of the body.

[1]Raap G: A position of value in studying the pelvis and its contents, *South Med J* 44:95, 1951.
[2]Cimmino CV: Radiography of the sigmoid flexure with the Chassard-Lapiné projection, *Med Radiogr Photogr* 30:44, 1954.
[3]Ettinger A, Elkin M: Study of the sigmoid by special roentgenographic views, *AJR Am J Roentgenol* 72:199, 1954.

- Instruct the patient to abduct the thighs as far as the edge of the table permits, so that they do not interfere with flexion of the body.
- Center the IR to the midline of the pelvis, and ask the patient to lean directly forward as far as possible (Fig. 17-126).
- Have the patient grasp the ankles for support.
- *Respiration:* Suspend.

The exposure required for this projection is approximately the same as that required for a lateral projection of the pelvis.

Central ray

- Perpendicular through the lumbosacral region at the level of the greater trochanters

Collimation

- Adjust to 14 × 17 inches (35 × 43 cm) on the collimator.

Structures shown

The Chassard-Lapiné image shows the rectum, rectosigmoid junction, and sigmoid in the axial projection (Fig. 17-127).

EVALUATION CRITERIA

The following should be clearly shown:
- Evidence of proper collimation
- Rectosigmoid area in the center of the image
- Rectosigmoid area not obscured by superior area of colon
- Minimal superimposition of rectosigmoid area
- Penetration of the lumbosacral region and the barium

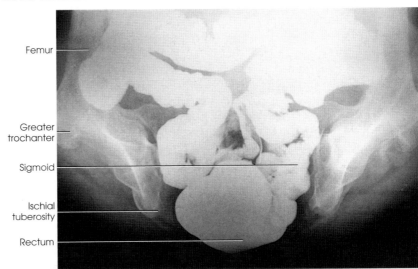
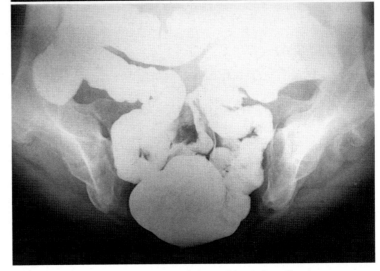

Fig. 17-127 Axial rectosigmoid: Chassard-Lapiné method.

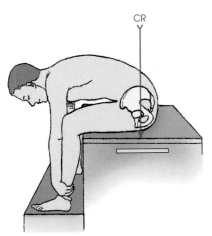

Fig. 17-126 Chassard-Lapiné method.

COLOSTOMY STUDIES

Enterostomy (Greek *enteron*, "intestine" + *stoma*, "opening") is the general term applied to the surgical procedure of forming an artificial opening to the intestine, usually through the abdominal wall, for fecal passage. The regional terms are *colostomy, cecostomy, ileostomy,* and *jejunostomy.*

The colon is the most common site of disease in the large intestine, and surgical procedures are often performed on this structure. Loop colostomy is sometimes performed to divert the fecal column, temporarily or permanently, from areas of diverticulitis or ulcerative colitis. Most colostomies are performed because of malignancies of the lower bowel and rectum. When a tumor is present, the lower carcinomatous part of the bowel is resected, and the end of the remaining part of the bowel is brought to the surface through the abdominal wall. This passage, or *stoma,* has no sphincter.

Preparation of intestinal tract

Postoperative contrast enema studies are performed at suitable intervals to allow the clinician to determine the efficacy of treatment in a patient with diverticulitis or ulcerative colitis and to detect new or recurrent lesions in a patient who has had a tumor. Adequate cleansing of the bowel, which is as important in the presence of a colostomy as otherwise, is crucial to show polyps and other intraluminal lesions. In a patient with a colostomy, the usual preparation is irrigation of the stoma the night before the study and again on the morning of the examination.

Colostomy enema equipment

Although equipment must be scrupulously clean, and nondisposable items must be sterilized after each use, sterile technique is not required because the stoma is part of the intestinal tract. Except for a suitable device to prevent stomal leakage of contrast material, the equipment used in a patient with a colostomy is the same as that used in routine contrast enema studies. The same barium sulfate formula is used, and gas studies are made. Opaque and double-contrast studies can be performed in a single-stage examination with use of a disposable enema kit.

A device must be used to prevent spillage of contrast enema material in a patient with a colostomy. Otherwise, because of the absence of sphincter control, the contrast enema may escape through the colostomy almost as rapidly as it is injected. If this happens, bowel filling is unsatisfactory, and shadows cast by barium soilage of the abdominal wall and the examining table obscure areas of interest. Abdominal stomas must be effectively occluded for studies made by retrograde injection, and leakage around the stomal catheter must be prevented for studies made by injection into an abdominal or a perineal colostomy. Numerous devices are available for this purpose.

DIAGNOSTIC ENEMA

Diagnostic enemas may be given through a colostomy stoma with the use of tips and adhesive disks designed for the patient's use in irrigating the colostomy (Fig. 17-128). These tips are available in four sizes to accommodate the usual sizes of colostomy stomas. The tips usually have a flange to prevent them from slipping through the colostomy opening. An adhesive disk is placed over the flange to minimize reflux soilage. The enema tubing is attached directly to the tip, which the patient holds in position to prevent the weight of the tubing from displacing the tip to an angled position. In addition to keeping a set of Laird tips on hand, it is recommended that the patient be asked to bring an irrigation device.

Retention catheters are also used in colostomy studies. Some radiologists use them alone, and others insert them through a device to prevent slipping and to collect leakage. Colostomy stomas are fragile and are subject to perforation by any undue pressure or trauma. Perforations have occurred during insertion of an inflated bulb into a blind pouch and as the result of overdistention of the stoma.

Preparation of patient

If the patient uses a special dressing, colostomy pouch, or stomal seal, he or she should be advised to bring a change for use after the examination. When fecal emission is such that a pouch is required, the patient should be given a suitable dressing to place over the stoma after the device has been removed.

The radiographer observes the following steps:
- Clothe the patient in a kimono type of gown that opens in front or back, depending on the location of the colostomy.
- Place the patient on the examining table in the supine position if he or she has an abdominal colostomy and in the prone position if he or she has a perineal colostomy.
- Before taking the preliminary image and while wearing disposable gloves, remove and discard any dressing.
- Cleanse the skin around the stoma appropriately.
- Place a gauze dressing over the stoma to absorb any seepage until the physician is ready to start the examination.
- Lubricate the stomal catheter or tube well (but not excessively) with a water-soluble lubricant. The catheter should be inserted by the physician or the patient. If a catheter is forced through a stoma, the colon may be perforated.

Spot images are taken during the examination. Postfluoroscopy images are taken as needed. The projections requested depend on the location of the stoma and the anatomy to be shown (Figs. 17-129 to 17-132).

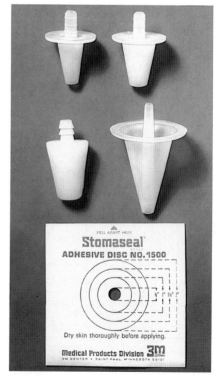

Fig. 17-128 Laird colostomy irrigation tips and Stomaseal disks.

Digestive System

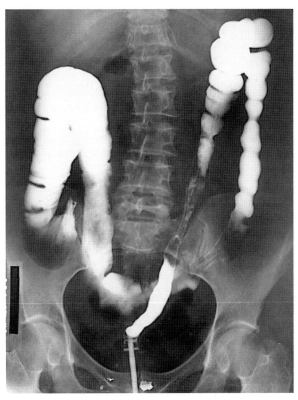

Fig. 17-129 Opaque colon via perineal colostomy.

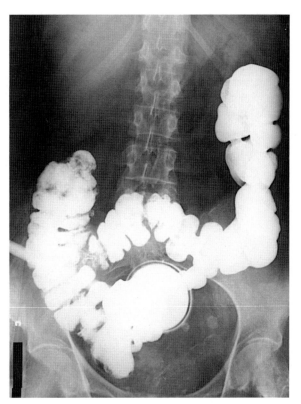

Fig. 17-130 Opaque colon via abdominal colostomy.

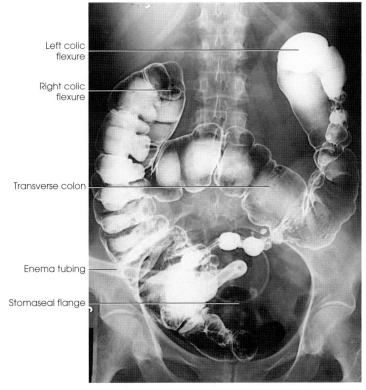

Left colic flexure

Right colic flexure

Transverse colon

Enema tubing

Stomaseal flange

Fig. 17-131 Double-contrast colon in patient with abdominal colostomy.

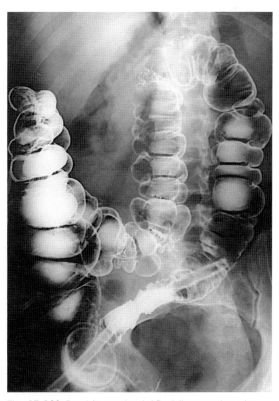

Fig. 17-132 Double-contrast AP oblique colon via abdominal colostomy.

DEFECOGRAPHY

Defecography, evacuation proctography, or *dynamic rectal examination* is a radiologic procedure performed on patients with defecation dysfunction. No preparation of the patient is necessary, and cleansing enemas are not recommended because water remaining in the rectum dilutes the contrast medium.

Early investigators[1] mixed a diluted suspension of barium sulfate, heated it, and added potato starch to form a smooth barium paste that was semisolid and malleable.[2,3] Barium manufacturers now package prepared barium products (100% weight/volume barium sulfate paste) with a special injector mechanism to instill barium directly into the rectum. In addition, viscous barium may be introduced into the vagina and the bladder filled with aqueous iodinated contrast media.

[1]Burhenne HJ: Intestinal evacuation study: a new roentgenologic technique, *Radiol Clin (Basel)* 33:79, 1964.

[2]Mahieu P et al: Defecography: I. Description of a new procedure and results in normal patients, *Gastrointest Radiol* 9:247, 1984.

[3]Mahieu P et al: Defecography: II. Contribution to the diagnosis of defecation disorders, *Gastrointest Radiol* 9:253, 1984.

After the contrast medium is instilled, the patient is usually seated in the lateral position on a commercially available radiolucent commode in front of a fluoroscopic unit. A special commode chair is recommended so that the anorectal junction and the zone of interest on the image are not overexposed. Lateral projections are obtained during defecation by spot imaging at the approximate rate of 1 to 2 frames per second. Video recording of the defecation process may be used, but the special equipment necessary to interpret the images is not always available, and a hard copy of the images is unavailable.[1] The resulting images are then evaluated (Fig. 17-133). This evaluation includes measurements of the anorectal angle and the angle between the long axes of the anal canal and rectum. These measurements are compared with normal values. In addition, changes in proximity of the rectum to the vagina and bladder during defecation are assessed when these structures have been filled with contrast media (Fig. 17-134).

[1]Mahieu PHG: Defecography. In Margulis AR, Burhenne H, editors: *Alimentary tract radiology,* vol 1, ed 4, St Louis, 1989, Mosby.

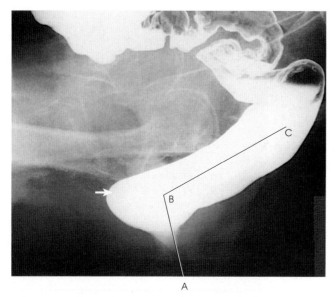

Fig. 17-133 Defecography. Lateral anus and rectum spot image showing long axis of anal canal (*line A-B*) and long axis of rectal canal (*line B-C*) in a patient with anorectal angle of 114 degrees. Anterior rectocele (*arrow*) also is shown.

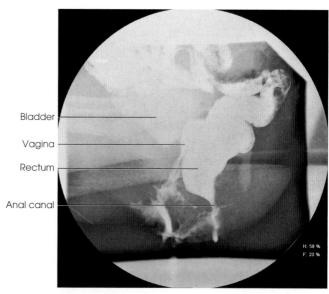

Fig. 17-134 Defecography. Lateral anal canal and rectum, vagina, and urinary bladder shown during patient straining.

(Courtesy Michelle Alting, AS, RT(R).)

Biliary Tract and Gallbladder

Several techniques can be used to examine the gallbladder and the biliary ductal system. In many institutions, sonography is the modality of choice. This section of the atlas discusses the radiographic techniques currently available.

Table 17-1 lists some of the prefixes associated with the biliary system. *Cholegraphy* is the general term for a radiographic study of the biliary system. More specific terms can be used to describe the portion of the biliary system under investigation. *Cholecystography* is the radiographic investigation of the gallbladder, and *cholangiography* is the radiographic study of the biliary ducts.

Advances in sonography, CT, MRI, and nuclear medicine have reduced the radiographic examination of the biliary tract primarily to direct injection procedures including percutaneous transhepatic cholangiography (PTC), postoperative (T-tube) cholangiography, and endoscopic retrograde cholangiopancreatography (ERCP). The contrast agent selected for use in direct-injection techniques may be any one of the water-soluble iodinated compounds employed for intravenous urography.

TABLE 17-1

Biliary system combining forms

Root forms	Meaning
Chole-	Relationship with bile
Cysto-	Bag or sac
Choledocho-	Common bile duct
Cholangio-	Bile ducts
Cholecyst-	Gallbladder

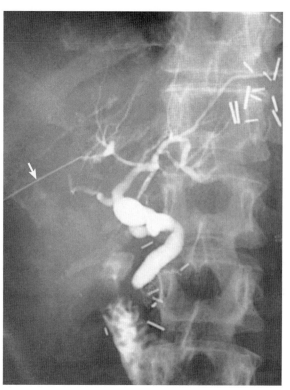

Fig. 17-135 PTC with Chiba needle (*arrow*) in position, showing dilated biliary ducts.

Percutaneous Transhepatic Cholangiography

PTC[1] is another technique employed for preoperative radiologic examination of the biliary tract. This technique is used for patients with jaundice when the ductal system has been shown to be dilated by CT or sonography but the cause of the obstruction is unclear. Performance of this examination has greatly increased because of the availability of the Chiba ("skinny") needle. In addition, PTC is often used to place a drainage catheter for treatment of obstructive jaundice. When a drainage catheter is used, diagnostic and drainage techniques are performed at the same time.

[1]Evans JA et al: Percutaneous transhepatic cholangiography, *Radiology* 78:362, 1962.

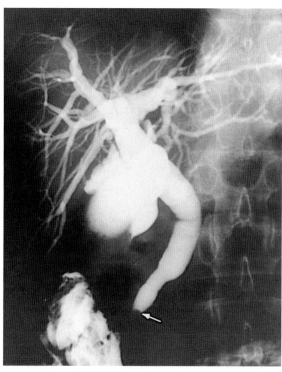

Fig. 17-136 PTC showing obstruction stone at ampulla (*arrow*).

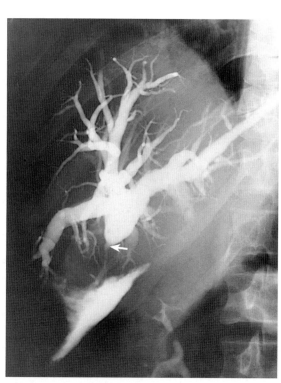

Fig. 17-137 PTC showing stenosis (*arrow*) of common hepatic duct caused by trauma.

PTC is performed by placing the patient on the radiographic table in the supine position. The patient's right side is surgically prepared and appropriately draped. After a local anesthetic is administered, the Chiba needle is held parallel to the floor and inserted through the right lateral intercostal space and advanced toward the liver hilum. The stylet of the needle is withdrawn, and a syringe filled with contrast medium is attached to the needle. Under fluoroscopic control, the needle is slowly withdrawn until contrast medium is seen to fill the biliary ducts. In most instances, the biliary tree is readily located because the ducts are generally dilated. After the biliary ducts are filled, the needle is completely withdrawn, and serial or spot AP projections of the biliary area are taken (Figs. 17-135 to 17-137).

BILIARY DRAINAGE PROCEDURE AND STONE EXTRACTION

If dilated biliary ducts are identified by CT, PTC, or sonography, the radiologist, after consultation with the referring physician, may elect to place a drainage catheter in the biliary duct.[1,2] A needle larger than the Chiba needle used in the PTC procedure is inserted through the lateral abdominal wall and into the biliary duct. A guidewire is passed through the lumen of the needle, and the needle is removed. After the catheter is passed over the guidewire, the wire is removed, leaving the catheter in place.

The catheter can be left in place for prolonged drainage, or it can be used for attempts to extract retained stones if they are identified. Retained stones are extracted using a wire basket and a small balloon catheter under fluoroscopic control. This extraction procedure is usually attempted after the catheter has been in place for some time (Figs. 17-138 and 17-139).

[1]Molnar W, Stockum AE: Relief of obstructive jaundice through percutaneous transhepatic catheter—a new therapeutic method, *AJR Am J Roentgenol* 122:356, 1974.
[2]Hardy CH et al: Percutaneous transhepatic biliary drainage, *Radiol Technol* 56:8, 1984.

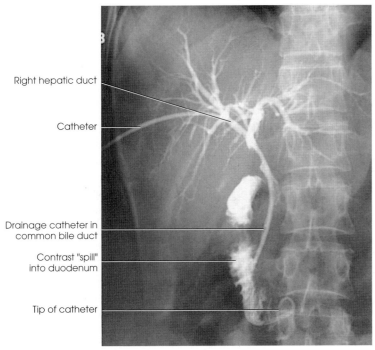

Right hepatic duct

Catheter

Drainage catheter in common bile duct

Contrast "spill" into duodenum

Tip of catheter

Fig. 17-138 PTC with drainage catheter in place.

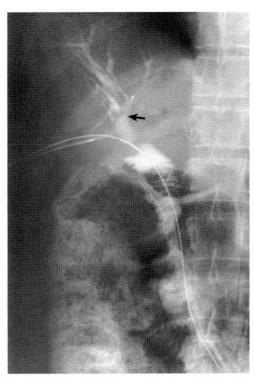

Fig. 17-139 Post-PTC image showing wire basket (*arrow*) around retained stone.

Postoperative (T-Tube) Cholangiography

Postoperative, delayed, and *T-tube cholangiography* are radiologic terms applied to the biliary tract examination that is performed via a T-shaped or pigtail-shaped catheter left in the common hepatic and common bile ducts for postoperative drainage (Fig. 17-140). A pigtail catheter is required for laparoscopic biliary procedures because it can be placed percutaneously. The T-tube catheter can be placed only during an open surgical procedure. This examination is performed to show the caliber and patency of the ducts, the status of the sphincter of the hepatopancreatic ampulla, and the presence of residual or previously undetected stones or other pathologic conditions.

Postoperative cholangiography is performed in the radiology department. Preliminary preparation usually consists of the following:

1. The drainage tube is clamped the day before the examination to let the tube fill with bile as a preventive measure against air bubbles entering the ducts, where they would simulate cholesterol stones.
2. The preceding meal is withheld.
3. When indicated, a cleansing enema is administered about 1 hour before the examination. Premedication is not required.

The contrast agent used is one of the water-soluble iodinated contrast media. The density of the contrast medium used in postoperative cholangiograms is recommended to be no greater than 25% to 30% because small stones may be obscured with a higher concentration.

After a preliminary image of the abdomen has been obtained, the patient is adjusted in the RPO position (AP oblique projection) with the RUQ of the abdomen centered to the midline of the grid (Fig. 17-141).

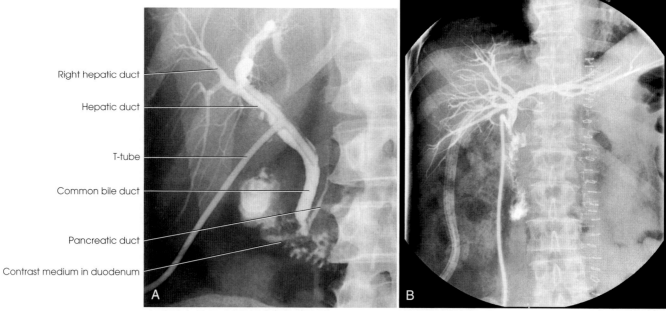

Right hepatic duct

Hepatic duct

T-tube

Common bile duct

Pancreatic duct

Contrast medium in duodenum

Fig. 17-140 A, Postoperative cholangiogram with T-tube catheter. **B,** Postoperative cholangiogram with pigtail catheter.

With universal precautions employed, the contrast medium is injected under fluoroscopic control, and spot and conventional images are made as indicated. Otherwise, 10×12-inch (24×30-cm) IRs are exposed serially after each of several fractional injections of the medium and then at specified intervals until most of the contrast solution has entered the duodenum.

Stern et al.[1] stressed the importance of obtaining a lateral projection to show ana-tomic branching of the hepatic ducts in this plane and to detect any abnormality not otherwise shown (Fig. 17-142). The clamp generally is not removed from the T-tube before the examination is completed. The patient may be turned onto the right side for this study.

---

[1]Stern WZ et al: The significance of the lateral view in T-tube cholangiography, *AJR Am J Roentgenol* 87:764, 1962.

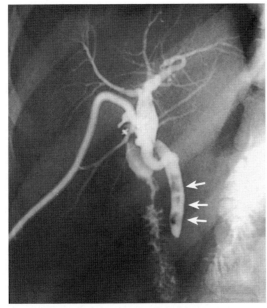

Fig. 17-141 AP oblique postoperative cholangiogram, RPO position, showing multiple stones in common bile duct (*arrows*).

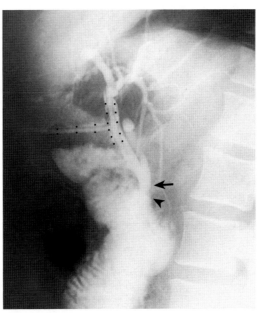

Fig. 17-142 Right lateral cholangiogram showing AP location of T-tube (*dots*), common bile duct (*arrow*), and hepatopancreatic ampulla (duct of Vater) (*arrowhead*).

Endoscopic Retrograde Cholangio-pancreatography

ERCP is a procedure used to diagnose biliary and pancreatic pathologic conditions. ERCP is a useful diagnostic method when the biliary ducts are not dilated and when no obstruction exists at the ampulla.

ERCP is performed by passing a fiberoptic endoscope through the mouth into the duodenum under fluoroscopic control. To ease passage of the endoscope, the patient's throat is sprayed with a local anesthetic. Because this causes temporary pharyngeal paresis, food and drink are usually prohibited for at least 1 hour after the examination. Food may be withheld for 10 hours after the procedure to minimize irritation to the stomach and small bowel.

After the endoscopist locates the hepatopancreatic ampulla (ampulla of Vater), a small cannula is passed through the endoscope and directed into the ampulla (Fig. 17-143). When the cannula is properly placed, contrast medium is injected into the common bile duct. The patient may then be moved, fluoroscopy performed, and spot images taken (Figs. 17-144 and 17-145). Oblique spot images may be taken to prevent overlap of the common bile duct and the pancreatic duct. Because the injected contrast material should drain from normal ducts within approximately 5 minutes, images must be exposed immediately.

The contrast medium that is used depends on the preference of the radiologist or gastroenterologist. Dense contrast agents opacify small ducts well, but they may obscure small stones. If small stones are suspected, use of a more dilute contrast medium is suggested.[1] A history of patient sensitivity to an iodinated contrast medium in another examination (e.g., intravenous urography) does not contraindicate its use for ERCP. The patient must be watched carefully, however, for a reaction to the contrast medium during ERCP.

ERCP is often indicated when clinical and radiographic findings indicate abnormalities in the biliary system or pancreas. Sonography of the upper part of the abdomen before endoscopy is often recommended to assure the physician that no pancreatic pseudocysts are present. This step is important because contrast medium injected into pseudocysts may lead to inflammation or rupture.

[1]Cotton P, William C: *Practical gastrointestinal endoscopy,* Oxford, England, 1980, Blackwell.

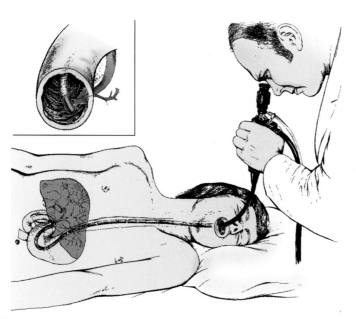

Fig. 17-143 Cannulation procedure. Procedure is begun with the patient in left lateral position. This schematic diagram gives an overview of location of the examiner and position of scope and its relationship to various internal organs. *Inset:* Magnified view of tip of scope with cannula in papilla.

(From Stewart ET et al: *Atlas of endoscopic retrograde cholangiopancreatography,* St Louis, 1977, Mosby.)

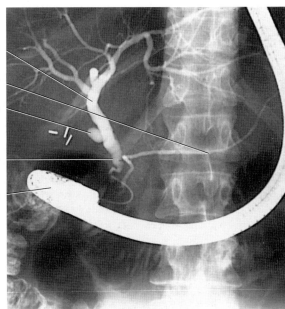
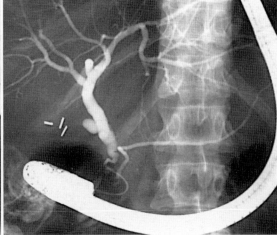

Common hepatic duct

Pancreatic duct

Cystic stump

Common bile duct

Endoscope

Fig. 17-144 ERCP spot image, PA projection.

Pancreatic duct

Cannula

Fig. 17-145 ERCP spot image, PA projection.

Abdominal Fistulae and Sinuses

To show radiographically the origin and extent of fistulae (abnormal passages, usually between two internal organs) and sinuses (abnormal channels leading to abscesses), the following steps are taken:

- Fill the tract with a radiopaque contrast medium, usually under fluoroscopic control.

- Obtain right-angle projections. Oblique projections are occasionally required to show the full extent of a sinus tract.
- To explore fistulae and sinuses in the abdominal region, have the intestinal tract as free of gas and fecal material as possible.
- Unless the injection is made under fluoroscopic control, take a scout image of the abdomen to check the condition of the intestinal tract before beginning the examination.
- When more than one sinus opening is present, occlude each accessory opening with sterile gauze packing to prevent reflux of the contrast substance and to identify every opening with a specific lead marker placed over the dressing (Figs. 17-146 to 17-148).
- Dress and identify the primary sinus opening in a similar manner if the catheter is removed after the injection.
- When reflux of contrast medium occurs, cleanse the skin thoroughly before making an exposure.

- When fluoroscopy is not employed, place the patient in position for the first projection before the injection to prevent drainage of the opaque substance by unnecessary movement. An initial image is taken and evaluated before the examination is started or the patient's position is changed.

To show a fistula involving the colon, barium is instilled by enema. If a fistula involving the small bowel is suspected, the patient ingests a thin barium suspension, which is followed by fluoroscopy or radiography until it reaches the suspected region. The bladder is filled with iodinated contrast media when involvement of this structure is evaluated. Cutaneous fistulae and sinus tracts are opacified by introduction of an iodinated contrast medium through a small-diameter catheter. The procedures are performed using fluoroscopic observation, with images taken as indicated.

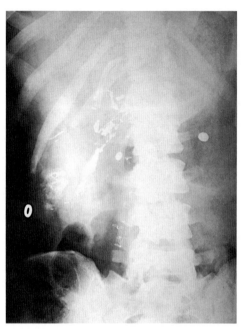

Fig. 17-146 AP abdomen showing contrast media–filled sinus tract with lead circular ring on body surface.

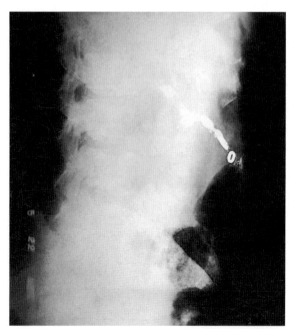

Fig. 17-147 Lateral abdomen showing sinus tract with lead circular ring on body surface.

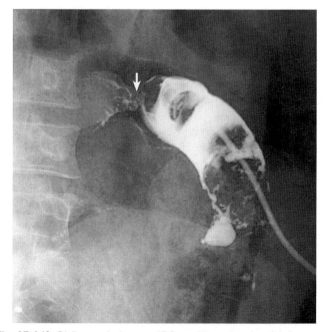

Fig. 17-148 Oblique abdomen, LPO position, showing fistula (*arrow*).

18

URINARY SYSTEM AND VENIPUNCTURE

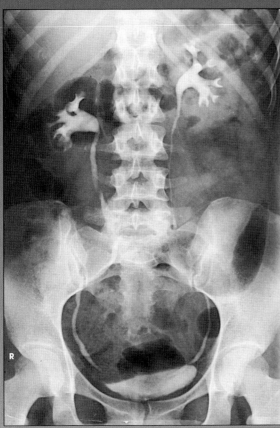

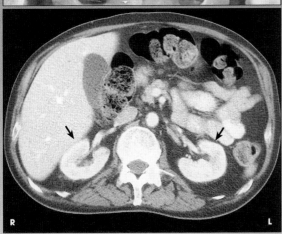

SUMMARY OF PROJECTIONS

PROJECTIONS, POSITIONS, AND METHODS

Page	Essential	Anatomy	Projection	Position	Method
204	♠	Urinary system	AP		
206	♠	Urinary system	AP oblique	RPO and LPO	
207	♠	Urinary system	Lateral	R or L	
208	♠	Urinary system	Lateral	Dorsal decubitus	
209		Renal parenchyma	AP		
212	♠	Pelvicaliceal system and ureters: *retrograde urography*	AP		
216	♠	Urinary bladder	AP axial or PA axial		
218	♠	Urinary bladder	AP oblique	RPO or LPO	
220	♠	Urinary bladder	Lateral	R or L	
221	♠	Male cystourethrography	AP oblique	RPO or LPO	
222		Female cystourethrography	AP		INJECTION

Icons in the Essential column indicate projections frequently performed in the United States and Canada. Students should be competent in these projections.

Urinary System

The *urinary system* includes two *kidneys,* two *ureters,* one *urinary bladder,* and one *urethra* (Figs. 18-1 and 18-2). The functions of the kidneys include removing waste products from the blood, maintaining fluid and electrolyte balance, and secreting substances that affect blood pressure and other important body functions. The kidneys normally excrete 1 to 2 L of urine per day. Urine is expelled from the body via the *excretory system,* as the urinary system is often called. The excretory system consists of the following:

- A variable number of urine-draining branches in the kidney called the *calyces* and an expanded portion called the *renal pelvis,* which together are known as the *pelvicaliceal system*
- Two long tubes called *ureters,* with one ureter extending from the pelvis of each kidney
- A saclike portion, the *urinary bladder,* which receives the distal portion of the ureters and serves as a reservoir
- A third and smaller tubular portion, the *urethra,* which conveys the urine to the exterior of the body

Suprarenal Glands

Closely associated with the urinary system are the two *suprarenal,* or *adrenal, glands.* These ductless endocrine glands have no functional relationship with the urinary system but are included in this chapter because of their anatomic relationship with the kidneys. Each suprarenal gland consists of a small, flattened body composed of an internal *medullary portion* and an outer *cortical portion.* Each gland is enclosed in a fibrous sheath and is situated in the retroperitoneal tissue in close contact with the fatty capsule overlying the medial and superior aspects of the upper pole of the kidney. The suprarenal glands furnish two important substances: (1) epinephrine, which is secreted by the medulla; and (2) cortical hormones, which are secreted by the cortex. These glands are subject to malfunction and numerous diseases. They are not usually shown on preliminary images but are delineated when computed tomography (CT) is used. The suprarenal circulation may be shown by selective catheterization of a suprarenal artery or vein in angiographic procedures.

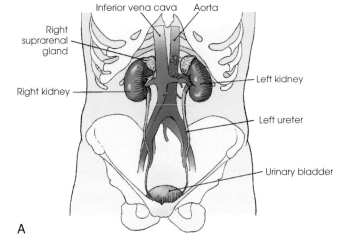

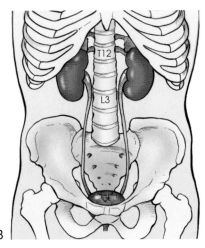

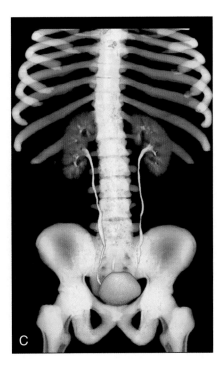

Fig. 18-1 Anterior aspect of urinary system in relation to surrounding structures. **A,** Abdominal structures. **B,** Bony structures. **C,** Three-dimensional CT image of urinary system in relation to bony structures.

Kidneys

The *kidneys* are bean-shaped bodies. The lateral border of each kidney is convex, and the medial border is concave. They have slightly convex anterior and posterior surfaces, and they are arbitrarily divided into upper and lower poles. The kidneys are approximately $4\frac{1}{2}$ inches (11.5 cm) long, 2 to 3 inches (5 to 7.6 cm) wide, and about $1\frac{1}{4}$ inches (3 cm) thick. The left kidney usually is slightly longer and narrower than the right kidney.

The kidneys are situated behind the peritoneum (retroperitoneal) and are in contact with the posterior wall of the abdominal cavity, one kidney lying on each side of and in the same coronal plane with L3. The superior aspect of the kidney lies more posterior than the inferior aspect (see Fig. 18-2). Each kidney lies in an oblique plane and is rotated about 30 degrees anteriorly toward the aorta, which lies on top of the vertebral body (Fig. 18-3). This natural anatomic position is the basis for the 30-degree rotation of the AP oblique projections (RPO and LPO positions). In AP oblique projections, the elevated kidney is demonstrated without distortion, as the 30-degree rotation orients the upper kidney parallel to the IR plane. The dependent kidney is positioned almost perpendicular to the IR plane, so the lower kidney is oriented to demonstrate the anterior and posterior surfaces in the oblique positions.

The kidneys normally extend from the level of the superior border of T12 to the level of the transverse processes of L3 in sthenic individuals; they are higher in individuals with a hypersthenic habitus and lower in persons with an asthenic habitus. Because of the large space occupied by the liver, the right kidney is slightly lower than, or caudal to, the left kidney.

The outer covering of the kidney is called the *renal capsule.* The capsule is a semitransparent membrane that is continuous with the outer coat of the ureter. Each kidney is embedded in a mass of fatty tissue called the *adipose capsule.* The capsule and kidney are enveloped in a sheath of superficial fascia, the *renal fascia,* which is attached to the diaphragm, lumbar vertebrae, peritoneum, and other adjacent structures. The kidneys are supported in a fairly fixed position, partially through the fascial attachments and partially by the surrounding organs. They have respiratory movement of approximately 1 inch (2.5 cm) and normally drop no more than 2 inches (5 cm) in the change from supine to upright position.

The concave medial border of each kidney has a longitudinal slit, or *hilum,* for transmission of the blood and lymphatic vessels, nerves, and ureter (Fig. 18-4). The hilum expands into the body of the kidney to form a central cavity called the *renal sinus.* The renal sinus is a fat-filled space surrounding the renal pelvis and vessels.

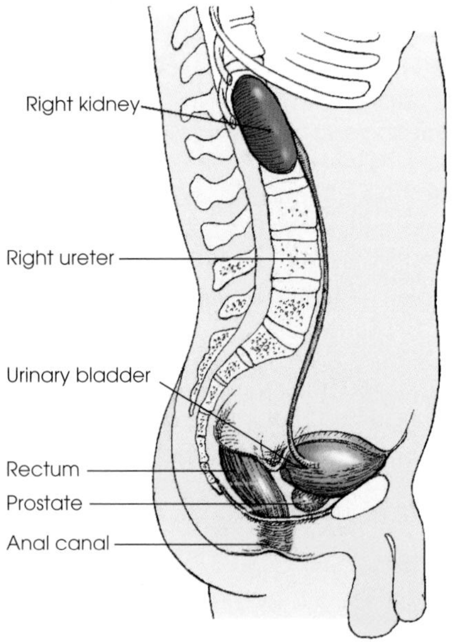

Fig. 18-2 Lateral aspect of male urinary system in relation to surrounding structures.

Right kidney

Right ureter

Urinary bladder

Rectum

Prostate

Anal canal

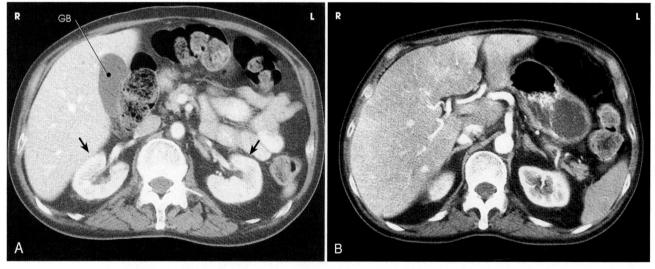

Fig. 18-3 A, Axial CT image through center of kidney. Note 30-degree anterior angulation of kidneys (*arrows*). *GB,* gallbladder. **B,** Axial CT image of upper abdomen. Note superior aspect of right kidney and midportion of left kidney showing lower placed left kidney.

(From Kelley LL, Petersen CM: *Sectional anatomy for imaging professionals,* ed 2, St Louis, 2007, Mosby.)

Each kidney has an outer renal cortex and an inner *renal medulla*. The renal medulla, composed mainly of the collecting tubules that give it a striated appearance, consists of 8 to 15 cone-shaped segments called the *renal pyramids*. The apices of the segments converge toward the renal sinus to drain into the pelvicaliceal system. The more compact renal cortex lies between the periphery of the organ and the bases of the medullary segments and extends medially between the pyramids to the renal sinus. These extensions of the cortex are called *renal columns*.

The essential microscopic components of the parenchyma of the kidney are called *nephrons* (Fig. 18-5). Each kidney contains approximately 1 million of these tubular structures. The individual nephron is composed of a *renal corpuscle* and a *renal tubule*. The renal corpuscle consists of a double-walled membranous cup called the *glomerular capsule* (Bowman capsule) and a cluster of blood capillaries called the *glomerulus*. The glomerulus is formed by a minute branch of the renal artery entering the capsule and dividing into capillaries. The capillaries turn back and, as they ascend, unite to form a single vessel leaving the capsule.

The vessel entering the capsule is called the *afferent arteriole,* and the one leaving the capsule is termed the *efferent arteriole.* After exiting the glomerular capsules, the efferent arterioles form the capillary network surrounding the straight and convoluted tubules, and these capillaries reunite and continue on to communicate with the renal veins.

The thin inner wall of the capsule closely adheres to the capillary coils and is separated by a comparatively wide space from the outer layer, which is continuous with the beginning of a renal tubule. The glomerulus serves as a filter for the blood, permitting water and finely dissolved substances to pass through the walls of the capillaries into the capsule. The change from filtrate to urine is caused in part by the water and the usable dissolved substances being absorbed through the epithelial lining of the tubules into the surrounding capillary network.

Each *renal tubule* continues from a glomerular capsule in the cortex of the kidney and then travels a circuitous path through the cortical and medullary substances, becoming the *proximal convoluted tubule,* the *nephron loop* (loop of Henle), and the *distal convoluted tubule*. The distal convoluted tubule opens into the collecting ducts that begin in the cortex. The *collecting ducts* converge toward the renal pelvis and unite along their course, so that each group within the pyramid forms a central tubule that opens at a *renal papilla* and drains its tributaries into the minor calyx.

The *calyces* are cup-shaped stems arising at the sides of the papilla of each renal pyramid. Each calyx encloses one or more papillae, so that there are usually fewer calyces than pyramids. The beginning branches are called the *minor calyces* (numbering from 4 to 13), and they unite to form two or three larger tubes called the *major calyces*. The major calyces unite to form the expanded, funnel-shaped renal pelvis. The wide upper portion of the *renal pelvis* lies within the hilum, and its tapering lower part passes through the hilum to become continuous with the ureter. This area, where the renal pelvis transitions to the ureter, is called the *ureteropelvic junction* (UPJ).

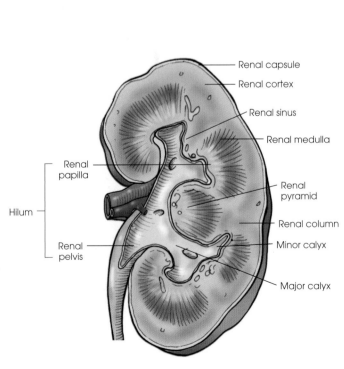

Fig. 18-4 Midcoronal section of kidney.

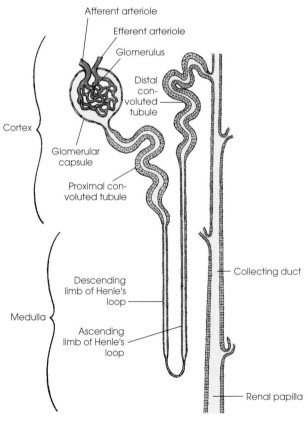

Fig. 18-5 Diagram of nephron and collecting duct.

Ureters

Each *ureter* is 10 to 12 inches (25 to 30 cm) long. The ureters descend behind the peritoneum and in front of the psoas muscle and the transverse processes of the lumbar vertebrae, pass inferiorly and posteriorly in front of the sacral wing, and then curve anteriorly and medially to enter the posterolateral surface of the urinary bladder at approximately the level of the ischial spine. The ureters convey the urine from the renal pelves to the bladder by slow, rhythmic peristaltic contractions.

Urinary Bladder

The *urinary bladder* is a musculomembranous sac that serves as a reservoir for urine. The bladder is situated immediately posterior and superior to the pubic symphysis and is directly anterior to the rectum in the male and anterior to the vaginal canal in the female. The *apex* of the bladder is at the anterosuperior aspect and is adjacent to the superior aspect of the pubic symphysis. The most fixed part of the bladder is the neck, which rests on the prostate in the male and on the pelvic diaphragm in the female.

The bladder varies in size, shape, and position according to its content. It is freely movable and is held in position by folds of the peritoneum. When empty, the bladder is located in the pelvic cavity. As the bladder fills, it gradually assumes an oval shape while expanding superiorly and anteriorly into the abdominal cavity. The adult bladder can hold approximately 500 mL of fluid when completely full. The urge for *micturition* (urination) occurs when about 250 mL of urine is in the bladder.

The ureters enter the posterior wall of the bladder at the lateral margins of the superior part of its *base* and pass obliquely through the wall to their respective internal orifices (Fig. 18-6). This portion of each ureter, where it joins the bladder, is called the *ureterovesical junction* (UVJ). These two openings are about 1 inch (2.5 cm) apart when the bladder is empty and about 2 inches (5 cm) apart when the bladder is distended. The openings are equidistant from the internal urethral orifice, which is situated at the neck (lowest part) of the bladder. The triangular area between the three orifices is called the *trigone*. The mucosa over the trigone is always smooth, whereas the remainder of the lining contains folds, called *rugae*, when the bladder is empty.

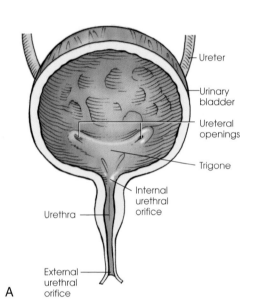
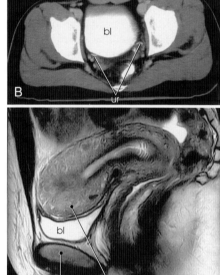

Fig. 18-6 A, Anterior view of urinary bladder. **B,** Axial CT image of pelvis showing contrast medium–filled bladder (bl) and ureters (ur). **C,** Sagittal MRI of female pelvis showing contrast medium–filled bladder (bl) and relationship to uterus (ut) and pubis (pub).

(**B** and **C,** From Kelley LL, Petersen CM: *Sectional anatomy for imaging professionals,* ed 2, St Louis, 2007, Mosby.)

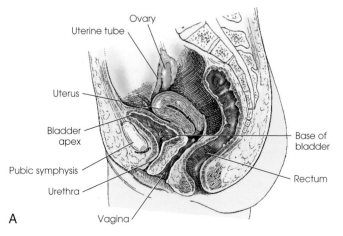
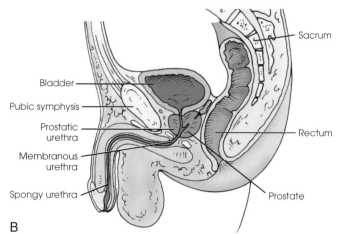

Fig. 18-7 A, Midsagittal section through female pelvis. **B,** Male pelvis.

Urethra

The *urethra,* which conveys the urine out of the body, is a narrow, musculomembranous tube with a sphincter type of muscle at the neck of the bladder. The urethra arises at the internal urethral orifice in the urinary bladder and extends about 1½ inches (3.8 cm) in the female and 7 to 8 inches (17.8 to 20 cm) in the male.

The female urethra passes along the thick anterior wall of the vagina to the external urethral orifice, which is located in the vestibule about 1 inch (2.5 cm) anterior to the vaginal opening (see Fig. 18-6). The male urethra extends from the bladder to the end of the penis and is divided into *prostatic, membranous,* and *spongy* portions (Fig. 18-7). The prostatic portion is about 1 inch (2.5 cm) long, reaches from the bladder to the floor of the pelvis, and is completely surrounded by the prostate. The membranous portion of the canal passes through the urogenital diaphragm; it is slightly constricted and about ½ inch (1.3 cm) long. The spongy portion passes through the shaft of the penis, extending from the floor of the pelvis to the external urethral orifice. The distal prostatic, membranous, and spongy parts of the male urethra also serve as the excretory canal of the reproductive system.

Prostate

The *prostate,* a small glandular body surrounding the proximal part of the male urethra, is situated just posterior to the inferior portion of the pubic symphysis. The prostate is considered part of the male reproductive system, but because of its close proximity to the bladder, it is commonly described with the urinary system. The conical base of the prostate is attached to the inferior surface of the urinary bladder, and its apex is in contact with the pelvic diaphragm. The prostate measures about 1½ inches (3.8 cm) transversely and ¾ inch (1.9 cm) anteroposteriorly at its base; vertically the prostate is approximately 1 inch (2.5 cm) long. The prostate gland secretes a milky fluid that combines with semen from the seminal vesicles and vas deferens. These secretions enter the urethra via ducts in the prostatic urethra.

SUMMARY OF ANATOMY

Urinary system (excretory system)
Kidneys (R and L)
Ureters (R and L)
Urinary bladder
Urethra

Suprarenal glands (adrenal glands)
Medullary portion
Cortical portion

Kidneys
Adipose capsule
Renal fascia
Hilum
Renal capsule
Renal sinus
Renal cortex
   Renal columns
Renal medulla
   Renal pyramids
Nephrons
   Renal corpuscle
      Glomerular capsule (Bowman capsule)
      Glomerulus
      Afferent arteriole
      Efferent arteriole
   Renal tubule
      Proximal convoluted tubule
      Nephron loop (loop of Henle)
      Distal convoluted tubule
      Collecting ducts
      Renal papilla
  Calyces
     Minor calyces
     Major calyces
     Renal pelvis

Urinary bladder
Apex
Base
Neck
Trigone
Rugae

Urethra
Male urethra
Prostatic
Membranous
Spongy

Prostate

SUMMARY OF PATHOLOGY

Condition	Definition
Benign prostatic hyperplasia (BPH)	Enlargement of prostate
Calculus	Abnormal concretion of mineral salts, often called a stone
Carcinoma	Malignant new growth composed of epithelial cells
Bladder	Carcinoma located in the bladder
Renal cell	Carcinoma located in the kidney
Congenital anomaly	Abnormality present at birth
Duplicate collecting system	Two renal pelves or ureters from the same kidney
Horseshoe kidney	Fusion of the kidneys, usually at the lower poles
Pelvic kidney	Kidney that fails to ascend and remains in the pelvis
Cystitis	Inflammation of the bladder
Fistula	Abnormal connection between two internal organs or between an organ and the body surface
Glomerulonephritis	Inflammation of the capillary loops in the glomeruli of the kidney
Hydronephrosis	Distention of renal pelvis and calyces with urine
Nephroptosis	Excessive inferior displacement of the kidneys or kidney prolapse
Phleboliths	Pelvic vein calcifications
Polycystic kidney	Massive enlargement of the kidney with the formation of many cysts
Pyelonephritis	Inflammation of the kidney and renal pelvis
Renal hypertension	Increased blood pressure to the kidneys
Renal obstruction	Condition preventing normal flow of urine through the urinary system
Stenosis	Narrowing or contraction of a passage
Tumor	New tissue growth where cell proliferation is uncontrolled
Wilms	Most common pediatric abdominal neoplasm affecting the kidney
Ureterocele	Ballooning of the lower end of the ureter into the bladder
Vesicoureteral reflux	Backward flow of urine from the bladder into the ureters

SAMPLE EXPOSURE TECHNIQUE CHART ESSENTIAL PROJECTIONS

These techniques were accurate for the equipment used to produce each exposure. However, use caution when applying them in your department because generator output characteristics and IR energy sensitivities vary widely.[1]

This chart was created in collaboration with Dennis Bowman, AS, RT(R), Clinical Instructor, Community Hospital of the Monterey Peninsula, Monterey, CA. http://digitalradiographysolutions.com/

URINARY SYSTEM

Part	cm	kVp*	SID†	Collimation	CR‡ mAs	CR‡ Dose (mGy)‖	DR§ mAs	DR§ Dose (mGy)‖
Urinary system (urography)								
AP¶	21	80	40″	14″ × 17″ (35 × 43 cm)	40**	5.480	16**	2.188
AP oblique¶	24	80	40″	14″ × 17″ (35 × 43 cm)	56**	8.250	25**	3.660
Lateral¶	27	80	40″	12″ × 17″ (30 × 43 cm)	100**	15.89	40**	6.320
Urinary bladder								
AP and PA axial¶	18	80	40″	9″ × 9″ (23 × 23 cm)	56**	6.790	22**	2.670
AP oblique¶	21	80	40″	9″ × 9″ (23 × 23 cm)	65**	8.510	28**	3.660
Lateral¶	31	85	40″	8″ × 9″ (20 × 23 cm)	110**	20.41	45**	8.300

[1]ACR-AAPM-SIMM Practice Guidelines for Digital Radiography, 2007.
*kVp values are for a high-frequency generator.
†40 inch minimum; 44 to 48 inches recommended to improve spatial resolution (mAs increase needed, but no increase in patient dose will result).
‡AGFA CR MD 4.0 General IP, CR 75.0 reader, 400 speed class, with 6:1 (178LPI) grid when needed.
§GE Definium 8000, with 13:1 grid when needed.
‖All doses are skin entrance for an average adult (160 to 200 pound male, 150 to 190 pound female) at part thickness indicated.
¶Bucky/Grid.
**Large focal spot.

ABBREVIATIONS USED IN CHAPTER 18

ACR	American College of Radiology
ASRT	American Society of Radiologic Technologists
BPH	Benign prostatic hyperplasia
BUN	Blood urea nitrogen
CDC	U.S. Centers for Disease Control and Prevention
GFR	Glomerular filtration rate
IV	Intravenous
IVP	Intravenous pyelogram
UPJ	Ureteropelvic junction
VCUG	Voiding cystourethrogram

See Addendum B for a summary of all abbreviations used in Volume 2.

Prostate

Overview

Radiographic examination of the urinary system involves the use of a water-soluble iodinated contrast medium to allow visualization of the pertinent anatomy and, frequently, to evaluate physiologic function. The role of radiography in evaluation of the urinary system has changed because of the increased use of multiplanar imaging modalities such as computed tomography (CT), magnetic resonance imaging (MRI), and ultrasonography (US). Multidetector CT, with three-dimensional reconstruction capabilities, has improved visualization of small pathologies that were difficult or impossible to see on radiographic images. Despite the decreased use of contrast urography, the American College of Radiology (ACR) specifies that excretory urography is particularly useful in demonstrating the collecting system and ureters and in evaluating ureteral obstruction, compression, and displacement. Additionally, contrast urography can be tailored to provide diagnostic information at a lower radiation dose than can be provided by helical multidetector CT.[1]

[1]*ACR Practice Guideline for the Performance of Excretory Urography, revised 2009.*

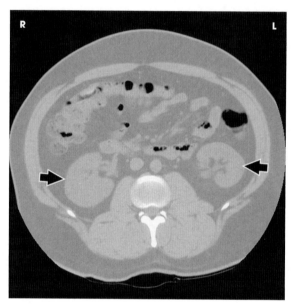

Fig. 18-8 CT of abdomen without contrast media showing parenchyma and renal pelvis of both kidneys (*arrows*).

(Courtesy Karl Mockler, RT(R).)

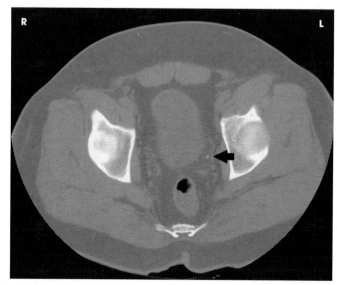

Fig. 18-9 CT "stone protocol" without contrast media showing renal calculus in left distal ureter (*arrow*).

(Courtesy Karl Mockler, RT(R).)

The specialized radiography procedures are preceded by a plain, or scout, image of the abdominopelvic areas for detection of abnormalities that can be shown on plain radiography. The preliminary examination may consist of only a KUB. Oblique or lateral projections, or both, may be obtained to localize calcifications, such as urinary calculi or phleboliths, and tumor masses. An upright position may be used to show the mobility of the kidneys and to demonstrate nephroptosis.

Preliminary radiography can usually show the position and mobility of the kidneys and usually their size and shape because of the contrast furnished by the radiolucent fatty capsule surrounding the kidneys. In addition, properly selected CT soft tissue windows can show the renal parenchyma without contrast media (Fig. 18-8). Visualization of the thin-walled drainage, or collecting, system (calyces and pelves, ureters, urinary bladder, and urethra) requires that the canals be filled with a contrast medium. The urinary bladder is outlined when it is filled with urine, but it is not adequately shown. The ureters and the urethra cannot be distinguished on preliminary images. A CT "stone protocol" without contrast medium can clearly show calcified renal stones (Fig. 18-9).

CONTRAST STUDIES

To delineate and differentiate cysts and tumor masses situated within the kidney, the renal parenchyma is opacified by an intravenously introduced organic, iodinated contrast medium and then radiographed by tomography (Fig. 18-10) or CT (Fig. 18-11). The contrast solution may be introduced into the vein by rapid bolus injection or by infusion.

Angiographic procedures are used to investigate the blood vessels of the kidneys and the suprarenal glands (see Chapter 23, Volume 3). An example of the direct injection of contrast medium into the renal artery is shown in Fig. 18-12.

Radiologic investigations of the renal drainage, or collecting, system are performed by various procedures classified under the general term *urography*. This term embraces two regularly used techniques for filling the urinary canals with a contrast medium. Imaging of cutaneous urinary diversions has been described by Long.[1]

[1]Long BW: Radiography of cutaneous urinary diversions, *Radiol Technol* 60:109, 1988.

Urinary System and Venipuncture

Antegrade filling

Antegrade filling techniques allow the contrast medium to enter the kidney in the normal direction of blood flow. In selective patients, this is done by introducing the contrast material directly into the kidney through a percutaneous puncture of the renal pelvis—a technique called *percutaneous antegrade urography.* Much more commonly used is the physiologic technique, in which the contrast agent is generally administered intravenously. This technique is called *excretory* or *intravenous urography* (EU or IVU) and is shown in Fig. 18-13.

IVU is used in examinations of the upper urinary tract in infants and children and is generally considered to be the preferred technique in adults unless use of the retrograde technique is definitely indicated. Because the contrast medium is administered intravenously and all parts of the urinary system are normally shown, the excretory technique is correctly referred to as IVU. The term *pyelography* refers to the radiographic demonstration of the renal pelves and calyces. This examination has been erroneously called an intravenous pyelogram (IVP).

After the opaque contrast medium enters the bloodstream, it is conveyed to the renal glomeruli and is discharged into the capsules with the glomerular filtrate, which is excreted as urine. With the reabsorption of water, the contrast material becomes sufficiently concentrated to render the urinary canals radiopaque. The urinary bladder is well outlined by this technique, and satisfactory voiding urethrograms may be obtained.

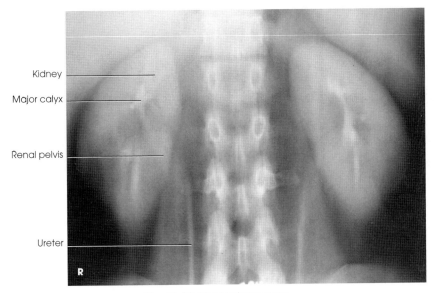

Kidney

Major calyx

Renal pelvis

Ureter

Fig. 18-10 Nephrotomogram.

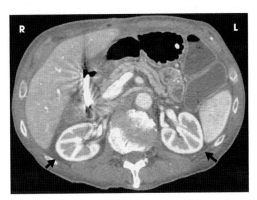

Fig. 18-11 CT image of abdomen with contrast media showing early filling of both kidneys (*arrows*).

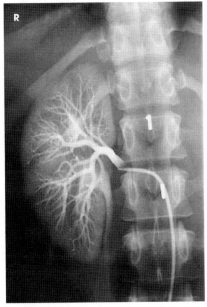

Fig. 18-12 Selective right renal arteriogram.

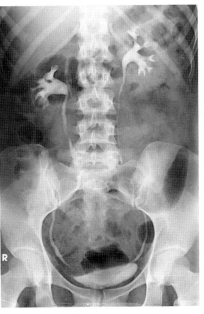

Fig. 18-13 Excretory urogram.

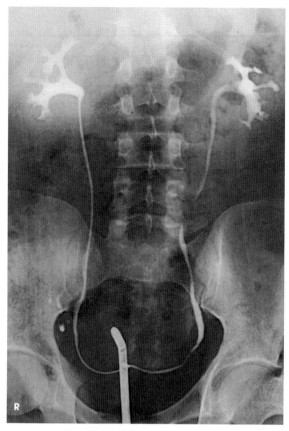

Fig. 18-14 Retrograde urogram.

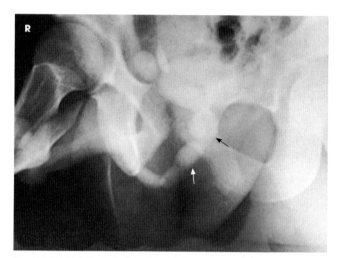

Fig. 18-15 Voiding study after routine injection IVU. Dilation of proximal urethra (*arrows*) is the result of urethral stricture.

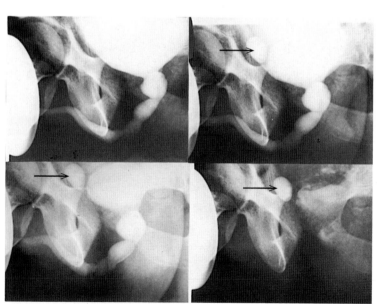

Fig. 18-16 Voiding studies of same patient as in Fig. 18-15 after infusion nephrourography. Note increase in opacification of contrast medium–filled cavities by this method and bladder diverticulum (*arrows*).

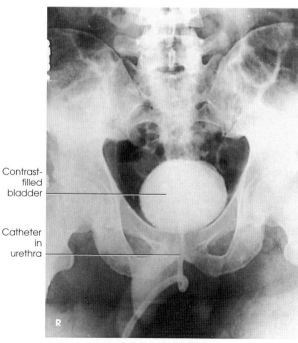

Contrast-filled bladder

Catheter in urethra

Fig. 18-17 Cystogram.

Retrograde filling

In some procedures involving the urinary system, the contrast material is introduced against the normal flow. This is called *retrograde urography* (Fig. 18-14). The contrast medium is injected directly into the canals via ureteral catheterization for contrast filling of the upper urinary tract and via urethral catheterization for contrast filling of the lower part of the urinary tract. Cystoscopy is required to localize the vesicoureteral orifices for the passage of ureteral catheters.

Retrograde urographic examination of the proximal urinary tract is primarily a urologic procedure. Catheterization and contrast filling of the urinary canals are performed by the attending urologist in conjunction with a physical or endoscopic examination. This technique enables the urologist to obtain catheterized specimens of urine directly from each renal pelvis. Because the canals can be fully distended by direct injection of the contrast agent, the retrograde urographic examination sometimes provides more information about the anatomy of the different parts of the collecting system than can be obtained by the excretory technique. For the retrograde procedure, an evaluation of kidney function depends on an intravenously administered dye substance to stain the color of the urine that subsequently trickles through the respective ureteral catheters. The antegrade and retrograde techniques of examination are occasionally required for a complete urologic study.

Investigations of the lower urinary tract—bladder, lower ureters, and urethra—are usually done by the retrograde technique, which requires no instrumentation beyond passage of a urethral catheter. Investigations may also be done by the physiologic technique (Figs. 18-15 and 18-16). Bladder examinations are usually denoted by the general term *cystography* (Fig. 18-17). A procedure that includes inspection of the lower ureters is *cystoureterography* (Fig. 18-18), and a procedure that includes inspection of the urethra is *cystourethrography* (Fig. 18-19).

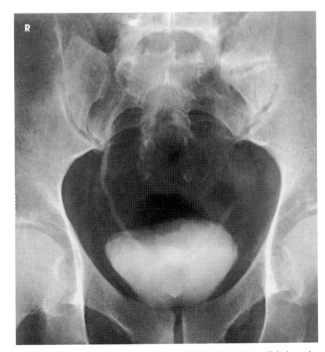

Fig. 18-18 Cystoureterogram: AP bladder showing distal ureters.

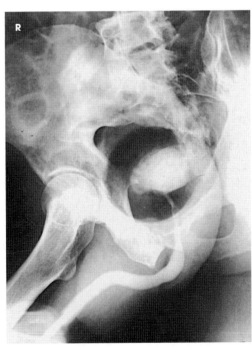

Fig. 18-19 Injection cystourethrogram showing urethra in a male patient.

Contrast media

Retrograde urography (Figs. 18-20 and 18-21) was first performed in 1904 with the introduction of air into the urinary bladder. In 1906, retrograde urography and cystography were performed with the first opaque medium, a colloidal silver preparation that is no longer used. Silver iodide, which is a nontoxic inorganic compound, was introduced in 1911. Sodium iodide and sodium bromide, also inorganic compounds, were first used for retrograde urography in 1918. The bromides and iodides are no longer widely used for examinations of the renal pelves and ureters because they irritate the mucosa and commonly cause considerable patient discomfort.

Because a large quantity of solution is required to fill the urinary bladder, iodinated salts in concentrations of 30% or less are used in cystography. A large selection of commercially available contrast media may be used for all types of radiographic examinations of the urinary system. It is important to review the product insert packaged with every contrast agent.

Excretory urography (Figs. 18-22 and 18-23) was first reported by Rowntree et al. in 1923.[1] These investigators used a 10% solution of chemically pure sodium iodide as the contrast medium. This agent was excreted too slowly, however, to show the renal pelves and ureters satisfactorily, and it proved too toxic for functional distribution. Early in 1929, Roseno and Jepkins[2] introduced a compound containing sodium iodide and urea. The latter constituent, which is one of the nitrogenous substances removed from the blood and eliminated by the kidneys, served to accelerate excretion and to fill the renal pelves with opacified urine quickly. Although satisfactory renal images were obtained with this compound, patients experienced considerable distress as a result of its toxicity.

---

[1]Rowntree LG et al: Roentgenography of the urinary tract during excretion of sodium iodide, *JAMA* 8:368, 1923.
[2]Roseno A, Jepkins H: Intravenous pyelography, *Fortschr Roentgenstr* 39:859, 1929. Abstract: *AJR Am J Roentgenol* 22:685, 1929.

In 1929, Swick developed the organic compound Uroselectan, which had an iodine content of 42%. Present-day ionic contrast media for excretory urography are the result of extensive research by many investigators. These media are available under various trade names in concentrations ranging from approximately 50% to 70%. Sterile solutions of the media are supplied in dose-size ampules or vials.

In the early 1970s, research was initiated to develop nonionic contrast media. Development progressed, and several nonionic contrast agents are currently available for urographic, vascular, and intrathecal injection. Although nonionic contrast media are less likely to cause a reaction in the patient, they are twice as expensive as ionic agents.

Many institutions have developed criteria to determine which patient receives which contrast medium. The choice of whether to use an ionic or nonionic contrast medium depends on patient risk and economics.

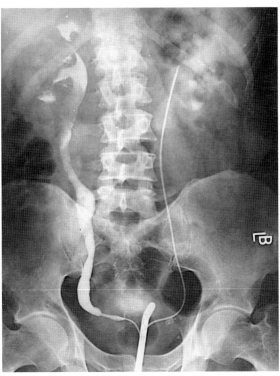

Fig. 18-20 Retrograde urogram with contrast medium–filled right renal pelvis and catheter in left renal pelvis.

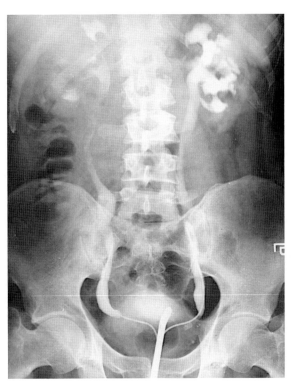

Fig. 18-21 Retrograde urogram.

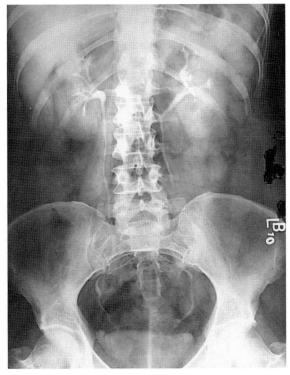

Fig. 18-22 Excretory urogram, 10 minutes after injection of contrast medium.

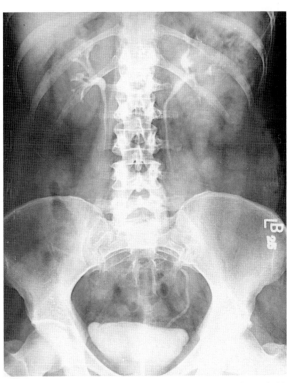

Fig. 18-23 Excretory urogram on same patient as in Fig. 18-22, 25 minutes after contrast medium injection.

Adverse reactions to iodinated media

The iodinated organic preparations that are compounded for urologic examinations are of low toxicity. Consequently, adverse reactions are usually mild and of short duration. Common reactions include a feeling of warmth and flushing. Occasionally, nausea, vomiting, a few hives, and edema of the respiratory mucous membrane result. Severe and serious reactions occur only rarely but are always a possibility. The clinical history of each patient must be carefully checked, and the patient must be kept under careful observation for any sign of systemic reactions. According to the 2013 version of the American College of Radiology (ACR) Manual on Contrast Media, "nearly all life-threatening contrast reactions occur within the first 20 minutes after contrast medium injection." The patient should not be left unattended during this time period. Emergency equipment and medication (diphenhydramine, epinephrine) to treat adverse reactions must be readily available. The ACR additionally states that the radiologist, or his or her qualified designee, who is on-site during the procedure must be prepared and able to treat these reactions.

Preparation of intestinal tract

Although unobstructed visualization of the urinary tracts requires that the intestinal tract be free of gas and solid fecal material (Fig. 18-24), bowel preparation is not attempted in infants and children. Use of cleansing measures in adults depends on the condition of the patient. Gas (particularly swallowed air, which is quickly dispersed through the small bowel) rather than fecal material usually interferes with the examination.

Hope and Campoy[1] recommended that infants and children be given a carbonated soft drink to distend the stomach with gas. By this maneuver, the gas-containing intestinal loops are usually pushed inferiorly, and the upper urinary tracts, particularly on the left side of the body, are clearly visualized through the outline of the gas-filled stomach. Hope and Campoy stated that the aerated drink should be given in an amount adequate to inflate the stomach fully: at least 2 oz. is required for a newborn infant, and 12 oz. is required for a 7-year-old child. In conjunction with the carbonated drink, Hope and Campoy recommended using a highly concentrated contrast medium. A gas-distended stomach is shown in Fig. 18-25.

---

[1]Hope JW, Campoy F: The use of carbonated beverages in pediatric excretory urography, *Radiology* 64:66, 1955.

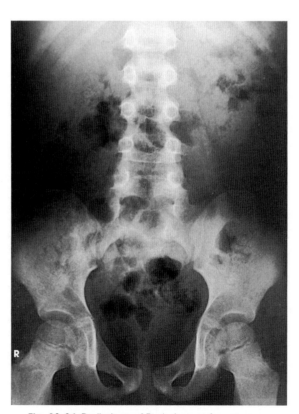

Fig. 18-24 Preliminary AP abdomen for urogram.

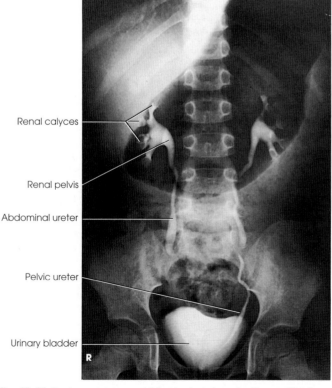

Renal calyces

Renal pelvis

Abdominal ureter

Pelvic ureter

Urinary bladder

Fig. 18-25 Supine urogram at 15-minute interval with gas-filled stomach.

Berdon et al.[2] stated that the prone position resolves the problem of obscuring gas in most patients (Figs. 18-26 and 18-27). It is unnecessary to inflate the stomach with air alone or with air as part of an aerated drink. By exerting pressure on the abdomen, the prone position moves the gas laterally away from the pelvicaliceal structures. Gas in the antral portion of the stomach is displaced into its fundic portion, gas in the transverse colon shifts into the ascending and descending segments, and gas in the sigmoid colon shifts into the descending colon and rectum. These investigators noted, however, that the prone position occasionally fails to produce the desired result in small infants when the small intestine is dilated. Gastric inflation also fails in these patients because the dilated small intestine merely elevates the gas-filled stomach and does not improve visualization. They recommended examination of such infants *after* the intestinal gas has passed.

[2]Berdon WE et al: Prone radiography in intravenous pyelography in infants and children, *AJR Am J Roentgenol* 103:444, 1968.

Preparation of patient

Medical opinion concerning patient preparation varies widely. With modifications as required, the following procedure seems to be in general use:

- When time permits, have the patient follow a low-residue diet for 1 to 2 days to prevent gas formation caused by excessive fermentation of the intestinal contents.
- Have the patient eat a light evening meal on the day before the examination.
- When indicated by costive bowel action, administer a non–gas-forming laxative the evening before the examination.
- Have the patient take nothing by mouth after midnight on the day of the examination. The patient should not be dehydrated, however. Patients with multiple myeloma, high uric acid levels, or diabetes must be well hydrated before IVU is performed; these patients are at increased risk for contrast medium–induced renal failure if they are dehydrated.

- In preparation for *retrograde urography,* have the patient drink a large amount of water (4 or 5 cups) several hours before the examination to ensure excretion of urine in an amount sufficient for bilateral catheterized specimens and renal function tests.
- No patient preparation is usually necessary for examination of the lower urinary tract.

Outpatients should be given explicit directions regarding any order from the physician pertaining to diet, fluid intake, and laxatives or other medication. The patient should also be given a suitable explanation for each preparative measure to ensure cooperation.

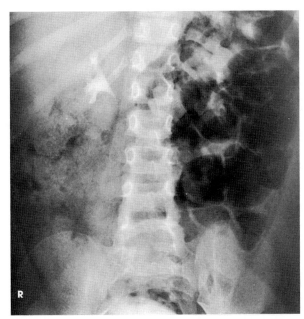

Fig. 18-26 Urogram: supine position. Intestinal gas obscuring left kidney.

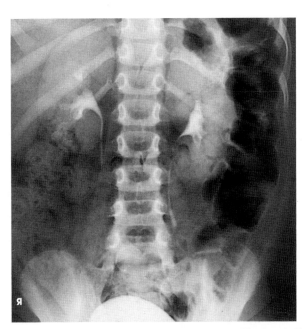

Fig. 18-27 Urogram: prone position, in the same patient as in Fig. 18-26. Visualization of left kidney and ureter is markedly improved.

EQUIPMENT

Any standard radiographic table is suitable to perform preliminary excretory urography and most retrograde studies of the bladder and urethra. A combination cystoscopic-radiographic unit facilitates retrograde urographic procedures requiring cystoscopy. The cystoscopic unit is also used for IVU and retrograde bladder and urethra studies; however, for the patient's comfort, the table should have an extensible leg rest.

Infusion nephrourography requires a table equipped with tomographic apparatus. Tomography should be performed when intestinal gas obscures some of the underlying structures, or when hypersthenic patients are being examined (Figs. 18-28 to 18-30).

For the patient's comfort and to prevent delays during the examination, all preparations for the examination should be completed before the patient is placed on the table. In addition to an identification and side marker, excretory urographic studies require a time interval marker for each postinjection study. Body position markers (supine, prone, upright or semi-upright, Trendelenburg, decubitus) should also be used.

Some institutions perform excretory urograms (proximal urinary tract studies) using a 10 × 12-inch (24 × 30-cm) IR placed crosswise, but these studies can also be made on 14 × 17-inch (35 × 43-cm) IRs placed lengthwise. The upright study is made on a 14 × 17-inch (35 × 43-cm) IR because it is taken to show the mobility of the kidneys, to demonstrate nephroptosis, and to outline the lower ureters and bladder. Studies of the bladder before and after voiding are usually taken on 10 × 12-inch (24 × 30-cm) IRs.

The following guidelines are observed in preparing additional equipment for the examination:

- Have an emergency cart fully equipped and conveniently placed.
- Arrange the instruments for injection of the contrast agent on a small, movable table or on a tray.
- Have frequently used sterile items readily available. Disposable syringes and needles are available in standard sizes and are widely used in this procedure.
- Have required nonsterile items available: a tourniquet, a small waste basin, an emesis basin, general disposable wipes, one or two bottles of contrast medium, and a small prepared dressing for application to the puncture site.
- Have iodine or alcohol wipes available.
- Provide a folded towel or a small pillow that can be placed under the patient's elbow to relieve pressure during the injection.

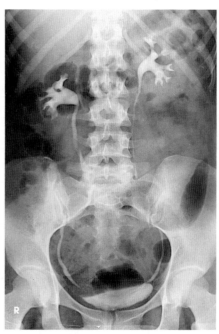

Fig. 18-28 Urogram: AP projection.

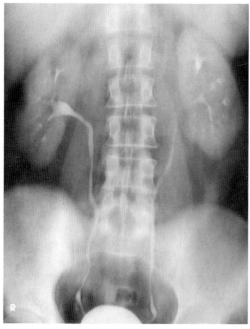

Fig. 18-29 Urogram: AP projection using tomography.

PROCEDURE

Image quality and exposure technique

Urograms should have the same contrast, density, and degree of soft tissue density as abdominal images. The images must show a sharply defined outline of the kidneys, lower border of the liver, and lateral margin of the psoas muscles. The amount of bone detail visible in these studies varies according to the thickness of the abdomen (Fig. 18-31).

Motion control

An immobilization band usually is not applied over the upper abdomen in urographic examinations because the resultant pressure may interfere with the passage of fluid through the ureters and may cause distortion of the canals. The elimination of motion in urographic examinations depends on exposure time and on securing the full cooperation of the patient.

The examination procedure should be explained so that the adult patient is prepared for any transitory distress caused by injection of contrast solution or by the cystoscopic procedure. The patient should be assured that everything possible will be done for the patient's comfort. The success of the examination depends in large part on the ability of the radiographer to gain the confidence of the patient.

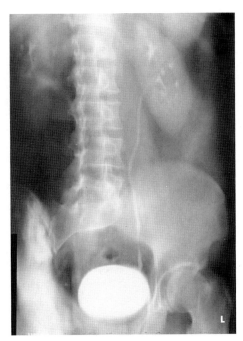

Fig. 18-30 Urogram: AP oblique projection, LPO position, using tomography. Note that left kidney is perpendicular to IR.

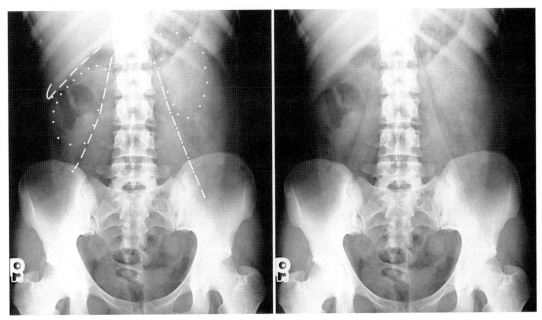

Fig. 18-31 AP abdomen showing margins of kidney (*dots*), liver (*dashes*), and psoas muscles (*dot-dash lines*).

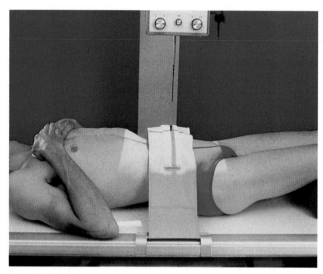

Fig. 18-32 Ureteral compression device in place for urogram.

Ureteral compression

In excretory urography, compression is sometimes applied over the distal ends of the ureters. This compression is applied to retard flow of the opacified urine into the bladder and to ensure adequate filling of the renal pelves and calyces. If compression is used, it must be placed so that the pressure over the distal ends of the ureters is centered at the level of the anterior superior iliac spine (ASIS). As much pressure as the patient can comfortably tolerate is applied with the immobilization band (Figs. 18-32 and 18-33). This pressure should be released slowly when the compression device is removed to reduce pain caused by rapid changes in intra-abdominal pressure. Compression is generally contraindicated if a patient has urinary stones, an abdominal mass or aneurysm, a colostomy, a suprapubic catheter, traumatic injury, or recent abdominal surgery.

As a result of improvements in contrast agents, ureteral compression is not routinely used in most health care facilities. With the increased doses of contrast medium now employed, most of the ureteral area is usually shown over a series of images. In addition, a prone image is an adequate substitute for ureteral compression for filling the pyelocalyceal system and mid-ureters.

Respiration

For purposes of comparison, all exposures are made at the end of the same phase of breathing—at the *end of expiration* unless otherwise requested. Because the normal respiratory excursion of the kidneys varies from $\frac{1}{2}$ to $1\frac{1}{2}$ inches (1.3 to 3.8 cm), it is occasionally possible to differentiate renal shadows from other shadows by making an exposure at a different phase of arrested respiration. When an exposure is made at a respiratory phase different from what is usually used, the image should be so marked.

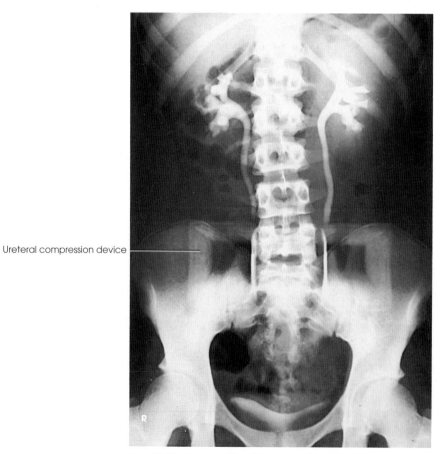

Ureteral compression device

Fig. 18-33 Urogram showing ureteral compression device in proper position over distal ureters.

PRELIMINARY EXAMINATION

A preliminary examination of the abdomen is made before a specialized investigation of the urinary tract is conducted. This examination sometimes reveals extrarenal lesions that are responsible for the symptoms attributed to the urinary tract and renders the urographic procedure unnecessary. An upright AP projection may also be required to show the mobility of the kidneys. An oblique or lateral projection, or both, in the dorsal decubitus position may be required to localize a tumor mass or to differentiate renal stones from gallstones or calcified mesenteric nodes.

The scout image—an AP projection with the patient recumbent—shows the contour of the kidneys; their location in the supine position; and the presence of renal calculi or calcifications outside the renal collecting system, such as phleboliths, which are small calcifications in the wall of pelvic veins (see Fig. 18-31). This image also serves to check the preparation of the gastrointestinal tract and to enable the radiographer to make any necessary alterations to exposure factors.

Radiation Protection

It is the responsibility of the radiographer to observe the following guidelines concerning radiation protection:

- Apply a gonadal shield if it does not overlap the area under investigation.
- Restrict radiation to the area of interest by close collimation.
- Work carefully so that repeat exposures are unnecessary.

- Shield males for all examinations except examinations of the urethra by using a shadow shield or by placing a piece of lead just below the pubic symphysis.
- When excretory urography IRs are centered to the kidneys, place lead over the female pelvis for shielding. Unless the procedure is considered an emergency, perform radiography of the abdomen and pelvis only if there is no chance of patient pregnancy. For most projections in this chapter, females generally cannot be shielded without obscuring a portion of the urinary system. (Gonad shielding is not shown on the patient images in this atlas for illustrative purposes.) Carefully follow department guidelines regarding gonad shielding.

Intravenous Urography

IVU shows the function and structure of the urinary system. *Function* is shown by the ability of the kidneys to filter contrast medium from the blood and concentrate it with the urine. Anatomic *structures* are usually visualized as the contrast material follows the excretion route of the urine. The primary application of IVU is to evaluate the suspected or continued presence of ureteral obstruction.

The *ACR Practice Guideline for the Performance of Excretory Urography* (2009) emphasizes that an evaluation of the merits and availability of cross-sectional imaging modalities should be performed before IVU is performed. Indications for IVU include, but are not limited to, the following:

- Evaluation of abdominal masses, renal cysts, and renal tumors
- Urolithiasis—calculi or stones of the kidneys or urinary tract
- Pyelonephritis—infection of the upper urinary tract, which can be acute or chronic
- Hydronephrosis—abnormal dilation of the pelvicaliceal system (urography is used to help determine the cause of the dilation)
- Assessment of the effects of trauma and therapeutic interventions
- Preoperative evaluation of the function, location, size, and shape of the kidneys and ureters
- Renal hypertension (urography is commonly performed to evaluate functional symmetry of the renal collecting systems)

The most common contraindications for IVU relate to (1) the ability of the kidneys to filter contrast medium from the blood and (2) the patient's allergic history. Some contraindications can be overcome by the use of nonionic contrast agents. Patients with conditions in which the kidneys are unable to filter waste or excrete urine (renal failure, anuria) should have the kidneys evaluated by some technique other than excretory urography. Older patients and patients with any of the following risk factors are strong candidates to receive a nonionic contrast medium or should be examined using another modality: asthma, previous contrast media reaction, circulatory or cardiovascular disease, elevated creatinine level, sickle cell disease, diabetes mellitus, or multiple myeloma.

RADIOGRAPHIC PROCEDURE

Before the procedure begins, the patient should be instructed to empty the bladder and change into an appropriate radiolucent gown. Emptying the bladder prevents dilution of the contrast medium with urine. The patient's clinical history, allergic history, and blood creatinine levels should be reviewed. The normal creatinine level is 0.6 to 1.2 mg/100 mL. The glomerular filtration rate (GFR), a calculation that uses the creatinine level (plus age, race, gender, and body size), is the best overall index of kidney function. The National Kidney Foundation considers a normal GFR range to be 120 to 125 mL/min and a value of 90 mL/min or less as an indicator of renal dysfunction. A below-normal GFR should be reviewed by the radiologist or the physician before the contrast media procedure is continued. The radiographer then takes the following steps:

- Place the patient on the table in the supine position, and adjust the patient to center the midsagittal plane of the body to the midline of the grid.
- Place a support under the patient's knees to reduce the lordotic curvature of the lumbar spine and to provide greater comfort for the patient (Fig. 18-34).

- Attach the footboard in preparation for a possible upright or semi-upright position.
- If the head of the table is to be lowered farther to enhance pelvicaliceal filling, attach the shoulder support and adjust it to the patient's height.
- When ureteric compression is to be used, place the compression device so that it is ready for immediate application at the specified time.
- Obtain a preliminary, or scout, image of the abdomen. Then prepare for the first postinjection exposure before the contrast medium is injected.
- Place the IR in the Bucky tray; position identification, side, and time interval markers; and make any change in centering or exposure technique as indicated by the scout image.
- Have ready a folded towel or other suitable support and the tourniquet for placement under the selected elbow.
- Prepare the contrast medium for injection using aseptic technique.
- According to the preference of the examining physician, administer 30 to 100 mL of the contrast medium to an adult patient of average size. The dose administered to infants and children is regulated according to age and weight.

- Produce images at specified intervals from the time of *completion of the injection* of contrast medium. (This may depend on the protocol of the department.) These time intervals must be included on each image. Depending on the patient's hydration status and the speed of the injection, the contrast agent normally begins to appear in the pelvicaliceal system within 2 to 8 minutes.

Uptake of contrast medium is seen in the nephrons of the kidney if an image is exposed as the kidneys start to filter the contrast medium from the blood. The initial contrast "blush" of the kidney is termed the *nephrogram phase*. Nephrotomography, if a component of the routine IVU procedure, is usually performed during the nephrogram phase. As the kidneys continue to filter and concentrate the contrast medium, it is directed to the pelvicaliceal system. The greatest concentration of contrast medium in the kidneys normally occurs 15 to 20 minutes after injection. Immediately after each IR is exposed, it is processed and reviewed to determine, according to the kidney function of the individual patient, the time intervals at which the most intense kidney image can be obtained.

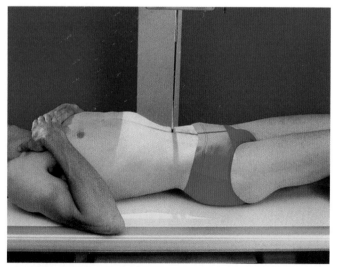

Fig. 18-34 Patient in supine position for urogram, AP projection. Note support under knees.

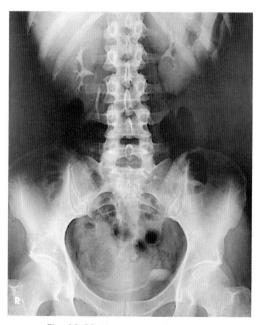

Fig. 18-35 Urogram at 3 minutes.

The most commonly recommended radiographic images for IVU are AP projections at time intervals ranging from 3 to 20 minutes (Figs. 18-35 to 18-37). Some physicians prefer bolus injection of the contrast medium followed by a 30-second image to obtain a nephrogram. AP oblique projections (30-degree) may be taken at 5- to 10-minute intervals. In some patients, supplemental images are required to show better all parts of the urinary system and to differentiate normal anatomy from pathologic conditions. These may include an AP projection with the patient in the Trendelenburg or upright position, oblique or lateral projections, or a lateral projection with the patient in the dorsal or ventral decubitus position.

Unless further study of the bladder is indicated or voiding urethrograms are to be made, the patient is sent to the lavatory to void. A postvoid image of the bladder (Figs. 18-38 and 18-39) may be taken to detect, by the presence of residual urine, conditions such as small tumor masses or enlargement of the prostate gland in men. When all necessary images have been obtained, the patient is released from the imaging department. Any contrast medium remaining in the body is filtered from the blood by the kidneys and eventually is excreted in the urine. Some physicians suggest having the patient drink extra fluids for a few days to help flush out the contrast medium.

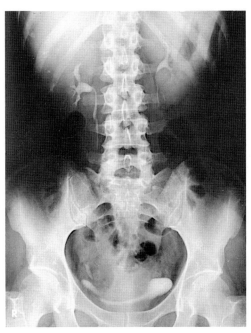

Fig. 18-36 Urogram at 6 minutes.

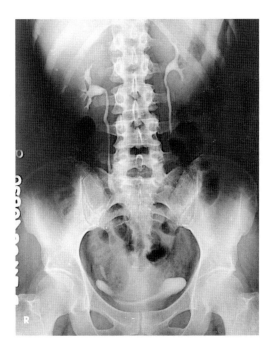

Fig. 18-37 Urogram at 9 minutes.

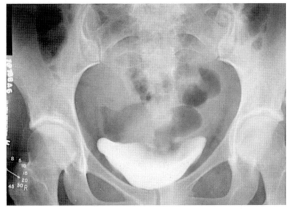

Fig. 18-38 Prevoiding filled bladder.

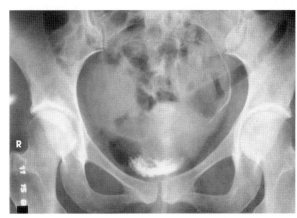

Fig. 18-39 Postvoiding emptied bladder.

▲ AP PROJECTION

Image receptor: 14 × 17 inch (35 × 43 cm) lengthwise

Position of patient
- Place the patient supine on the radiographic table for the AP projection of the urinary system. Preliminary (scout) and postinjection images are most commonly obtained with the patient supine (Fig. 18-40).
- Place a support under the patient's knees to relieve strain on the back.
- Place the patient in an upright or a semi-upright position for an AP projection to show the opacified bladder and the mobility of the kidneys (Fig. 18-41).

- To show the lower ends of the ureters, it may be helpful to use the Trendelenburg position and an AP projection with the head of the table lowered 15 to 20 degrees and the central ray directed perpendicular to the IR. In this angled position, the weight of the contained fluid stretches the bladder fundus superiorly, providing an unobstructed image of the lower ureters and the vesicoureteral orifice areas.
- If needed, apply ureteral compression (see Fig. 18-32).

Position of part
- Center the midsagittal plane of the patient's body to the midline of the grid device.
- Place the patient's arms out of the collimated field.
- Center the IR at the level of the iliac crests. If the patient is too tall to include the entire urinary system, take a second exposure on a 10 × 12-inch (24 × 30-cm) IR centered to the bladder. The 10 × 12-inch (24 × 30-cm) IR is placed crosswise and centered 2 to 3 inches (5 to 7.6 cm) above the upper border of the pubic symphysis.
- *Shield gonads.*
- *Respiration:* Suspend at the end of expiration.

Central ray
- Perpendicular to the IR at the level of the iliac crests

Collimation
- Adjust to 14 × 17 inches (35 × 43 cm) on the collimator.

Structures shown
AP projection of the urinary system shows the kidneys, ureters, and bladder filled with contrast medium (Figs. 18-42 to 18-44).

NOTE: The prone position may be recommended to show the ureteropelvic region and to fill the obstructed ureter in the presence of hydronephrosis. The ureters fill better in the prone position, which reverses the curve of their inferior course. The kidneys are situated obliquely, slanting anteriorly in the transverse plane, so the opacified urine tends to collect in and distend the dependent part of the pelvicaliceal system. The supine position allows the more posteriorly placed upper calyces to fill more readily, and the anterior and inferior parts of the pelvicaliceal system fill more easily in the prone position.

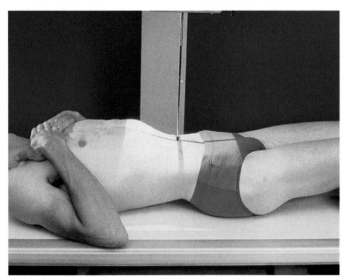

Fig. 18-40 Supine urogram: AP projection.

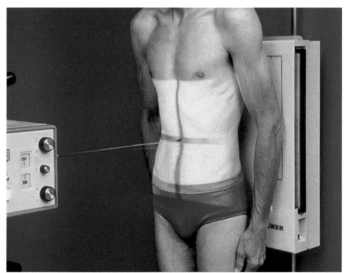

Fig. 18-41 Upright urogram: AP projection.

EVALUATION CRITERIA

The following should be clearly shown:
- Evidence of proper collimation

AP and PA Projections

- Entire renal outlines
- Bladder and pubic symphysis (a separate image of the bladder area is needed if the bladder was not included)
- No motion
- Exposure technique clearly showing contrast medium in the renal area, ureters, and bladder
- Compression devices, if used, centered over the upper sacrum and resulting in good renal filling
- Vertebral column centered on the image
- No artifacts from elastic in the patient's underclothing
- Prostatic region inferior to the pubic symphysis on older male patients
- Time marker
- PA projection showing the lower kidneys and entire ureters (bladder included if patient size permits)
- Superimposing intestinal gas in the AP projection moved for the PA projection

AP Bladder

- Bladder
- No rotation of the pelvis
- Prostate area in male patients
- Postvoid images clearly labeled and showing only residual contrast medium

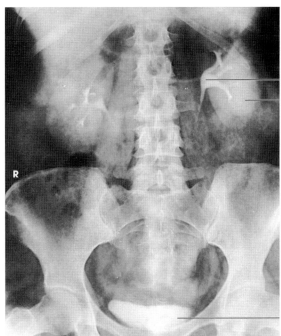

Fig. 18-42 Semi-upright urogram: AP projection. Note mobility of kidneys.

Renal pelvis
Left kidney
Bladder

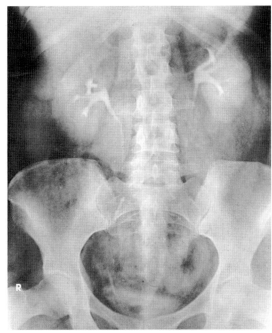

Fig. 18-43 Supine urogram: AP projection.

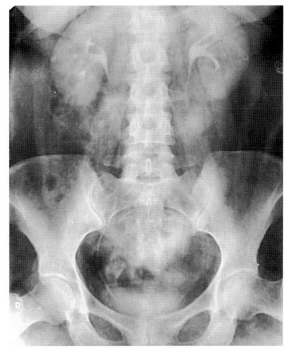

Fig. 18-44 Trendelenburg position urogram: AP projection.

⚜ AP OBLIQUE PROJECTION
RPO and LPO positions

Image receptor: 14 × 17 inch (35 × 43 cm) lengthwise

Position of patient

- Place the patient supine on the radiographic table for oblique projections of the urinary system. The kidneys are situated obliquely, slanting anteriorly in the transverse plane.
- When performing AP oblique projections, remember that the kidney closer to the IR is *perpendicular* to the plane of the IR and the kidney farther from the IR is *parallel* with this plane.

Position of part

- Turn the patient so that the midcoronal plane forms an angle of 30 degrees from the IR plane.
- Adjust the patient's shoulders and hips so that they are in the same plane, and place suitable supports under the elevated side as needed.
- Place the arms so that they are not superimposed on the urinary system.
- Center the spine to the grid (Fig. 18-45).
- Center the IR at the level of the iliac crests.
- *Shield gonads.*
- *Respiration:* Suspend at the end of expiration.

Central ray

- Perpendicular to the center of the IR at the level of the iliac crests, entering approximately 2 inches (5 cm) lateral to the midline on the elevated side

Collimation

- Adjust to 14 × 17 inches (35 × 43 cm) on the collimator.

Structures shown

An AP oblique projection of the urinary system shows the kidneys, ureters, and bladder filled with contrast medium. The elevated kidney is parallel with the IR, and the down-side kidney is perpendicular with the IR (Fig. 18-46).

The following should be clearly shown:
- Evidence of proper collimation
- Patient rotated approximately 30 degrees
- No superimposition of the kidney remote from the IR on the vertebrae
- Entire down-side kidney
- Bladder and lower ureters on 14 × 17-inch (35 × 43-cm) IRs if patient size permits
- Exposure technique that shows the anatomy
- Time marker

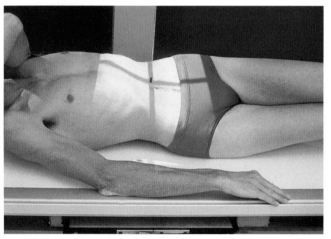

Fig. 18-45 Urogram: AP oblique projection, 30-degree RPO position.

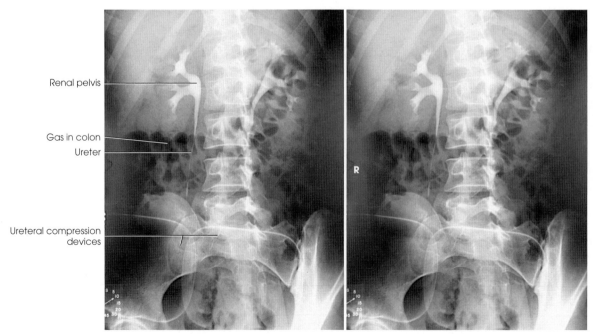

Renal pelvis

Gas in colon
Ureter

Ureteral compression devices

R

Fig. 18-46 Urogram at 10 minutes: AP oblique projection, RPO position.

⚜ LATERAL PROJECTION
R or L position

Image receptor: 14 × 17 inch (35 × 43 cm) lengthwise

Position of patient
- Turn the patient to a lateral recumbent position on the right or left side, as indicated.

Position of part
- Flex the patient's knees to a comfortable position, and adjust the body so that the midcoronal plane is centered to the midline of the grid.
- Place supports between the patient's knees and ankles.
- Flex the patient's elbows, and place the hands under the patient's head (Fig. 18-47).
- Center the IR at the level of the iliac crests.
- *Shield gonads.*
- *Respiration:* Suspend at the end of expiration.

Central ray
- Perpendicular to the IR, entering the midcoronal plane at the level of the iliac crest

Collimation
- Adjust to 14 × 17 inches (35 × 43 cm) on the collimator.

Structures shown
A lateral projection of the abdomen shows the kidneys, ureters, and bladder filled with contrast material. Lateral projections are used to show conditions such as rotation or pressure displacement of a kidney and to localize calcareous areas and tumor masses (Fig. 18-48).

EVALUATION CRITERIA
The following should be clearly shown:
- Evidence of proper collimation
- Entire urinary system
- Bladder and pubic symphysis
- Exposure technique clearly showing contrast medium in the renal area, ureters, and bladder
- No rotation of the patient (check pelvis and lumbar vertebrae)
- Time marker

Urinary System

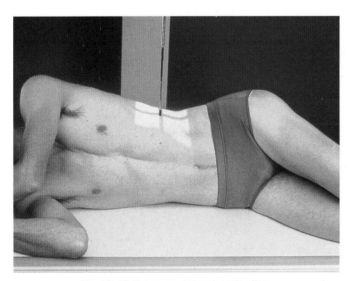

Fig. 18-47 Urogram: lateral projection.

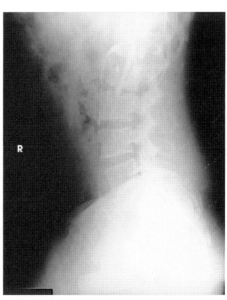

Fig. 18-48 Urogram: lateral projection.

⚕ LATERAL PROJECTION
Dorsal decubitus position

Image receptor: 14 × 17 inch (35 × 43 cm)

Position of patient
- Place the patient in the supine position on a radiographic cart with the side in question in contact with the vertical grid device. Ensure that the wheels are *locked.*
- Place the patient's arms across the upper chest to ensure that they are not projected over any abdominal contents, or place them behind the head.
- Flex the patient's knees slightly to relieve strain on the back.

Position of part
- Adjust the height of the vertical grid device so that the long axis of the IR is centered to the midcoronal plane of the patient's body.
- Position the patient so that a point approximately at the level of the iliac crests is centered to the IR (Fig. 18-49).
- Adjust the patient to ensure that no rotation from the supine or prone position is present.
- *Shield gonads.*
- *Respiration:* Suspend at the end of expiration.

Central ray
- *Horizontal* and perpendicular to the center of the IR, entering the midcoronal plane at the level of the iliac crests

Collimation
- Adjust to 14 × 17 inches (35 × 43 cm) on the collimator.

Structures shown
Rolleston and Reay[1] recommended the ventral decubitus position to show the UPJ in the presence of hydronephrosis. Cook et al.[2] advocated this position to determine whether an extrarenal mass in the flank is intraperitoneal or extraperitoneal, and they stated that the position makes it easy to screen kidneys and ureters for abnormal anterior displacement (Fig. 18-50).

[1]Rolleston GL, Reay ER: The pelvi-ureteric junction, *Br J Radiol* 30:617, 1957.
[2]Cook IK et al: Determination of the normal position of the upper urinary tract in the lateral abdominal urogram, *Radiology* 99:499, 1971.

The following should be clearly shown:
- Evidence of proper collimation
- Entire urinary system
- Bladder and pubic symphysis
- Exposure technique clearly showing contrast medium in the renal area, ureters, and bladder
- No rotation of the patient (check pelvis and lumbar vertebrae)
- Time marker
- Patient elevated so that entire abdomen is visible

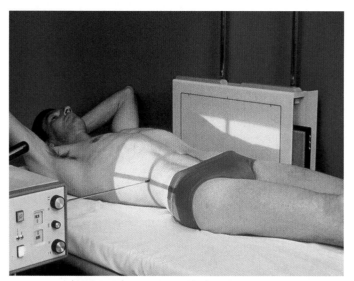

Fig. 18-49 Urogram: lateral projection, dorsal decubitus position.

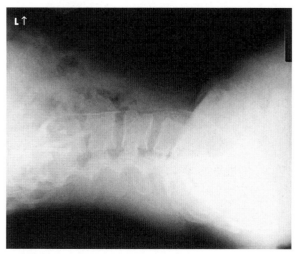

Fig. 18-50 Urogram: lateral projection, dorsal decubitus position.

Nephrotomography
AP PROJECTION

The renal parenchyma (nephrons and collecting tubes) is best visualized by performing tomography immediately after the introduction of contrast medium. Evans et al.,[1,2] who introduced nephrotomography, found that by using tomography rather than stationary projections, they could eliminate superimpositions of intestinal contents and more clearly define small intrarenal lesions.

Indications and contraindications

The use of nephrotomography has dramatically declined because of the availability of sectional imaging modalities with greater specificity for renal disease. The ACR states that "nephrotomography may be useful to help distinguish renal calculi from intestinal contents."[3] Contraindications are mainly related to renal failure and contrast media sensitivity, as noted for IVU.

[1]Evans JA et al: Nephrotomography, *AJR Am J Roentgenol* 71:213, 1954.
[2]Evans JA: Nephrotomography in the investigation of renal masses, *Radiology* 69:684, 1957.
[3]ACR Appropriateness Criteria: Acute onset flank pain—suspicious of stone disease. Retrieved on December 20, 2013, from http://www.acr.org/~/media/ACR/Documents/AppCriteria/Diagnostic/AcuteOnsetFlankPainSuspicionStoneDisease.pdf.

Examination procedure

After contrast medium has been injected for IVU, the first AP projection of the abdomen is performed during the arterial phase of opacification (Fig. 18-51), and multiple tomograms of the upper abdomen are obtained during the nephrographic phase after the renal parenchyma becomes opacified—hence the term *nephrotomography* (Fig. 18-52). The nephrotic phase normally occurs within 5 minutes after completion of injection or infusion.

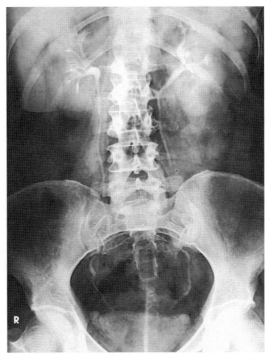

Fig. 18-51 Nephrourogram: AP projection, arterial phase.

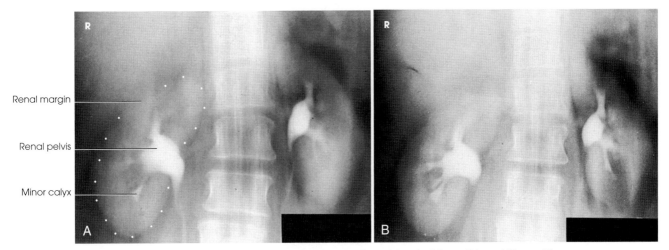

Renal margin

Renal pelvis

Minor calyx

Fig. 18-52 Nephrotomogram: **A** and **B**, AP projection at level of 9 cm (**A**) and 10 cm (**B**) in the same patient as in Fig. 18-51.

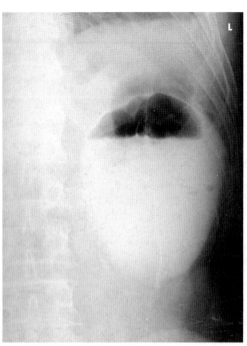

Fig. 18-53 Upright AP left kidney: percutaneous injection of iodinated contrast material and gas into renal cyst.

PERCUTANEOUS RENAL PUNCTURE

Percutaneous renal puncture, as introduced by Lindblom,[1,2] is a radiologic procedure for the investigation of renal masses. Specifically, it is used to differentiate cysts and tumors of the renal parenchyma. This procedure is performed by direct injection of a contrast medium into the cyst under fluoroscopic control (Figs. 18-53 and 18-54). Ultrasonography of the kidney has practically eliminated the need for percutaneous renal puncture. Most masses that are clearly diagnosed as cystic by ultrasound examination are not surgically managed.

[1]Lindblom K: Percutaneous puncture of renal cysts and tumors, *Acta Radiol* 27:66, 1946.
[2]Lindblom K: Diagnostic kidney puncture in cysts and tumors, *AJR Am J Roentgenol* 68:209, 1952.

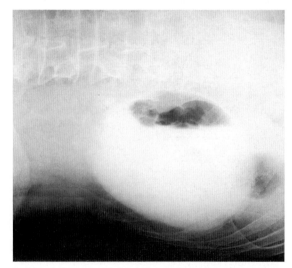

Fig. 18-54 AP projection left kidney, left lateral decubitus position, in the same patient as in Fig. 18-53.

In a similar procedure, the renal pelvis is entered percutaneously for direct contrast filling of the pelvicaliceal system in selected patients with hydronephrosis.[1-3] This procedure, called *percutaneous antegrade pyelography*[3] to distinguish it from the retrograde technique of direct pelvicaliceal filling, is usually restricted to the investigation of patients with marked hydronephrosis and patients with suspected hydronephrosis, for whom conclusive information is not gained by excretory or retrograde urography (Fig. 18-55). This procedure may also be called a *nephrostogram* because the contrast media injection is frequently made through a percutaneous nephrostomy catheter. Normally, AP abdominal images are obtained for this procedure, although other projections may be requested.

[1]Wickbom I: Pyelography after direct puncture of the renal pelvis, *Acta Radiol* 41:505, 1954.
[2]Weens HS, Florence TJ: The diagnosis of hydronephrosis by percutaneous renal puncture, *J Urol* 72:589, 1954.
[3]Casey WC, Goodwin WE: Percutaneous antegrade pyelography and hydronephrosis, *J Urol* 74:164, 1955.

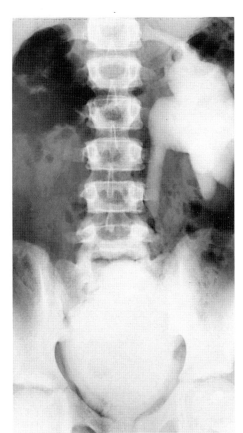

Fig. 18-55 AP projection left kidney, left lateral decubitus position, in the same patient as in Fig. 18-53.

Retrograde Urography

⚹ AP PROJECTION

Retrograde urography requires that the ureters be catheterized so that a contrast agent can be injected directly into the pelvicaliceal system. This technique provides improved opacification of the renal collecting system but little physiologic information about the urinary system.

Indications and contraindications

Retrograde urography is indicated for evaluation of the collecting system in patients who have renal insufficiency or who are allergic to iodinated contrast media. Because the contrast medium is not introduced into the circulatory system, the incidence of reactions is reduced.

Examination procedure

Similar to all examinations requiring instrumentation, retrograde urography is classified as an operative procedure. This combined urologic-radiologic examination is performed under careful aseptic conditions by the attending urologist with the assistance of a nurse and radiographer. The procedure is performed in a specially equipped cystoscopic-radiographic examining room, which, because of its collaborative nature, may be located in the urology department or the radiology department. A nurse is responsible for preparation of the instruments and for care and draping of the patient. A responsibility of the radiographer is to ensure that overhead parts of the radiographic equipment are free of dust for protection of the operative field and the sterile layout.

The radiographer positions the patient on the cystoscopic table with knees flexed over the stirrups of the adjustable leg supports (Fig. 18-56). This is a modified lithotomy position; the true lithotomy position requires acute flexion of the hips and knees.

If a general anesthetic is not used, the radiographer explains the breathing procedure to the patient and checks the patient's position on the table. The kidneys and the full extent of the ureters in patients of average height are included on a 14 × 17-inch (35 × 43-cm) IR when the third lumbar vertebra is centered to the grid.

If elevation of the thighs does not reduce the lumbar curve, a pillow is adjusted under the patient's head and shoulders so that the back is in contact with the table. Most cystoscopic-radiographic tables are equipped with an adjustable leg rest to permit extension of the patient's legs for certain radiographic studies.

The urologist performs catheterization of the ureters through a ureterocystoscope, which is a cystoscope with an arrangement that aids insertion of the catheters into the vesicoureteral orifices. After the endoscopic examination, the urologist passes a ureteral catheter well into one or both ureters (Fig. 18-57) and, while leaving the catheters in position, usually withdraws the cystoscope.

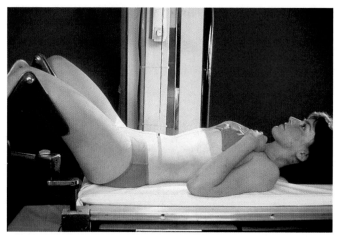

Fig. 18-56 Patient positioned on table for retrograde urography, modified lithotomy position.

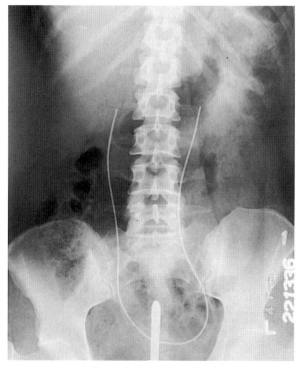

Fig. 18-57 Retrograde urogram with catheters in proximal ureters: AP projection.

After taking two catheterized specimens of urine from each kidney for laboratory tests—one specimen for culture and one for microscopic examination—the urologist tests kidney function. For this test, a color dye is injected intravenously, and the function of each kidney is determined by the specified time required for the dye substance to appear in the urine as it trickles through the respective catheters.

Immediately after the kidney function test, the radiographer rechecks the position of the patient and exposes the preliminary IR (if this has not been done previously) so that the images are ready for inspection by the time the kidney function test has been completed. After reviewing the image, the urologist injects contrast medium and proceeds with the urographic examination. When a bilateral examination is to be performed, both sides are filled simultaneously to avoid subjecting the patient to unnecessary radiation exposure. Additional studies in which only one side is refilled may be performed as indicated.

The most commonly used retrograde urographic series usually consists of three AP projections: the preliminary image showing the ureteral catheters in position (see Fig. 18-57), the pyelogram, and the ureterogram. Some urologists recommend that the head of the table be lowered 10 to 15 degrees for the pyelogram to prevent the contrast solution from escaping into the ureters. Other urologists recommend that pressure be maintained on the syringe during the pyelographic exposure to ensure complete filling of the pelvicaliceal system. The head of the table may be elevated 35 to 40 degrees for the ureterogram to show any tortuosity of the ureters and mobility of the kidneys.

Filling of the average normal renal pelvis requires 3 to 5 mL of contrast solution; however, a larger quantity is required when the structure is dilated. The best index of complete filling, and the one most commonly used, is an indication from the patient as soon as a sense of fullness is felt in the back.

When both sides are to be filled, the urologist injects the contrast solution through the catheters in an amount sufficient to fill the renal pelves and calyces. When signaled by the physician, the patient suspends respiration at the end of expiration, and the exposure for the pyelogram is made (Fig. 18-58).

After the pyelographic exposure, the IR is quickly changed, and the head of the table may be elevated in preparation for the ureterogram. For this exposure, the patient is instructed to inspire deeply and then to suspend respiration at the end of full expiration. Simultaneously with the breathing procedure, the catheters are slowly withdrawn to the lower ends of the ureters as the contrast solution is injected into the canals. At a signal from the urologist, the ureterographic exposure is made (Fig. 18-59).

Additional projections are sometimes required. RPO or LPO (AP oblique) projections are often necessary. Occasionally, a lateral projection, with the patient turned onto the affected side, is performed to show anterior displacement of a kidney or ureter and to delineate a perinephric abscess. Lateral projections with the patient in the ventral or dorsal decubitus position (as required) are also useful, showing the ureteropelvic region in patients with hydronephrosis.

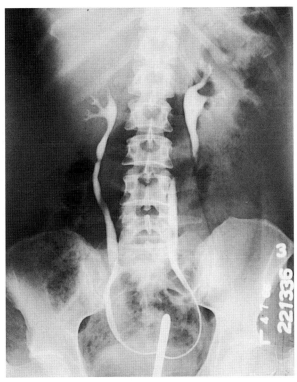

Fig. 18-58 Retrograde urogram with renal pelves filled: AP projection.

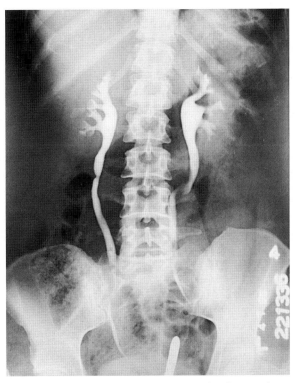

Fig. 18-59 Retrograde urogram showing renal pelves and contrast medium–filled ureters: AP projection.

Urinary Bladder, Lower Ureters, Urethra, and Prostate

With few exceptions, radiologic examinations of the lower urinary tract are performed with the retrograde technique of introducing contrast material. These examinations are identified, according to the specific purpose of the investigation, by the terms *cystography, cystoureterography, cystourethrography,* and *prostatography.* Most often, they are denoted by the general term *cystography.* Cystoscopy is not required before retrograde contrast filling of the lower urinary canals, but when both examinations are indicated, they are usually performed in a single-stage procedure to spare the patient preparation and instrumentation for separate examinations. When cystoscopy is not indicated, these examinations are best carried out on an all-purpose radiographic table unless the combination table is equipped with an extensible leg rest.

Indications and contraindications

Retrograde studies of the lower urinary tract are indicated for vesicoureteral reflux, recurrent lower urinary tract infection, neurogenic bladder, bladder trauma, lower urinary tract fistulae, urethral stricture, and posterior urethral valves. Contraindications to lower urinary tract studies are related to catheterization of the urethra.

Contrast media

The contrast agents used for contrast studies of the lower urinary tracts are ionic solutions of sodium or meglumine diatrizoates or the newer nonionic contrast media mentioned previously. These are the same organic compounds used for IVU, but their concentration is reduced, usually to 30%, for retrograde urography.

Injection equipment

Examinations are performed under careful aseptic conditions. Infants, children, and, usually, adults may be catheterized before they are brought to the radiology department. When the patient is to be catheterized in the radiology department, a sterile catheterization tray must be set up to specifications. Because of the danger of contamination in transferring a sterile liquid from one container to another, the use of commercially available premixed contrast solutions is recommended.

Preliminary preparations

The following guidelines are observed in preparing the patient for the examination:

- Protect the examination table from urine soilage with radiolucent plastic sheeting and disposable underpadding. Correctly arranged disposable padding does much to reduce soilage during voiding studies and consequently eliminates the need for extensive cleaning between patients. A suitable disposal receptacle should be available.
- A few minutes before the examination, accompany the patient to a lavatory. Give the patient supplies for perineal care, and instruct the patient to empty the bladder.
- When the patient is prepared, place the patient on the examination table for the catheterization procedure.

Patients are usually tense, primarily because of embarrassment. It is important that they be given as much privacy as possible. Only required personnel should be present during the examination, and patients should be properly draped and covered according to room temperature.

Contrast injection

For retrograde cystography (Figs. 18-60 and 18-61), cystourethrography, and voiding cystourethrography, the contrast material is introduced into the bladder by injection or infusion through a catheter passed into position via the urethral canal. A small, disposable Foley catheter is used to occlude the vesicourethral orifice in the examination of infants and children, and this catheter may be used in the examination of adults when interval studies are to be made for the detection of delayed ureteral reflux.

Studies are made during voiding to delineate the urethral canal and to detect ureteral reflux, which may occur only during urination (Fig. 18-62). When urethral studies are to be made during injection of contrast material, a soft rubber urethral-orifice acorn is fitted directly onto a contrast-loaded syringe for female patients and is usually fitted onto a cannula attached to a clamp device for male patients.

RETROGRADE CYSTOGRAPHY
Contrast injection technique

In preparing for this examination, the following steps are taken:

- With the urethral catheter in place, adjust the patient in the supine position for a preliminary image and the first cystogram.
- Usually, take cystograms of adult patients on 10 × 12-inch (24 × 30-cm) IRs placed lengthwise.
- Center the IR at the level of the soft tissue depression just above the most prominent point of the greater trochanters. This centering coincides with the middle area of a filled bladder of average size. The 12-inch (30-cm) IR includes the region of the distal end of the ureters to show ureteral reflux and the prostate and proximal part of the male urethra.
- Have large IRs nearby for use when ureteral reflux is shown. Some radiologists request studies during contrast filling of the bladder and during voiding.

After the preliminary image is taken, the physician removes the catheter clamp, and the bladder is drained in preparation for the introduction of contrast material. After introducing the contrast agent, the physician clamps the catheter and tapes it to the thigh to keep it from being displaced during position changes.

The initial cystographic images generally consist of four projections: one AP, two AP oblique, and one lateral. Additional studies, including voiding cystourethrograms, are obtained as indicated. The Chassard-Lapiné method (see Chapter 17, Volume 2), is sometimes used to obtain an axial projection of the posterior surface of the bladder and the lower end of the ureters when they are opacified. These projections of the bladder are also made when it is opacified by the excretory technique of urography.

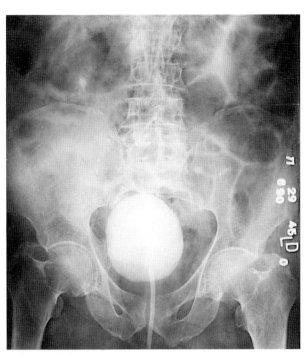

Fig. 18-60 Retrograde cystogram after introduction of contrast medium: AP projection.

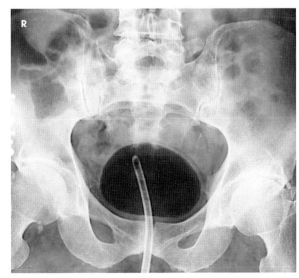

Fig. 18-61 Retrograde cystogram after introduction of air: AP projection.

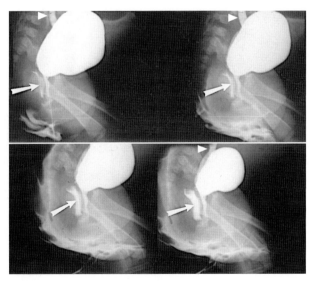

Fig. 18-62 Serial (polygraphic) voiding cystourethrograms in an infant girl with bilateral ureteral reflux (*arrowheads*). Urethra is normal. Vaginal reflux (*arrows*) is a normal finding.

✦ AP AXIAL OR PA AXIAL PROJECTION

Image receptor: 10 × 12 inch (24 × 30 cm) lengthwise

Position of patient

• Place the patient supine on the radiographic table for the AP projection of the urinary bladder.

NOTE: Preliminary (scout) and postinjection images are most commonly obtained with the patient supine. The prone position is sometimes used to image areas of the bladder not clearly seen on the AP axial projection. An AP axial projection using the Trendelenburg position at 15 to 20 degrees and with the central ray directed vertically is sometimes used to show the distal ends of the ureters. In this angled position, the weight of the contained fluid stretches the bladder fundus superiorly, giving an unobstructed projection of the lower ureters and the vesicoureteral orifice areas.

Position of part

• Center the midsagittal plane of the patient's body to the midline of the grid device.
• Adjust the patient's shoulders and hips so that they are equidistant from the IR.
• Place the patient's arms where they do not cast shadows on the IR.
• If the patient is positioned for a supine image, have the patient's legs extended so that the lumbosacral area of the spine is arched enough to tilt the anterior pelvic bones inferiorly. In this position, the pubic bones can more easily be projected below the bladder neck and proximal urethra (Fig. 18-63).
• Center the IR 2 inches (5 cm) above the upper border of the pubic symphysis (or at the pubic symphysis for voiding studies).
• *Respiration:* Suspend at the end of expiration.

Central ray

AP

• Angled 10 to 15 degrees caudal to the center of the IR. The central ray should enter 2 inches (5 cm) above the upper border of the pubic symphysis. When the bladder neck and proximal urethra are the main areas of interest, 5-degree caudal angulation of the central ray is usually sufficient to project the pubic bones below them. More or less angulation may be necessary, depending on the amount of lordosis of the lumbar spine. With greater lordosis, less angulation may be needed (see Fig. 18-63).

PA

• When performing PA axial projections of the bladder, direct the central ray through the region of the bladder neck at an angle 10 to 15 degrees cephalad, entering about 1 inch (2.5 cm) distal to the tip of the coccyx and exiting a little above the superior border of the pubic symphysis. If the prostate is the area of interest, the central ray is directed 20 to 25 degrees cephalad to project it above the pubic bones. For PA axial projections, the IR is centered to the central ray.
• Perpendicular to the pubic symphysis for voiding studies

Collimation

• Adjust to 10 × 12 inches (24 × 30 cm) on the collimator.

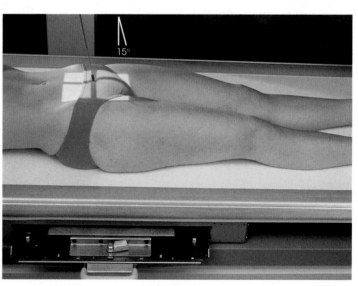

Fig. 18-63 Retrograde cystogram. AP axial bladder with 15-degree caudal angulation of central ray.

Structures shown

AP axial and PA axial projections show the bladder filled with contrast medium (Figs. 18-64 and 18-65). If reflux is present, the distal ureters are also visualized.

EVALUATION CRITERIA

The following should be clearly shown:
■ Evidence of proper collimation
■ Regions of the distal end of the ureters, bladder, and proximal portion of the urethra
■ Pubic bones projected below the bladder neck and proximal urethra
■ Exposure technique clearly showing contrast medium in the bladder, distal ureters, and proximal urethra

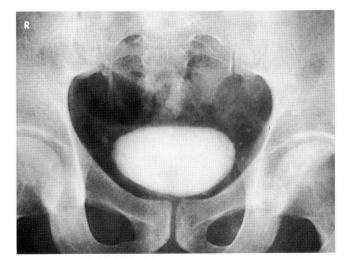

Fig. 18-64 Excretory cystogram: AP axial projection.

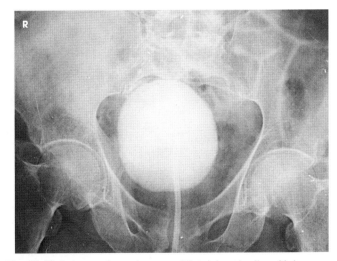

Fig. 18-65 Retrograde cystogram: AP axial projection. Note catheter in bladder.

✦ AP OBLIQUE PROJECTION
RPO or LPO position

Image receptor: 10×12 inch (24×30 cm) lengthwise

Position of patient
- Place the patient in the supine position on the radiographic table.

Position of part
- Rotate the patient 40 to 60 degrees RPO or LPO, according to the preference of the examining physician (Fig. 18-66).
- Adjust the patient so that the pubic arch closest to the table is aligned over the midline of the grid.
- Extend and abduct the uppermost thigh enough to prevent its superimposition on the bladder area.
- Center the IR 2 inches (5 cm) above the upper border of the pubic symphysis and approximately 2 inches (5 cm) medial to the upper ASIS (or at the pubic symphysis for voiding studies).
- *Respiration:* Suspend at the end of expiration.

Central ray
- Perpendicular to the center of the IR. The central ray falls 2 inches (5 cm) above the upper border of the pubic symphysis and 2 inches (5 cm) medial to the upper ASIS. When the bladder neck and proximal urethra are the main areas of interest, 10-degree caudal angulation of the central ray is usually sufficient to project the pubic bones below them.
- Perpendicular at the level of the pubic symphysis for voiding studies

Collimation
- Adjust to 10×12 inches (24×30 cm) on the collimator.

Structures shown
Oblique projections show the bladder filled with contrast medium. If reflux is present, the distal ureters are also visualized (Figs. 18-67 and 18-68).

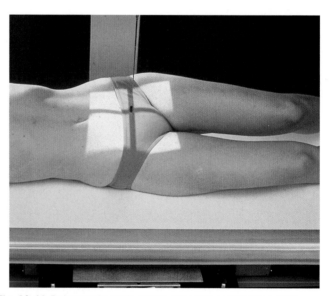

Fig. 18-66 Retrograde cystogram: AP oblique bladder, RPO position.

EVALUATION CRITERIA

The following should be clearly shown:

- Evidence of proper collimation
- Regions of the distal ends of the ureters and bladder, and the proximal portion of the urethra
- Pubic bones projected below the bladder neck and the proximal urethra
- Exposure technique clearly showing contrast medium in the bladder, distal ureters, and proximal urethra
- No superimposition of the bladder by the uppermost thigh

Voiding studies

- Entire urethra visible and filled with contrast medium
- Urethra overlapping the thigh on oblique projections for improved visibility
- Urethra lying posterior to the superimposed pubic and ischial rami on the side down in oblique projections

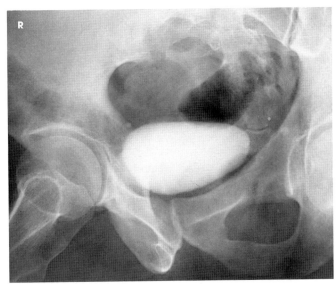

Fig. 18-67 Excretory cystogram: AP oblique bladder, RPO position.

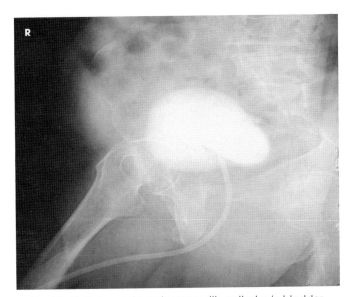

Fig. 18-68 Retrograde cystogram with catheter in bladder.

⚹ LATERAL PROJECTION
R or L position

Image receptor: 10 × 12 inch (24 × 30 cm) lengthwise

Position of patient
- Place the patient in the lateral recumbent position on the right or the left side, as indicated.

Position of part
- Slightly flex the patient's knees to a comfortable position, and adjust the body so that the midcoronal plane is centered to the midline of the grid.
- Flex the patient's elbows, and place the hands under the head (Fig. 18-69).
- Center the IR 2 inches (5 cm) above the upper border of the pubic symphysis at the midcoronal plane.
- *Respiration:* Suspend at the end of expiration.

Central ray
- Perpendicular to the IR and 2 inches (5 cm) above the upper border of the pubic symphysis at the midcoronal plane

Collimation
- Adjust to 10 × 12 inches (24 × 30 cm) on the collimator.

Structures shown
A lateral image shows the bladder filled with contrast medium. If reflux is present, the distal ureters are also visualized. Lateral projections show the anterior and posterior bladder walls and the base of the bladder (Fig. 18-70).

The following should be clearly shown:
- Evidence of proper collimation
- Regions of the distal end of the ureters, bladder, and proximal portion of the urethra
- Exposure technique clearly showing contrast medium in the bladder, distal ureters, and proximal urethra
- Bladder and distal ureters visible through the pelvis
- Superimposed hips and femur

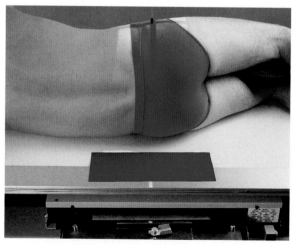

Fig. 18-69 Cystogram: lateral projection.

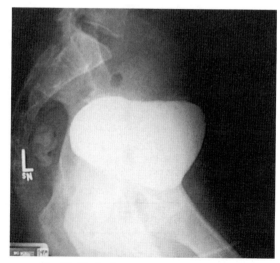

Fig. 18-70 Cystogram: lateral projection.

♠ AP OBLIQUE PROJECTION
RPO or LPO position

Male cystourethrography may be preceded by an endoscopic examination, after which the bladder is catheterized so that it can be drained just before contrast material is injected.

The following steps are taken:
- Use 10 × 12-inch (24 × 30-cm) IRs placed lengthwise for cystourethrograms in men.
- The patient is adjusted on the combination table so that the IR can be centered at the level of the superior border of the pubic symphysis. This centering coincides with the root of the penis, and a 12-inch (30-cm) IR includes the bladder and the external urethral orifice.
- After inspecting the preliminary image, the physician drains the bladder and withdraws the catheter.
- The supine patient is adjusted in an oblique position so that the bladder neck and the entire urethra are delineated as free of bony superimposition as possible. Rotate the patient's body 35 to 40 degrees, and adjust it so that the elevated pubis is centered to the midline of the grid. The superimposed pubic and ischial rami of the down-side and the body of the elevated pubis usually are projected anterior to the bladder neck, proximal urethra, and prostate (Fig. 18-71).

- The patient's lower knee is flexed only slightly to keep the soft tissues on the medial side of the thigh as near to the center of the IR as possible.
- The elevated thigh is extended and retracted enough to prevent overlapping.
- With the patient in the correct position, the physician inserts the contrast medium–loaded urethral syringe or the nozzle of a device such as the Brodney clamp into the urethral orifice. The physician extends the penis along the soft tissues of the medial side of the lower thigh to obtain a uniform density of the deep and cavernous portions of the urethral canal.

- At a signal from the physician, instruct the patient to hold still; make the exposure while injection of contrast material is continued to ensure filling of the entire urethra (Fig. 18-72).
- The bladder may be filled with a contrast material so that a voiding study can be performed (Fig. 18-73). This is usually done without changing the patient's position. When a standing-upright voiding study is required, the patient is adjusted before a vertical grid device and is supplied with a urinal. (Further information on positioning is provided on pp. 216-220 of this volume.)

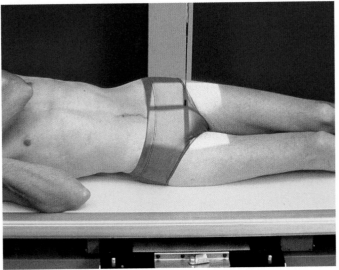

Fig. 18-71 Cystourethrogram: AP oblique projection, RPO position.

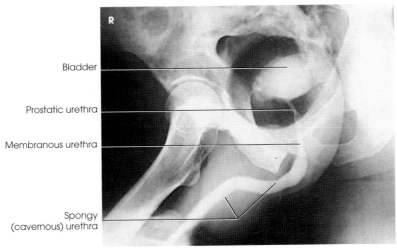

Bladder

Prostatic urethra

Membranous urethra

Spongy (cavernous) urethra

Fig. 18-72 Injection cystourethrogram: AP oblique urethra, RPO position.

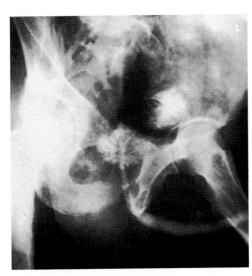

Fig. 18-73 Voiding cystourethrogram: AP oblique urethra, LPO position.

AP PROJECTION

INJECTION METHOD

The female urethra averages $1\frac{1}{2}$ inches (3.5 cm) in length. Its opening into the bladder is situated at the level of the superior border of the pubic symphysis. From this point, the vessel slants obliquely inferiorly and anteriorly to its termination in the vestibule of the vulva, about 1 inch (2.5 cm) anterior to the vaginal orifice. The female urethra is subject to conditions such as tumors, abscesses, diverticula, dilation, and strictures. It is also subject to urinary incontinence during the stress of increased intra-abdominal pressure, as occurs during sneezing or coughing. In the investigation of abnormalities other than stress incontinence, contrast studies are made during injection of contrast medium or during voiding.

Cystourethrography is usually preceded by an endoscopic examination. For this reason, it may be performed by the attending urologist or gynecologist with the assistance of a nurse and a radiographer.

The following steps are observed:

- After the physical examination, the cystoscope is removed, and a catheter is inserted into the bladder so that the bladder can be drained just before injection of the contrast solution.
- The patient is adjusted in the supine position on the table.

- An 8 × 10-inch (18 × 24-cm) or 10 × 12-inch (24 × 30-cm) IR is placed lengthwise and centered at the level of the superior border of the pubic symphysis.
- A 5-degree caudal angulation of the central ray is usually sufficient to free the bladder neck of superimposition.
- After inspecting the preliminary image, the physician drains the bladder and withdraws the catheter. The physician uses a syringe fitted with a blunt-nosed, soft rubber acorn, which is held firmly against the urethral orifice to prevent reflux as the contrast solution is injected during exposure.
- Oblique projections may be required in addition to the AP projection. For oblique projections, the patient is rotated 35 to 40 degrees so that the urethra is posterior to the pubic symphysis. The uppermost thigh is extended and abducted enough to prevent overlapping.
- Further information on positioning is provided on p. 218 of this volume.
- The physician fills the bladder for each voiding study to be made.

- For an AP projection (Figs. 18-74 and 18-75), the patient is maintained in the supine position, or the head of the table is elevated enough to place the patient in a semi-seated position.
- A lateral voiding study of the female vesicourethral canal is performed with the patient recumbent or upright. In either case, the IR is centered at the level of the superior border of the pubic symphysis.

Metallic bead chain cystourethrography

The metallic bead chain technique of investigating anatomic abnormalities responsible for stress incontinence in women was described by Stevens and Smith[1] in 1937 and by Barnes[2] in 1940. This technique is used to delineate anatomic changes that occur in the shape and position of the bladder floor, in the

---

[1]Stevens WE, Smith SP: Roentgenological examination of the female urethra, *J Urol* 37:194, 1937.
[2]Barnes AC: A method for evaluating the stress of urinary incontinence, *Am J Obstet Gynecol* 40:381, 1940.

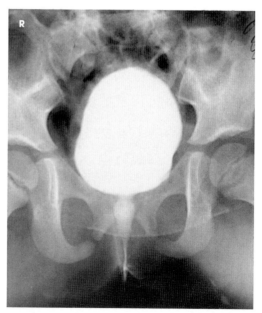

Fig. 18-74 Voiding cystourethrogram: AP projection.

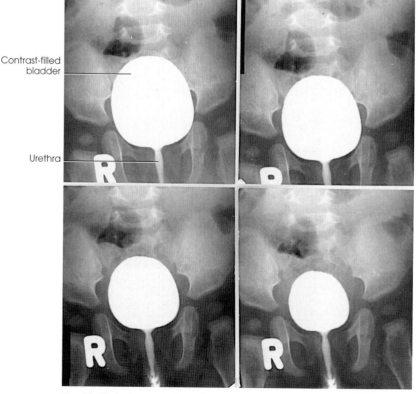

Contrast-filled bladder

Urethra

Fig. 18-75 Serial voiding images showing four stages of bladder emptying.

posterior urethrovesical angle, in the position of the proximal urethral orifice, and in the angle of inclination of the urethral axis under the stress of increased intra-abdominal pressure as exerted by the Valsalva maneuver.

Comparison AP and lateral projections are made with the patient standing at rest (Figs. 18-76 and 18-77) and straining (Figs. 18-78 and 18-79).

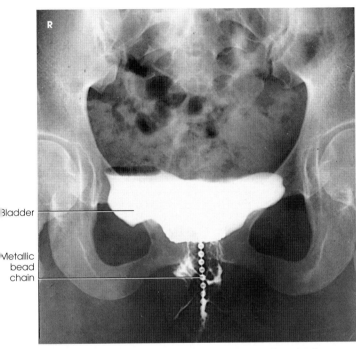

Bladder

Metallic bead chain

Fig. 18-76 Upright cystourethrogram: resting AP projection.

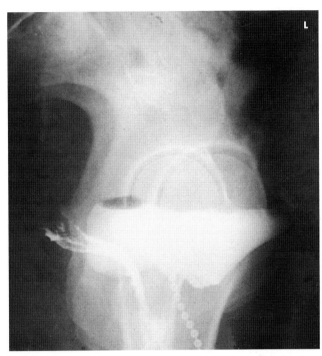

Fig. 18-77 Upright cystourethrogram: resting lateral projection.

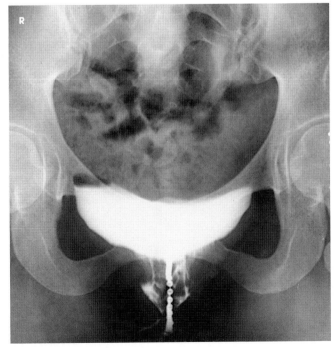

Fig. 18-78 Upright cystourethrogram: stress AP projection in the same patient as in Fig. 18-76.

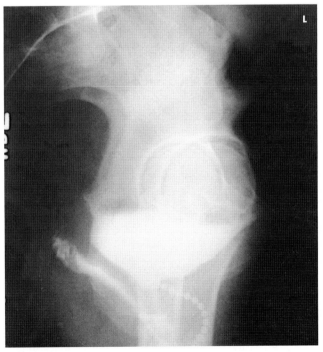

Fig. 18-79 Upright cystourethrogram: stress lateral projection.

For this examination, the physician extends a flexible metallic bead chain through the urethral canal. The proximal portion of the chain rests within the bladder, and the distal end is taped to the thigh. To show the length of the urethra, a small metal marker is attached with a piece of tape to the vaginal mucosa just lateral to the urethral orifice. After instillation of the metallic chain, a catheter is passed into the bladder, the contents of the bladder are drained, and an opaque contrast solution is injected. The catheter is removed for the imaging procedure.

Hodgkinson et al.[1] recommended the upright position, which uses gravity and simulates normal body activity. Two sets of images (AP and lateral projections) are obtained, and the rest of the studies *must* be exposed before the stress studies are made because the bladder does not immediately return to its normal resting position after straining.

After the metallic chain and contrast solution are instilled, the patient is usually prepared for upright images. The examining room should be readied in advance so that the patient, who will be uncomfortable, can be given immediate attention. The patient must be given kind reassurance and must be examined in privacy. Klawon[1] found that fear of involuntary voiding can be relieved by placing a folded towel or disposable pad between the patient's thighs before stress images are taken. Thus protected, the patient willingly applies full pressure during stress studies.

The IR size and centering point are the same as for other female cystourethrograms. (Further information on positioning of the lower urinary tract is provided on p. 218 of this volume.)

[1]Hodgkinson CP et al: Urethrocystograms: metallic bead chain technique, *Clin Obstet Gynecol* 1:668, 1958.

[1]Klawon MM: Urethrocystography and urinary stress incontinence in women, *Radiol Technol* 39:353, 1968.

Radiologic technologists may perform venipuncture and administer medications by physician order for specific indications in certain types of IV therapy related to radiographic procedures. Most commonly, this medication consists of some type of radiographic contrast medium.[1] For this reason, this chapter provides additional information on the professional and legal considerations of IV access and medication administration, common medications in the imaging department, patient education and assessment, infection control, venipuncture equipment and procedure, contrast reactions, and documentation.

Professional and Legal Considerations

Because of patient risk and legal liabilities, the radiologic technologist must follow professional recommendations, state regulations, and institutional policies for administration of medications. The information presented in this section is meant to be an introduction to IV therapy. Competency in this area requires the completion of a formal course of instruction with supervised clinical practice and evaluation.

The American Society of Radiologic Technologists (ASRT) includes venipuncture and IV medication administration in the curriculum guidelines for educational opportunities offered to technologists. Additional support for administration of medications and venipuncture as part of the technologist's scope of practice is found in the ACR's 1987 Resolution No. 27 and *Manual on Contrast Media*

[1]Tortorici M: *Administration of imaging pharmaceuticals,* Philadelphia, 1996, Saunders.

(2013).[1,2] These documents support the injection of contrast materials and diagnostic levels of radiopharmaceuticals within specific established guidelines by certified or licensed radiologic technologists. The ASRT Standards of Practice for Radiography also support the administration of medication by technologists.

Technologists who perform venipuncture and contrast media administration must be knowledgeable about the specific state regulations and facility policies that govern these activities. Technologists also are responsible for professional decisions and actions in their practice. Competency in the skills of venipuncture and contrast media administration are based on cognitive knowledge, proficiency in psychomotor skills, positive affective values, and validation in a clinical setting.

Medications

Medications for a specific procedure are prescribed by a physician, who is also responsible for obtaining informed consent for the procedure. A technologist may administer medications for radiographic procedures, which can require medications for sedation, pain management, contrast media administration, and emergencies.[3] Technologists must have extensive knowledge of all medications used in the radiology department. IV medications are administered into the body via the vascular system; when administered, they cannot be retrieved. Before administering any medication, the technologist must know the medication's name, dosages, indications, contraindications, and possible adverse reactions (Table 18-1).

[1]Tortorici M: *Administration of imaging pharmaceuticals,* Philadelphia, 1996, Saunders.
[2]*ACR Manual on Contrast Media, v.9, 2013, p. 13.*
[3]Kowalczyk N, Donnett K: *Integrated patient care for the imaging professional,* St Louis, 1996, Mosby.

Patient Education

The manner in which the technologist approaches the patient can have a direct influence on the patient's response to the procedure. Although the technologist may consider the procedure routine, the patient may be totally unfamiliar with its specifics. Apprehension experienced by the patient can cause vasoconstriction, making venipuncture more difficult and more painful.[1] Careful explanation and a confident, sympathetic attitude can help the patient relax.

The technologist must provide information about the procedure in terms the patient can understand. The patient's questions must be answered in "layman's" language. By explaining the details of the procedure, the technologist can help alleviate fears and solicit cooperation from the patient. It is important to explain the steps in the procedure, its expected duration, and any limitations or restrictions associated with its performance. The patient may have heard an inaccurate "horror" story about the procedure from a neighbor or friend. The technologist may need to correct misconceptions and provide accurate information.

For simple procedures, the patient must be reassured that the process is relatively straightforward and causes only slight discomfort. For more complex and longer procedures, the technologist must gain the patient's cooperation by providing appropriate, factual information and offering support. *The patient should never be told that insertion of the needle used in venipuncture does not hurt.* After all, a foreign object is going to be inserted through the patient's skin, which has myriad nerves that may be aggravated by insertion of a needle. The technologist must tell the truth and explain that the amount of pain experienced varies with each patient.[2]

[1]*Managing IV therapy: skillbuilders,* Springhouse, PA, 1991, Springhouse.
[2]Hoeltke L: *The complete textbook of phlebotomy,* ed 3, Albany, NY, 2006, Delmar.

TABLE 18-1

Medications commonly used in an imaging department

Generic name	Brand name	Indications	Action	Adverse reactions
Atropine sulfate	Atropine *How supplied:* injection, tablets	Symptomatic bradycardia, bradyarrhythmia	Inhibits acetylcholine at parasympathetic neuroeffector junction, enhancing and increasing heart rate	Bradycardia, headache, dry mouth, nausea, vomiting
Diphenhydramine hydrochloride	Benadryl *How supplied:* tablets, capsules, elixir, syrup, injection	Allergic reactions, sedation	Competes with histamine for special receptors on effector cells; prevents but does not reverse histamine-mediated responses	Seizures, sleepiness, insomnia, incoordination, restlessness, nausea, vomiting, diarrhea
Meperidine hydrochloride	Demerol *How supplied:* tablets, syrup, injection	Mild to moderate pain; adjunct to anesthesia	Binds with opiate receptors of CNS	Seizures, cardiac arrest, shock, respiratory depression
Dopamine hydrochloride	Dopamine *How supplied:* injection	Shock, increase cardiac output, correct hypotension	Stimulates dopaminergic and α and β receptors of sympathetic nervous system	Tachycardia, hypotension, nausea, vomiting, anaphylactic reactions
Adrenaline	Epinephrine *How supplied:* injection, inhaler	Restore cardiac rhythm in cardiac arrest; bronchospasm; anaphylaxis	Relaxes bronchial smooth muscle by stimulating β_2 receptors and α and β receptors in sympathetic nervous system	Palpations, ventricular fibrillation, shock, nervousness
Glucagons	Glucagon *How supplied:* injection	Hypoglycemia	Increases blood glucose level by promoting catalytic depolymerization of hepatic glycogen to glucose	Bronchospasm, hypotension, nausea, vomiting
Morphine sulfate	Morphine *How supplied:* tablets, syrup, oral suspension, injection	Severe pain	Binds with opiate receptors of CNS	Bradycardia, shock, cardiac arrest, apnea, respiratory depression, respiratory arrest
Chloral hydrate	Noctec *How supplied:* capsules, syrup, suppositories	Sedation	Unknown, sedative effects may be caused by its primary metabolite	Drowsiness, nightmares, hallucinations, nausea, vomiting, diarrhea
Promethazine hydrochloride	Phenergan *How supplied:* tablets, syrup, injection, suppositories	Nausea, sedation	Competes with histamine for special receptors on effector cells; prevents but does not reverse histamine-mediated responses	Dry mouth
Diazepam	Valium *How supplied:* tablets, capsules, oral solutions, injections	Anxiety	Unknown; probably depresses CNS at limbic and subcortical levels	Cardiovascular collapse, bradycardia, respiratory depression, acute withdrawal syndrome
Midazolam hydrochloride	Versed *How supplied:* injection	Preoperative sedation (to induce sleepiness or drowsiness and relieve apprehension)	Unknown; thought to depress CNS at limbic and subcortical levels	Apnea, depressed respiratory rate, nausea, vomiting, hiccups, pain at injection site
Hydroxyzine hydrochloride	Vistaril *How supplied:* tablets, syrup, capsules, injection	Nausea and vomiting, anxiety, preoperative and postoperative adjunctive therapy	Unknown; actions may be due to suppression of activity in key regions of subcortical area of CNS	Dry mouth, dyspnea, wheezing, chest tightness

Data from *Nursing 2006 drug handbook*, Ambler, PA, 2006, Lippincott Williams & Wilkins.

Interactions	Effects on diagnostic imaging procedures	Contraindications	Patient care considerations
May increase anticholinergic drug effects; use together cautiously	None known	Patients with obstructive disease of gastrointestinal tract, paralytic ileus, toxic megacolon, tachycardia, myocardia or ischemia, or asthma	Watch for tachycardia in cardiac patients; may lead to ventricular fibrillation
Increased effects when used with other CNS depressants	None known	Hypersensitivity to drug during acute asthmatic attacks and in newborns or premature neonates and breastfeeding women	Use with extreme caution in patients with angle-closure glaucoma, asthma, COPD
May be incompatible when mixed in same IV container	None known	Patients with hypersensitivity to drug and patients who have received MAO inhibitors within past 14 days	Give slowly by direct IV injection; oral dose is less than half as effective as parenteral dose; compatible with most IV solutions
α and β blockers may antagonize effects	None known	Patients with uncorrected tachycardia, pheochromocytoma, or ventricular fibrillation	During infusion, frequently monitor ECG, blood pressure, cardiac output, central venous pressure, pulse rate, urine output, and color and temperature of limbs
Avoid using with α blockers (may cause hypotension)	None known	Patients with shock, organic brain damage, cardiac dilation, arrhythmias, coronary insufficiency, or cerebral arteriosclerosis	Drug of choice in emergency treatment of acute anaphylactic reactions; avoid IM use of parenteral suspension into buttocks
Inhibits glucagon-induced insulin release	None known	Patients with hypersensitivity to drug or with pheochromocytoma	Arouse patient from coma as quickly as possible and give additional carbohydrates orally to prevent secondary hypoglycemic reactions
In combination with other depressants and narcotics, use with extreme caution	None known	Patients with hypersensitivity to drug or conditions that would preclude administration of IV opioids	Use with extreme caution in patients with head injuries or increased intracranial pressure and in elderly patients
Alkaline solutions incompatible with aqueous solutions of chloral hydrate	None known	Patients with hepatic or renal impairment, severe cardiac disease, or hypersensitivity to drug	Note two strengths of oral liquid form; double-check dose, especially when administering to children
Increased effects when used with other CNS depressants	Discontinue drug 48 hr before myelogram because of high risk of seizures	Patients with hypersensitivity to drug; intestinal obstruction, prostatic hyperplasias	Do not administer subcutaneously
Other CNS depressants	May cause minor changes in ECG patterns	Patients with hypersensitivity to drug or soy protein, shock, coma, or acute alcohol intoxication	Monitor respirations and have emergency resuscitation equipment available before administering
CNS depressants may increase risk of apnea	None known	Patients with hypersensitivity to drug, acute angle-closure glaucoma, shock, coma, or acute alcohol intoxication	Use cautiously in patients with uncompensated acute illness and in elderly patients; have emergency resuscitation equipment available before administering
Can increase CNS depression	None known	Hypersensitivity to drug, during pregnancy, and in breastfeeding women	If used in conjunction with other CNS medication, observe for oversedation

Patient Assessment

The patient must be assessed before any medication is administered. A thorough patient history must be obtained, including any allergies the individual may have. It is essential to determine whether the patient has any known allergies to foods, medications, environmental agents, or other substances. Before venipuncture is performed, the technologist needs to be aware of the potential for an allergic reaction to the iodine tincture used in puncture site preparation or an adverse reaction to the medication being injected.

Other assessment criteria include the patient's current medications. Knowledge of some common medication actions can help the radiologic technologist evaluate changes in a patient's condition during a procedure. Certain diabetic medications interact adversely with contrast media. The interaction of medications must be assessed before the procedure is performed.

During the physical evaluation, it is important to determine whether the patient has previously undergone surgical procedures that might affect site selection for venipuncture (e.g., a mastectomy with resultant compromised lymph nodes and vascular abnormalities, such as atrioventricular shunts). To determine the appropriate type and amount of medication to be administered, the physician requires information about the patient's past and current disease processes, such as hypertension and renal disease. Evaluation of the glomerular filtration rate (GFR) (normal range 120-125 ml/min), blood urea nitrogen (BUN) level (average range 10 to 20 mg/dL), and the creatinine level (average range 0.05 to 1.2 mg/dL) should be included among the assessment criteria.

Infection Control

Each time the body system is entered, the potential for contamination exists.[1] Strict aseptic techniques and universal precautions must always be used when medications are administered with a needle.[2] If a medication is injected incorrectly, a microorganism may enter the body and cause an infection or other complications. The U.S. Centers for Disease Control and Prevention (CDC) has developed specific guidelines to prevent the transmission of infection during preparation and administration of medications. These guidelines are part of the standard precautions used by every health care facility, and the technologist must strictly adhere to the guidelines when performing radiologic procedures.

Studies using IV filters have shown a significant reduction in infusion phlebitis. Filters are devices located within the tubing used for IV administration. Filters prevent injection of particulate and microbial matter into the circulatory system. Use of a filter for a bolus injection reduces the rate at which medication can be injected. In addition, the viscosity of a medication may determine whether a filter is used and the rate of injection. Although a filter helps in reducing the possibility of bacteria being introduced into the blood, its use creates additional factors of risks versus benefits. The physician or health care facility should have policies to address these issues.

[1]Smith S et al: *Clinical nursing skills: basic to advanced skills,* ed 6, Stamford, CT, 2003, Appleton & Lange.
[2]Adler AM, Carlton RR: *Introduction to radiography and patient care,* ed 4, Philadelphia, 2007, Saunders.

Venipuncture Supplies and Equipment
NEEDLES AND SYRINGES

The technologist assembles the proper syringe and needle for the planned injection. The syringe may be glass or plastic. Plastic syringes are disposed of after only one use; glass syringes may be cleaned and must be sterilized before they are used again. The syringe has three parts: the *tip,* where the needle attaches to the syringe; the *barrel,* which includes the calibration markings; and the *plunger,* which fits snugly inside the barrel and allows the user to instill the medication (Fig. 18-80). The tip of the syringe for an IV injection has a locking device to hold the needle securely. The size of the syringe depends on the volume of material to be injected. The technologist should select a syringe one size larger than the volume desired. This larger syringe maximizes the accuracy of the dose by allowing the total amount of medication to be drawn into one syringe.

All needles used in venipuncture are disposable and are used only once. During preparation and administration of contrast media, the technologist may use several types of needles, including a hypodermic needle, a butterfly set, and an over-the-needle cannula (Fig. 18-81).

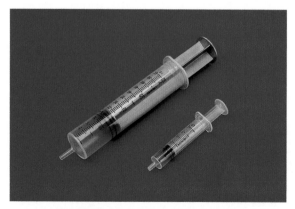

Fig. 18-80 Plastic disposable syringes.

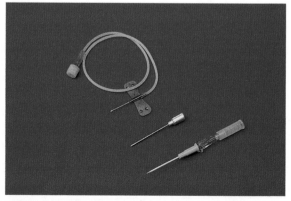

Fig. 18-81 Types of needles: over-the-cannula needle, or angiocatheter (*bottom*); hypodermic needle (*center*); and metal butterfly needle (*top*).

Hypodermic needles vary in gauge and length (see Fig. 18-81). Needle *gauge* refers to the *diameter* of the needle bore, with the gauge increasing as the diameter of the bore decreases. An 18-gauge needle is larger than a 22-gauge needle. As the bore of the needle increases, a given volume of fluid may be administered more rapidly. If bore size is reduced and fluid volume and rate of administration remain constant, the pressure (force) of the injection increases. The *length* of a needle is measured in inches and may range from ½ inch (1.3 cm) (used for intradermal injections) to 4½ inches (11.5 cm) (used for intrathecal [spinal] injections). Generally, needles 1 to 1½ inches (2.5 to 3.8 cm) long are most commonly used for IV injections. The needle has three parts: the *hub*, which is the part that attaches to the syringe; the *cannula* or *shaft*, which is the length of the needle; and the *bevel*, which is the slanted portion of the needle tip. Needles should be visually examined before and after use to determine whether any structural defects, such as nonbeveled points or bent shafts, are present.[1]

Butterfly sets or *angiocatheters* are preferable to a conventional hypodermic needle for most radiographic IV therapies. The butterfly set consists of a stainless steel needle with plastic appendages on either side and approximately 6 inches of plastic tubing that ends with a connector. The plastic appendages, often called wings, aid in inserting the needle and stabilizing the needle after venous patency has been confirmed.

The *over-the-needle cannula* is a device in which, after the venipuncture is made, the catheter is slipped off the needle into the vein and the steel needle is removed. This type of needle is recommended for long-term therapy or for rapid infusions, such as infusions that use an automated power injector. The choice of needle should be based on assessment of the patient, institutional policy, and technologist preference.

MEDICATION PREPARATION

Although IV drug administration offers the most immediate results in terms of effect, certain safety precautions must be followed. The technologist must identify the correct patient before medication is

administered. During preparation and again before administration, the medication in the container also must be verified.

If medication is supplied in a bottle or vial, the preparation procedure has several variations. First, the solution must be evaluated for contamination. Discoloration and dissolution are the most common signs of contamination. If either of those is observed, the solution should not be used. Then the protective cap is removed, with care taken not to contaminate the underlying surface. Containers have rubber stoppers through which a hypodermic needle can be inserted. If a single-dose vial is being used, and no contamination has occurred, the rubber stopper requires no additional cleansing. Multiple-dose vial stoppers must be cleaned with an alcohol wipe.

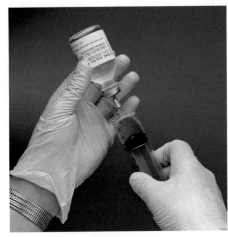

Fig. 18-82 Place tip of needle above level of fluid before injection of air to decrease air bubbles in solution.

For a closed system to be maintained and to reduce the chance of possible infection, a volume of air equal to the amount of desired fluid must be injected into the bottle. The plunger of the syringe is pulled back to the level of the desired amount of medication. The shaft of the plunger must not be contaminated at any time during preparation of the medication. The needle on the syringe is inserted into the rubber stopper, all the way to the hub of the needle. Then the vial is inverted by placing the end of the needle above the fluid level in the bottle (Fig. 18-82). Next, a small amount of air is *slowly* injected into the vial *above* the level of the fluid. This technique helps to decrease air bubbles in the solution. After the air has been injected, the vial and syringe are held inverted and perpendicular to a horizontal plane, and the tip of the needle is pulled *below* the fluid level. The desired amount of medication is aspirated into the syringe by pulling down on the plunger of the syringe. This procedure may have to be repeated several times to expel all of the medication. If air bubbles cling to the syringe casing, the syringe may be lightly tapped to release them. A one-handed method is used to recap the syringe (Fig. 18-83).

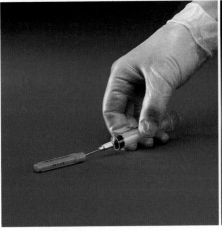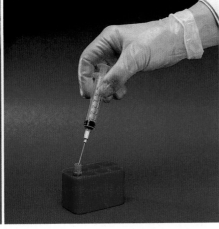

Fig. 18-83 When recapping a syringe, use a one-handed method.

[1]Strasinger S, DiLorenzo M: *Phlebotomy workbook for the multiskilled healthcare professional,* ed 2, Philadelphia, 2003, FA Davis.

Preparation of an infusion from a glass bottle or plastic bag begins with identification and verification of the solution and its expiration date (Fig. 18-84). The solution should not contain any visible particles. The tubing used for the infusion is determined by the method of injection and the type of container. Electronic infusion devices require different tubing than gravity infusion devices. A glass container necessitates vented tubing (Fig. 18-85), whereas a plastic container requires non-vented tubing (Fig. 18-86).

To prepare for drip infusion of a medication, the technologist removes the tubing from the sterile package and closes the clamp (Fig. 18-87). Failure to close the clamp may result in loss of the vacuum in the solution container. The protective coverings are removed from the port of the solution and the tubing spike. Then the fill chamber of the tubing is squeezed, and the spike is inserted into the solution. The solution is then inverted, and the chamber is released. The solution should fill the chamber to the measurement line. The tubing is primed by opening the clamp, which allows the solution to travel the length of the tubing, expelling any air. The tube is filled with solution, the clamp is closed, and the protective covering is secured. The solution is then ready for administration.

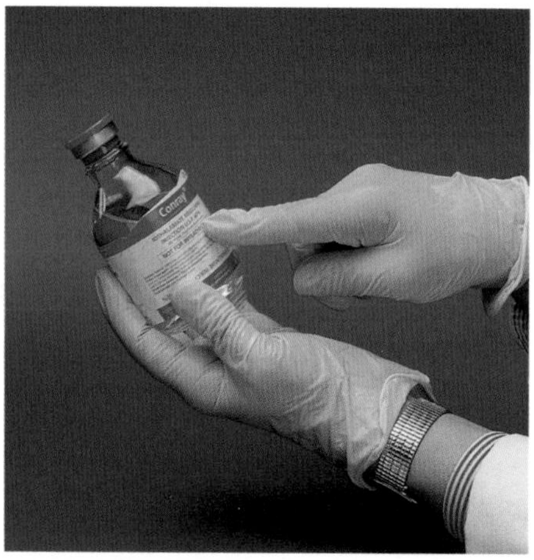

Procedure
SITE SELECTION

Selection of an appropriate vein for venipuncture is crucial. Finding the vein is sometimes difficult, and the most visible veins are not always the best choice.[1] Technologists administer IV medication and contrast media via the venous system. If a pulse is palpated during assessment for a puncture site, that vessel must *not* be used because it is an *artery*. The prime factors to consider in selecting a vein are (1) suitability of location, (2) condition of the vein, (3) purpose of the infusion, and (4) duration of therapy. The veins most often used in establishing IV access are the basilic or cephalic veins on the back of the hand, the basilic vein on the medial, anterior forearm and elbow and the cephalic vein on the lateral, anterior forearm and elbow. The anterior surface of the elbow is also referred to as the *antecubital* space[2] (Fig. 18-88).

A general rule is to select the most distal site that can accept the desired-size needle and tolerate the injection rate and solution. Although the veins located at the antecubital space may be the most accessible, the largest, and the easiest to puncture, they may not be the best choice. Because of their convenient location, these sites may be overused and can become scarred or sclerotic. Antecubital accesses are located over an area of joint flexion; any motion can dislodge the cannula, causing infiltration or resulting in mechanical phlebitis. A flexible IV catheter is the needle of choice for placement of a venous access in the antecubital space. The patient's arm should be immobilized to inhibit the ability to flex the elbow.

[1]Steele J: *Practical IV therapy,* Springhouse, PA, 1988, Springhouse.
[2]Jensen S, Peppers M: *Pharmacology and drug administration for imaging technologists,* ed 2, St Louis, 2006, Elsevier/Mosby.

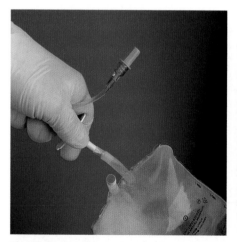

Fig. 18-84 Identify the correct solution and expiration date.

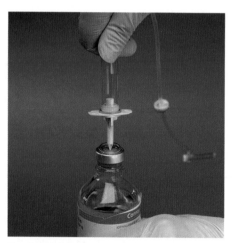

Fig. 18-85 Vented tubing is required for glass bottle containers.

Fig. 18-86 Solutions in plastic bags require nonvented tubing.

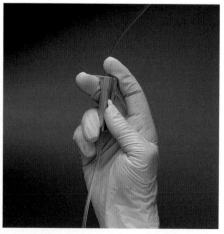

Fig. 18-87 Close tubing clamp before inserting spike into container of solution.

The condition of the vein must also be considered in the selection of an appropriate puncture site. The selected vein must be able to tolerate the needed or desired cannula size. The vein should have resilience qualities and be anchored by surrounding supportive tissues to prevent rolling.

Another consideration in vein selection is the rate of flow required for the procedure and the viscosity and amount of medication to be administered. Because the purpose of the infusion determines the rate of flow, the solution to be infused should be evaluated during the site selection process. Larger veins should be selected for infusions of large quantities or for rapid infusions. Large veins are also used for the infusion of highly viscous solutions or solutions that are irritating to vessels.[1]

The expected duration of the therapy and the patient's comfort are other factors that must be considered in selecting a venipuncture site. If a prolonged course of therapy is anticipated, areas over flexion joints should be avoided, and the dorsal surfaces of the upper limbs should be carefully examined. Venous access in these locations provides greater freedom and comfort to the patient.

[1]Adler AM, Carlton RR: *Introduction to radiologic sciences and patient care,* ed 5, St Louis, 2012, Elsevier/Saunders.

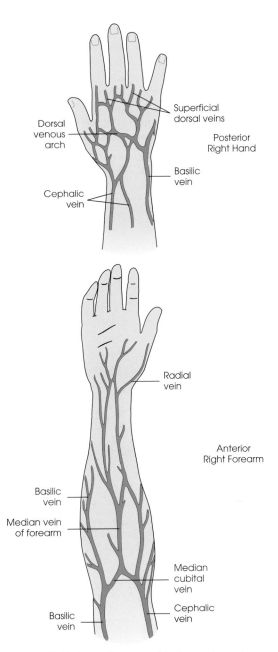

Fig. 18-88 Veins easily accessible for venipuncture.

SITE PREPARATION

The surface of the skin must be prepared and cleaned. If the area selected for venipuncture is hairy, the hair should be clipped to permit better cleansing of the skin and visualization of the vein; this also makes removal of the cannula less painful when the infusion is terminated. Shaving is not recommended. The skin is cleansed with an antiseptic, which should remain in contact with the skin for at least 30 seconds. The preferred solution is iodine tincture 1% to 2%. Isopropyl alcohol 70% is recommended if the patient is sensitive to iodine. The skin should be cleaned in a *circular motion from the center of the injection site* to approximately a 2-inch circle. When the swab has been placed on the skin, it should not be lifted from the surface until the cleansing process is complete (Fig. 18-89).

Many facilities have a policy that provides the patient an opportunity to request a local anesthetic for IV infusion catheter placement. This technique reduces the pain felt by the patient during insertion of an angiocatheter or needle. The local anesthetic can be administered topically or by injection.

A facility's procedure for local anesthetic determines the specific criteria for that institution. Commonly accepted guidelines are as follows: First, 0.1 to 0.2 mL of 1% lidocaine without epinephrine or sterile saline is prepared in a tuberculin or insulin syringe with a 23- to 25-gauge needle. The site for injection is selected and prepared. Then the anesthetic is injected subcutaneously (beneath the skin, into the soft tissue) or intradermally (immediately under the skin in the dermal layer) at the venipuncture site. Topical anesthesia is achieved by applying 5 g of eutectic mixture of local anesthetic cream and covering the area with an occlusive dressing. Maximal effects are achieved in 45 to 60 minutes.

The medication to be injected should already be prepared, and any tubing should be primed with the solution to prevent injection of air into the vascular system.

VENIPUNCTURE

After the solution has been prepared, the site has been selected, and the type of syringe and the needle to be used have been determined, the technologist is ready to perform the venipuncture.

Techniques for venipuncture follow one of two courses: (1) the *direct,* or *one-step,* entry method or (2) the *indirect* method. The *direct,* or *one-step,* method is performed by thrusting the cannula through the skin and into the vein in one quick motion. The needle and cannula enter the skin directly over the vein. This technique is excellent as long as large veins are available.[1] The *indirect* method is a two-step technique. First, the over-the-needle cannula is inserted through the skin adjacent to or below the point where the vein is visible. The cannula is advanced and maneuvered to pierce the vein. For the actual venipuncture procedure, the technologist washes the hands. The patient is identified. Next, the technologist instructs the patient about the procedure. The technologist performs the following steps:

---

[1]Weinstein SM: *Plumer's principles and practice of intravenous therapy,* ed 8, Boston, 2006, Little, Brown.

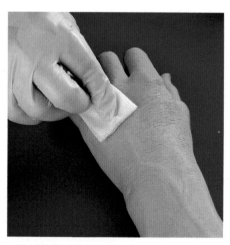

Fig. 18-89 Prepare site for venipuncture.

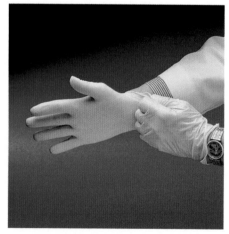

Fig. 18-90 Put on clean gloves.

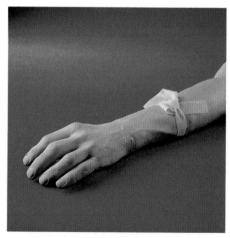

Fig. 18-91 Apply tourniquet 6 to 8 inches above intended venipuncture site, with free end directed superiorly.

1. The technologist puts on gloves and cleans the area in accordance with facility protocol (Fig. 18-90).
2. A local anesthetic is administered according to facility policy (optional).
3. A tourniquet is placed 6 to 8 inches (15 to 20 cm) above the intended site of puncture. The tourniquet should be tight enough to distend the vessels but not occlude them. The loose ends of the tourniquet should be placed away from the injection site to prevent contamination of the aseptic area (Fig. 18-91).

4. The technologist holds the patient's limb with the nondominant hand, using that thumb to stabilize and anchor the selected vein. The best method of accessing the vein—direct or indirect technique—is determined.
5. Using the dominant hand, the technologist places the needle bevel up at a 45-degree angle to the skin's surface. The bevel-up position produces less trauma to the skin and vein (Fig. 18-92).

6. The technologist uses a quick, sharp darting motion to enter the skin with the needle. On entering the skin, the technologist decreases the angle of the needle to 15 degrees from the long axis of the vessel. Using an indirect method, the technologist slowly proceeds with a downward motion on the hub or wings of the needle; while raising the point of the needle, the technologist advances the needle parallel and then punctures the vein. The needle may have to be maneuvered slightly to facilitate actual venous puncture. If the direct method of access is used, the needle is placed on the skin directly over the vein, and entry into the vein is accomplished in one movement of the needle through the skin and vein. When the vein is entered, a backflow of blood may occur—this indicates a successful venipuncture.
7. After the vein is punctured and blood return is noted, the cannula is advanced cautiously up the lumen of the vessel for approximately $\frac{3}{4}$ inch (1.9 cm).
8. Release the tourniquet (Fig. 18-93).
9. If a backflow of blood does not occur, verify venous access before injecting the medication. Aspiration of blood directly into the syringe of medication verifies placement before injection. Another method of placement verification is to attach a syringe of normal saline to the hub of the needle before aspirating for blood. The advantage of this method is that only saline, an isotonic solution, is injected if the needle is not in place and extravasation occurs. A successful venipuncture does not guarantee a successful injection. If a bolus injection is desired, the tourniquet may not be released until the injection has been completed. If this technique is used, the protocol must be included in the facility's policies and procedures.
10. Anchor the needle with tape and a dressing, as required by policy (Fig. 18-94). Then administer the medication (Fig. 18-95).

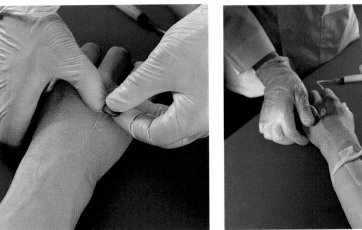

Fig. 18-92 Stabilize vein and enter skin with needle at 45-degree angle.

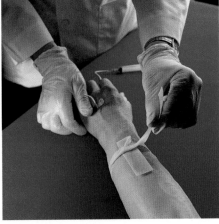

Fig. 18-93 Release tourniquet after venous access has been obtained. Do not permit tourniquet to touch needle.

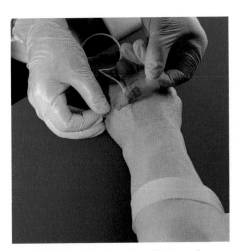

Fig. 18-94 Anchor needle with tape to secure placement.

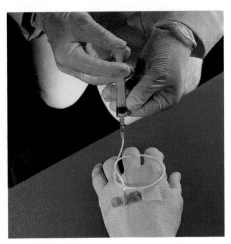

Fig. 18-95 Administer medication.

With experience, a technologist's fingers become sensitive to the sensation of the needle entering the vein—the resistance encountered as the needle penetrates the wall of the vein and the "pop" felt at the loss of resistance as the cannula enters the lumen. If both walls of the vein are punctured with a needle, the vessel develops a hematoma. The cannula should be removed immediately, and direct pressure should be applied to the puncture site. If a venipuncture attempt is unsuccessful with an over-the-needle cannula, and the needle has been removed from the cannula, the needle should not be reinserted into the catheter. Reinserting the needle into the cannula can shear a portion of the catheter.

ADMINISTRATION

The technologist should administer the medication or contrast medium at the established rate. During the injection process, the injection site should be observed and palpated proximal to the puncture for signs of infiltration. An infiltration, or extravasation, is a process whereby fluid passes into the tissue instead of the vein.

A patient may have a venous access that was established before the radiologic procedure. Careful assessment of site and medication compatibility must be performed before the existing IV line can be used. (Compatibility is the ability of one medication to mix with another.) Special precautions should be taken with a patient who is currently receiving cardiac, blood pressure, heparin, or diabetes medications. The physician, nurse, or pharmacist should be consulted before medication is administered to such a patient. Verification must be obtained to ensure that the medication being infused through the established IV line is compatible with the *contrast medium* to be administered. Before the contrast medium is injected, the infusion should be stopped, and the line should be flushed with normal saline through the port nearest the insertion site. The *contrast medium* is then administered, and the line is flushed again with normal saline. The amount of normal saline used depends on the facility's policies and procedures. After the contrast medium has been administered, the IV infusion solution is restarted.

Heparin or saline locks allow intermittent injections through a port. The port is a small adapter with an access that is attached to an IV catheter when more than one injection is anticipated.[1] As determined by procedure criteria, the cannula is flushed with heparin and saline to maintain patency during dormant periods.

The patency (open, unobstructed flow) of the intermittent device is verified by aspirating blood and injecting normal saline without infiltration. Then the medication is administered. Finally, the medication is flushed through the device with saline. Depending on protocols, the device may then be flushed with heparin or normal saline.

After the medication has been administered and the radiologic procedure has been completed, the venous access may be discontinued. The radiologic technologist should carefully remove any tape or protective dressing covering the puncture site. Using a 2 × 2-inch (6 × 6-cm) gauze pad at the injection site, the technologist removes the needle by pulling it straight from the vein. Direct pressure on the site is applied with the gauze only after the needle has been removed (Fig. 18-96). The technologist then puts the contaminated gloves, needles, and gauze in appropriate disposal containers (Fig. 18-97).

[1]Ehrlich R, Coakes D: *Patient care in radiography,* ed 8, St Louis, 2013, Elsevier/Mosby.

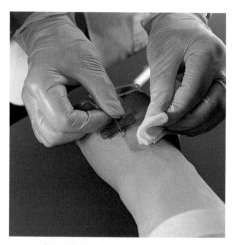

Fig. 18-96 Remove IV access.

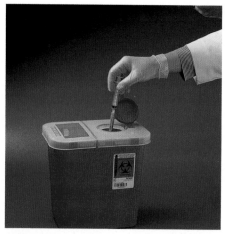

Fig. 18-97 Discard needles in puncture-resistant containers.

Reactions and Complications

Any *medication* has the potential to be harmful if it is not administered properly.[1] Technologists must be aware of possible untoward medication reactions and be able to recognize and report signs and symptoms of side effects as they occur.[2] The technologist who prepares a medication should also perform the administration.

Reactions can be mild, moderate, or severe. Mild reactions can include a sensation of warmth, a metallic taste, or sneezing. Moderate reactions can manifest as nausea, vomiting, or itching. Finally, a severe, or *anaphylactic,* reaction can cause a respiratory or cardiac crisis. The treatment for each category of reaction should be established in the procedures of each facility or department. The role of the radiologic technologist in the case of a reaction should also be defined in these documents. Competent professional standards of practice for the technologist include monitoring the patient's vital signs before, during, and after injection of a contrast medium or certain types of medications. The specific monitoring criteria should be established by institutional policy. If an untoward event should occur, responding personnel would have access to important information about the patient's condition before the event occurred.

Every health care provider should be familiar with emergency procedures in the work environment. Emergency crash carts contain many medications and pieces of equipment that require regular review. Proficiency in operation of equipment and administration of medications must be maintained. The technologist must have the knowledge, proficiency, and confidence to manage crisis situations.

[1]Kowalczyk N, Donnett K: *Integrated patient care for the imaging professional,* St Louis, 1996, Mosby.
[2]Adler AM, Carlton RR: *Introduction to radiography and patient care,* ed 3, Philadelphia, 2003, Saunders.

Infiltration, or *extravasation,* is another complication associated with the administration of contrast media or medications. This complication occurs when the medication or contrast material enters the soft tissue instead of the vein.[1] Signs include swelling, redness, burning, and pain. The most common cause of extravasation is needle displacement. If infiltration occurs, the procedure should be stopped immediately, and venous access should be discontinued. The physician must be notified, and specific treatment instructions must be requested. Although the ACR reports no clear consensus on the most effective treatment for extravasation, common therapies are (1) cold compress to alleviate pain at the injection site and (2) warm compress to increase blood flow to the site for more rapid absorption of the extravasated contrast.[1] The incident should be charted in the manner specified by department protocol.

Documentation

In the administration of any medication, the radiologic technologist should always observe five "rights of medication administration":

- The right patient
- The right medication
- The right route
- The right amount
- The right time

The *right patient* must receive the medication. The identity of the patient must be confirmed before the medication is administered. Methods of patient identification include checking the patient's wristband and asking the patient to restate his or her name. If the patient is unable to speak, seek assistance in identifying the patient from a family member or significant other. Ensuring that the *right medication* is administered requires that the name of the medication be verified at least three times: during the selection process, during preparation, and immediately before administration. The amount of medication is determined by the physician or by departmental protocols. The *right route, right amount,* and *right time* are determined by the physician, the type of medication, and the procedure.

[1]ACR Committee on Drugs and Contrast Media: *ACR manual on contrast media,* version 9, 2013, Reston, VA, 2013, American College of Radiology, ACR Committee on Drugs and Contrast Media.

Documentation of the five rights of medication administration should be included in every patient's permanent medical record. In addition to these five rights, the documentation should include the size, type, and location of the needle; the number of venipuncture attempts; and the identity of the health care personnel who performed the procedure. Information about how the patient responded to the procedure should also be documented. The following is an example of correct documentation technique for a technologist performing venipuncture and administering a medication:

> 4-15-99 at 0900 a venous access on Mr. John Q Public was performed using an 18-gauge angiocatheter. The access was established in the dorsum of the left hand after one attempt. Then 100 mL of [the specific name of the medication] was administered by IV push via the access. The patient tolerated the injection procedure and medication without complaints of pain or discomfort and with no unexpected side effects. (Sandy R. Ray, RT)

The objective of medication therapy and administration is to provide maximal benefit to the patient with minimal harm. Medications are intended to help maintain health, treat or prevent disease, relieve symptoms, alter body processes, and diagnose disease. All medications are not ideal in their effects on the human body. It is important that health care providers understand their role and responsibilities in the administration of medications. Because the medications used by the radiologic technologist are imperfect, caution for the patient's well-being and skill in the administration of medications are priorities. Patients have the right to expect that the personnel who administer medications are informed about dosages, actions, indications, adverse reactions, interactions, contraindications, and special considerations. Education, training, licensing, and experience are crucial in establishing competency in this area of practice.

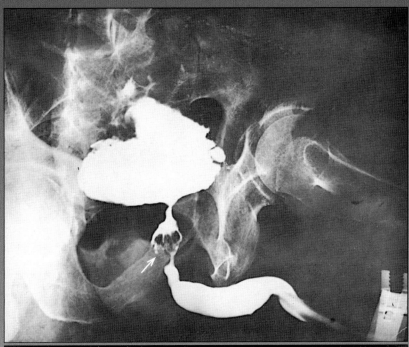

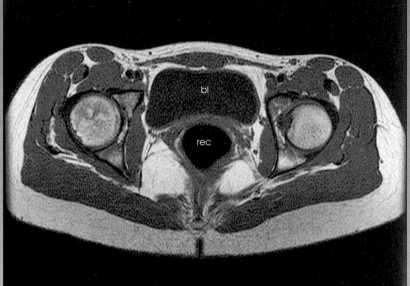

SUMMARY OF PROJECTIONS

PROJECTIONS, POSITIONS, AND METHODS

Page	Essential	Anatomy	Projection	Position	Method
246		Hysterosalpingography	AP, lateral, axial, oblique		
253		Seminal ducts	AP or AP oblique		

Female Reproductive System

The female reproductive system consists of an internal and an external group of organs, connected by the vaginal canal. This chapter does not address the anatomy of the external genitalia because those structures do not require radiographic demonstration. The internal genital organs consist of the female gonads, or *ovaries,* which are two glandular bodies homologous to the male testes, and a system of canals composed of the *uterine tubes, uterus,* and *vagina.*

OVARIES

The two ovaries are small, glandular organs with an internal secretion that controls the menstrual cycle and an external secretion containing the *ova,* or female reproductive cells (Fig. 19-1). Each ovary is shaped approximately like an almond. The ovaries lie one on each side, inferior and posterior to the uterine tube and near the lateral wall of the pelvis. They are attached to the posterior surface of the broad ligament of the uterus by the *mesovarium.*

The ovary has a core of vascular tissue, the *medulla,* and an outer portion of glandular tissue termed the *cortex.* The cortex contains *ovarian follicles* in all stages of development, and each follicle contains one ovum. A fully developed ovarian follicle is referred to as a *graafian follicle.* As the minute ovum matures, the size of the follicle and its fluid content increase so that the wall of the follicle's sac approaches the surface of the ovary and in time ruptures, liberating the ovum and follicular fluid into the peritoneal cavity. Extrusion of an ovum by the rupture of a follicle is called *ovulation* and usually occurs one time during the menstrual cycle. When the ovum is in the pelvic cavity, it is drawn toward the uterine tube.

UTERINE TUBES

The two *uterine tubes,* or fallopian tubes, arise from the lateral angle of the uterus, pass laterally above the ovaries, and open into the peritoneal cavity. These tubes collect ova released by the ovaries and convey the cells to the uterine cavity. Each tube is 3 to 5 inches (7.6 to 13 cm) long (Fig. 19-2) and has a small diameter at its uterine end, which opens into the cavity of the uterus by a minute orifice. The tube itself is divided into three parts: the isthmus, the ampulla, and the infundibulum. The *isthmus* is a short segment near the uterus. The *ampulla* comprises most of the tube and is wider than the isthmus. The terminal and lateral portion of the tube is the *infundibulum* and is flared in appearance. The infundibulum ends in a series of irregular prolonged processes called *fimbriae.* One of the fimbriae is attached to or near the ovary.

The mucosal lining of the uterine tube contains hairlike projections called *cilia.* The lining is arranged in folds that increase in number and complexity as they approach the fimbriated extremity of the tube. The cilia draw the ovum into the tube, which then conveys it to the uterine cavity by peristaltic movements. Passage of the ovum through the tube requires several days. Fertilization of the cell occurs in the outer part of the tube, and the fertilized ovum migrates to the uterus for implantation.

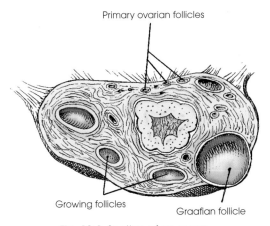

Primary ovarian follicles

Growing follicles

Graafian follicle

Fig. 19-1 Section of an ovary.

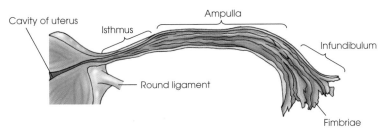

Cavity of uterus

Isthmus

Ampulla

Infundibulum

Round ligament

Fimbriae

Fig. 19-2 Section of left uterine tube.

UTERUS

The *uterus* is a pear-shaped, muscular organ (Figs. 19-3 and 19-4). Its primary functions are to receive and retain the fertilized ovum until development of the fetus is complete and, when the fetus is mature, to expel it during birth.

The uterus consists of four parts: fundus, body, isthmus, and cervix. The *fundus* is the bluntly rounded, superiormost portion of the uterus. The *body* narrows from the fundus to the isthmus and is the point of attachment for the ligaments that secure the uterus within the pelvis. The *isthmus* (superior part of the cervix), a constricted area between the body and the cervix, is approximately ½ inch (1.3 cm) long. The *cervix,* the cylindric vaginal end of the uterus, is approximately 1 inch (2.5 cm) long. The vagina is attached around the circumference of the cervix.

The *nulliparous* uterus (i.e., the uterus of a woman who has not given birth) is approximately 3 inches (7.6 cm) in length, almost half of which represents the length of the cervix. The cervix is approximately ¾ inch (1.9 cm) in diameter. During pregnancy, the body of the uterus gradually expands into the abdominal cavity, reaching the epigastric region in the 8th month. After parturition, the organ shrinks to almost its original size but undergoes characteristic changes in shape.

The uterus is situated in the central part of the pelvic cavity, where it lies posterior and superior to the urinary bladder and anterior to the rectal ampulla. The long axis, which is slightly concave anteriorly, is directed inferiorly and posteriorly at a near right angle to the axis of the vaginal canal into which the lower end of the cervix projects.

The cavity of the body of the uterus, or the uterine cavity proper, is triangular in shape when viewed in the frontal plane. The canal of the cervix is dilated in the center and constricted at each extremity. The proximal end of the canal is continuous with the canal of the isthmus. The distal orifice is called the *uterine ostium.*

The mucosal lining of the uterine cavity is called the *endometrium.* This lining undergoes cyclic changes, called the *menstrual cycle,* at about 4-week intervals from puberty to menopause. During each premenstrual period, the endometrium is prepared for implantation and nutrition of the fertilized ovum. If fertilization has not occurred, the menstrual flow of blood and necrosed particles of uterine mucosa ensues.

VAGINA

The *vagina* is a muscular structure with walls and a canal lying posterior to the urinary bladder and urethra and anterior to the rectum. Averaging about 3 inches (7.6 cm) in length, the vagina extends inferiorly and anteriorly from the uterus to the exterior. The *mucosa* of the vagina is continuous with that of the uterus. The space between the labia minora, which is known as the *vaginal vestibule,* contains the *vaginal orifice* and the *urethral orifice.*

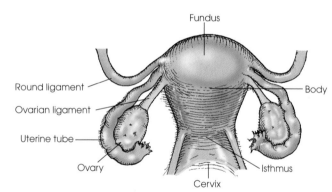

Fig. 19-3 Superoposterior view of uterus, ovaries, and uterine tubes.

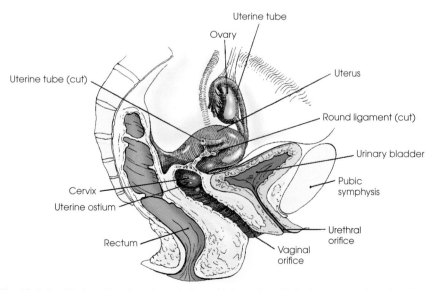

Fig. 19-4 Sagittal section showing relation of internal genitalia to surrounding structures.

FETAL DEVELOPMENT

During the *implantation* process, the fertilized ovum, called a *zygote,* is passed from the uterine tube into the uterine cavity, where it adheres to and becomes embedded in the uterine lining. About 2 weeks after fertilization of the ovum, the *embryo* begins to appear. The embryo becomes a fetus 9 weeks after fertilization and assumes a human appearance (Fig. 19-5).

During the first 2 weeks of embryonic development, the growing fertilized ovum is primarily concerned with establishment of its nutritive and protective covering, the *chorion* and the *amnion.* As the chorion develops, it forms (1) the outer layer of the protective membranes enclosing the embryo and (2) the embryonic portion of the *placenta,* by which the umbilical cord is attached to the mother's uterus, and through which food is supplied to and waste is removed from the fetus. The amnion, often referred to as the "bag of water" by the laity, forms the inner layer of the fetal membranes and contains amniotic fluid in which the fetus floats. After birth, the uterine lining is expelled with the fetal membranes and the placenta, constituting the afterbirth. A new endometrium is then regenerated.

The fertilized ovum usually becomes embedded near the fundus of the uterine cavity, most frequently on the anterior or posterior wall. Implantation occasionally occurs so low, however, that the fully developed placenta encroaches on or obstructs the cervical canal. This condition results in premature separation of the placenta, termed *placenta previa* (Fig. 19-6).

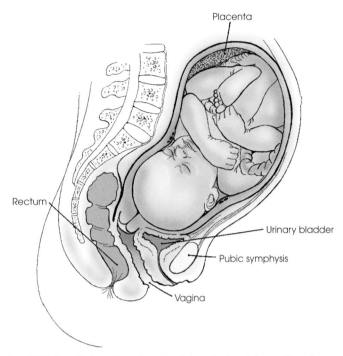

Fig. 19-5 Sagittal section showing fetus of about 7 months of age.

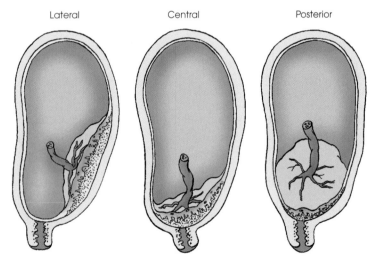

Fig. 19-6 Schematic drawings of several placental sites in low implantation.

Male Reproductive System

The male genital system consists of a pair of male *gonads*, the *testes*, which produce spermatozoa; two excretory channels, the *ductus deferens* (vas deferens); the *prostate;* the ejaculatory ducts; the *seminal vesicles;* and a pair of *bulbourethral glands*, which produce secretions that are added to the secretions of the testes and ductal mucosa to constitute the final product of seminal fluid. The *penis*, the *scrotum*, and the structures enclosed by the scrotal sac (testes, epididymides, spermatic cords, and part of the ductus deferens) are the external genital organs.

TESTES

The *testes* are ovoid bodies averaging $1\frac{1}{2}$ inches (3.8 cm) in length and about 1 inch (2.5 cm) in width and depth (Fig. 19-7). Each testis is divided into 200 to 300 partial compartments that constitute the glandular substance of the testis. Each compartment houses one or more convoluted, germ cell–producing tubules. These tubules converge and unite to form 15 to 20 ductules that emerge from the testis to enter the head of the epididymis.

The *epididymis* is an oblong structure that is attached to the superior and lateroposterior aspects of the testis. The ductules leading out of the testis enter the head of the epididymis to become continuous with the coiled and convoluted ductules that make up this structure. As the ductules pass inferiorly, they progressively unite to form the main duct, which is continuous with the ductus deferens.

DUCTUS DEFERENS

The *ductus deferens* is 16 to 18 inches (40 to 45 cm) long and extends from the tail of the epididymis to the posteroinferior surface of the urinary bladder. Only its first part is convoluted. From its beginning, the ductus deferens ascends along the medial side of the epididymis on the posterior surface of the testis to join the other constituents of the spermatic cord, with which it emerges from the scrotal sac and passes into the pelvic cavity through the inguinal canal (Fig. 19-8). Near its termination, the duct expands into an *ampulla* for storage of seminal fluid and then ends by uniting with the duct of the seminal vesicle.

SEMINAL VESICLES

The two *seminal vesicles* are sacculated structures about 2 inches (5 cm) long (Fig. 19-9). They are situated obliquely on the lateroposterior surface of the bladder, where, from the level of the ureterocystic junction, each slants inferiorly and medially to the base of the prostate. Each ampulla of the ductus deferens lies along the medial border of the seminal vesicle to form the ejaculatory duct.

EJACULATORY DUCTS

The *ejaculatory ducts* are formed by the union of the ductus deferens and the duct of the seminal vesicle. The ejaculatory ducts average about $\frac{1}{2}$ inch (1.3 cm) in length and originate behind the neck of the bladder. The two ducts enter the base of the prostate and, passing obliquely inferiorly through the substance of the gland, open into the prostatic urethra at the lateral margins of the prostatic utricle. These ducts eject sperm into the urethra before ejaculation.

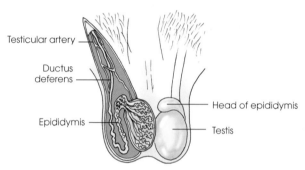

Fig. 19-7 Frontal section of testes and ductus deferens.

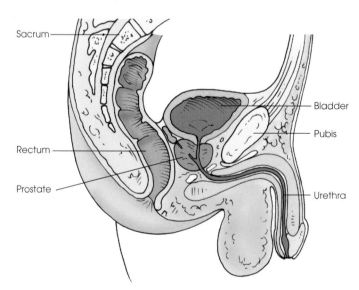

Fig. 19-8 Sagittal section showing male genital system.

PROSTATE

The *prostate,* an accessory genital organ, is a cone-shaped organ that averages 1¼ inches (3.2 cm) in length. The prostate encircles the proximal portion of the male urethra and, extending from the bladder neck to the pelvic floor, lies in front of the rectal ampulla approximately 1 inch (2.5 cm) posterior to the lower two thirds of the pubic symphysis (see Fig. 19-9). The prostate comprises muscular and glandular tissue. The ducts of the prostate open into the prostatic portion of the urethra.

Because of advances in diagnostic ultrasound imaging, radiographic examinations of the male reproductive system are performed less often than in the past. The prostate can be ultrasonically imaged through the urine-filled bladder or by using a special rectal transducer. The seminal ducts can be imaged when the rectum is filled with an ultrasound gel and a special rectal transducer is used. Testicular ultrasonic scans are performed to evaluate a palpable mass or an enlarged testis and to check for metastasis. Most testicular scans are performed because of a palpable mass or an enlarged testis.

> **PROCEDURES REMOVED**
>
> The following procedures have been removed from this edition of the atlas. See previous editions of the atlas for a description of these procedures.
> • Pelvimetry

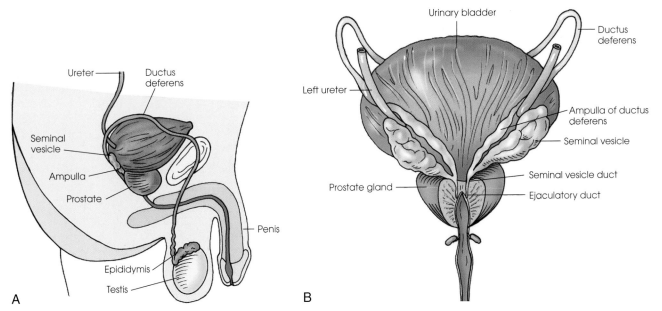

A

B

Fig. 19-9 A, Sagittal section through male pelvis. **B,** Posterior view of male reproductive organs.

SUMMARY OF ANATOMY TERMS

Female reproductive system
Ovaries
Uterine tubes
Uterus
Vagina

Ovaries
Ova
Mesovarium
Medulla
Cortex
Ovarian follicles
Graafian follicle
Ovulation

Uterine tubes (fallopian tubes)
Isthmus
Ampulla
Infundibulum
Fimbriae
Cilia

Uterus
Fundus
Body
Isthmus
Cervix
Uterine ostium
Endometrium

Vagina
Mucosa
Vaginal vestibule
Vaginal orifice
Urethral orifice

Fetal development
Zygote
Embryo
Fetus
Placenta

Male reproductive system
Testes

Ductus deferens
(vas deferens)
Prostate
Ejaculatory ducts
Seminal vesicles
Bulbourethral glands
Penis
Scrotum

Testes
Epididymis

Ductus deferens
Ampulla

SUMMARY OF PATHOLOGY

Condition	Definition
Adhesion	Union of two surfaces that are normally separate
Cryptorchidism	Condition of undescended testis
Endometrial polyp	Growth or mass protruding from endometrium
Epididymitis	Inflammation of the epididymis
Uterine tube obstruction	Condition preventing normal flow through uterine tube
Fistula	Abnormal connection between two internal organs or between an organ and the body surface
Testicular torsion	Twisting of the testis at its base, causing acute ischemia
Tumor	New tissue growth where cell proliferation is uncontrolled
Dermoid cyst	Tumor of the ovary filled with sebaceous material and hair
Prostate cancer	Second most common malignancy in men
Seminoma	Most common type of testicular tumor
Uterine fibroid	Smooth muscle tumor of the uterus

ABBREVIATIONS USED IN CHAPTER 19

HSG   Hysterosalpingography
IUD   Intrauterine device

See Addendum B for a summary of all abbreviations used in Volume 2.

Reproductive System

Female Radiography
NONPREGNANT PATIENT

Radiologic investigations of the nonpregnant uterus, accessory organs, and vagina are denoted by the terms *hysterosalpingography* (HSG), *pelvic pneumography,* and *vaginography*. Each procedure requires the use of contrast medium and should be performed under aseptic conditions. *HSG* involves the introduction of a radiopaque contrast medium through a uterine cannula. The procedure is performed to determine the size, shape, and position of the uterus and uterine tubes; to delineate lesions such as polyps, submucous tumor masses, or fistulous tracts; and to investigate the patency of the uterine tubes in patients who have been unable to conceive (Fig. 19-10).

Pelvic pneumography, which requires the introduction of a gaseous contrast medium directly into the peritoneal cavity, is now rarely performed because of the development of ultrasound techniques for evaluating the pelvic cavity. *Vaginography* is performed to investigate congenital abnormalities, vaginal fistulae, and other pathologic conditions involving the vagina.

Contrast media

Various opaque media are used in examinations of the female genital passages. The water-soluble contrast media employed for intravenous urography are widely used for HSG and vaginography.

Preparation of intestinal tract

Preparation of the intestinal tract for any of these examinations usually consists of the following:
1. A non–gas-forming laxative is administered on the preceding evening if the patient is constipated.
2. Before reporting for the examination, the patient receives cleansing enemas until the return flow is clear.
3. The meal preceding the examination is withheld.

Appointment date and care of patient

Gynecologic examinations should be scheduled approximately 10 days after the onset of menstruation. This is the interval during which the endometrium is least congested. More important, because this time interval is a few days before ovulation normally occurs, there is little danger of irradiating a recently fertilized ovum.

The relatively minor instrumentation required for the introduction of contrast medium in these examinations normally necessitates neither hospitalization nor premedication. Some patients experience unpleasant but transitory aftereffects. The radiology department should have facilities in which an outpatient can rest in the recumbent position before returning home.

The patient is requested to empty her bladder completely immediately before the examination; this prevents pressure displacement and superimposition of the bladder on the pelvic genitalia. In addition, the patient's vagina is irrigated just before the examination. At this time, the patient should be given the necessary supplies and instructed to cleanse the perineal region.

Radiation protection

To deliver the least possible amount of radiation to the gonads, the radiologist restricts fluoroscopy and imaging to the minimum required for a satisfactory examination.

Hysterosalpingography

HSG is performed by a physician, with spot images made while the patient is in the supine position on a fluoroscopic table. The examination may also be performed by the physician with conventional radiographic images obtained using an overhead tube. When fluoroscopy is used, spot images may be the only images obtained. Preparation of the patient for the examination includes the following steps:
- After irrigation of the vaginal canal, complete emptying of the bladder, and perineal cleansing, place the patient on the examining table.
- Adjust the patient in the lithotomy position, with the knees flexed over leg rests.
- When a combination table is used, adjust the patient's position to permit the IRs to be centered to a point 2 inches (5 cm) proximal to the pubic symphysis; lengthwise 10 × 12-inch (24 × 30-cm) IRs or collimated field sizes are used for all studies.

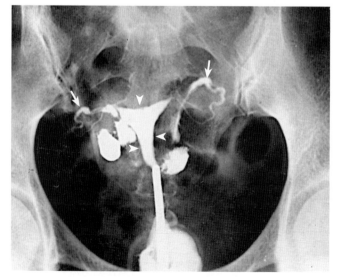

Fig. 19-10 HSG reveals bilateral hydrosalpinx of uterine tubes (*arrows*). Contrast medium–filled uterine cavity is normal (*arrowheads*).

After inspection of the preliminary image and with a vaginal speculum in position, the physician inserts a uterine cannula through the cervical canal; fits the attached rubber plug, or acorn, firmly against the external cervical os; applies counterpressure with a tenaculum to prevent reflux of the contrast medium; and withdraws the speculum unless it is radiolucent. An opaque or a gaseous contrast medium may be injected via the cannula into the uterine cavity. The contrast material flows through patent uterine tubes and "spills" into the peritoneal cavity (Figs. 19-11 to 19-13). Patency of the uterine tubes can be determined by transuterine gas insufflation (Rubin test), but the length, position, and course of the ducts can be shown only by opacifying the lumina.

Free-flowing, iodinated organic contrast agents are usually injected at room temperature. These agents pass through patent uterine tubes quickly, and the resultant peritoneal spill is absorbed and eliminated via the urinary system, usually within 2 hours.

The contrast medium may be injected with a pressometer or a syringe. Intrauterine pressure is maintained for radiographic studies by closing the cannular valve. In the absence of fluoroscopy, the contrast medium is introduced in two to four fractional doses so that excessive peritoneal spillage does not occur. Each fractional dose is followed by a radiographic study to determine whether the filling is adequate as shown by the peritoneal spill.

The images may consist of no more than a single AP projection taken at the end of each fractional injection. Other projections (oblique, axial, and lateral) are taken as indicated.

EVALUATION CRITERIA

The following should be clearly shown:
- The pelvic region 2 inches (5 cm) above the pubic symphysis centered on the image
- All contrast media visible, including any "spill" areas
- Brightness and contrast sufficient to show soft tissues and contrast media

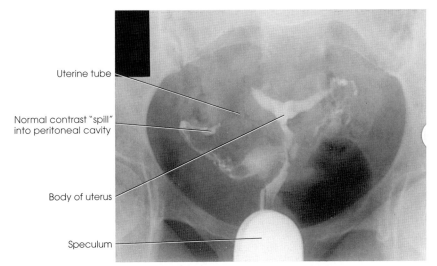

Uterine tube

Normal contrast "spill" into peritoneal cavity

Body of uterus

Speculum

Fig. 19-11 Hysterosalpingogram, AP projection, showing normal uterus and uterine tubes.

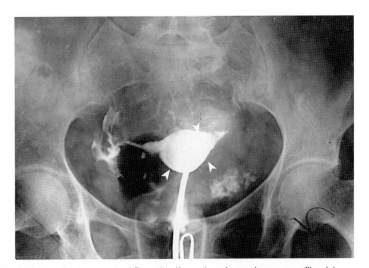

Fig. 19-12 Hysterosalpingogram, AP projection, showing submucous fibroid occupying entire uterine cavity (*arrowheads*).

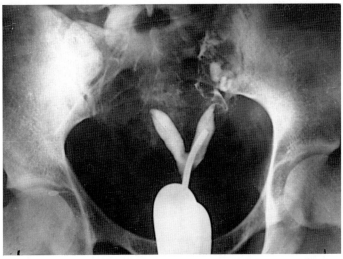

Fig. 19-13 Hysterosalpingogram, AP projection, revealing uterine cavity as bicornuate in outline.

Imaging of female contraceptive devices

HSG is performed about three months after insertion of the permanent type of intrauterine device (IUD) (Fig. 19-14). Additionally, HSG and other imaging modalities, such as ultrasound, may also be used to check for proper placement of temporary IUDs and in cases of suspected displacement. For these reasons, radiographers should be acquainted with the appearance of IUDs in images. IUDs have

been used for contraception for many decades. Currently, there are only two forms of temporary IUDs and one for permanent contraception (Figs. 19-15 and 19-16). IUD insertion is usually performed in an out-patient procedure in a physician's office; however, conscious sedation is required to insert the permanent IUD.[1]

---

[1]Wittmer M et al: Hysterosalpingography for assessing efficacy of Essure microinsert permanent birth control device, *AJR Am J Roentgenol* 187:955, 2006.

While an HSG is required to insure that the permanent IUD is properly functioning, insertion of this device is much less invasive than the other permanent sterility option, tubal ligation.

AP and lateral projections of the abdomen are suggested for IUD localization. Occasionally, oblique projections are indicated. Most IUDs are radiopaque because of their metallic composition. Radiography alone is *not* a reliable method of extrauterine localization of an IUD.

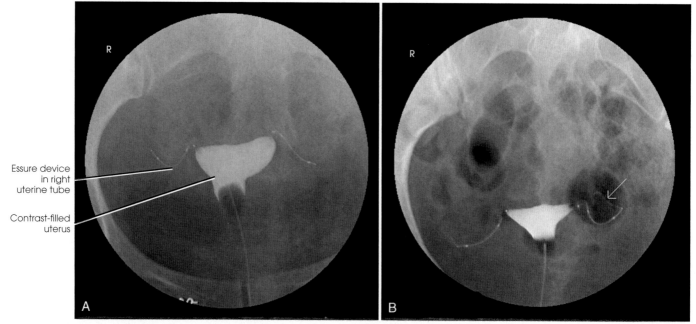

Essure device in right uterine tube

Contrast-filled uterus

Fig. 19-14 Hysterosalpingogram three-months post Essure® insertion. (Essure confirmation test). **A,** HSG spot image confirms occlusion of uterine tubes. **B,** HSG spot demonstrates failure of left uterine tube occlusion (arrow points to contrast spill into peritoneum).

(Images courtesy of NEA Baptist Memorial Hospital, Jonesboro, AR.)

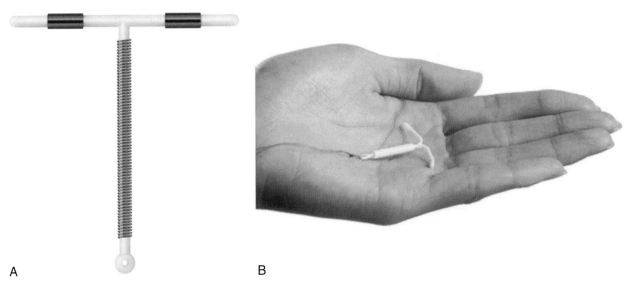

A

B

Fig. 19-15 Temporary intrauterine contraceptive device (IUD). **A,** ParaGard (intrauterine copper contraceptive) manufactured by Teva Women's Health, Inc. Actual size is 32 × 36 mm. **B,** Mirena (levonorgestrel-releasing intrauterine system) manufactured by Bayer Healthcare Pharmaceuticals.

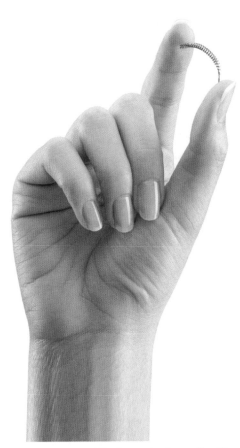

Fig. 19-16 Permanent contraceptive IUD, Essure by Bayer Healthcare Pharmaceuticals.

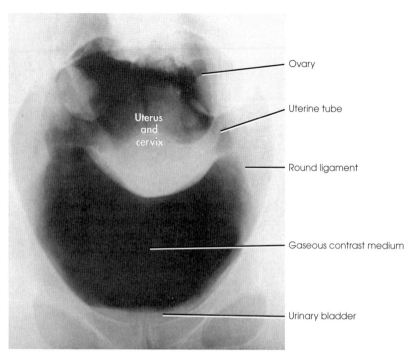

Fig. 19-17 Normal pelvic pneumogram. (See Fig. 19-3 for correlation with image.)

Pelvic pneumography

Pelvic pneumography, gynecography, and *pangynecography* are the terms used to denote radiologic examinations of the female pelvic organs via intraperitoneal gas insufflation (Fig. 19-17). These procedures have essentially been replaced by ultrasonography and other diagnostic techniques. (Pelvic pneumography is described in Volume 3 of the fourth edition of this atlas.)

Vaginography

Vaginography is used in the investigation of congenital malformations and pathologic conditions such as vesicovaginal and enterovaginal fistulae. The examination is performed by introducing a contrast medium into the vaginal canal. Lambie et al.[1] recommended using a thin barium sulfate mixture to investigate fistulous communications with the intestine. At the end of the examination, the patient is instructed to expel as much of the barium mixture as possible, and the canal is cleansed by vaginal irrigation. For investigation of other conditions, Coe[2] advocated the use of an iodinated organic compound.

A rectal retention tube is employed to introduce the contrast medium so that the moderately inflated balloon can be used to prevent reflux. In one technique, the physician inserts only the tip of the tube into the vaginal orifice. The patient is requested to extend the thighs and to hold them in close approximation to keep the inflated balloon pressed firmly against the vaginal entrance. In another technique, the tube is inserted far enough to place the deflated balloon within the distal end of the vagina, and the balloon is inflated under fluoroscopic observation. The barium mixture is introduced with the usual enema equipment. The water-soluble medium is injected with a syringe.

Vaginography is performed on a combination fluoroscopic-radiographic table. Contrast medium is injected under fluoroscopic control, and spot images are exposed as indicated during the filling (Fig. 19-18).

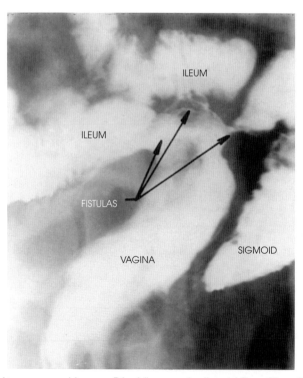

Fig. 19-18 Vaginogram, spot image, PA oblique projection, LAO position. Sigmoid fistula and two ileum fistulae are shown.

[1]Lambie RW et al: Demonstration of fistulae by vaginography, *AJR Am J Roentgenol* 90:717, 1963.
[2]Coe FO: Vaginography, *AJR Am J Roentgenol* 90:721, 1963.

The images in Figs. 19-19 to 19-21 were taken with the central ray directed perpendicular to the midpoint of the IR. For localized studies, the central ray is centered at the level of the superior border of the pubic symphysis.

In each examination, the radiographic projections required are determined by the radiologist according to fluoroscopic findings. Low rectovaginal fistulae are best shown in the lateral projection, and fistulous communications with the sigmoid or ileum or both are best shown in oblique projections.

EVALUATION CRITERIA

The following should be clearly shown:
- Superior border of the pubic symphysis centered on the image
- Any fistulae in their entirety
- Pelvis on oblique projections not superimposed by the proximal thigh
- Superimposed hips and femora in the lateral image
- Exposure sufficient to demonstrate the vagina and any fistula

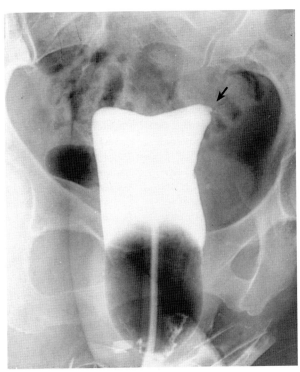

Fig. 19-19 Vaginogram, AP projection, showing small fistulous tract (*arrow*) projecting laterally from apex of vagina and ending in abscess.

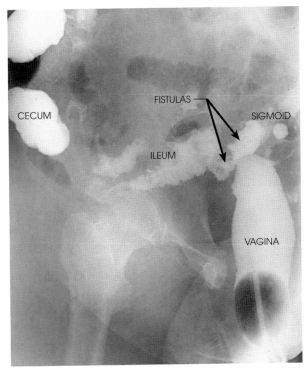

Fig. 19-20 Vaginogram, AP oblique projection, RPO position. Fistulae to ileum and sigmoid are shown.

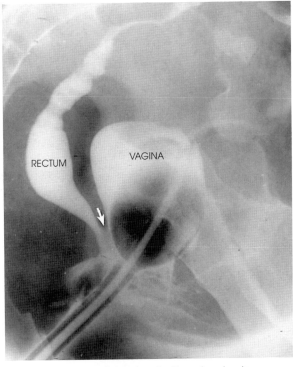

Fig. 19-21 Vaginogram, lateral projection, showing low rectovaginal fistula.

PREGNANT PATIENT

Ultrasonography provides visualization of the fetus and placenta with no apparent risk to the patient or fetus. Diagnostic sonography is the preferred diagnostic tool for examination of a pregnant woman. For informational purposes, the following radiographic procedures are defined:

- *Fetography*—radiographic examination of the fetus in utero.
  - This examination should be performed after the 18th week of gestation because of the danger of radiation-induced fetal malformations.
  - Fetography is employed to detect suspected abnormalities of development, to confirm suspected fetal death, to determine the presentation and position of the fetus, and to determine whether the pregnancy is single or multiple (Fig. 19-22).
- *Pelvimetry*—radiographic examination to demonstrate the architecture of the maternal pelvis to compare with the size of the fetal head
  - This examination was performed to determine the necessity of a cesarean section
- *Placentography*—radiographic examination to demonstrate the walls of the uterus for localization of the placenta in cases of suspected placenta previa.

For more detailed information on the above procedures, refer to the 12th and earlier editions of this atlas.

Radiation protection

Radiologic examinations of pregnant patients are performed only when required information can be obtained in no other way. In addition to the danger of genetic changes that may result from reproductive cell irradiation is the danger of radiation-induced malformations of the developing fetus. When possible, radiation for any purpose is avoided during pregnancy, especially during the first trimester of gestation. If examination of the abdominopelvic region is necessary, it is restricted to the absolute minimum number of images. The radiographer's responsibility is to perform the work carefully and thoughtfully so that repeat exposures are unnecessary.

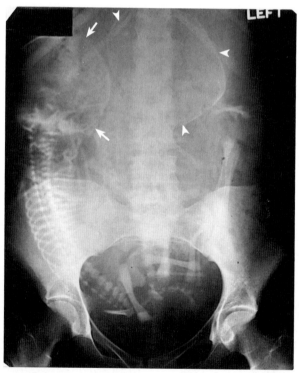

Fig. 19-22 Fetography, PA projection. Twin pregnancy showing two fetal heads (*arrows and arrowheads*).

Male Radiography

SEMINAL DUCTS

Radiologic examinations of the seminal ducts[1-3] are performed to investigate certain genitourinary abnormalities, such as cysts, abscesses, tumors, inflammation, and sterility. The regional terms applied to these examinations are *vesiculography,*

[1]Boreau J et al: Epididymography, *Med Radiogr Photogr* 29:63, 1953.
[2]Boreau J: *L'étude radiologique des voies séminales normales et pathologiques,* Paris, 1953, Masson & Cie.
[3]Vasselle B: *Etude radiologique des voies séminales de l'homme,* Thesis, Paris, 1953.

epididymography, and, when combined, *epididymovesiculography.*

The water-soluble, iodinated compounds used for intravenous urography are also employed as contrast media for these procedures. A gaseous contrast medium can be injected into each scrotal sac to improve contrast in the examination of extrapelvic structures.

The seminal vesicles are sometimes opacified directly by urethroscopic catheterization of the ejaculatory ducts. More frequently, the entire duct system is inspected by introducing contrast solution into the canals via the ductus deferens. Small bilateral incisions in the upper part of the scrotum are required for exposure

and identification of these ducts. The needle that is used to inject the contrast medium is inserted into the duct in the direction of the portion of the tract under investigation—distally for study of the extrapelvic ducts, then proximally for study of the intrapelvic ducts.

A nongrid exposure technique is used to delineate extrapelvic structures (Figs. 19-23 to 19-25). The examining urologist places the IR and adjusts the position of the testes for desired projections of the ducts. A grid technique is used to show the intrapelvic ducts (Figs. 19-24 to 19-28). AP and oblique projections are made using 8 × 10-inch (18 × 24-cm) or 10 × 12-inch (24 × 30-cm) lengthwise IRs or collimated field sizes and centered at the level of the superior border of the pubic symphysis.

EVALUATION CRITERIA

The following should be clearly shown:
- Evidence of proper collimation

AP Projection
- IR centered at the level of the superior border of the pubic symphysis
- No rotation of the patient
- Exposure sufficient to demonstrate all structures of interest

Oblique Projection
- Region of interest in the center of the collimated field
- No superimposition of the seminal ducts by the ilia
- No overlap of the region of the prostate or urethra by the uppermost thigh

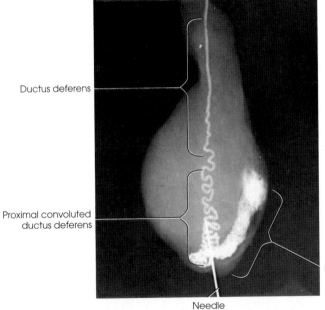

Fig. 19-23 Epididymogram showing normal epididymis and origin of ductus deferens. The needle is at the epididymovasal kink, which can be palpated.

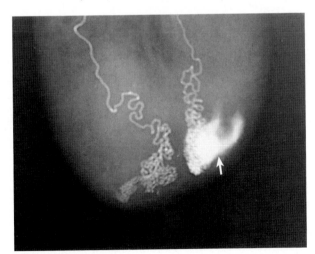

Fig. 19-24 Epididymogram showing tuberculosis (cold abscess) of epididymis (*arrow*).

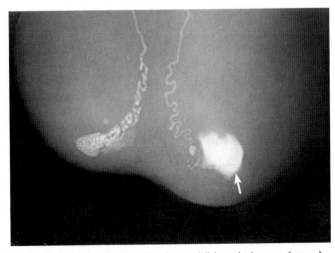

Fig. 19-25 Epididymogram showing epididymal abscess (*arrow*) observed during acute orchitis (third relapse). Epididymovasal kink is atrophic.

PROSTATE

Prostatography is a term applied to investigation of the prostate by radiographic, cystographic, or vesiculographic procedures. It is seldom performed today because of advances in diagnostic ultrasonography. Radiographic examination of the prostate gland was described in the 8th and earlier editions of this atlas.

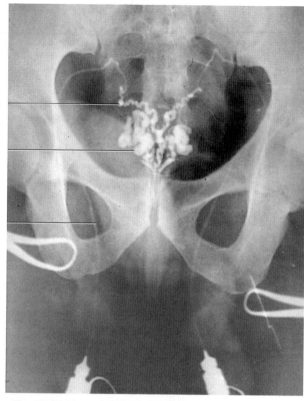

Distal ductus deferens

Seminal vesicle

Proximal ductus deferens

Fig. 19-26 Normal vesiculogram.

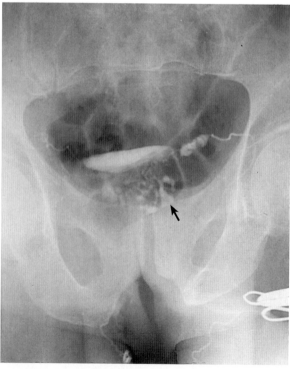

Fig. 19-27 Vesiculogram of tuberculous seminal vesicle associated with deferentitis, showing small abscesses, ampullitis, and considerable vesiculitis on left (*arrow*).

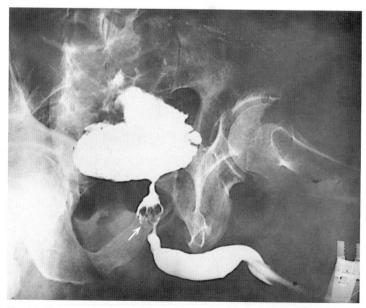

Fig. 19-28 Vesiculogram showing beginning (budding) metastasis of crista urethralis (*arrow*) discovered 2 years after prostatectomy for cancer of the prostate.

20

SKULL, FACIAL BONES, AND PARANASAL SINUSES

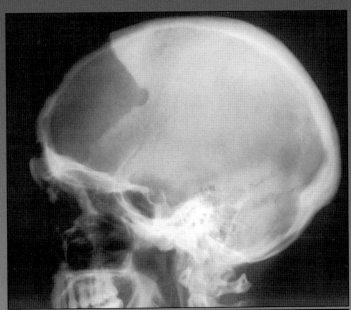

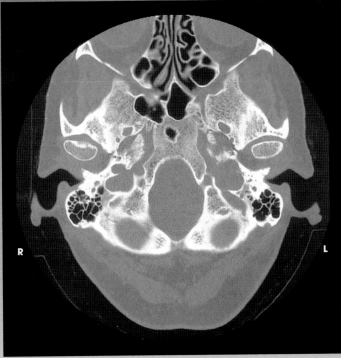

SUMMARY OF PROJECTIONS

PROJECTIONS, POSITIONS, AND METHODS

Page	Essential	Anatomy	Projection	Position	Method
291	🌲	Cranium	Lateral	R or L	
294	🌲	Cranium	Lateral	R or L dorsal decubitus	
294	🌲	Cranium	Lateral	R or L supine lateral	
296	🌲	Cranium	PA		
296	🌲	Cranium	PA axial		CALDWELL
300	🌲	Cranium	AP		
300	🌲	Cranium	AP axial		
302	🌲	Cranium	AP axial		TOWNE
308	🌲	Cranium	PA axial		HAAS
310	🌲	Cranial base	Submentovertical (SMV)		SCHÜLLER
317		Eye	Lateral	R or L	
318		Eye	PA axial		
319		Eye	Parietoacanthial		MODIFIED WATERS
320	🌲	Facial bones	Lateral	R or L	
323	🌲	Facial bones	Parietoacanthial		WATERS
325		Facial bones	Modified parietoacanthial		MODIFIED WATERS
327	🌲	Facial bones	Acanthioparietal		REVERSE WATERS
329	🌲	Facial bones	PA axial		CALDWELL
331	🌲	Nasal bones	Lateral	R and L	
333	🌲	Zygomatic arches	Submentovertical		
335	🌲	Zygomatic arch	Tangential		
337	🌲	Zygomatic arches	AP axial		MODIFIED TOWNE
339	🌲	Mandibular rami	PA		
340	🌲	Mandibular rami	PA axial		
341		Mandibular body	PA		
342		Mandibular body	PA axial		
343	🌲	Mandible	Axiolateral, axiolateral oblique		
346		Mandible	Submentovertical		
347	🌲	TMJs	AP axial		
349		TMJs	Axiolateral	R and L	
351	🌲	TMJs	Axiolateral oblique	R and L	
353		Mandible	Panoramic		TOMOGRAPHY
358	🌲	Paranasal sinuses	Lateral	R or L upright	
360	🌲	Frontal and anterior ethmoidal sinuses	PA axial	Upright	CALDWELL
362	🌲	Maxillary sinuses	Parietoacanthial	Upright	WATERS
364	🌲	Maxillary and sphenoidal sinuses	Parietoacanthial	Upright with open mouth	WATERS
366	🌲	Ethmoidal and sphenoidal sinuses	Submentovertical	Upright	

Icons in the Essential column indicate projections frequently performed in the United States and Canada. Students should be competent in these projections.

Skull

The *skull* rests on the superior aspect of the vertebral column. It is composed of 22 separate bones divided into two distinct groups: 8 *cranial* bones and 14 *facial* bones. The cranial bones are divided further into the *calvaria* and the *floor* (Box 20-1). The cranial bones form a protective housing for the brain. The facial bones provide structure, shape, and support for the face. They also form a protective housing for the upper ends of the respiratory and digestive tracts and, with several of the cranial bones, form the orbital sockets for protection of the organs of sight. The *hyoid bone* is commonly discussed with this group of bones.

The bones of the skull are identified in Figs. 20-1 to 20-3. The 22 primary bones of the skull should be located and recognized in the different views before they are studied in greater detail.

BOX 20-1
Skull bones

Cranial bones (8)		Facial bones (14)	
Calvaria		Nasal (right and left)	2
Frontal	1	Lacrimal (right and left)	2
Occipital	1	Maxillary (right and left)	2
Right parietal	1	Zygomatic (right and left)	2
Left parietal	1	Palatine (right and left)	2
		Inferior nasal conchae (right and left)	2
Floor		Vomer	1
Ethmoid	1	Mandible	1
Sphenoid	1		
Right temporal	1		
Left temporal	1		

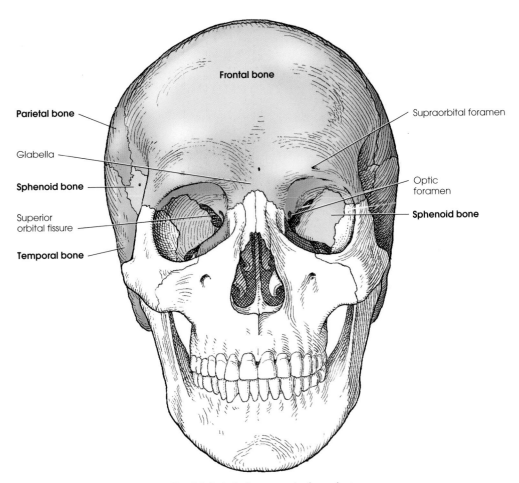

Fig. 20-1 Anterior aspect of cranium.

Labels: Frontal bone, Parietal bone, Glabella, Sphenoid bone, Superior orbital fissure, Temporal bone, Supraorbital foramen, Optic foramen, Sphenoid bone

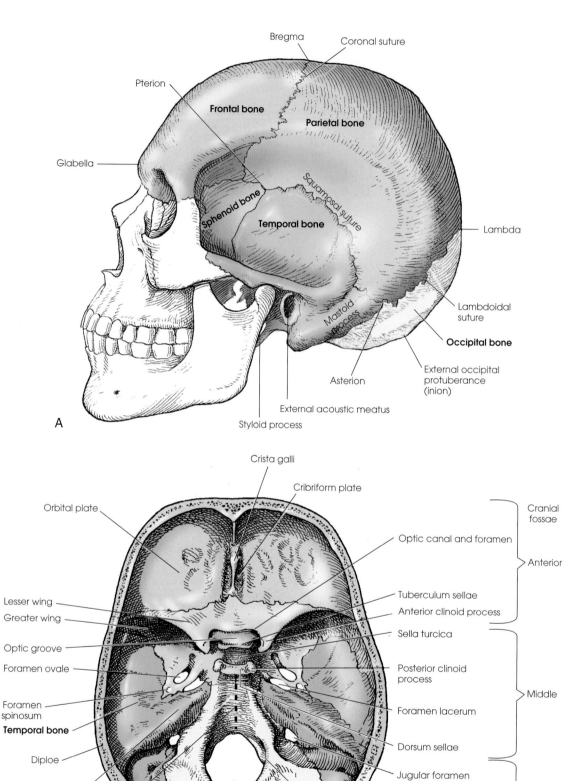

Fig. 20-2 A, Lateral aspect of cranium. **B,** Superior aspect of cranial base.

The bones of the cranial vault are composed of two plates of compact tissue separated by an inner layer of spongy tissue called *diploë*. The outer plate, or table, is thicker than the inner table over most of the vault, and the thickness of the layer of spongy tissue varies considerably.

Except for the mandible, the bones of the cranium and face are joined by fibrous joints called *sutures*. The sutures are named *coronal, sagittal, squamosal,* and *lambdoidal* (see Figs. 20-1 and 20-2). The *coronal suture* is found between the frontal and parietal bones. The *sagittal suture* is located on the top of the head between the two parietal bones and just behind the coronal suture line (not visible in Figs. 20-1 and 20-2). The junction of the coronal and sagittal sutures is the *bregma*. Between the temporal bones and the parietal bones are the *squamosal sutures*. Between the occipital bone and the parietal bones is the *lambdoidal suture*.

The *lambda* is the junction of the lambdoidal and sagittal sutures. On the lateral aspect of the skull, the junction of the parietal bone, squamosal suture, and greater wing of the sphenoid is the *pterion,* which overlies the middle meningeal artery. At the junction of the occipital bone, parietal bone, and mastoid portion of the temporal bone is the *asterion.*

In a newborn infant, the bones of the cranium are thin and not fully developed. They contain a small amount of calcium,

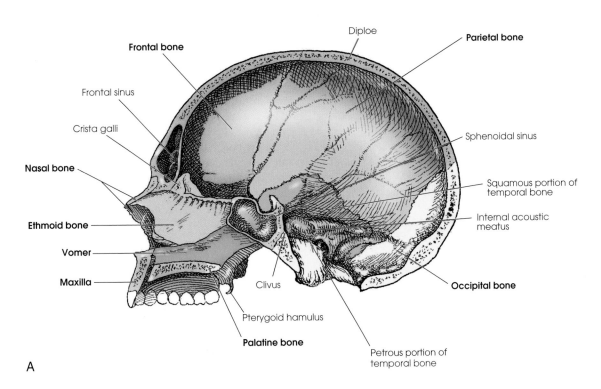

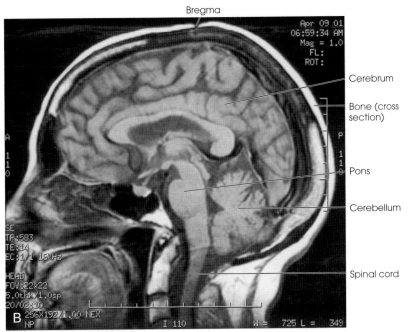

Fig. 20-3 A, Lateral aspect of interior of cranium. **B,** Sagittal MRI of cranium showing contents and position of brain. Note bony protective housing.

are indistinctly marked, and present six areas of incomplete ossification called *fontanels,* often spelled *fontenelles* (Fig. 20-4). Two of the fontanels are situated in the midsagittal plane at the superior and posterior angles of the parietal bones. The *anterior fontanel* is located at the junction of the two parietal bones and the one frontal bone at the bregma. Posteriorly and in the midsagittal plane is the *posterior fontanel,* located at the point labeled *lambda* in Fig. 20-2. Two fontanels are also on each side at the inferior angles of the parietal bones. Each *sphenoidal fontanel* is found at the site of the pterion; the *mastoid fontanels* are found at the asteria. The posterior and sphenoidal fontanels normally close in the 1st and 3rd months after birth, and the anterior and mastoid fontanels close during the 2nd year of life.

The cranium develops rapidly in size and density during the first 5 or 6 years, after which a gradual increase occurs until adult size and density are achieved, usually by the age of 12 years. The thickness and degree of mineralization in normal adult crania show comparatively little difference in radiopacity from person to person, and the atrophy of old age is

less marked than in other regions of the body.

Internally, the cranial floor is divided into three regions: anterior, middle, and posterior cranial fossae (see Fig. 20-2, *B*). The *anterior cranial fossa* extends from the anterior frontal bone to the lesser wings of the sphenoid. It is associated mainly with the frontal lobes of the cerebrum. The *middle cranial fossa* accommodates the temporal lobes and associated neurovascular structures and extends from the lesser wings of the sphenoid bone to the apices of petrous portions of the temporal bones. The deep depression posterior to the petrous ridges is the *posterior cranial fossa,* which protects the cerebellum, pons, and medulla oblongata (see Fig. 20-3, *B*).

The average or so-called normal cranium is more or less oval in shape, wider in back than in front. The average cranium measures approximately 6 inches (15 cm) at its widest point from side to side, 7 inches (17.8 cm) at its longest point from front to back, and 9 inches (22 cm) at its deepest point from the vertex to the submental region. Crania vary in size and shape, with resultant vari-

ation in the position and relationship of internal parts.

Internal deviations from the norm are usually indicated by external deviations and can be estimated with a reasonable degree of accuracy. The length and width of the normally shaped head vary by 1 inch (2.5 cm). Any deviation from this relationship indicates a comparable change in the position and relationship of the internal structures. If the deviation involves more than a 5-degree change, it must be compensated for by a change in part rotation or central ray angulation. This "rule" applies to all images except direct lateral projections. A ½-inch (1.3 cm) change in the 1-inch (2.5-cm) width-to-length measurement indicates an approximately 5-degree change in the direction of the internal parts with reference to the midsagittal plane.

It is important for the radiographer to understand cranial anatomy from the standpoint of the size, shape, position, and relationship of component parts of the cranium, so that estimations and compensations can be made for deviations from the norm.

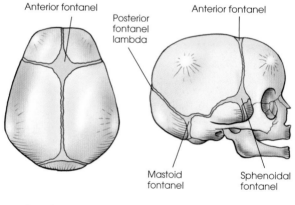

Superior aspect   Lateral aspect

Fig. 20-4 Fontanels of a newborn.

Cranial Bones
FRONTAL BONE

The *frontal bone* has a vertical portion and horizontal portions. The vertical portion, called the *frontal squama,* forms the forehead and the anterior part of the vault. The horizontal portions form the orbital plates (roofs of the orbits), part of the roof of the nasal cavity, and the greater part of the anterior cranial fossa (Figs. 20-5 to 20-7).

On each side of the midsagittal plane of the superior portion of the squama is a rounded elevation called the *frontal eminence.* Below the frontal eminences, just above the *supraorbital margins,* are two arched ridges that correspond in position to the eyebrows. These ridges are called the *superciliary arches.* In the center of the supraorbital margin is an opening for nerves and blood vessels called the *supraorbital foramen.* The smooth elevation between the superciliary arches is termed the *glabella.*

The *frontal sinuses* (Fig. 20-8) are situated between the two tables of the squama on each side of the midsagittal plane. These irregularly shaped sinuses are separated by a bony wall, which may be incomplete and usually deviates from the midline.

The squama articulates with the parietal bones at the coronal suture, the greater wing of the sphenoid bone at the frontosphenoidal suture, and the nasal bones at the frontonasal suture. The midpoint of the frontonasal suture is termed the *nasion.*

The frontal bone articulates with the right and left parietals, the sphenoid, and the ethmoid bones of the cranium.

The *orbital plates* of the horizontal portion of the frontal bone are separated by a notch called the *ethmoidal notch.* This notch receives the cribriform plate of the ethmoid bone. At the anterior edge of the ethmoidal notch is a small inferior projection of bone, the *nasal spine,* which is the superiormost component of the bony nasal septum. The posterior margins of the orbital plates articulate with the lesser wings of the sphenoid bone.

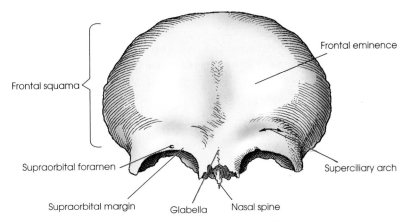

Fig. 20-5 Anterior aspect of frontal bone.

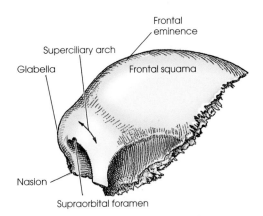

Fig. 20-6 Lateral aspect of frontal bone.

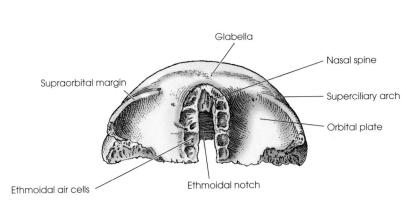

Fig. 20-7 Inferior aspect of frontal bone.

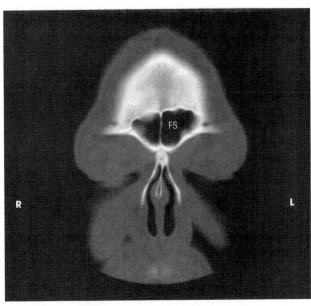

Fig. 20-8 Coronal CT image of frontal sinuses (*FS*).

(From Kelley LL, Petersen CM: *Sectional anatomy for imaging professionals,* ed 2, St Louis, 2007, Mosby.)

ETHMOID BONE

The *ethmoid bone* is a small, cube-shaped bone that consists of a horizontal plate; a vertical plate; and two light, spongy lateral masses called *labyrinths* (Figs. 20-9 to 20-12). Situated between the orbits, the ethmoid bone forms part of the anterior cranial fossa, the nasal cavity and orbital walls, and the bony nasal septum.

The horizontal portion of the ethmoid bone, called the *cribriform plate,* is received into the ethmoidal notch of the frontal bone. The cribriform plate is perforated by many foramina for the transmission of olfactory nerves. The plate also has a thick, conical process, the *crista galli,* which projects superiorly from its anterior midline and serves as the anterior attachment for the falx cerebri.

The vertical portion of the ethmoid bone is called the *perpendicular plate.* This plate is a thin, flat bone that projects inferiorly from the inferior surface of the cribriform plate and, with the nasal spine, forms the superior portion of the bony septum of the nose.

The *labyrinths* contain the *ethmoidal sinuses,* or air cells. The cells of each side are arbitrarily divided into three groups: the *anterior, middle,* and *posterior ethmoidal air cells* (see Fig. 20-12, *A* and *B*). The walls of the labyrinths form part of the medial walls of the orbits and part of the lateral walls of the nasal cavity. Projecting inferiorly from each medial wall of the labyrinths are two thin, scroll-shaped processes called the *superior* and *middle nasal conchae.*

The ethmoid bone articulates with the frontal and sphenoid bones of the cranium.

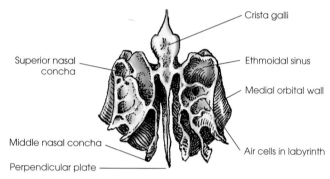

Fig. 20-9 Anterior aspect of ethmoid bone.

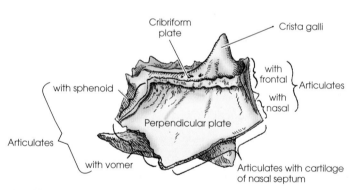

Fig. 20-10 Lateral aspect of ethmoid bone with labyrinth removed.

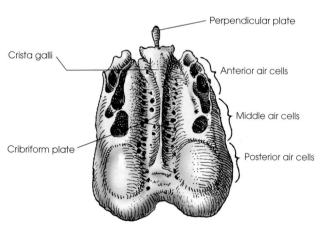

Fig. 20-11 Superior aspect of ethmoid bone.

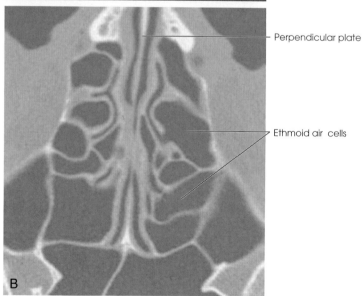

Fig. 20-12 A, Coronal CT image of ethmoidal sinuses (*Ets*). **B,** Axial CT scan of ethmoidal sinus and perpendicular plate.

(**A,** From Kelley LL, Petersen CM: *Sectional anatomy for imaging professionals,* ed 2, St Louis, 2007, Mosby.)

PARIETAL BONES

The two *parietal bones* are square and have a convex external surface and a concave internal surface (Figs. 20-13 and 20-14). The parietal bones form a large portion of the sides of the cranium. They also form the posterior portion of the cranial roof by their articulation with each other at the sagittal suture in the midsagittal plane.

Each parietal bone presents a prominent bulge, called the *parietal eminence,* near the central portion of its external surface. In radiography, the width of the head should be measured at this point because it is the widest point of the head.

Each parietal bone articulates with the frontal, temporal, occipital, sphenoid, and opposite parietal bones of the cranium.

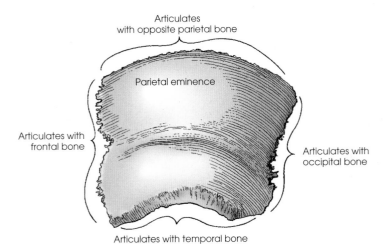

Fig. 20-13 External surface of parietal bone.

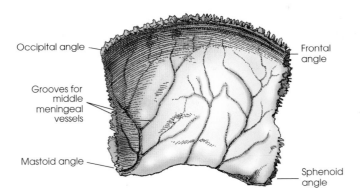

Fig. 20-14 Internal surface of parietal bone.

SPHENOID BONE

The *sphenoid bone* is an irregularly wedge-shaped bone that resembles a bat with its wings extended. It is situated in the base of the cranium anterior to the temporal bones and basilar part of the occipital bone (Figs. 20-15 to 20-17). The sphenoid bone consists of a body; two lesser wings and two greater wings, which project laterally from the sides of the body; and two pterygoid processes, which project inferiorly from each side of the inferior surface of the body.

The *body* of the sphenoid bone contains the two *sphenoidal sinuses,* which are incompletely separated by a median septum (see Fig. 20-15, *B,* and 20-17). The anterior surface of the body forms the posterior bony wall of the nasal cavity. The superior surface presents a deep depression called the *sella turcica* and contains a gland called the *pituitary gland.* The sella turcica lies in the midsagittal plane of the cranium at a point ¾ inch (1.9 cm) anterior and ¾ inch (1.9 cm) superior to the level of the *external acoustic meatus*

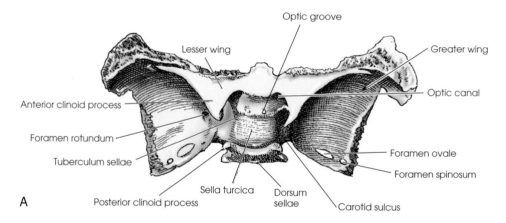

A

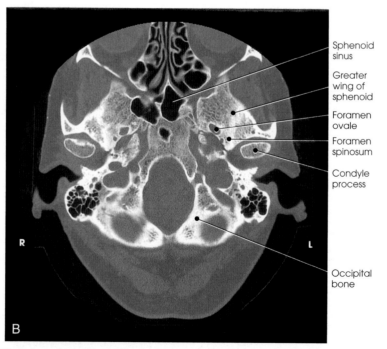

B

Fig. 20-15 A, Superior aspect of sphenoid bone. **B,** Axial CT scan of sphenoid bone.

(**B,** From Kelley LL, Petersen CM: *Sectional anatomy for imaging professionals,* ed 2, St Louis, 2007, Mosby.)

(EAM). The sella turcica is bounded anteriorly by the *tuberculum sellae* and posteriorly by the *dorsum sellae,* which bears the *posterior clinoid processes* (see Fig. 20-16, *B*). The slanted area of bone posterior and inferior to the dorsum sellae is continuous with the basilar portion of the occipital bone and is called the *clivus.* The clivus supports the pons. On either side of the sella turcica is a groove, the *carotid sulcus,* in which the internal carotid artery and the cavernous sinus lie.

The *optic groove* extends across the anterior portion of the tuberculum sellae. The groove ends on each side at the *optic canal.* The optic canal is the opening into the apex of the orbit for the transmission of the optic nerve and ophthalmic artery. The actual opening is called the *optic foramen.*

The *lesser wings* are triangular in shape and nearly horizontal in position. They arise, one on each side, from the anterosuperior portion of the body of the sphenoid bone and project laterally, ending in sharp points. The lesser wings form the posteromedial portion of the roofs of the orbits, the posterior portion of the anterior cranial fossa, the upper margin of the *superior orbital fissures,* and the optic canals. The medial ends of their posterior borders form the *anterior clinoid processes.* Each process arises from two roots. The anterior (superior) root is thin and flat, and the posterior (inferior) root, referred to as the *sphenoid strut,* is thick and rounded. The circular opening between the two roots is the *optic canal.*

The *greater wings* arise from the sides of the body of the sphenoid bone and curve laterally, posteriorly, anteriorly, and superiorly. The greater wings form part of the middle cranial fossa, the posterolateral walls of the orbits, the lower margin of the superior orbital sulci, and the greater part of the posterior margin of the inferior orbital sulci. The *foramina rotundum, ovale,* and *spinosum* are paired and are situated in the greater wings. Because these foramina transmit nerves and blood vessels, they are subject to radiologic investigation for the detection of erosive lesions of neurogenic or vascular origin.

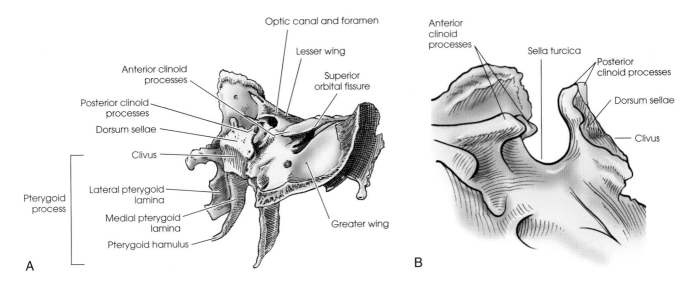

Fig. 20-16 A, Oblique aspect of upper and lateroposterior aspects of sphenoid bone (right lateral pterygoid lamina removed). **B,** Sella turcica of sphenoid bone, lateral view.

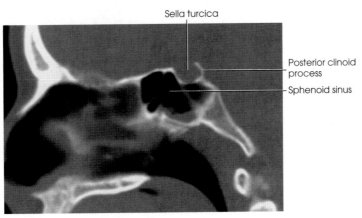

Fig. 20-17 Sagittal CT scan of sella turcica and sphenoid sinus.

The *pterygoid processes* arise from the lateral portions of the inferior surface of the body of the sphenoid bone and the medial portions of the inferior surfaces of the greater wings. These processes project inferiorly and curve laterally. Each pterygoid process consists of two plates of bone, the *medial* and *lateral pterygoid laminae*, which are fused at their supero-anterior parts. The inferior extremity of the medial lamina possesses an elongated, hook-shaped process, the *pterygoid hamulus*, which makes it longer and narrower than the lateral lamina. The pterygoid processes articulate with the palatine bones anteriorly and with the wings of the vomer, where they enter into the formation of the nasal cavity.

The sphenoid bone articulates with each of the other seven bones of the cranium.

OCCIPITAL BONE

The *occipital bone* is situated at the posteroinferior part of the cranium. It forms the posterior half of the base of the cranium and the greater part of the posterior cranial fossa (Figs. 20-18 to 20-20). The occipital bone has four parts: the *squama,* which is saucer-shaped, being convex externally; *two occipital condyles,* which extend anteriorly, one on each side of the foramen magnum; and the *basilar portion.* The occipital bone also has a large aperture, the *foramen magnum,*

through which the inferior portion of the medulla oblongata passes as it exits the cranial cavity and joins the spinal cord.

The *squama* curves posteriorly and superiorly from the foramen magnum and is curved from side to side. It articulates with the parietal bones at the lambdoidal sutures and with the mastoid portions of the temporal bones at the occipitomastoid sutures. On the external surface of the squama, midway between its summit and the foramen magnum, is a prominent process termed the *external occipital protuberance,* or *inion,* which corresponds in position with the *internal occipital protuberance.*

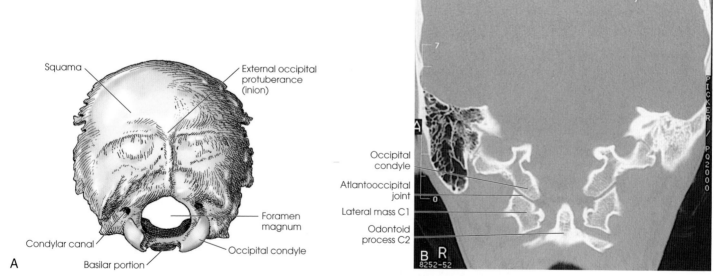

Squama — External occipital protuberance (inion) — Condylar canal — Basilar portion — Foramen magnum — Occipital condyle

Occipital condyle — Atlantooccipital joint — Lateral mass C1 — Odontoid process C2

A

Fig. 20-18 A, External surface of occipital bone. **B,** Coronal CT showing atlantooccipital joint.

(**B,** Courtesy Siemens Medical Systems, Iselin, NJ.)

The *occipital condyles* project anteriorly, one from each side of the squama, for articulation with the atlas of the cervical spine. Part of each lateral portion curves medially to fuse with the basilar portion and complete the foramen magnum, and part of it projects laterally to form the jugular process. On the inferior surface of the curved parts, extending from the level of the middle of the foramen magnum anteriorly to the level of its anterior margin, reciprocally shaped condyles articulate with superior facets of the atlas. These articulations, known as the *occipitoatlantal joints,* are the only bony articulations between the skull and the neck. The *hypoglossal canals* are found at the anterior ends of the condyles and transmit the hypoglossal nerves. At the posterior end of the condyles are the *condylar canals,* through which the emissary veins pass. The anterior portion of the occipital bone contains a deep notch that forms a part of the *jugular foramen* (see Fig. 20-2, *B*). The jugular foramen is an important large opening in the skull for two reasons: It allows blood to drain from the brain via the internal jugular vein, and it lets three cranial nerves pass through it.

The *basilar portion* of the occipital bone curves anteriorly and superiorly to its junction with the body of the sphenoid. In an adult, the basilar part of the occipital bone fuses with the body of the sphenoid bone, resulting in the formation of a continuous bone. The sloping surface of this junction between the dorsum sellae of the sphenoid bone and the basilar portion of the occipital bone is called the *clivus.*

The occipital bone articulates with the two parietals, the two temporal bones and the sphenoid of the cranium, and the first cervical vertebra.

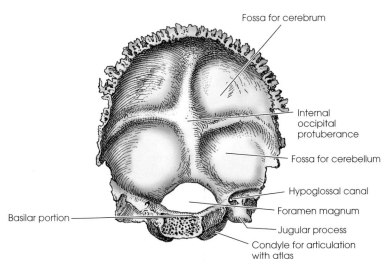

Fig. 20-19 Internal surface of occipital bone.

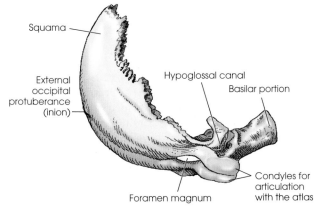

Fig. 20-20 Lateroinferior aspect of occipital bone.

TEMPORAL BONES

The temporal bones are irregular in shape and are situated on each side of the base of the cranium between the greater wings of the sphenoid bone and the occipital bone (Figs. 20-21 to 20-25). The temporal bones form a large part of the middle fossa of the cranium and a small part of the posterior fossa. Each temporal bone consists of a squamous portion, a tympanic portion, a styloid process, a zygomatic process, and a petromastoid portion (the mastoid and petrous portions) that contains the organs of hearing and balance.

The *squamous portion* is the thin upper portion of the temporal bone. It forms a part of the side wall of the cranium and has a prominent arched process, the *zygomatic process,* which projects anteriorly to articulate with the zygomatic bone of the face and complete the zygomatic arch. On the inferior border of the zygomatic process is a rounded eminence, the *articular tubercle,* which forms the anterior boundary of the *mandibular fossa.* The mandibular fossa receives the condyle of the mandible to form the *temporomandibular joint* (TMJ).

The *tympanic portion* is situated below the squama and in front of the mastoid and petrous portions of the temporal bone. This portion forms the anterior wall, the inferior wall, and part of the posterior walls of the EAM. The EAM is approximately ½ inch (1.3 cm) in length and projects medially, anteriorly, and slightly superiorly.

The *styloid process,* a slender, pointed bone of variable length, projects inferiorly, anteriorly, and slightly medially from the inferior portion of the tympanic part of the temporal bone.

Petromastoid portion

The petrous and mastoid portions together are called the *petromastoid portion.* The mastoid portion, which forms the inferior, posterior part of the temporal bone, is prolonged into the conical *mastoid process* (see Figs. 20-23 and 20-25).

The *mastoid portion* articulates with the parietal bone at its superior border through the parietomastoid suture and with the occipital bone at its posterior border through the occipitomastoid suture, which is contiguous with the lambdoidal suture. The *mastoid process* varies considerably in size, depending on its pneumatization, and is larger in males than in females.

The first of the *mastoid air cells* to develop is situated at the upper anterior part of the process and is termed the *mastoid antrum.* This air cell is quite large and communicates with the tympanic cavity. Shortly before or after birth, smaller air cells begin to develop around the mastoid antrum and continue to increase in number and size until around puberty. The air cells vary considerably in size and number. Occasionally, they are absent altogether, in which case the mastoid process is solid bone and is usually small.

The *petrous portion,* often called the *petrous pyramid,* is conical or pyramidal and is the thickest, densest bone in the cranium. This part of the temporal bone contains the organs of hearing and balance. From its base at the squamous and mastoid portions, the petrous portion projects medially and anteriorly between the greater wing of the sphenoid bone and the occipital bone to the body of the sphenoid bone, with which its apex articulates. The internal carotid artery in the *carotid canal* enters the inferior aspect of the petrous portion, passes superior to the cochlea, then passes medially to exit the *petrous apex.* Near the petrous apex is a ragged foramen called the *foramen lacerum.* The carotid canal opens into this foramen, which contains the internal carotid artery (see Fig. 20-2, *B*). At the center of the posterior aspect of the petrous portion is the *internal acoustic meatus* (IAM), which transmits the vestibulocochlear and facial nerves. The upper border of the petrous portion is commonly referred to as the *petrous ridge.* The top of the ridge lies approximately at the level of an external radiography landmark called the *top of ear attachment* (TEA).

The temporal bone articulates with the parietal, occipital, and sphenoid bones of the cranium.

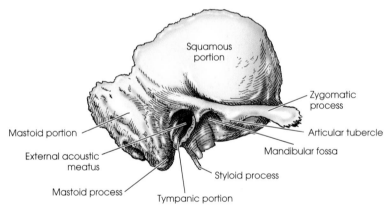

Fig. 20-21 Lateral aspect of temporal bone.

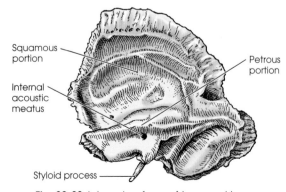

Fig. 20-22 Internal surface of temporal bone.

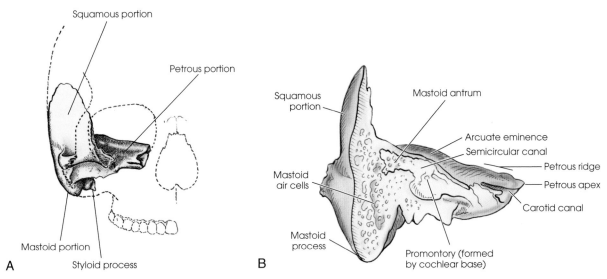

Squamous portion

Petrous portion

Mastoid portion

Styloid process

A

Squamous portion

Mastoid antrum

Arcuate eminence

Semicircular canal

Petrous ridge

Petrous apex

Carotid canal

Mastoid air cells

Mastoid process

Promontory (formed by cochlear base)

B

Fig. 20-23 A, Anterior aspect of temporal bone in relation to surrounding structures.
B, Coronal section through mastoid and petrous portions of temporal bone.

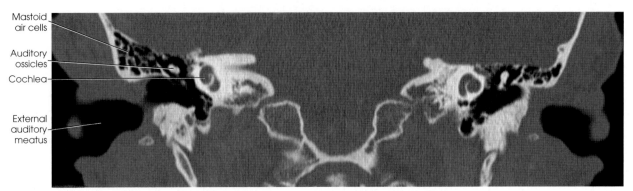

Mastoid air cells

Auditory ossicles

Cochlea

External auditory meatus

Fig. 20-24 Coronal CT scan through temporal bones.

(Courtesy Karl Mockler, RT(R).)

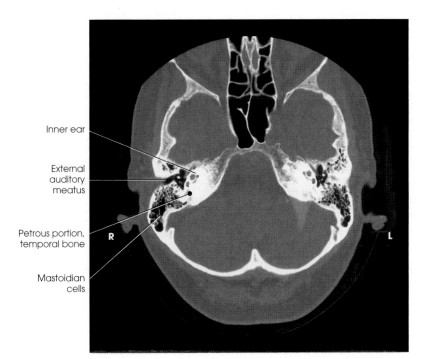

Inner ear

External auditory meatus

Petrous portion, temporal bone

Mastoidian cells

R

L

Fig. 20-25 Axial CT scan of petrous portion at level of external auditory meatus.

(From Kelley LL, Petersen CM: *Sectional anatomy for imaging professionals,* ed 2, St Louis, 2007, Mosby.)

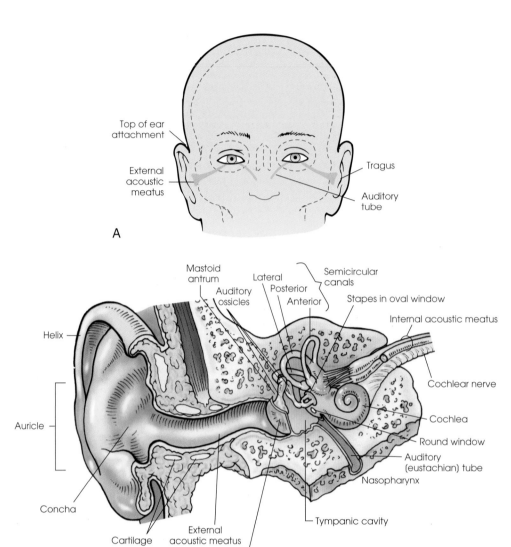

Fig. 20-26 A, Frontal view of face showing internal structures of the ear (*shaded area*). **B,** External, middle, and internal ear.

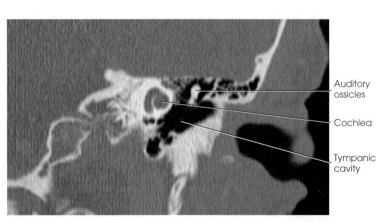

Fig. 20-27 Coronal CT scan through petrous portion of temporal bone showing middle and inner ear.

(Courtesy Karl Mockler, RT(R).)

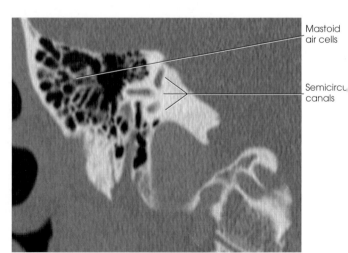

Fig. 20-28 Coronal CT scan of petromastoid portion of temporal bone showing semicircular canals and mastoid air cells.

(Courtesy Karl Mockler, RT(R).)

Ear

The ear is the organ of hearing and balance (Fig. 20-26). The essential parts of the ear are housed in the petrous portion of the temporal bone. The organs of hearing and equilibrium consist of three main divisions: external ear, middle ear, and internal ear.

EXTERNAL EAR

The *external ear* consists of two parts: (1) the *auricle,* the oval-shaped, fibrocartilaginous, sound-collecting organ situated on the side of the head, and (2) the *external acoustic meatus (EAM),* a sound-conducting canal. The superior attachment of the auricle is the top of ear attachment (TEA). The TEA is a reference point for positioning the lateral cervical spine. The auricle has a deep central depression, the *concha,* the lower part of which leads into the EAM. At its anterior margin, the auricle has a prominent cartilaginous lip, the *tragus,* which projects posteriorly over the entrance of the meatus. The outer rim of the ear is the *helix.* The EAM is about 1 inch (2.5 cm) long. The outer third of the canal wall is cartilaginous, and the inner two thirds is osseous. From the meatal orifice, the canal forms a slight curve as it passes medially and anteriorly in line with the axis of the IAM. The EAM ends at the tympanic membrane of the middle ear.

MIDDLE EAR

The *middle ear* is situated between the external ear and the internal ear. The middle ear proper consists of (1) the *tympanic membrane* (or eardrum); (2) an irregularly shaped, air-containing compartment called the *tympanic cavity;* and (3) three small bones called the *auditory ossicles* (see Figs. 20-25 and 20-26). The middle ear communicates with the mastoid antrum and auditory eustachian tube.

The *tympanic membrane* is a thin, concavoconvex, membranous disk with an elliptic shape. The disk, the convex surface of which is directed medially, is situated obliquely over the medial end of the EAM and serves as a partition between the external ear and the middle ear. The function of the tympanic membrane is the transmission of sound vibrations.

The *tympanic cavity* is a narrow, irregularly shaped chamber that lies just posterior and medial to the mandibular fossa. The cavity is separated from the external ear by the tympanic membrane and from the internal ear by the bony labyrinth. The tympanic cavity communicates with the nasopharynx through the *auditory (eustachian) tube,* a passage by which air pressure in the middle ear is equalized with the pressure in the outside air passages. The auditory tube is about $1\frac{1}{4}$ inches (3 cm) long. From its entrance into the tympanic cavity, the auditory tube passes medially and inferiorly to its orifice on the lateral wall of the nasopharynx.

The mastoid antrum is the large air cavity situated in the temporal bone above the mastoid air cells and immediately behind the posterior wall of the middle ear.

The *auditory ossicles,* named for their shape, are the *malleus* (hammer), *incus* (anvil), and *stapes* (stirrup). These three delicate bones are articulated to permit vibratory motion. They bridge the middle ear cavity for the transmission of sound vibrations from the tympanic membrane to the internal ear. The handle of the malleus (the outermost ossicle) is attached to the tympanic membrane, and its head articulates with the incus (the central ossicle). The head of the stapes (the innermost ossicle) articulates with the incus, and its base is fitted into the oval window of the inner ear.

INTERNAL EAR

The *internal ear* contains the essential sensory apparatus of hearing and equilibrium and lies on the densest portion of the petrous portion immediately below the arcuate eminence. Composed of an irregularly shaped bony chamber called the *bony labyrinth,* the internal ear is housed within the bony chamber and is an intercommunicating system of ducts and sacs known as the *membranous labyrinth.* The bony labyrinth consists of three distinctly shaped parts: (1) a spiral-coiled, tubular part called the *cochlea,* which communicates with the middle ear through the membranous covering of the *round window* (Fig. 20-27); (2) a small, ovoid central compartment behind the cochlea, known as the *vestibule,* which communicates with the middle ear via the *oval window;* and (3) three unequally sized *semicircular canals* that form right angles to one another and are called, according to their positions, the *anterior, posterior,* and *lateral semicircular canals* (Fig. 20-28). From its cranial orifice, the internal acoustic meatus (IAM) passes inferiorly and laterally for a distance of about $\frac{1}{2}$ inch (1.3 cm). Through this canal, the cochlear and vestibular nerves pass from their fibers in the respective parts of the membranous labyrinth to the brain. The cochlea is used for hearing, and the vestibule and semicircular canals are involved with equilibrium.

Facial Bones
NASAL BONES

The two small, thin *nasal bones* vary in size and shape in different individuals (Figs. 20-29 and 20-30). They form the superior bony wall (called the *bridge* of the nose) of the nasal cavity. The nasal bones articulate in the midsagittal plane, where at their posterosuperior surface they also articulate with the perpendicular plate of the ethmoid bone. They articulate with the frontal bone above and with the maxillae at the sides.

LACRIMAL BONES

The two *lacrimal bones,* which are the smallest bones in the skull, are very thin and are situated at the anterior part of the medial wall of the orbits between the labyrinth of the ethmoid bone and the maxilla (see Figs. 20-29 and 20-30). Together with the maxillae, the lacrimal bones form the lacrimal fossae, which accommodate the lacrimal sacs. Each lacrimal bone contains a *lacrimal foramen* through which a tear duct passes. Each lacrimal bone articulates with the frontal and ethmoid cranial bones and the maxilla and inferior nasal concha facial bones. The lacrimal bones can be seen on PA and lateral projections of the skull.

MAXILLARY BONES

The two *maxillary bones* are the largest of the immovable bones of the face (see Figs. 20-29 and 20-30). Each articulates with all other facial bones except the mandible. Each also articulates with the frontal and ethmoid bones of the cranium. The maxillary bones form part of the lateral walls and most of the floor of the nasal cavity, part of the floor of the orbital cavities, and three fourths of the roof of the mouth. Their zygomatic processes articulate with the zygomatic bones and assist in the formation of the prominence of the cheeks. The body of each maxilla contains a large, pyramidal cavity called the *maxillary sinus,* which empties into the nasal cavity. An *infraorbital foramen* is located under each orbit and serves as a passage through which the infraorbital nerve and artery reach the nose.

At their inferior borders, the maxillae possess a thick, spongy ridge called the *alveolar process,* which supports the roots of the teeth. In the anterior midsagittal plane at their junction with each other, the maxillary bones form a pointed, forward-projecting process called the *anterior nasal spine.* The midpoint of this prominence is called the *acanthion.*

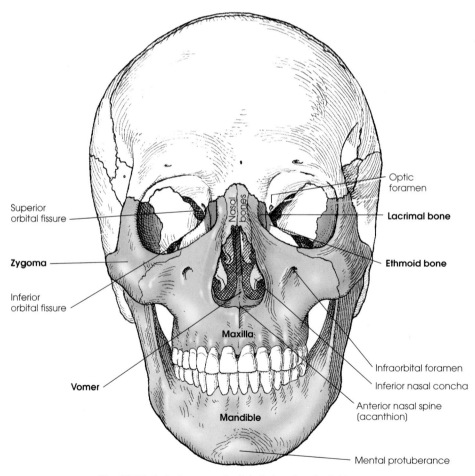

Fig. 20-29 Anterior aspect of skull showing facial bones.

ZYGOMATIC BONES

The zygomatic bones form the prominence of the cheeks and a part of the side wall and floor of the orbital cavities (see Figs. 20-29 and 20-30). A posteriorly extending *temporal process* unites with the zygomatic process of the temporal bone to form the *zygomatic arch*. The zygomatic bones articulate with the frontal bone superiorly, with the zygomatic process of the temporal bone at the side, with the maxilla anteriorly, and with the sphenoid bone posteriorly.

PALATINE BONES

The two palatine bones are L-shaped bones composed of *vertical* and *horizontal plates*. The horizontal plates articulate with the maxillae to complete the posterior fourth of the bony palate, or roof of the mouth (see Fig. 20-3). The vertical portions of the palatine bones extend upward between the maxillae and the pterygoid processes of the sphenoid bone in the posterior nasal cavity. The superior tips of the vertical portions of the palatine bones assist in forming the posteromedial bony orbit.

INFERIOR NASAL CONCHAE

The inferior nasal conchae extend diagonally and inferiorly from the lateral walls of the nasal cavity at approximately its lower third (see Fig. 20-29). They are long, narrow, and extremely thin; they curl laterally, which gives them a scroll-like appearance.

The upper two nasal conchae are processes of the ethmoid bone. The three nasal conchae project into and divide the lateral portion of the respective sides of the nasal cavity into superior, middle, and inferior meatus. They are covered with a mucous membrane to warm, moisten, and cleanse inhaled air.

VOMER

The *vomer* is a thin plate of bone situated in the midsagittal plane of the floor of the nasal cavity, where it forms the inferior part of the *nasal septum* (see Fig. 20-29). The anterior border of the vomer slants superiorly and posteriorly from the anterior nasal spine to the body of the sphenoid bone, with which its superior border articulates. The superior part of its anterior border articulates with the perpendicular plate of the ethmoid bone; its posterior border is free.

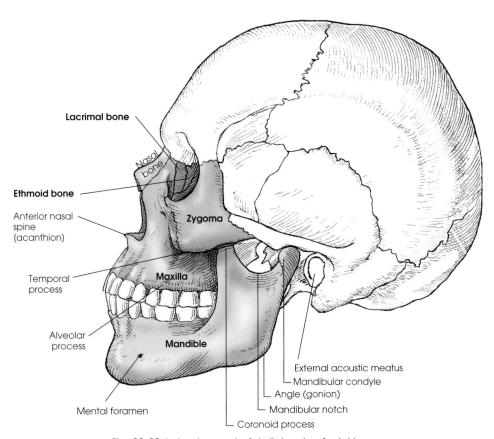

Fig. 20-30 Lateral aspect of skull showing facial bones.

Lacrimal bone
Nasal bone
Ethmoid bone
Anterior nasal spine (acanthion)
Zygoma
Temporal process
Maxilla
Alveolar process
Mandible
Mental foramen
Coronoid process
Mandibular notch
Angle (gonion)
Mandibular condyle
External acoustic meatus

MANDIBLE

The *mandible,* the largest and densest bone of the face, consists of a curved horizontal portion, called the *body,* and two vertical portions, called the *rami,* which unite with the body at the *angle* of the mandible, or *gonion* (Fig. 20-31). At birth, the mandible consists of bilateral pieces held together by a fibrous symphysis that ossifies during the first year of life. At the site of ossification is a slight ridge that ends below in a triangular prominence, the *mental protuberance.* The *symphysis* is the most anterior and central part of the mandible. This is where the left and right halves of the mandible have fused.

The superior border of the body of the mandible consists of spongy bone, called the *alveolar portion,* which supports the roots of the teeth. Below the second premolar tooth, approximately halfway between the superior and inferior borders of the bone, is a small opening on each side for the transmission of nerves and blood vessels. These two openings are called the *mental foramina.*

The rami project superiorly at an obtuse angle to the body of the mandible, and their broad surface forms an angle of approximately 110 to 120 degrees. Each ramus presents two processes at its upper extremity—one coronoid and one condylar—which are separated by a concave area called the *mandibular notch.* The anterior process, the *coronoid process,* is thin and tapered and projects to a higher level than the posterior process. The *condylar process* consists of a constricted area, the *neck,* above which is a broad, thick, almost transversely placed *condyle* that articulates with the mandibular fossa of the temporal bone (Fig. 20-32). This articulation, the TMJ, slants posteriorly approximately 15 degrees and inferiorly and medially approximately 15 degrees. Radiographic projections, produced from the opposite side, must reverse these directions. In other words, the central ray angulation must be superior and anterior to coincide with the long axis of the joint. The TMJ is situated immediately in front of the EAM.

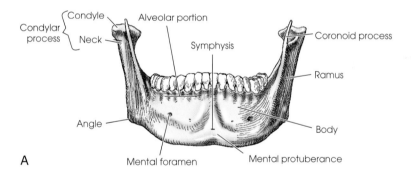

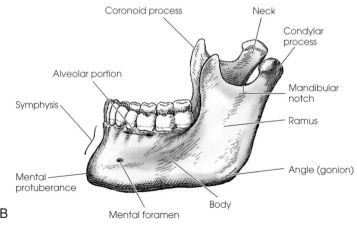

Fig. 20-31 A, Anterior aspect of mandible. **B,** Lateral aspect of mandible.

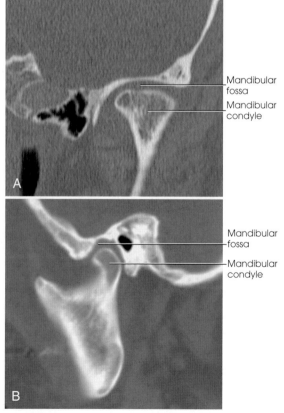

Fig. 20-32 CT scan of mandibular condyle situated in mandibular fossa. **A,** Coronal. **B,** Sagittal.

(Courtesy Karl Mockler, RT(R).)

HYOID BONE

The *hyoid bone* is a small, U-shaped structure situated at the base of the tongue, where it is held in position in part by the stylohyoid ligaments extending from the styloid processes of the temporal bones (Fig. 20-33). Although the hyoid bone is an accessory bone of the axial skeleton, it is described in this chapter because of its connection with the temporal bones. The hyoid is the only bone in the body that does not articulate with any other bone.

The hyoid bone is divided into a *body,* two *greater cornua,* and two *lesser cornua.* The bone serves as an attachment for certain muscles of the larynx and tongue and is easily palpated just above the larynx.

ORBITS

Each orbit is composed of *seven* different bones (Fig. 20-34). Three of these are cranial bones: *frontal, sphenoid,* and *ethmoid.* The other four bones are the facial bones: *maxilla, zygoma, lacrimal,* and *palatine.* The circumference of the orbit, or outer rim area, is composed of three of the seven bones—frontal, zygoma, and maxilla. The remaining four bones compose most of the posterior aspect of the orbit.

Articulations of the Skull

The sutures of the skull are connected by toothlike projections of bone interlocked with a thin layer of fibrous tissue. These articulations allow no movement and are classified as *fibrous* joints of the *suture* type. The articulations of the facial bones, including the joints between the roots of the teeth and the jawbones, are *fibrous gomphoses.* The exception is the point at which the rounded condyle of the mandible articulates with the mandibular fossa of the temporal bone to form the TMJ. The TMJ articulation is a *synovial* joint of the *hinge* and *gliding* type. The atlantooccipital joint is a *synovial ellipsoidal* joint that joins the base of the skull (occipital bone) with the atlas of the cervical spine. The seven joints of the skull are summarized in Table 20-1.

TABLE 20-1
Joints of the skull

| Joint | Structural classification | | Movement |
	Tissue	Type	
Coronal suture	Fibrous	Suture	Immovable
Sagittal suture	Fibrous	Suture	Immovable
Lambdoidal suture	Fibrous	Suture	Immovable
Squamosal suture	Fibrous	Suture	Immovable
Temporomandibular	Synovial	Hinge and gliding	Freely movable
Alveolar sockets	Fibrous	Gomphosis	Immovable
Atlantooccipital	Synovial	Ellipsoidal	Freely movable

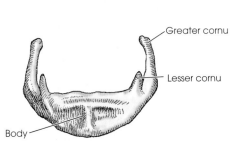

Fig. 20-33 Anterior aspect of hyoid.

Greater cornu

Lesser cornu

Body

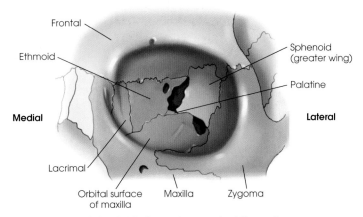

Frontal

Ethmoid

Sphenoid (greater wing)

Palatine

Medial

Lateral

Lacrimal

Orbital surface of maxilla

Maxilla

Zygoma

Fig. 20-34 Orbit. Seven bones of orbit are shown.

Sinuses

The air-containing cavities situated in the frontal, ethmoidal, and sphenoidal bones of the cranium and the maxillary bones of the face are called the *paranasal sinuses* because of their formation from the nasal mucosa and their continued communication with the nasal fossae (Fig. 20-35). Although the functions of the sinuses are not agreed on by all anatomists, these cavities are believed to do the following:

- Serve as a resonating chamber for the voice
- Decrease the weight of the skull by containing air
- Help warm and moisten inhaled air
- Act as shock absorbers in trauma (as airbags do in automobiles)
- Possibly control the immune system

The sinuses begin to develop early in fetal life, at first appearing as small sacculations of the mucosa of the nasal meatus and recesses. As the pouches, or sacs, grow, they gradually invade the respective bones to form the air sinuses and cells. The maxillary sinuses are usually sufficiently well developed and aerated at birth to be shown radiographically. The other groups of sinuses develop more slowly; by age 6 or 7 years, the frontal and sphenoidal sinuses are distinguishable from the ethmoidal air cells, which they resemble in size and position. The ethmoidal air cells develop during puberty, and the sinuses are not completely developed until age 17 or 18 years. When fully developed, each of the sinuses communicates with the others and with the nasal cavity.

An understanding of the actual size, shape, and position of the sinuses within the skull is made possible by studying the sinuses on computed tomography (CT) head images (Fig. 20-36).

MAXILLARY SINUSES

The largest sinuses, the maxillary sinuses, are paired and are located in the body of each maxilla (see Figs. 20-35 and 20-36). Although the maxillary sinuses appear rectangular in the lateral image, they are approximately pyramidal in shape and have only three walls. The apices are directed inferiorly and laterally. The two maxillary sinuses vary considerably in size and shape but are usually symmetric. In adults, each maxillary sinus is approximately $1\frac{1}{2}$ inches (3.5 cm) high and 1 to $1\frac{1}{3}$ inches (2.5 to 3 cm) wide. The sinus is often divided into subcompartments by partial septa, and occasionally it is divided into two sinuses by a complete septum. The sinus floor presents several elevations that correspond to the roots of the subjacent teeth. The maxillary sinuses communicate with the middle nasal meatus at the superior aspect of the sinus.

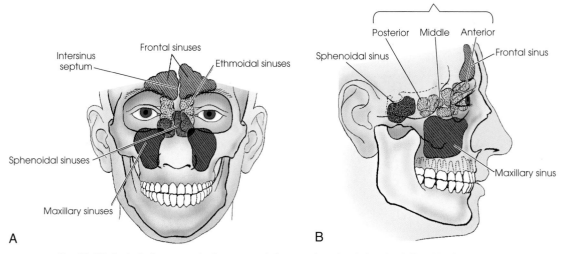

Fig. 20-35 A, Anterior aspect of paranasal sinuses, showing lateral relationship to each other and to surrounding parts. **B,** Schematic drawing of paranasal sinuses, showing AP relationship to each other and surrounding parts.

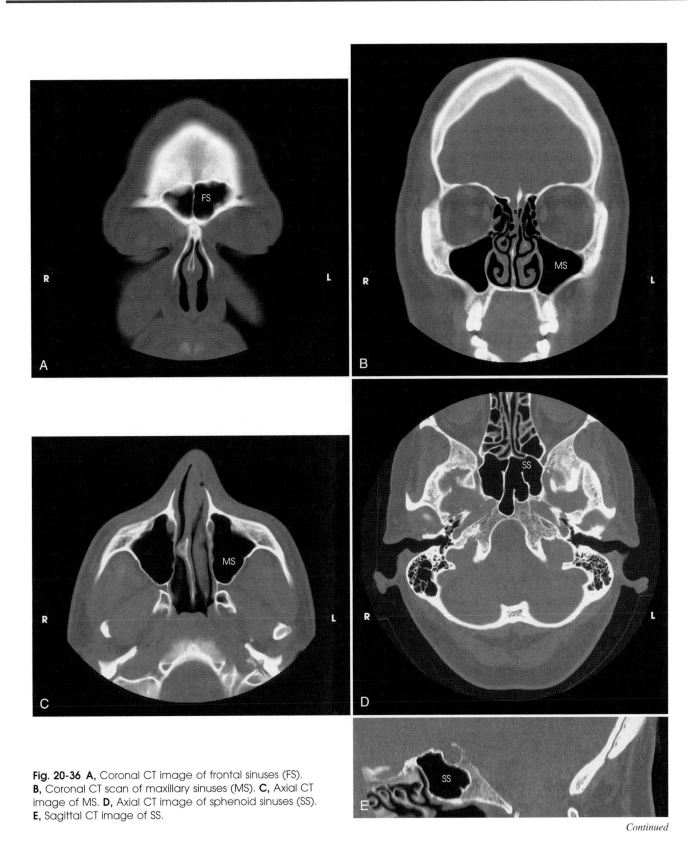

Fig. 20-36 A, Coronal CT image of frontal sinuses (FS).
B, Coronal CT scan of maxillary sinuses (MS). **C,** Axial CT
image of MS. **D,** Axial CT image of sphenoid sinuses (SS).
E, Sagittal CT image of SS.

Continued

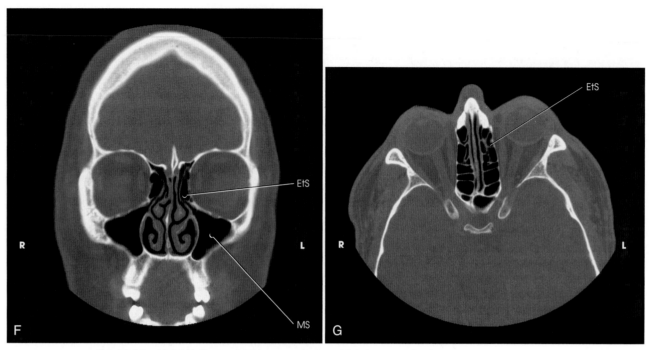

Fig. 20-36, cont'd F, Coronal CT image of ethmoidal sinuses (EtS). **G,** Axial CT image of EtS.

(From Kelley LL, Petersen CM: *Sectional anatomy for imaging professionals,* ed 2, St Louis, 2007, Mosby.)

FRONTAL SINUSES

The frontal sinuses, the second largest sinuses, are paired and are normally located between the tables of the vertical plate of the frontal bone (see Figs. 20-35 and 30-36). The frontal sinuses vary greatly in size and form. Occasionally they are absent. One or both may be approximately ¾ to 1 inch (2 to 2.5 cm) in the vertical or lateral dimension. The sinuses often extend beyond the frontal region of the bone, most frequently into the orbital plates. The *intersinus septum* is usually deviated from the midline; for this reason, the frontal sinuses are rarely symmetric. Multiple septa are sometimes present. Similar to maxillary sinuses, the frontal sinuses drain into the middle nasal meatus.

ETHMOIDAL SINUSES

The two ethmoidal sinuses are located within the lateral masses of the labyrinths of the ethmoid bone. They are composed of a varying number of air cells that are divided into three main groups: anterior, middle, and posterior (see Figs. 20-35 and 20-36). The anterior and middle ethmoidal cells range in number from two to eight, and each group opens into the middle nasal meatus. The posterior cells range in number from two to six or more and drain into the superior nasal meatus.

SPHENOIDAL SINUSES

The sphenoidal sinuses are normally paired and occupy the body of the sphenoid bone (see Figs. 20-35 and 20-36). Anatomists state that often only one sphenoidal sinus is present; however, more than two sphenoidal sinuses are never present. The sphenoidal sinuses vary considerably in size and shape and are usually asymmetric. They lie immediately below the sella turcica and extend between the dorsum sellae and the posterior ethmoidal air cells. The sphenoidal sinuses open into the sphenoethmoidal recess of the nasal cavity.

Text continued on p. 285.

Sinuses

SUMMARY OF ANATOMY

Skull
Cranial bones (8)
Facial bones (14)

Cranial bones
Calvaria
  Frontal
  Right parietal
  Left parietal
  Occipital
Floor
  Right temporal
  Left temporal
  Sphenoid
  Ethmoid
Diploë

Sutures
Coronal suture
Sagittal suture
Squamosal sutures
Lambdoidal suture
Bregma
Lambda
Pterion
Asterion

Fontanels
Anterior fontanel
Posterior fontanel
Sphenoidal fontanels (2)
Mastoid fontanels (2)

Fossae
Anterior cranial fossa
Middle cranial fossa
Posterior cranial fossa

Frontal bone
Frontal squama
Frontal eminence
Supraorbital margins
Superciliary arches
Supraorbital foramen
Glabella
Frontal sinuses
Nasion
Orbital plates
  Ethmoidal notch
  Nasal spine

Ethmoid bone
Cribriform plate
  Crista galli
Perpendicular plate
Labyrinths
  Anterior air cells
  Middle air cells
  Posterior air cells
  Ethmoidal sinuses
  Superior nasal conchae
  Middle nasal conchae

Parietal bones (R & L)
Parietal eminence

Sphenoid bone
Body
  Sphenoidal sinuses
  Sella turcica
    Tuberculum sellae
    Dorsum sellae
    Posterior clinoid processes
  Clivus
Carotid sulcus
Optic groove
  Optic canals
  Optic foramen
Lesser wings
  Superior orbital fissures
  Anterior clinoid processes
  Sphenoid strut
Greater wings
  Foramen rotundum
  Foramen ovale
  Foramen spinosum
  Pterygoid processes
    Medial pterygoid lamina
      pterygoid hamulus
    Lateral pterygoid lamina

Occipital bone
Foramen magnum
Squama
  External occipital
    protuberance (inion)
  Internal occipital
    protuberance
  Occipital condyles
    Hypoglossal canals
    Condylar canals
    Jugular foramen
  Basilar portion
    Clivus

Temporal bones (R & L)
Squamous portions
  Zygomatic process
  Articular tubercle
  Mandibular fossa
Tympanic portions
  External acoustic meatus
    (EAM)
  Styloid process
Petromastoid portions
  Mastoid portions
    Mastoid process
    Mastoid antrum
    Mastoid air cells
  Petrous portions (petrous
    pyramids)
    Carotid canals
    Petrous apex
    Foramen lacerum
    Internal acoustic meatus
      (IAM)
    Petrous ridge
    Top of ear attachment (TEA)

Ear
External ear
  Auricle
    Concha
    Tragus
    Helix
  EAM
Middle ear
  Tympanic membrane
  Tympanic cavity
  Auditory (eustachian)
  tube
Auditory ossicles
  Malleus
  Incus
  Stapes
Internal ear
  Arcuate eminence
  Bony labyrinth
    Cochlea
    Round window
    Vestibule
    Oval window
    Semicircular canals
      Anterior
      Posterior
      Lateral
  Membranous labyrinth

Facial bones (14)
Nasal (R & L)
Lacrimal (R & L)
Maxillary (R & L)
Zygomatic (R & L)
Palatine (R & L)
Inferior nasal conchae
  (R & L)
Vomer (1)
Mandible (1)
Hyoid bone
Diploë

Lacrimal bones (R & L)
Lacrimal foramen

Maxillary bones (R & L)
Maxillary sinuses
Infraorbital foramen
Alveolar process
Anterior nasal spine
Acanthion

Zygomatic bones (R & L)
Temporal process
Zygomatic arch

Palatine bones (R & L)
Vertical plates
Horizontal plates

Inferior nasal conchae (R & L)

Vomer (1)
Nasal septum

Mandible (1)
Body
  Alveolar portion
  Mental foramina
Angle (gonion)
Rami
  Coronoid process
  Condylar process
    Condyle
    Neck
    Temporomandibular joint
      (TMJ)
  Mandibular notch
Mental protuberance
  (mentum)
Symphysis

Hyoid bone
Body
Greater cornua
Lesser cornua

Paranasal sinuses
Maxillary sinuses
Frontal sinuses
  Intersinus septum
Ethmoidal sinuses
  Anterior ethmoidal cells
  Middle ethmoidal cells
  Posterior ethmoidal cells
Sphenoidal sinuses

Articulations
Coronal suture
Sagittal suture
Lambdoidal sutures
Squamosal sutures
Temporomandibular (TMJ)
Alveolar sockets
Atlantooccipital

Morphology
Mesocephalic
Brachycephalic
Dolichocephalic

Orbit
Base
Apex
Optic foramen
Superior orbital fissures
Inferior orbital fissures

Eye
Eyeball
Conjunctiva
Sclera
Cornea
Retina
  Rods
  Cones

Sinuses

SUMMARY OF PATHOLOGY

Condition	Definition
Fracture	Disruption in continuity of bone
Basal	Fracture located at the base of the skull
Blowout	Fracture of the floor of the orbit
Contre-coup	Fracture to one side of a structure caused by trauma to the other side
Depressed	Fracture causing a portion of the skull to be pushed into the cranial cavity
Le Fort	Bilateral horizontal fractures of the maxillae
Linear	Irregular or jagged fracture of the skull
Tripod	Fracture of the zygomatic arch and orbital floor or rim and dislocation of the frontozygomatic suture
Mastoiditis	Inflammation of the mastoid antrum and air cells
Metastasis	Transfer of cancerous lesion from one area to another
Osteomyelitis	Inflammation of bone due to a pyogenic infection
Osteopetrosis	Increased density of atypically soft bone
Osteoporosis	Loss of bone density
Paget disease	Thick, soft bone marked by bowing and fractures
Polyp	Growth or mass protruding from a mucous membrane
Sinusitis	Inflammation of one or more of the paranasal sinuses
TMJ syndrome	Dysfunction of temporomandibular joint (TMJ)
Tumor	New tissue growth where cell proliferation is uncontrolled
Acoustic neuroma	Benign tumor arising from Schwann cells of eighth cranial nerve (also termed "schwannoma")
Multiple myeloma	Malignant neoplasm of plasma cells involving the bone marrow and causing destruction of the bone
Osteoma	Tumor composed of bony tissue
Pituitary adenoma	Tumor arising from the pituitary gland, usually in the anterior lobe

SAMPLE EXPOSURE TECHNIQUE CHART ESSENTIAL PROJECTIONS

These techniques were accurate for the equipment used to produce each exposure. However, use caution when applying them in your department because generator output characteristics and IR energy sensitivities vary widely.[1]

This chart was created in collaboration with Dennis Bowman, AS, RT(R), Clinical Instructor, Community Hospital of the Monterey Peninsula, Monterey, CA.

http://digitalradiographysolutions.com/

SKULL, FACIAL BONES, AND PARANASAL SINUSES

Part	cm	kVp*	SID[†]	Collimation	CR[‡] mAs	CR[‡] Dose (mGy)[∥]	DR[§] mAs	DR[§] Dose (mGy)[∥]
Cranium								
Lateral[¶]	15	85	40"	11" × 9" (28 × 23 cm)	6.3**	0.794	3.2**	0.399
PA[¶]	20	85	40"	8" × 10" (20 × 25 cm)	12.5**	1.781	6.3**	0.891
PA axial (Caldwell)[¶]	20	85	40"	8" × 11" (20 × 28 cm)	14**	2.008	7.1**	1.014
AP[¶]	20	85	40"	8" × 10" (20 × 25 cm)	12**	1.781	6.3**	0.893
AP axial[¶]	20	85	40"	8" × 11" (20 × 28 cm)	14**	2.005	7.1**	1.014
AP axial (Towne)[¶]	22	85	40"	8.5" × 12" (21.3 × 30 cm)	20[††]	3.030	10[††]	1.507
PA axial (Haas)[¶]	21	85	40"	8.5" × 12" (21.3 × 30 cm)	20[††]	2.950	10[††]	1.467
Cranial base								
SMV[¶]	23	85	40"	8" × 11" (20 × 28 cm)	28[††]	4.330	14[††]	2.169
Facial bones								
Lateral[¶]	15	80	40"	7" × 7" (18 × 18 cm)	6.3**	0.701	3.2**	0.354
Parietoacanthial (Waters)[¶]	24	85	40"	7.5" × 8" (18.8 × 20 cm)	16**	2.470	8**	1.231
Acanthioparietal (reverse Waters)[¶]	24	85	40"	7.5" × 8" (18.8 × 20 cm)	16**	2.470	8**	1.231
PA axial (Caldwell)[¶]	20	85	40"	7.5" × 8" (18.8 × 20 cm)	14**	1.958	7.1**	0.988
Nasal bones								
Lateral[‡‡]	6	70	40"	3" × 5" (8 × 13 cm)	5.0**	0.282	2.5**	1.408
Zygomatic arches								
SMV[¶]	23	80	40"	8" × 5" (20 × 13 cm)	16[††]	2.094	8[††]	1.041
Tangential[¶]	20	80	40"	3" × 5" (8 × 13 cm)	14[††]	1.294	7.1[††]	0.653
AP axial[¶]	17	80	40"	8.5" × 7" (21.3 × 18 cm)	20[††]	2.270	6.3[††]	1.126
Mandibular rami								
PA[¶]	17	80	40"	8" × 5" (20 × 13 cm)	12.5**	1.367	6.3**	0.686
PA axial[¶]	17	80	40"	8" × 5" (20 × 13 cm)	14**	1.532	7**	0.773
Mandible								
Axiolateral oblique[¶]	13	80	40"	8" × 6" (20 × 15 cm)	12.5**	1.266	6.3**	0.635

SKULL, FACIAL BONES, AND PARANASAL SINUSES

Part	cm	kVp*	SID†	Collimation	CR‡		DR§	
					mAs	Dose (mGy)‖	mAs	Dose (mGy)‖
TMJ								
AP axial¶	21	80	40″	8.5″ × 7″ (21.3 × 18 cm)	20**	2.480	10**	1.233
Axiolateral oblique¶	15	80	40″	4″ × 4″ (10 × 10 cm)	16††	1.501	8††	0.748
Paranasal sinuses								
Lateral¶	15	85	40″	6″ × 6″ (15 × 15 cm)	6.3**	0.721	3.2**	0.363
Frontal and anterior ethmoidal sinuses								
PA axial (Caldwell)¶	20	85	40″	6″ × 6″ (15 × 15 cm)	14**	1.807	7.1**	0.912
Maxillary sinuses								
Parietoacanthial (Waters)¶	24	85	40″	6″ × 6″ (15 × 15 cm)	16**	2.280	8**	1.133
Maxillary and sphenoidal sinuses								
Parietoacanthial (open-mouth Waters)¶	24	85	40″	6″ × 6.5″ (15 × 16.3 cm)	14**	2.003	7.1**	1.011
Ethmoidal and sphenoidal sinuses								
SMV¶	23	85	40″	6.5″ × 6.5″ (16.3 × 16.3 cm)	28††	3.900	14††	1.948

¹ACR-AAPM-SIMM Practice Guidelines for Digital Radiography, 2007.
*kVp values are for a high-frequency generator.
†40 inch minimum; 44 to 48 inches recommended to improve spatial resolution (mAs increase needed, but no increase in patient dose will result).
‡AGFA CR MD 4.0 General IP, CR 75.0 reader, 400 speed class, with 6:1 (178LPI) grid when needed.
§GE Definium 8000, with 13:1 grid when needed.
‖All doses are skin entrance for an average adult (160 to 200 pound male, 150 to 190 pound female) at part thickness indicated.
¶Bucky/Grid.
**Small focal spot.
††Large focal spot.
‡‡Nongrid.

ABBREVIATIONS USED IN CHAPTER 20

AML	Acanthiomeatal line
EAM	External acoustic meatus
GML	Glabellomeatal line
IAM	Internal acoustic meatus
IOML	Infraorbitomeatal line
IPL	Interpupillary line
MML	Mentomeatal line
OID	Object-to-IR distance
OML	Orbitomeatal line
TEA	Top of ear attachment
TMJ	Temporomandibular joint

See Addendum B for a summary of all abbreviations used in Volume 2.

Skull, Facial Bones, and Paranasal Sinuses

Skull Topography

The basic localization points and planes of the skull (all of which can be seen or palpated) used in radiographic positioning are illustrated in Figs. 20-37 and 20-38.

Accurate positioning of the skull requires a full understanding of these landmarks, *which should be studied thoroughly before positioning of the skull is learned.* The planes, points, lines, and abbreviations most frequently used in skull positioning are as follows:

- Midsagittal plane
- Interpupillary line
- Acanthion
- Outer canthus
- Infraorbital margin
- EAM
- Orbitomeatal line (OML)
- Infraorbitomeatal line (IOML)
- Acanthiomeatal line (AML)
- Mentomeatal line (MML)

In an adult, an average 7-degree angle difference exists between the OML and the IOML, and an average 8-degree angle difference exists between the OML and the glabellomeatal line. The degree difference between the cranial positioning lines must be recognized. Often the relationship of the patient, IR, and central ray is the same, but the angle that is described may vary depending on the cranial line of reference.

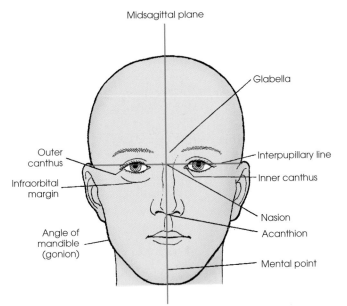

Fig. 20-37 Anterior landmarks.

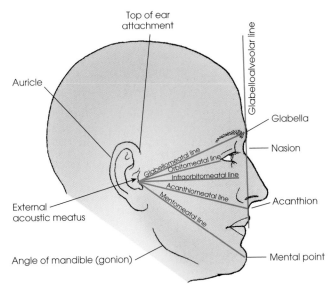

Fig. 20-38 Lateral landmarks.

Skull Morphology

All radiographic images of the skull are based on the normal size and shape of the cranium. Rules have been established for centering and adjustment of localization points and planes and for the exact degree of central ray angulation for each projection. Although the heads of many patients fall within the limits of normality and can be radiographed satisfactorily using established positions, numerous skulls vary enough in shape that the standard procedure must be adjusted to obtain an undistorted image.

In the typically shaped head (see Fig. 20-36), the petrous pyramids project anteriorly and medially at an angle of 47 degrees from the midsagittal plane of the skull. The superior borders of these structures are situated in the base of the cranium.

Depending on its shape, the atypical cranium requires more or less rotation of the head or an increase or decrease in angulation of the central ray compared with the typical, or *mesocephalic,* skull (Fig. 20-39). In the *brachycephalic* skull (Fig. 20-40), which is short from front to back, broad from side to side, and shallow from vertex to base, the internal structures are higher with reference to the IOML, and their long axes are more frontal in position (i.e., the petrous pyramids form a wider angle with the midsagittal plane). The petrous pyramids lie at an average angle of 54 degrees. In the *dolichocephalic* skull (Fig. 20-41), which is long from front to back, narrow from side to side, and deep from vertex to base, the internal structures are lower with reference to the IOML, and their long axes are less frontal in position (i.e., the petrous

pyramids form a narrower angle with the midsagittal plane). The petrous pyramids form an average angle of 40 degrees in the dolichocephalic skull.

Asymmetry must also be considered. The orbits are not always symmetric in size and shape, the lower jaw is often asymmetric, and the nasal bones and cartilage are frequently deviated from the midsagittal plane. Many deviations are not as obvious as these, but if the radiographer adheres to the fundamental rules of positioning, relatively little difficulty is encountered. Varying the position of the part or the degree of central ray angulation to compensate for structural variations becomes a simple procedure if care and precision are used initially.

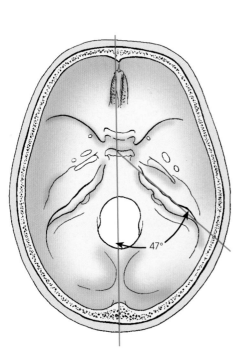

Fig. 20-39 Mesocephalic skull.

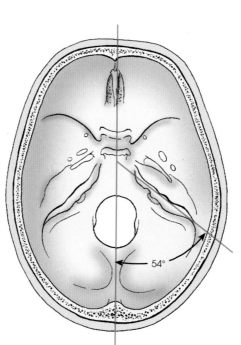

Fig. 20-40 Brachycephalic skull.

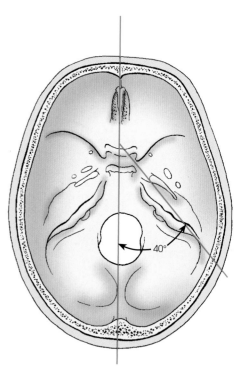

Fig. 20-41 Dolichocephalic skull.

If possible, the radiography student should obtain a dry skull specimen and image it in the standard positions. This is the best technique for studying the anatomy of different parts of the cranium from actual and radiographic standpoints. It is important to compare the actual structure (its position in the head, its relationship to adjacent structures in each radiographic position, and its relationship to the IR and the central ray angulation) with the resultant image. In this way, the radiographer can develop the ability to look at a head as though it were transparent—to visualize the location and direction of the internal parts according to the shape of the cranium. By studying the image cast by the part being examined with reference to its relationship to the images of adjacent structures, the radiographer learns to detect quickly and accurately any error in the image and any deviation from the normal cranium that requires compensation.

It is also advisable to keep a complete set of radiographic images of a normally shaped skull. These images can be used for comparison with atypical skulls in determining the deviation and the correct adjustment to make in the degree and direction of part rotation or central ray angulation. Radiographic examples of correct and incorrect skull rotation are shown in Figs. 20-42 and 20-43.

The radiographic positions depicted in Chapter 20 show the patient seated at the vertical grid device or lying on a radiographic table. Whether the radiographer elects to perform the examination with the patient in the recumbent or upright position depends on four variables: (1) the equipment available, (2) the age and condition of the patient, (3) the preference of the radiographer and/or radiologist, and (4) whether upright images would increase diagnostic value, such as showing air-fluid levels in paranasal sinuses.

With the exception of paranasal sinuses, which should be radiographed upright, the remaining radiographic positions are shown with the patient *either* upright or recumbent. Comparable images can usually be obtained with the patient either upright or recumbent. For example, a recumbent skull image can also be obtained with the patient upright as long as the OML and central ray angulation remain constant. Therefore unless specifically noted in the text, the photographic illustration does *not* constitute a recommendation for performing the examination with the patient in the upright or recumbent position. Line drawings illustrating both table and upright radiography are included for most radiographic positions in this chapter.

Skull Morphology

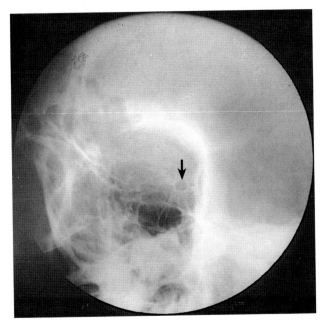

Fig. 20-42 Correct rotation clearly showing optic canal (*arrow*).

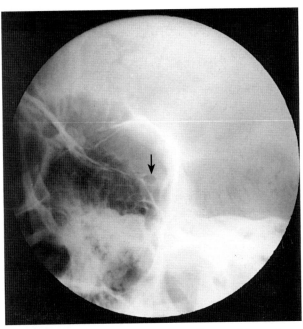

Fig. 20-43 Incorrect rotation for optic canal (*arrow*).

Technical Considerations

GENERAL BODY POSITION

The position of the body is important in radiography of the skull. Uncomfortable body position resulting in rotation or other motion is responsible for most repeat examinations. The radiographer, engrossed in adjusting the patient's head, may forget that the head is attached to a body. If the body is not correctly adjusted, this places so great a strain on the muscles that they cannot support the position. This is especially true when recumbent positions are used for skull radiography. Some guidelines to alleviate strain and facilitate accurate positioning are as follows:

- To prevent lateral rotation of the head, place the patient's body so that its long axis, depending on the image, either coincides with or is parallel to the midline of the radiographic table. To prevent superior or inferior pull on the head, resulting in longitudinal angulation or tilt, place the patient's body so that the long axis of the cervical vertebrae coincides with the level of the midpoint of the foramen magnum.
- Support any elevated part, such as the patient's shoulder or hip, on a pillow or sandbags to relieve strain.
- For examinations of hyposthenic or asthenic patients, elevate the patient's chest on a small pillow to raise the cervical vertebrae to the correct level for the lateral, PA, and oblique projections when the patient is recumbent.
- For examination of obese or hyposthenic patients, elevate the patient's head on a radiolucent pad to obtain the correct part-IR relationship if needed. An advantage of a head unit is that it simplifies handling of these patients.

- While adjusting the body, stand in a position that facilitates estimation of the approximate part position. For example, stand so that the longitudinal axis of the radiographic table is visible as the midsagittal plane of the body is being centered. This allows the anterior surface of the forehead to be viewed while the degree of body rotation for a lateral projection of the skull is adjusted. Therefore the body can be adjusted in such a way that it does not interfere with the final adjustment of the head, and the final position is comfortable for the patient.

When the body is correctly placed and adjusted so that the long axis of the cervical vertebrae is supported at the level of the foramen magnum, the final position of the head requires only minor adjustments. The average patient can maintain this relatively comfortable position without the aid of elaborate immobilization devices, although the following techniques may be helpful:

- If necessary, apply a head clamp with equal pressure on the two sides of the head.
- If such a clamp is not available, use a strip of adhesive tape where it will not be projected onto the image. The portion of the tape touching the hair should have the adhesive side covered with a second piece of tape so that the hairs are not pulled out when the tape is removed. Do not place adhesive tape directly on the patient's skin.
- When the area to be exposed is small, immobilize the head with sandbags placed against the sides or vertex.

Correct basic body positions and compensatory adjustments for recumbent radiography are illustrated in Figs. 20-44 to 20-51.

CLEANLINESS

The hair and face are naturally oily and leave a residue, even with the most hygienic patients. If the patient is sick, the residue is worse. During positioning of the skull, the patient's hair, mouth, nose, and eyes come in direct contact with the vertical grid device, tabletop, or IR. For medical asepsis, a paper towel or a cloth sheet may be placed between the imaging surface and the patient. As part of standard procedure, the contacted area should be cleaned with a disinfectant before and after positioning.

Radiation Protection

Protection of the patient from unnecessary radiation is a professional responsibility of the radiographer (see Chapter 1 for specific guidelines). In this chapter, radiation shielding of the patient is not specified or illustrated. The federal government has reported that placing a lead shield over a patient's pelvis does not significantly reduce gonadal exposure during imaging of the skull, facial bones, or sinuses.[1] Lead shields should be used to reassure the patient, however, and shielding the abdomen of a pregnant woman is recommended by the authors of this atlas.

Infants and children should receive radiation shielding of the thyroid and thymus glands and the gonads. The protective lead shielding used to cover the thyroid and thymus glands can also assist in immobilizing pediatric patients.

The most effective way to protect the patient from unnecessary radiation is to restrict the radiation beam by using *proper collimation*. Taking care to ensure that the patient is properly instructed and immobilized also reduces the likelihood of having to repeat the procedure, further limiting the radiation exposure received by the patient.

---

[1]HEW 76-8013 *Handbook of Selected Organ Doses.*

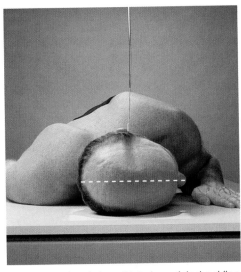

Fig. 20-44 Horizontal sagittal plane (*dashed lines*).

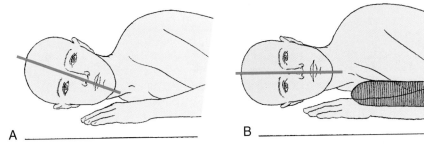

A _____ **B** _____

Fig. 20-45 Adjusting sagittal planes to horizontal position. **A,** Asthenic or hyposthenic patient. **B,** Angulation corrected.

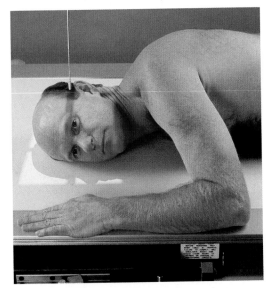

Fig. 20-46 Horizontal sagittal plane.

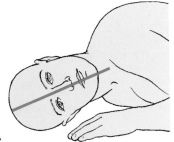

A **B**

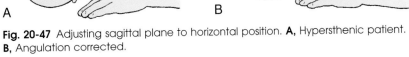

Fig. 20-47 Adjusting sagittal plane to horizontal position. **A,** Hypersthenic patient. **B,** Angulation corrected.

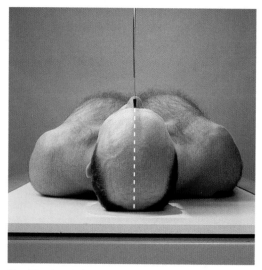

Fig. 20-48 Perpendicular sagittal plane (*dashed lines*).

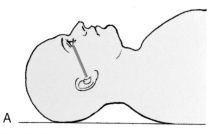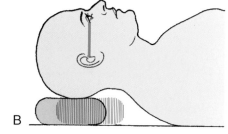

Fig. 20-49 Adjusting OML to vertical position. **A,** Hypersthenic or round-shouldered patient. **B,** Angulation corrected.

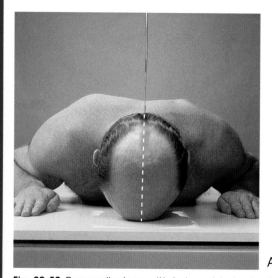

Fig. 20-50 Perpendicular sagittal plane (*dashed lines*).

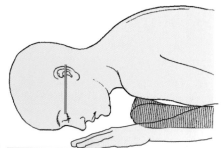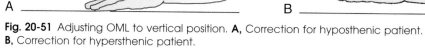

Fig. 20-51 Adjusting OML to vertical position. **A,** Correction for hyposthenic patient. **B,** Correction for hypersthenic patient.

♠ LATERAL PROJECTION
R or L position

Image receptor: 10×12 inch (24×30 cm) crosswise

Position of patient
- Place the patient in the anterior oblique position, seated upright or recumbent.
- If recumbent anterior oblique position is used, have the patient rest on the forearm and flex the knee of the elevated side.

Position of part
- With the side of interest closest to the IR, place one hand under the mandibular region and the opposite hand on the upper parietal region of the patient's head to help guide it into a true lateral position.

- Adjust the patient's head so that the midsagittal plane is parallel to the plane of the IR. If necessary, place a support under the side of the mandible to prevent it from sagging.
- Adjust the flexion of the patient's neck so that the IOML is perpendicular to the front edge of the IR. The IOML also should be parallel to the long axis of the IR.
- Check the head position so that the interpupillary line is perpendicular to the IR (Figs. 20-52 and 20-53).
- Immobilize the head.
- *Respiration:* Suspend.

Central ray
- Perpendicular, entering 2 inches (5 cm) superior to the EAM
- Center the IR to the central ray.

Collimation
- Adjust to 10×12 inches (24×30 cm) on the collimator.

Structures shown
This lateral image of the superimposed halves of the cranium shows the detail of the side adjacent to the IR. The sella turcica, anterior clinoid processes, dorsum sellae, and posterior clinoid processes are well shown in the lateral projection (Fig. 20-54).

EVALUATION CRITERIA
The following should be clearly shown:
- Evidence of proper collimation
- Entire cranium without rotation or tilt, demonstrated by:
  - Superimposed orbital roofs and greater wings of sphenoid
  - Superimposed mastoid regions and EAM
  - Superimposed TMJs
  - Sella turcica in profile
- Penetration of parietal region
- No overlap of cervical spine by mandible

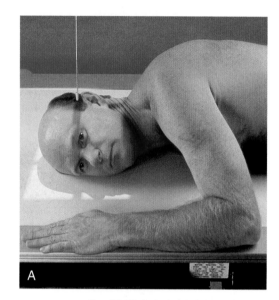
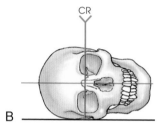

Fig. 20-52 A, Lateral skull, recumbent position. **B,** Table radiography diagram: lateral skull.

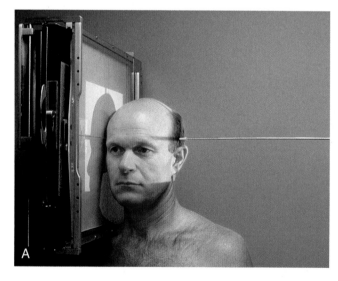
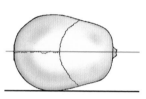
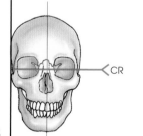
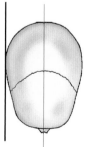

Fig. 20-53 A, Lateral skull, upright position. **B,** Upright radiography diagram: lateral skull.

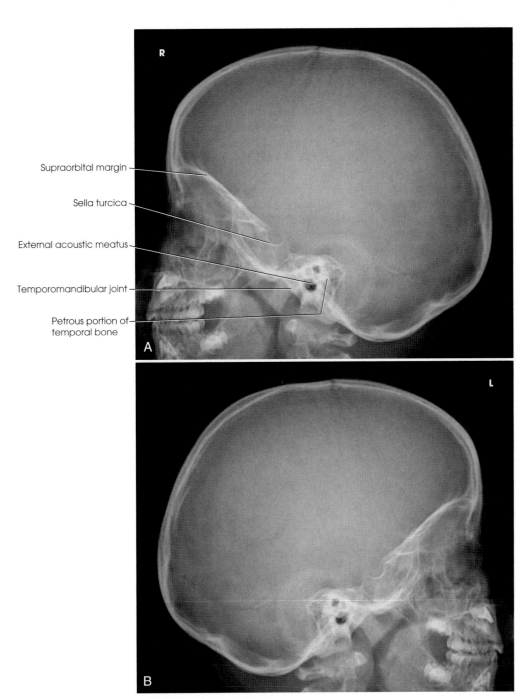

Supraorbital margin

Sella turcica

External acoustic meatus

Temporomandibular joint

Petrous portion of temporal bone

A

B

Fig. 20-54 A, Right lateral skull. **B,** Left lateral skull.

(Courtesy of St. Bernard's Medical Center, Jonesboro, AR.)

Cranium

♠ LATERAL PROJECTION
Dorsal decubitus or supine lateral position
R or L position

Dorsal decubitus

- With the patient supine, adjust the shoulders to lie in the same horizontal plane.
- After ruling out cervical injury, place the side of interest closest to the vertically placed grid IR. Elevate the patient's head enough to center it to the IR, and then support it on a radiolucent sponge.
- Adjust the patient's head so that the midsagittal plane is vertical and the interpupillary line is perpendicular to the IR (Fig. 20-55).
- Direct the central ray perpendicular to the IR, and center it 2 inches (5 cm) superior to the EAM.
- Robinson et al.[1] recommended using the dorsal decubitus lateral projection to show traumatic sphenoid sinus effusion (Fig. 20-56). They stated that this finding may be the only clue to the presence of a basal skull fracture.

---

[1]Robinson AE et al: Traumatic sphenoid sinus effusion, *AJR Am J Roentgenol* 101:795, 1967.

Supine lateral

- Place the patient in a supine or recumbent posterior oblique position, and turn the head toward the side being examined.
- Elevate and support the opposite shoulder and hip enough that the midsagittal plane of the head is parallel and the interpupillary line is perpendicular to the IR.
- Support the patient's head with a radiolucent sponge.
- Direct the central ray perpendicular to enter 2 inches (5 cm) superior to the EAM (Fig. 20-57).
- Center the IR to the central ray.

Structures shown

This lateral image of the superimposed halves of the cranium shows the detail of the side adjacent to the IR. The sella turcica, anterior clinoid processes, dorsum sellae, and posterior clinoid processes are well shown in the lateral projection (Fig. 20-58).

The following should be clearly shown:

- Evidence of proper collimation
- Entire cranium without rotation or tilt, demonstrated by:
  - ☐ Superimposed orbital roofs and greater wings of sphenoid
  - ☐ Superimposed mastoid regions and EAM
  - ☐ Superimposed TMJs
  - ☐ Sella turcica in profile
- Penetration of parietal region
- No overlap of cervical spine by mandible

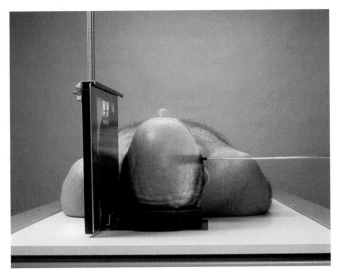

Fig. 20-55 Dorsal decubitus lateral skull.

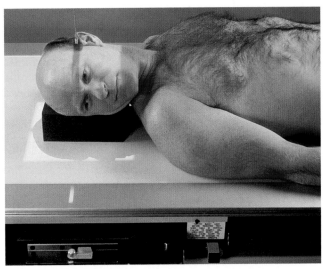

Fig. 20-57 Lateral skull with patient supine.

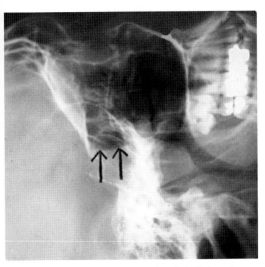

Fig. 20-56 Dorsal decubitus lateral skull showing sphenoid sinus effusion (*arrows*).

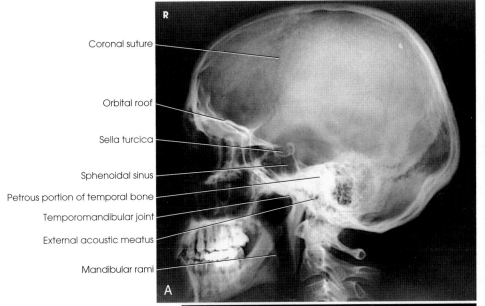

R

Coronal suture

Orbital roof

Sella turcica

Sphenoidal sinus

Petrous portion of temporal bone

Temporomandibular joint

External acoustic meatus

Mandibular rami

A

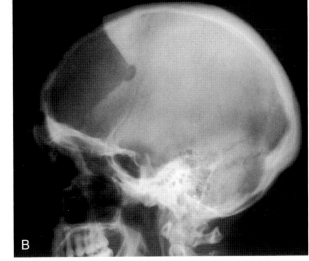

B

Fig. 20-58 A, Lateral skull. B, Lateral skull showing surgical removal of frontal bone.

⚜ PA PROJECTION
⚜ PA AXIAL PROJECTION
CALDWELL METHOD

Image receptor: 10 × 12 inch (24 × 30 cm) lengthwise

Position of patient
- Place the patient in a prone or seated position.
- Center the midsagittal plane of the patient's body to the midline of the grid.
- Rest the patient's forehead and nose on the table or against the upright Bucky.
- Flex the patient's elbows, and place the arms in a comfortable position.

Position of part
- Adjust the flexion of the patient's neck so that the OML is perpendicular to the plane of the IR.
- If the patient is recumbent, support the chin on a radiolucent sponge if needed.
- If the patient is obese or hypersthenic, a small radiolucent sponge may need to be placed under (or in front of) the forehead.
- Align the midsagittal plane perpendicular to the IR. This is accomplished by adjusting the lateral margins of the orbits or the EAM equidistant from the tabletop.
- Immobilize the patient's head, and center the IR to the nasion (Figs. 20-59 to 20-62).
- *Respiration:* Suspend.

Central ray
- For the PA projection, when the frontal bone is of primary interest, direct the central ray perpendicular to exit the nasion.
- For the Caldwell method, direct the central ray to exit the nasion at an angle of 15 degrees caudad.
- Center the IR to the central ray.
- To show the superior orbital fissures, direct the central ray through the mid-orbits at an angle of 20 to 25 degrees caudad.
- To show the rotundum foramina, direct the central ray to the nasion at an angle of 25 to 30 degrees caudad. (The Waters method, presented in the Sinus Radiography section is also used to show the rotundum foramina.)

Collimation
- Adjust to 10 × 12 inches (24 × 30 cm) on the collimator.

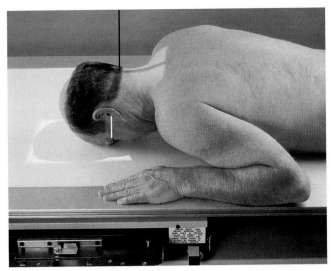

Fig. 20-59 PA skull: central ray angulation of 0 degrees for frontal bone.

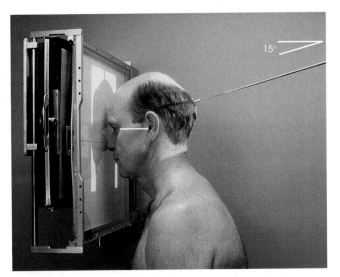

Fig. 20-60 PA axial skull: Caldwell method with central ray angulation of 15 degrees.

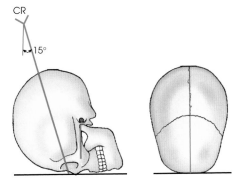

Fig. 20-61 Table radiography diagram: Caldwell method.

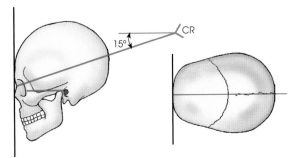

Fig. 20-62 Upright radiography diagram: Caldwell method.

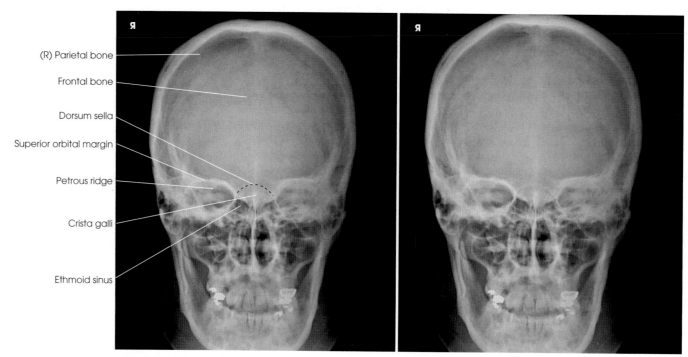

(R) Parietal bone

Frontal bone

Dorsum sella

Superior orbital margin

Petrous ridge

Crista galli

Ethmoid sinus

Fig. 20-63 PA skull with perpendicular central ray. (Courtesy of St. Bernard's Medical Center, Jonesboro, AR.)

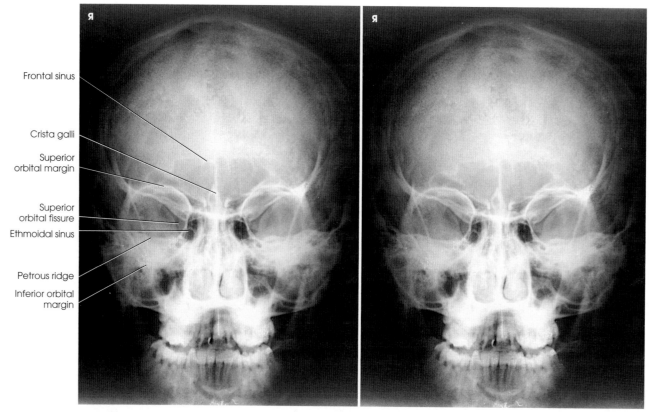

Frontal sinus

Crista galli

Superior orbital margin

Superior orbital fissure

Ethmoidal sinus

Petrous ridge

Inferior orbital margin

Fig. 20-64 PA axial skull: Caldwell method with 15-degree caudal central ray angulation.

Skull, Facial Bones, and Paranasal Sinuses

Structures shown

For the PA projection with a perpendicular central ray (Fig. 20-63), the orbits are filled by the margins of the petrous pyramids. Other structures shown include the posterior ethmoidal air cells, crista galli, frontal bone, and frontal sinuses. The dorsum sellae is seen as a curved line extending between the orbits, just above the ethmoidal air cells.

When the central ray is angled 15 degrees caudad to the nasion for the PA axial projection, Caldwell method, many of the same structures that appear in the PA projection are seen (Fig. 20-64); however, the petrous ridges are projected into the lower third of the orbits. The Caldwell method also shows the anterior ethmoidal air cells. Schüller,[1] who first described this positioning for the skull, recommended a caudal angle of 25 degrees.

---

[1]Schüller A: Die Schädelbasis im Rontgenbild, *Fortschr Roentgenstr* 11:215, 1905.

Stretcher and bedside examinations
Lateral decubitus position

- When the patient cannot be turned to the prone position for the PA or PA axial Caldwell projection, and cervical spinal injury has been ruled out, elevate one side enough to place the patient's head in a true lateral position, and support the shoulder and hip on pillows or sandbags if needed.
- Elevate the patient's head on a suitable support, and adjust its height to center the midsagittal plane of the head to a vertically positioned grid.
- Adjust the patient's head so that the OML is perpendicular to the plane of the IR (Fig. 20-65).
- Direct the *horizontal* central ray perpendicular, or 15 degrees caudad, to exit the nasion.

The following should be clearly shown:
- Evidence of proper collimation
- Entire cranium without rotation or tilt, demonstrated by:
  - Equal distances from lateral borders of skull to lateral borders of orbits on both sides
  - Symmetric petrous ridges
  - MSP of cranium aligned with long axis of collimated field
- PA axial (Caldwell) demonstrates petrous pyramids lying in lower third of orbit
- PA projection shows orbits filled by petrous ridges
- Entire cranial perimeter showing three distinct tables of squamous bone
- Penetration of frontal bone with appropriate brightness at lateral borders of skull

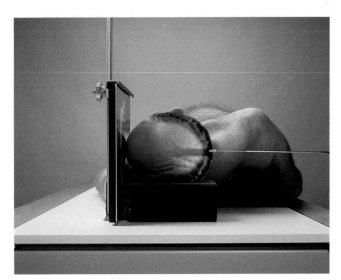

Fig. 20-65 PA skull with patient semi-supine.

✿ AP PROJECTION
✿ AP AXIAL PROJECTION

Image receptor: 10 × 12 inch (24 × 30 cm) lengthwise

When the patient cannot be positioned for a PA or PA axial projection, a similar but magnified image can be obtained with an AP projection.

Position of patient and part
- Position the patient supine with the midsagittal plane of the body centered to the grid.
- Ensure that the midsagittal plane and the OML are perpendicular to the IR.

Central ray
- Perpendicular (Fig. 20-66) or directed to the nasion at an angle 15 degrees cephalad (Fig. 20-67)
- Center IR to the central ray

Collimation
- Adjust to 10 × 12 inches (24 × 30 cm) on the collimator.

Structures shown
The structures shown on the AP projection are the same as the structures shown on the PA projection. On the AP projection (Fig. 20-68), the orbits are considerably magnified because of the increased object–to–image receptor distance (OID). Similarly, because of the magnification, the distance from the lateral margin of the orbit to the lateral margin of the temporal bone measures less on the AP projection than on the PA projection.

EVALUATION CRITERIA
The following should be clearly shown:
- Evidence of proper collimation
- Entire cranium without rotation or tilt, demonstrated by:
  - Equal distances from lateral borders of skull to lateral borders of orbits on both sides
  - Symmetric petrous ridges
  - MSP of cranium aligned with long axis of collimated field
- Petrous pyramids lying in lower third of orbit with a cephalad central ray angulation of 15 degrees and filling orbits with a 0-degree central ray angulation
- Entire cranial perimeter showing three distinct areas of squamous bone
- Penetration of frontal bone with appropriate brightness at lateral borders of skull

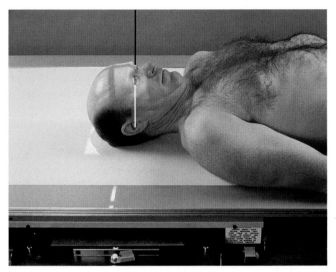

Fig. 20-66 AP skull.

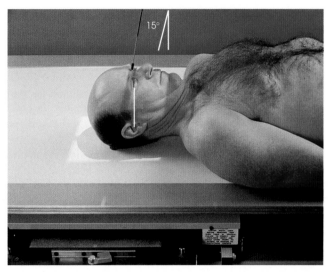

Fig. 20-67 AP axial skull with 15-degree cephalad central ray.

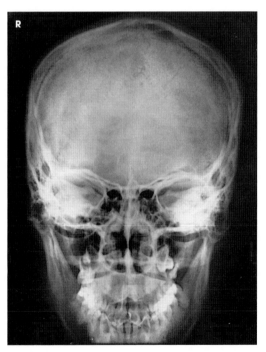

Fig. 20-68 AP skull with perpendicular central ray.

⚓ AP AXIAL PROJECTION
TOWNE METHOD

Image receptor: 10 × 12 inch (24 × 30 cm) lengthwise

NOTE: Although this technique is most commonly referred to as the Towne method,[1] numerous authors have described slightly different variations. In 1912, Grashey[2] published the first description of the AP axial projection of the cranium. In 1926, Altschul[3] and Towne[1] described the position. Altschul recommended strong depression of the chin and direction of the central ray through the foramen magnum at a caudal angle of 40 degrees. Towne (citing Chamberlain) recommended that with the patient's chin depressed, the central ray should be directed through the midsagittal plane from a point about 3 inches (7.6 cm) above the eyebrows to the foramen magnum. Towne gave no specific central ray angulation, but the angulation would depend on the flexion of the neck.

---

[1]Towne EB: Erosion of the petrous bone by acoustic nerve tumor, *Arch Otolaryngol* 4:515, 1926.
[2]Grashey R: Atlas typischer Röntgenbilder vom normalen Menschen. In *Lehmann's medizinische Atlanten,* ed 2, vol 5, Munich, 1912, JF Lehmann.
[3]Altschul W: Beiträg zur Röntgenologie des Gehörorganes, *Z Hals Nas Ohr* 14:335, 1926.

Position of patient
- With the patient supine or seated upright, center the midsagittal plane of the patient's body to the midline of the grid.
- Place the patient's arms in a comfortable position, and adjust the shoulders to lie in the same horizontal plane.
- To ensure the patient's comfort without increasing the IR distance, examine the hypersthenic or obese patient in the seated-upright position if possible.
- The skull can be brought closer to the IR by having the patient lean back lordotically and rest the shoulders against the vertical grid device. When this is impossible, the desired projection of the occipitobasal region may be obtained by using the PA axial projection described by Haas (pp. 308-309). The Haas method is the reverse of the AP axial projection and produces a comparable result.

Position of part
- Adjust the patient's head so that the midsagittal plane is perpendicular to the midline of the IR.
- Flex the patient's neck enough to place the OML perpendicular to the plane of the IR.
- When the patient cannot flex the neck to this extent, adjust the neck so that the IOML is perpendicular and then increase the central ray angulation by 7 degrees (Figs. 20-69 to 20-72).
- Position the IR so that its upper margin is at the level of the highest point of the cranial vertex. This places the center at or near the level of the foramen magnum.
- For a localized image of the dorsum sellae and petrous pyramids, adjust the IR so that its midpoint coincides with the central ray. The IR is centered at or slightly below the level of the occlusal plane.
- Recheck the position and immobilize the head.
- *Respiration:* Suspend.

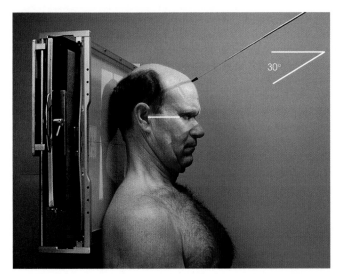

Fig. 20-69 AP axial skull: Towne method, upright position.

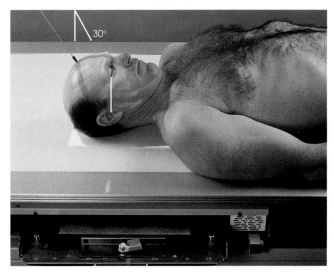

Fig. 20-70 AP axial skull: Towne method, supine position.

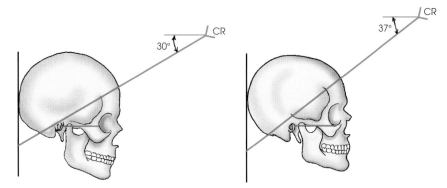

Fig. 20-71 Upright radiography diagram: AP axial skull: Towne method. Same radiographic result with central ray directed 30 degrees to OML or 37 degrees to IOML.

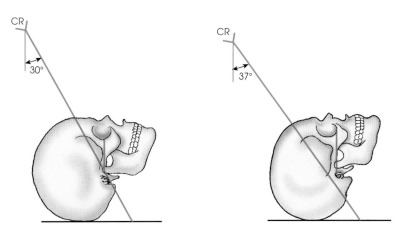

Fig. 20-72 Table radiography diagram: AP axial skull: Towne method.

Central ray

- Directed through the foramen magnum at a caudal angle of 30 degrees to the OML or 37 degrees to the IOML. The central ray enters approximately $2\frac{1}{2}$ inches (6.3 cm) above the glabella and passes through the level of the EAM.

Collimation

- Adjust to 10×12 inches (24×30 cm) on the collimator.

Structures shown

The AP axial projection shows a symmetric image of the petrous pyramids, the posterior portion of the foramen magnum, the dorsum sellae, and the posterior clinoid processes projected within the foramen magnum, the occipital bone, and the posterior portion of the parietal bones (Fig. 20-73). This projection is also used for tomographic studies of the ears, facial canal, jugular foramina, and rotundum foramina.

EVALUATION CRITERIA

The following should be clearly shown:

- Evidence of proper collimation
- Entire cranium, without rotation or tilt, demonstrated by:
  - □ Equal distances from lateral borders of skull to lateral margins of foramen magnum on both sides
  - □ Symmetric petrous pyramids
  - □ MSP of cranium aligned with long axis of collimated field
- Dorsum sellae and posterior clinoid processes visible within foramen magnum
- Penetration of occipital bone with appropriate brightness at lateral borders of skull

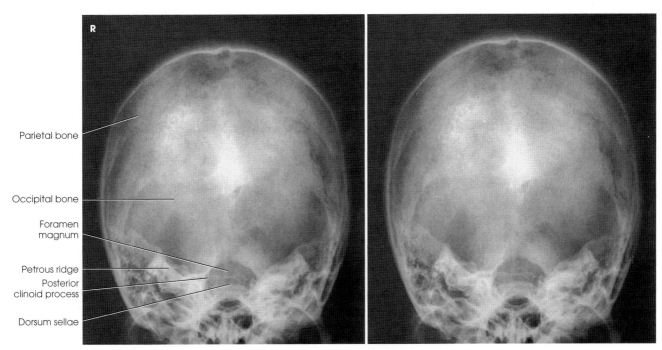

Parietal bone

Occipital bone

Foramen magnum

Petrous ridge

Posterior clinoid process

Dorsum sellae

Fig. 20-73 AP axial skull: Towne method with 30-degree central ray angulation to OML.

Pathologic condition or trauma

To show the entire foramen magnum, the caudal angulation of the central ray is increased from 40 to 60 degrees to the OML (Figs. 20-74 to 20-78).

Lateral decubitus position

For pathologic conditions, trauma, or a deformity such as a strongly accentuated dorsal kyphosis when the patient cannot be examined in a direct supine or prone position, the following steps should be taken:

- Adjust and support the body in a semi-recumbent position; this allows the head to be placed in a true lateral position.

- Immobilize the IR and grid in a vertical position behind the patient's occiput.
- Direct the *horizontal* central ray 30 degrees caudally to the OML (Fig. 20-79).

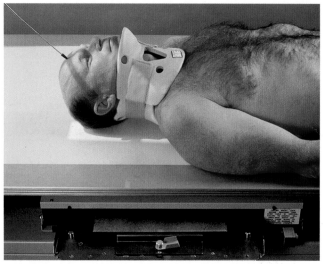

Fig. 20-74 AP axial skull, Towne method, on a trauma patient. OML and IOML lines are not perpendicular, which would require central ray angulation greater than 37 degrees.

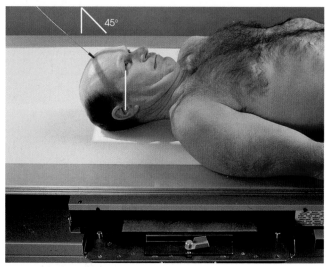

Fig. 20-75 AP axial skull: central ray angulation of 40 to 45 degrees.

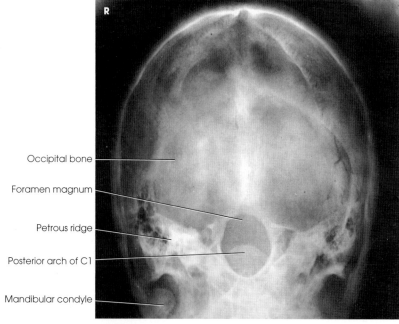

Occipital bone

Foramen magnum

Petrous ridge

Posterior arch of C1

Mandibular condyle

Fig. 20-76 AP axial skull: central ray angulation of 45 degrees.

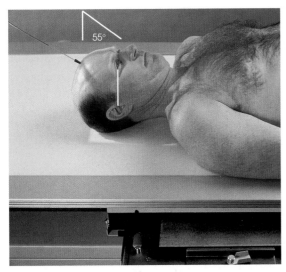

Fig. 20-77 AP axial foramen magnum, supine position.

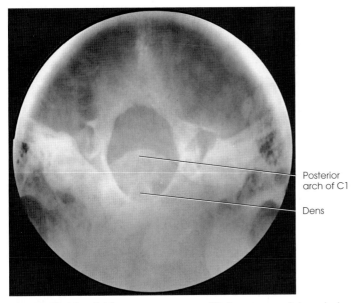

Posterior arch of C1

Dens

Fig. 20-78 AP axial foramen magnum: 55-degree caudal central ray.

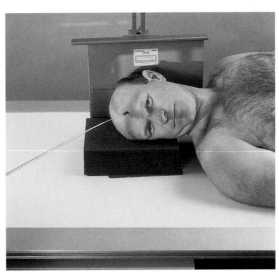

Fig. 20-79 AP axial skull, with the patient's head in lateral decubitus position and with IR and grid vertical.

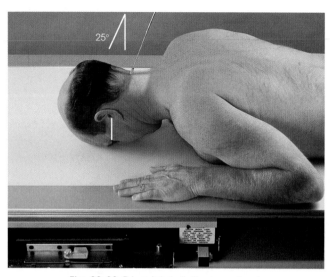

Fig. 20-80 PA axial skull: Haas method.

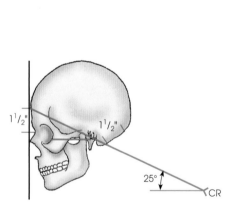

Fig. 20-81 Upright radiography diagram: PA axial skull: Haas method diagram.

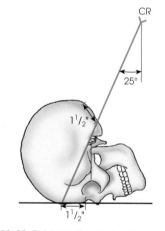

Fig. 20-82 Table radiography diagram: PA axial skull: Haas method diagram.

⚛ PA AXIAL PROJECTION
HAAS METHOD

Haas[1] devised this projection for obtaining an image of the sellar structures projected within the foramen magnum on hypersthenic, obese, or other patients who cannot be adjusted correctly for the AP axial (Towne) projection.

Image receptor: 10×12 inch (24×30 cm) lengthwise

Position of patient
- Adjust the patient in the prone or seated-upright position, and center the midsagittal plane of the body to the midline of the grid.
- Flex the patient's elbows, place the arms in a comfortable position, and adjust the shoulders to lie in the same horizontal plane.

Position of part
- Rest the patient's forehead and nose on the table, with the midsagittal plane perpendicular to the midline of the grid.
- Adjust the flexion of the neck so that the OML is perpendicular to the IR (see Figs. 20-80 to 20-82).
- Immobilize the head.
- For a localized image of the sellar region or the petrous pyramids, or both, adjust the position of the IR so that the midpoint coincides with the central ray; shift the IR cephalad approximately 3 inches (7.6 cm) to include the vertex of the skull. An 8×10-inch (18×24-cm) IR is recommended.
- *Respiration:* Suspend.

Central ray
- Directed at a cephalad angle of 25 degrees to the OML to enter a point $1\frac{1}{2}$ inches (3.8 cm) below the external occipital protuberance (inion) and to exit approximately $1\frac{1}{2}$ inches (3.8 cm) superior to the nasion. The central ray can be varied to show other cranial anatomy.

[1]Haas L: Verfahren zur sagittalen Aufnahme der Sellagegend, *Fortschr Roentgenstr* 36:1198, 1927.

Collimation

- Adjust to 10×12 inches (24×30 cm) on the collimator.

Structures shown

PA axial projection shows the occipital region of the cranium and shows a symmetric image of the petrous pyramids and the dorsum sellae and posterior clinoid processes within the foramen magnum (Figs. 20-83 and 20-84).

EVALUATION CRITERIA

The following should be clearly shown:
- Evidence of proper collimation
- Entire cranium, without rotation or tilt, demonstrated by:
  □ Equal distances from lateral borders of skull to lateral margins of foramen magnum on both sides
  □ Symmetric petrous pyramids
  □ MSP of cranium aligned with long axis of collimated field
- Dorsum sellae and posterior clinoid processes visible within foramen magnum
- Penetration of occipital bone with appropriate brightness at lateral borders of skull

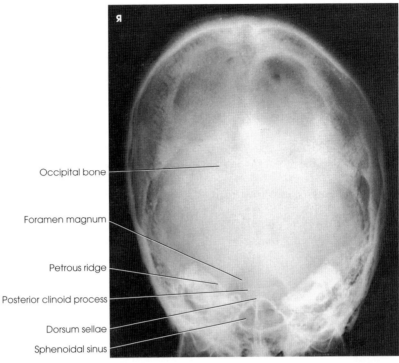

Occipital bone
Foramen magnum
Petrous ridge
Posterior clinoid process
Dorsum sellae
Sphenoidal sinus

Fig. 20-83 PA axial skull: Haas method, with 25-degree cephalad central ray.

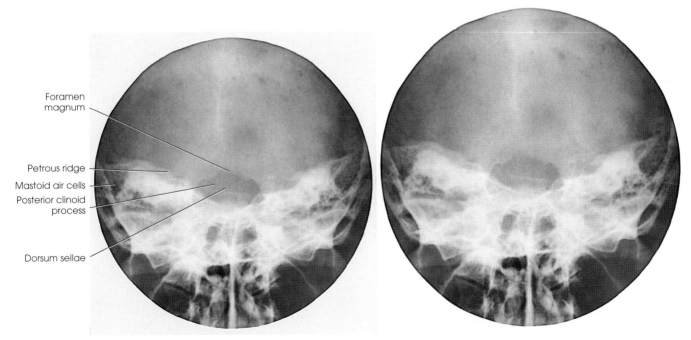

Foramen magnum
Petrous ridge
Mastoid air cells
Posterior clinoid process
Dorsum sellae

Fig. 20-84 PA axial sella turcica: Haas method, using cylindric extension cone that restricts collimation to small area. Beam restriction decreases scatter radiation and increases visibility of detail of sellar structures.

⚕ SUBMENTOVERTICAL PROJECTION
SCHÜLLER METHOD

Image receptor: 10 × 12 inch (24 × 30 cm) lengthwise

Position of patient
The success of the submentovertical (SMV) projection of the cranial base depends on placing the IOML as nearly parallel with the plane of the IR as possible and directing the central ray perpendicular to the IOML. The following steps are taken:

- Place the patient in the supine or the seated-upright position; the latter is more comfortable. If a chair that supports the back is used, the upright position allows greater freedom in positioning the patient's body to place the IOML parallel with the IR. If the patient is seated far enough away from the vertical grid device, the head can usually be adjusted without placing great pressure on the neck.
- When the patient is placed in the supine position, elevate the torso on firm pillows or a suitable pad to allow the head to rest on the vertex with the neck in hyperextension.
- Flex the patient's knees to relax the abdominal muscles.

- Place the patient's arms in a comfortable position, and adjust the shoulders to lie in the same horizontal plane.
- Do not keep the patient in the final adjustment longer than is absolutely necessary because the supine position places considerable strain on the neck.

Position of part
- With the midsagittal plane of the patient's body centered to the midline of the grid, extend the patient's neck to the greatest extent as can be achieved, placing the IOML as parallel as possible to the IR.
- Adjust the patient's head so that the midsagittal plane is perpendicular to the IR (Figs. 20-85 to 20-88).

NOTE: Patients placed in the supine position for the cranial base may have increased intracranial pressure. As a result, they may be dizzy or unstable for a few minutes after having been in this position. Use of the upright position may alleviate some of this pressure.

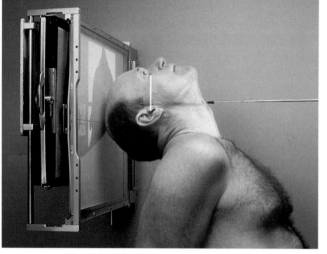

Fig. 20-85 SMV cranial base, patient upright.

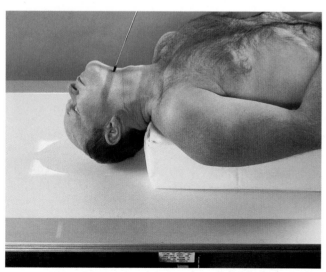

Fig. 20-87 SMV cranial base, patient supine.

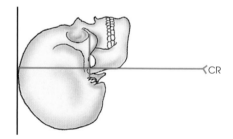

Fig. 20-86 Upright radiography diagram: SMV skull.

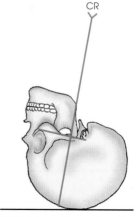

Fig. 20-88 Table radiography diagram: SMV skull.

- Immobilize the patient's head. In the absence of a head clamp, place a suitably backed strip of adhesive tape across the tip of the chin and anchor it to the sides of the radiographic unit if needed. (The part of the tape touching the skin should be covered.)
- *Respiration:* Suspend.

Central ray

- Directed through the sella turcica perpendicular to the IOML. The central ray enters the midsagittal plane of the throat between the angles of the mandible and passes through a point $\frac{3}{4}$ inch (1.9 cm) anterior to the level of the EAM.
- Center the IR to the central ray. The IR should be parallel to the IOML.

Collimation

- Adjust to 10×12 inches (24×30 cm) on the collimator.

Structures shown

SMV projection of the cranial base shows symmetric images of the petrosae, the mastoid processes, the foramina ovale and spinosum (which are best shown in this projection), the carotid canals, the sphenoidal and ethmoidal sinuses, the mandible, the bony nasal septum, the dens of the axis, and the occipital bone. The maxillary sinuses are superimposed over the mandible (Fig. 20-89).

SMV projection is also used for axial tomography of the orbits, optic canals, ethmoid bone, maxillary sinuses, and mastoid processes. With a decrease in the exposure factors, the zygomatic arches are also well shown in this position (see sections on Facial Bone Radiography and Sinus Radiography later in this chapter).

The following should be clearly shown:
- Evidence of proper collimation
- Entire cranium, without tilt, demonstrated by:
  - Equal distances from the lateral borders of the skull to the mandibular condyles on both sides
  - Symmetric petrosae
- IOML is parallel to IR (full neck extension), demonstrated by:
  - Mental protuberance superimposed over anterior frontal bone
  - Mandibular condyles anterior to petrosae
- Brightness and contrast sufficient to demonstrate cranial base anatomy

NOTE: Schüller[1] described and illustrated the basal projections—SMV and verticosubmental (VSM)—but Pfeiffer[2] gave specific directions for the central ray angulation.

[1]Schüller A: Die Schädelbasis im Rontgenbild, *Fortshr Reontgenstr* 11:215, 1905.
[2]Pfeiffer W: Beitrag zum Wert des axialen Schädelskiagrammes, *Arch Laryngol Rhinol* 30:1, 1916.

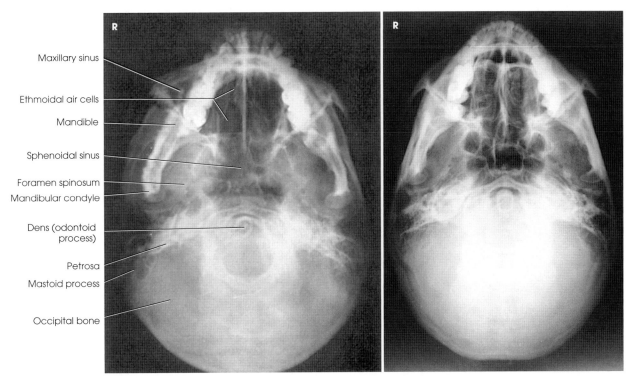

Maxillary sinus
Ethmoidal air cells
Mandible
Sphenoidal sinus
Foramen spinosum
Mandibular condyle
Dens (odontoid process)
Petrosa
Mastoid process
Occipital bone

Fig. 20-89 SMV cranial base.

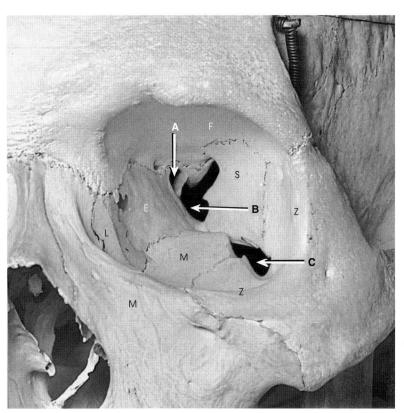

Fig. 20-90 Bones of left orbit of dry specimen. **A,** Optic canal and foramen. **B,** Superior orbital fissure. **C,** Inferior orbital fissure. *E,* ethmoid; *F,* frontal; *L,* lacrimal; *M,* maxilla; *S,* sphenoid; *Z,* zygomatic (palatine not shown).

Orbit

The orbits are cone-shaped, bony-walled cavities situated on each side of the midsagittal plane of the head (Fig. 20-90). They are formed by the seven previously described and illustrated bones of the cranium (frontal, ethmoid, and sphenoid) and the face (lacrimal, palatine, maxillary, and zygomatic). Each orbit has a roof, a medial wall, a lateral wall, and a floor. The easily palpable, quadrilateral-shaped anterior circumference of the orbit is called its *base*. The *apex* of the orbit corresponds to the *optic foramen*. The long axis of each orbit is directed obliquely, posteriorly, and medially at an average angle of 37 degrees to the midsagittal plane of the head and superiorly at an angle of about 30 degrees from the OML (Fig. 20-91).

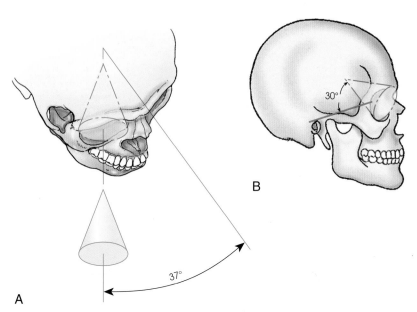

Fig. 20-91 Cone-shaped orbit. **A,** Average angle of 37 degrees from midsagittal plane. **B,** Average angle of 30 degrees superior to OML.

The orbits serve primarily as bony sockets for the eyeballs and the structures associated with them, but they also contain blood vessels and nerves that pass through openings in their walls to other regions. The major and frequently radiographed openings are the previously described optic foramina and the superior and inferior orbital sulci.

The *superior orbital fissure* is the cleft between the greater and lesser wings of the sphenoid bone. From the body of the sphenoid at a point near the orbital apex, this sulcus extends superiorly and laterally between the roof and the lateral wall of the orbit. The *inferior orbital fissure* is the narrow cleft extending from the lower anterolateral aspect of the sphenoid body anteriorly and laterally between the floor and lateral wall of the orbit. The anterior margin of the cleft is formed by the orbital plate of the maxilla, and its posterior margin is formed by the greater wing of the sphenoid bone and the zygomatic bone.

Because the walls of the orbits are thin, they are subject to fracture. When a person is forcibly struck squarely on the eyeball (e.g., by a fist, by a piece of sporting equipment), the resulting pressure directed to the eyeball forces the eyeball into the cone-shaped orbit and "blows out" the thin, delicate bony floor of the orbit (Figs. 20-92 and 20-93). The injury must be diagnosed and treated accurately so that the person's vision is not jeopardized. Blowout fractures may be shown using any combination of images obtained with the patient positioned for parietoacanthial projections (Waters method), radiographic tomography, or computed tomography (CT).

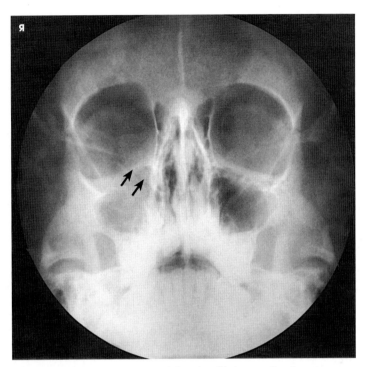

Fig. 20-92 Parietoacanthial orbits using Waters method and showing blowout fracture of orbit (*arrows*).

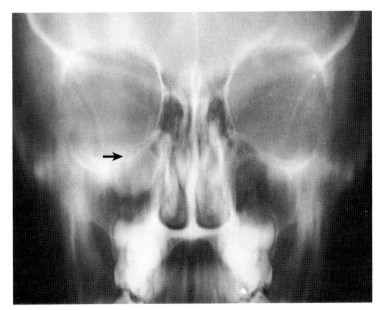

Fig. 20-93 Tomogram: AP projection showing fracture (*arrow*) in the same patient as in Fig. 20-92.

Eye

The organ of vision, or eye (Latin, *oculus;* Greek, *ophthalmos*), consists of the following: eyeball; optic nerve, which connects the eyeball to the brain; blood vessels; and accessory organs such as extrinsic muscles, lacrimal apparatus, and eyelids (Figs. 20-94 and 20-95).

The *eyeball* is situated in the anterior part of the orbital cavity. Its posterior segment (about two thirds of the bulb) is adjacent to the soft parts that occupy the remainder of the orbital cavity (chiefly muscles, fat, and connective tissue). The anterior portion of the eyeball is exposed and projects beyond the base of the orbit. Bone-free radiographic images of the ante-rior segment of the eye can be obtained. The exposed part of the eyeball is covered by a thin mucous membrane known as the *conjunctiva,* portions of which line the eyelids. The conjunctival membrane is kept moist by tear secretions from the lacrimal gland. These secretions prevent drying and friction irritation during movements of the eyeball and eyelids.

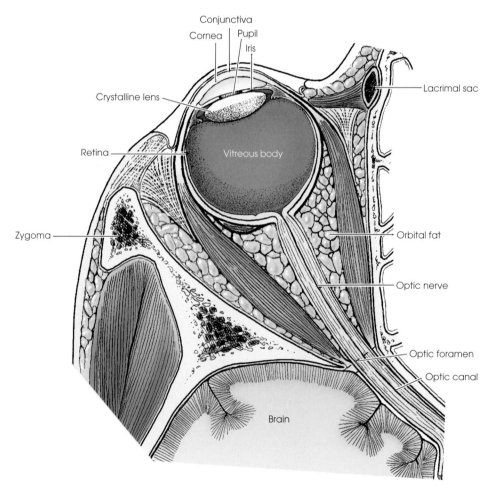

Fig. 20-94 Diagrammatic horizontal section of right orbital region: top-down view.

The outer, supporting coat of the eyeball is a firm, fibrous membrane consisting of a posterior segment called the *sclera* and an anterior segment called the *cornea*. The opaque, white sclera is commonly referred to as the "white of the eye." The cornea is situated in front of the *iris,* with its center point corresponding to the pupil. The corneal part of the membrane is transparent, allowing the passage of light into the eyeball, and it serves as one of the four refractive media of the eye.

The inner coat of the eyeball is called the *retina*. This delicate membrane is contiguous with the optic nerve. The retina is composed chiefly of nervous tissue and several million minute receptor organs, called *rods* and *cones,* which transmit light impulses to the brain. The rods and cones are important radiographically because they play a role in the ability of the radiologist or radiographer to see the fluoroscopic image. Their function is described in discussions of fluoroscopy in radiography physics and imaging textbooks.

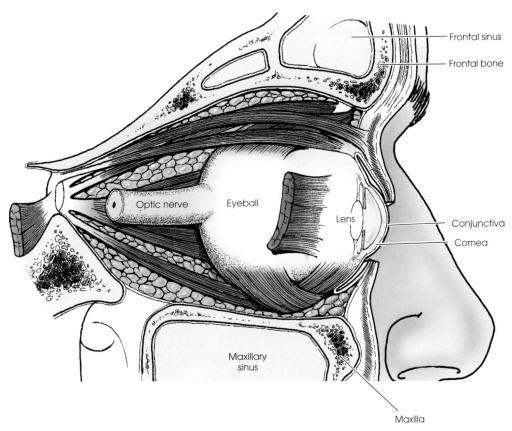

Fig. 20-95 Diagrammatic sagittal section of right orbital region.

LOCALIZATION OF FOREIGN BODIES WITHIN ORBIT OR EYE

Ultrasonography and CT (Fig. 20-96) have been increasingly used to locate foreign bodies in the eye. (Magnetic resonance imaging [MRI] is not used for foreign body localization because movement of a metallic foreign object by the magnetic field could lead to hemorrhage or other serious complications.) Whether an ultrasound or a radiographic approach is used, accurate localization of foreign particles lodged within the orbit or eye requires the use of a precision localization technique.

Localization methods removed

The *Vogt method, Sweet method, Pfeiffer-Comberg method,* and *parallax motion method* are sometimes used to localize foreign bodies in the eye. These methods were described briefly in the eighth edition of this atlas. Complete descriptions appeared in the seventh and earlier editions.

Image quality

Ultrafine recorded detail is essential for detecting and localizing minute foreign particles within the orbit or eyeball. The following are required:

1. The geometric unsharpness must be reduced as much as possible by the use of a close OID and a small, undamaged focal spot at a source–to–image receptor distance (SID) that is as long as is consistent with the exposure factors required.
2. Secondary radiation must be minimized by close collimation.
3. Motion must be eliminated by firmly immobilizing the patient's head and by having the patient gaze steadily at a fixed object, immobilizing the eyeballs.

An artifact can cast an image that simulates the appearance of a foreign body located within the orbit or eye. IRs and screens must be impeccably clean before each examination. In institutions and clinics that often perform these examinations, an adequate number of IR holders are kept in reserve for eye studies only. This measure protects them from the wear of routine use in less critical procedures.

PRELIMINARY EXAMINATION

Lateral projections, PA projections, and bone-free studies are performed to determine whether a radiographically demonstrable foreign body is present. For these images, the patient may be placed in the recumbent position or may be seated upright before a vertical grid device. These projections may be used for metallic foreign body screening before MRI procedures are performed.

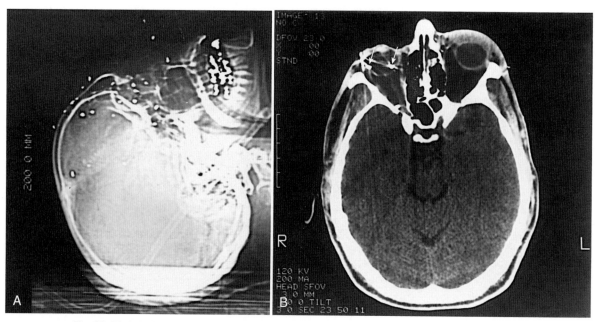

Fig. 20-96 A, Lateral localizer CT image showing multiple buckshot in the face. **B,** Axial CT image of same patient, showing shotgun pellets within the eye (*arrows*).

LATERAL PROJECTION

R or L position

A nongrid (very high-resolution) technique is recommended to reduce magnification and eliminate possible artifacts in or on the radiographic table and grid. The following steps are taken:

- With the patient semi-prone or seated upright, place the outer canthus of the affected eye adjacent to and centered over the midpoint of the IR.
- Adjust the patient's head to place the midsagittal plane parallel with the plane of the IR and the interpupillary line perpendicular to the IR plane.
- *Respiration:* Suspend.

Central ray

- Perpendicular through the outer canthus
- Instruct the patient to look straight ahead for the exposure (Figs. 20-97 and 20-98).

EVALUATION CRITERIA

The following should be clearly shown:

- Entire orbit(s)
- No rotation, demonstrated by:
  - Superimposed orbital roofs
- Close beam restriction centered to orbital region
- Brightness and contrast permitting optimal visibility of orbit and eye for localization of foreign bodies

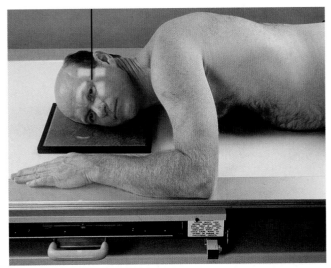

Fig. 20-97 Lateral projection for orbital foreign body localization.

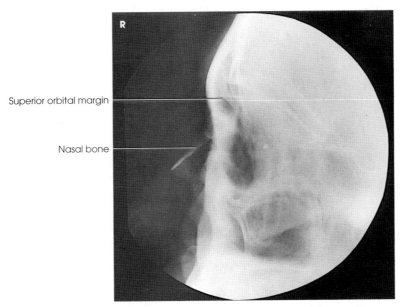

Superior orbital margin

Nasal bone

Fig. 20-98 Lateral projection showing foreign body (*white speck*).

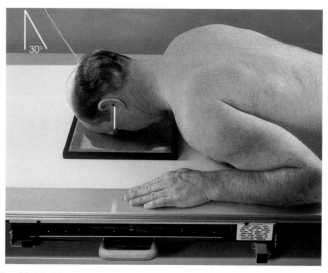

Fig. 20-99 PA axial projection for orbital foreign body localization.

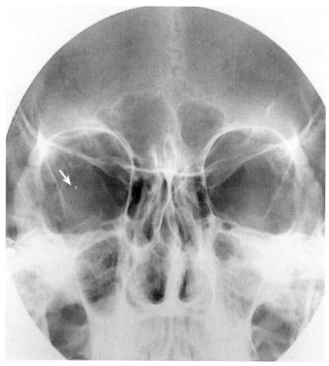

Fig. 20-100 PA axial projection showing foreign body (*arrow*) in the right eye.

PA AXIAL PROJECTION

A nongrid (very high-resolution) technique is recommended to reduce magnification and eliminate possible artifacts in or on the radiographic table and grid. The following steps are taken:

- Rest the patient's forehead and nose on the IR holder, and center the holder ¾ inch (1.9 cm) distal to the nasion.
- Adjust the patient's head so that the midsagittal plane and OML are perpendicular to the plane of the IR.
- *Respiration:* Suspend.

Central ray

- Directed through the center of the orbits at a caudal angulation of 30 degrees. This angulation is used to project the petrous portions of the temporal bones below the inferior margin of the orbits (Figs. 20-99 and 20-100).
- Instruct the patient to close the eyes and to concentrate on holding them still for the exposure.

EVALUATION CRITERIA

The following should be clearly shown:
- Entire orbit(s)
- Petrous pyramids lying below orbital shadows
- No rotation of cranium, demonstrated by:
  - Symmetric visualization of the orbits
- Close beam restriction centered to orbital region
- Brightness and contrast permitting optimal visibility of orbit and eye for localization of foreign bodies

PARIETOACANTHIAL PROJECTION
MODIFIED WATERS METHOD

Some physicians prefer to have the PA projection performed with the patient's head adjusted in a modified Waters position so that the petrous margins are displaced by part adjustment rather than by central ray angulation. The following steps are taken:

- With the IR centered at the level of the center of the orbits, rest the patient's chin on the IR holder.
- Adjust the patient's head so that the midsagittal plane is perpendicular to the plane of the IR.
- Adjust the flexion of the patient's neck so that the OML forms an angle of 50 degrees with the plane of the IR.
- *Respiration:* Suspend.

Central ray
- Perpendicular through the mid-orbits (Figs. 20-101 and 20-102)
- Instruct the patient to close the eyes and to concentrate on holding them still for the exposure.

EVALUATION CRITERIA

The following should be clearly shown:
- Entire orbit(s)
- Petrous pyramids lying well below orbital shadows
- No rotation, demonstrated by:
  - □ Symmetric visualization of orbits
- Close beam restriction centered to the orbital region
- Brightness and contrast permitting optimal visibility of orbit and eye for localization of foreign bodies

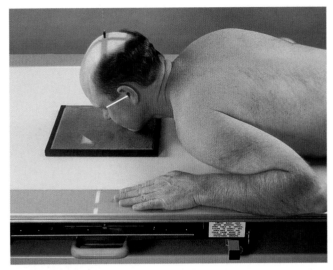

Fig. 20-101 Parietoacanthial projection, modified Waters method, for orbital foreign body localization.

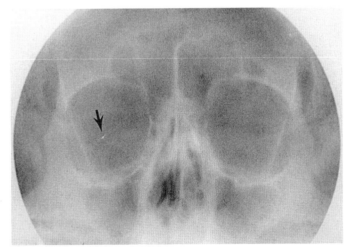

Fig. 20-102 Parietoacanthial projection, modified Waters method, showing foreign body (*arrow*).

⚚ LATERAL PROJECTION
R or L position

Image receptor: 8 × 10 inch (18 × 24 cm) lengthwise or 10 × 12 inch (24 × 30 cm) lengthwise, depending on availability

Position of patient
- Place the patient in a recumbent anterior oblique or seated anterior oblique position before a vertical grid device. This is the same basic position that is used for the lateral skull position.

Position of part
- Adjust the patient's head so that the midsagittal plane is parallel with the IR and the interpupillary line is perpendicular to the IR.
- Adjust the flexion of the patient's neck so that the infraorbitomeatal line (IOML) is perpendicular to the front edge of the IR (Figs. 20-103 to 105).
- Immobilize the head.
- *Respiration:* Suspend.

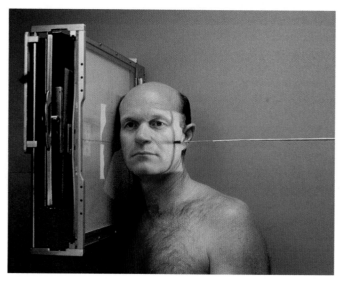

Fig. 20-103 Lateral facial bones.

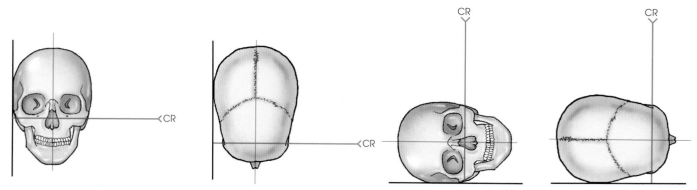

Fig. 20-104 Upright lateral facial bones diagram.

Fig. 20-105 Table radiography diagram: lateral facial bones.

Central ray

- Perpendicular and entering the lateral surface of the zygomatic bone halfway between the outer canthus and the external acoustic meatus (EAM)
- Center IR to the central ray.

Collimation

- Adjust to 6 × 10 inches (15 × 24 cm) on the collimator.

Structures shown

This projection shows a lateral image of the bones of the face, with the right and left sides superimposed (Fig. 20-106).

EVALUATION CRITERIA

The following should be clearly shown:

- Evidence of proper collimation
- All facial bones in their entirety, with the zygomatic bone in the center
- No rotation or tilt of the facial bones, demonstrated by:
  - □ Almost perfectly superimposed mandibular rami
  - □ Superimposed orbital roofs
  - □ Sella turcica in profile
- Brightness and contrast demonstrate soft tissue and bony trabecular detail

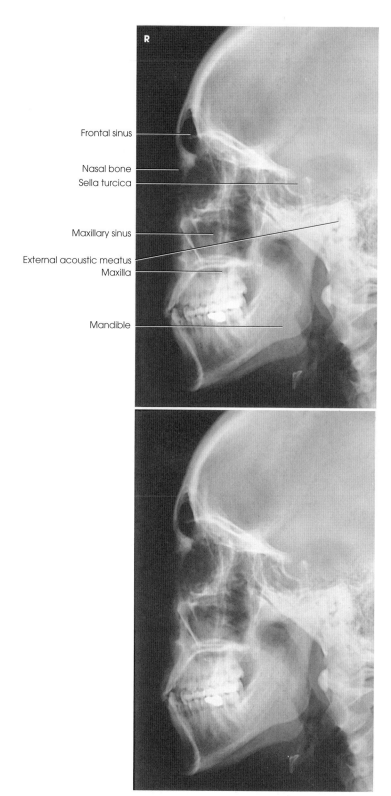

Frontal sinus

Nasal bone

Sella turcica

Maxillary sinus

External acoustic meatus

Maxilla

Mandible

Fig. 20-106 Lateral facial bones.

⚜ PARIETOACANTHIAL PROJECTION

WATERS METHOD[1]

Image receptor: 8 × 10 inch (18 × 24 cm) lengthwise or 10 × 12 inch (24 × 30 cm) lengthwise, depending on availability

Position of patient

- Place the patient in the prone or seated-upright position.

---

[1]Waters CA: Modification of the occipito-frontal position in roentgenography of the accessory nasal sinuses, *Arch Radiol Electrother* 20:15, 1915.

- Center the midsagittal plane of the patient's body to the midline of the grid device.

Position of part

- Rest the patient's head on the tip of the extended chin. Hyperextend the neck so that the orbitomeatal line (OML) forms a 37-degree angle with the plane of the IR.
- The mentomeatal line (MML) is approximately perpendicular to the plane of the IR; the average patient's nose is about ¾ inch (1.9 cm) away from the grid device.
- Adjust the head so that the midsagittal plane is perpendicular to the plane of the IR (Figs. 20-107 to 20-110).
- Center the IR at the level of the acanthion.
- Immobilize the head.
- *Respiration:* Suspend.

Central ray

- Perpendicular to exit the acanthion

Collimation

- Adjust to 8 × 10 inches (18 × 24 cm) on the collimator.

Structures shown

The parietoacanthial projection (Waters method) shows the orbits, maxillae, and zygomatic arches (see Fig. 20-110).

EVALUATION CRITERIA

The following should be clearly shown:

- ■ Evidence of proper collimation
- ■ Entire orbits and facial bones
- ■ No rotation or tilt, demonstrated by:
  - □ Distances between the lateral borders of the skull and the orbits equal on each side
  - □ MSP of head aligned with long axis of collimated field
- ■ Petrous ridges projected immediately below maxillary sinuses
- ■ Brightness and contrast demonstrate soft tissue and bony trabecular detail

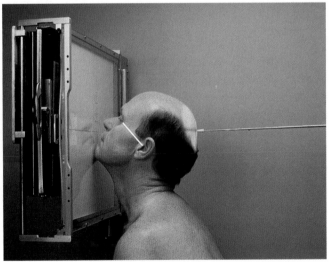

Fig. 20-107 Parietoacanthial facial bones: Waters method.

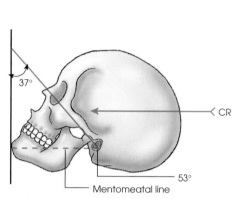

Fig. 20-108 Upright radiography diagram: parietoacanthial facial bones: Waters method.

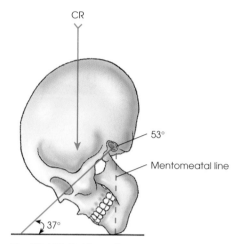

Fig. 20-109 Table radiography diagram: parietoacanthial facial bones: Waters method.

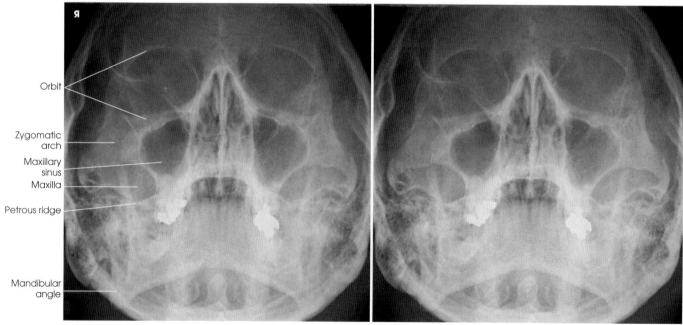

Orbit

Zygomatic arch

Maxillary sinus

Maxilla

Petrous ridge

Mandibular angle

Fig. 20-110 Parietoacanthial facial bones: Waters method.

(Courtesy of St. Bernard's Medical Center, Jonesboro, AR.)

MODIFIED PARIETOACANTHIAL PROJECTION

MODIFIED WATERS METHOD

Although the parietoacanthial projection (Waters method) is widely used, many institutions modify the projection by radiographing the patient using less extension of the patient's neck. This modification, although sometimes called a "shallow" Waters, actually increases the angulation of the OML by placing it more perpendicular to the plane of the IR. The patient's head is positioned as described using the Waters method, but the neck is extended to a lesser degree. In the modification, the OML is adjusted to form an approximately 55-degree angle with the plane of the IR (Figs. 20-111 to 20-113). The resulting radiographic image shows the facial bones with less axial angulation than with the Waters method (see Fig. 20-110). With the modified Waters method, the petrous ridges are projected immediately below the inferior border of the orbits at a level midway through the maxillary sinuses (Fig. 20-114).

The modified Waters method is a good projection to show blowout fractures. This method places the orbital floor perpendicular to the IR and parallel to the central ray, showing inferior displacement of the orbital floor and the commonly associated opacified maxillary sinus.

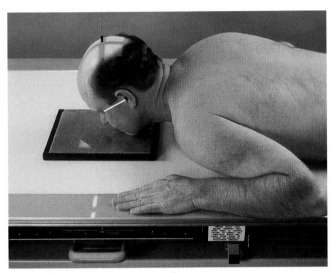

Fig. 20-111 Modified parietoacanthial facial bones: Waters method.

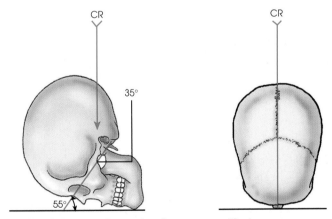

Fig. 20-112 Table radiography diagram, modified parietoacanthial facial bones: Waters method with OML adjusted to 55 degrees.

Facial Bones

325

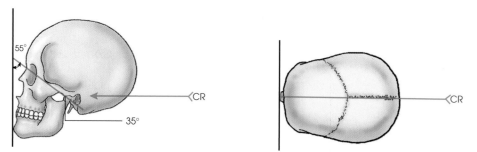

Fig. 20-113 Upright radiography diagram, modified parietoacanthial facial bones: Waters method with OML adjusted to 55 degrees.

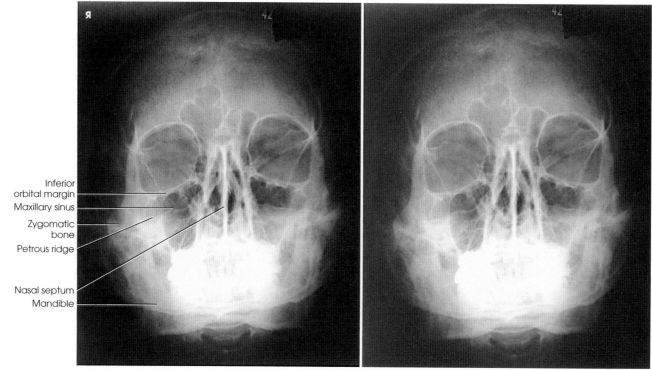

Inferior orbital margin

Maxillary sinus

Zygomatic bone

Petrous ridge

Nasal septum

Mandible

Fig. 20-114 Modified parietoacanthial facial bones: Waters method.

♠ ACANTHIOPARIETAL PROJECTION

REVERSE WATERS METHOD

Image receptor: 8 × 10 inch (18 × 24 cm) lengthwise or 10 × 12 inch (24 × 30 cm) lengthwise, depending on availability

The *reverse* Waters method is used to show the facial bones when the patient cannot be placed in the prone position.

Position of patient
- With the patient in the supine position, center the midsagittal plane of the body to the midline of the grid.

Position of part
- Bringing the patient's chin up, adjust the extension of the neck so that the OML forms a 37-degree angle with the plane of the IR (Fig. 20-115). If necessary, place a support under the patient's shoulders to help extend the neck.

- The MML is approximately perpendicular to the plane of the IR.
- Adjust the patient's head so that the midsagittal plane is perpendicular to the plane of the IR.
- Immobilize the head.
- *Respiration:* Suspend.

Central ray
- Perpendicular to enter the acanthion and centered to the IR

Collimation
- Adjust to 8 × 10 inches (18 × 24 cm) on the collimator.

Structures shown
The *reverse* Waters method shows the superior facial bones. The image is similar to that obtained with the Waters method, but the facial structures are considerably magnified (Fig. 20-116).

The following should be clearly shown:
- Evidence of proper collimation
- Entire orbits and facial bones
- No rotation or tilt, demonstrated by:
  - Distances between lateral borders of the skull and orbits equal on each side
  - MSP of head aligned with long axis of collimated field
- Petrous ridges projected below maxillary sinuses
- Brightness and contrast demonstrate soft tissue and bony trabecular detail

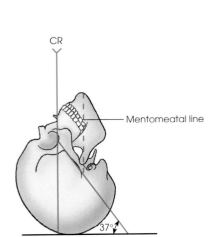

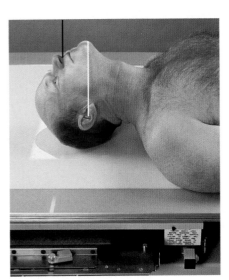

Fig. 20-115 Table radiography. Acanthioparietal facial bones: reverse Waters method with neck extended. MML is perpendicular to IR.

CR

Mentomeatal line

37°

Facial Bones

ACANTHIOPARIETAL PROJECTION FOR TRAUMA

Trauma patients are often unable to hyperextend the neck far enough to place the OML 37 degrees to the IR and the MML perpendicular to the plane of the IR. In these patients, the acanthioparietal projection, or the reverse Waters projection, can be achieved by adjusting the central ray so that it enters the acanthion while remaining parallel with the MML (Fig. 20-117).

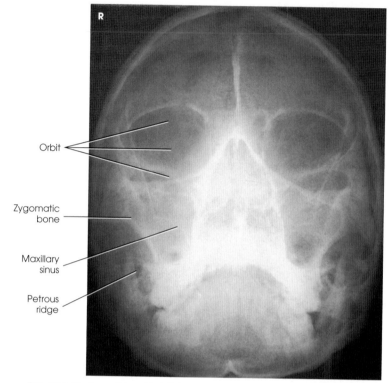

Fig. 20-116 Acanthioparietal facial bones: reverse Waters method.

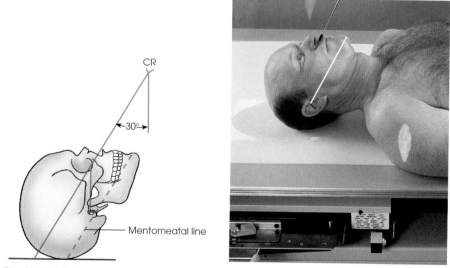

Fig. 20-117 Table radiography. Acanthioparietal facial bones: reverse Waters method with central ray parallel to MML.

⚘ PA AXIAL PROJECTION
CALDWELL METHOD

Image receptor: 8 × 10 inch (18 × 24 cm) lengthwise or 10 × 12 inch (24 × 30 cm) lengthwise, depending on availability

Position of patient
- Place the patient in a prone or a seated position.
- Center the midsagittal plane of the patient's body to the midline of the grid.
- Rest the patient's forehead and nose on the table or against the upright Bucky.
- Flex the patient's elbows, and place the arms in a comfortable position.

Position of part
- Adjust the flexion of the patient's neck so that the OML is perpendicular to the plane of the IR.
- If the patient is obese or hypersthenic, a small radiolucent sponge may need to be placed in front of the forehead.
- Align the midsagittal plane perpendicular to the IR by adjusting the lateral margins of the orbits or the EAM equidistant from the tabletop.
- Immobilize the patient's head, and center the IR to the nasion (Fig. 20-118).
- *Respiration:* Suspend.

Central ray
- Direct the central ray to exit the nasion at an angle of 15 degrees caudad.
- To show the orbital rims, in particular, the orbital floors, use a 30-degree caudal angle (sometimes referred to as the *exaggerated Caldwell*).
- Center the IR to the central ray.

Collimation
- Adjust to 8 × 10 inches (18 × 24 cm) on the collimator.

Structures shown
The PA axial projection, Caldwell method, shows the orbital rims, maxillae, nasal septum, zygomatic bones, and anterior nasal spine. When the central ray is angled 15 degrees caudad to the nasion, the petrous ridges are projected into the lower third of the orbits (Fig. 20-119). When the central ray is angled 30 degrees caudad, the petrous ridges are projected below the inferior margins of the orbits.

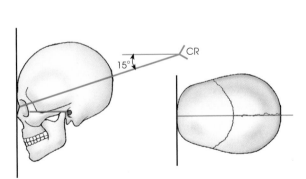
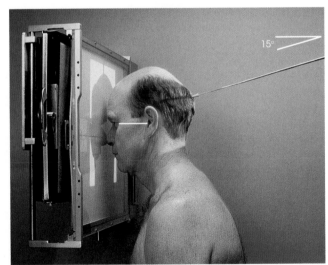

Fig. 20-118 Upright radiography, PA axial facial bones: Caldwell method.

EVALUATION CRITERIA

The following should be clearly shown:

- Evidence of proper collimation
- Entire orbits and facial bones
- No rotation or tilt, demonstrated by:
  - ☐ Equal distances from lateral borders of skull to lateral borders of orbits on both sides
  - ☐ MSP of head aligned with long axis of collimated field
- Symmetric petrous ridges lying in lower third of orbit
- Penetration of frontal bone with appropriate brightness at lateral borders of skull, which shows the facial bones

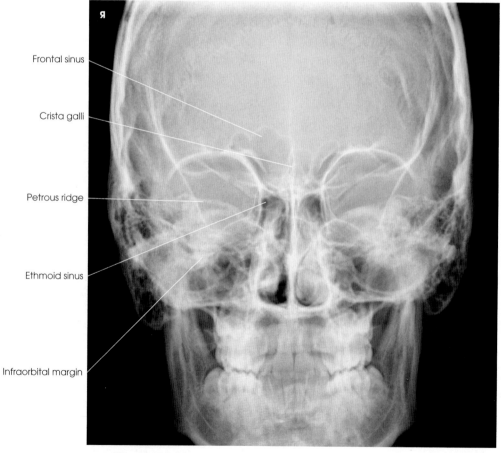

Fig. 20-119 PA axial facial bones: Caldwell method.

(Courtesy of St. Bernard's Medical Center, Jonesboro, AR.)

⚜ LATERAL PROJECTION
R and L positions

Image receptor: 8 × 10 inch (18 × 24 cm) lengthwise or 10 × 12 inch (24 × 30 cm), depending on availability, crosswise for two exposures on one IR

Position of patient
- With the patient in a recumbent or upright anterior oblique position, adjust the rotation of the body so that the midsagittal plane of the head can be placed horizontally.

Position of part
- Adjust the head so that the midsagittal plane is parallel with the tabletop and the interpupillary line is perpendicular to the tabletop.
- Adjust the flexion of the patient's neck so that the IOML is parallel with the transverse axis of the IR (Figs. 20-120 and 20-121).
- Support the mandible to prevent rotation.
- *Respiration:* Suspend.

Placement of IR
- When using an 8 × 10-inch (18 × 24-cm) IR, slide the unmasked half of the IR under the frontonasal region and center it to the nasion (see Fig. 20-120). This centering allows space for the identification marker to be projected across the upper part of the IR. Tape the side marker (R or L) in position.

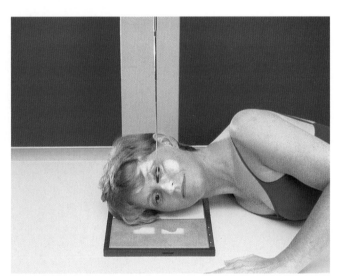

Fig. 20-120 Lateral nasal bones.

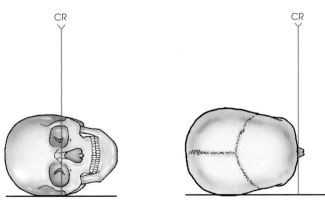

Fig. 20-121 Table radiography diagram: lateral nasal bones.

Central ray

• Perpendicular to the bridge of the nose at a point ½ inch (1.3 cm) distal to the nasion

Collimation

• Adjust to 3 × 3 inches (8 × 8 cm) on the collimator, with the field extending from the glabella to the acanthion and ½ inch (1.3 cm) beyond the tip of the nose.

Structures shown

The lateral images of the nasal bones show the side nearer the film or IR and the soft structures of the nose (Fig. 20-122). Both sides are examined for comparison.

EVALUATION CRITERIA

The following should be clearly shown:
■ Evidence of proper collimation
■ Nasal bones, anterior nasal spine, and frontonasal suture
■ No rotation of nasal bones and soft tissue
■ Brightness and contrast demonstrate soft tissue and bony trabecular detail

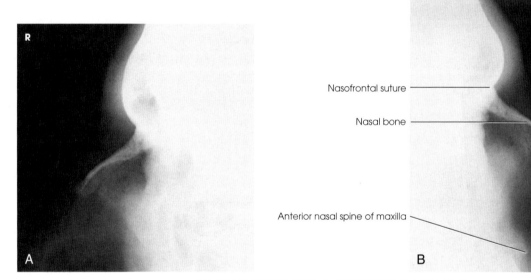

Nasofrontal suture

Nasal bone

Anterior nasal spine of maxilla

Fig. 20-122 Nasal bones. **A,** Right lateral. **B,** Left lateral.

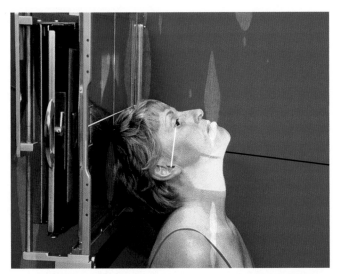

Fig. 20-123 SMV zygomatic arches, patient upright.

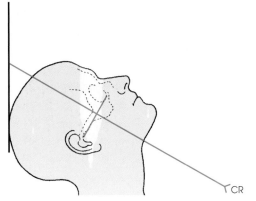

Fig. 20-124 Upright radiography diagram: SMV zygomatic arches.

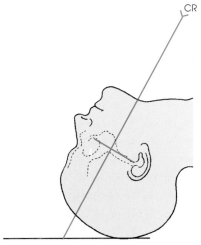

Fig. 20-125 Table radiography diagram: SMV zygomatic arches.

⚜ SUBMENTOVERTICAL PROJECTION

This projection is similar to the submentovertical (SMV) projection described in the Skull Radiography section.

> **Image receptor:** 8 × 10 inch (18 × 24 cm) or 10 × 12 inch (24 × 30 cm) crosswise, depending on availability

Position of patient
- Place the patient in a seated upright or supine position. A vertical head unit greatly assists a patient who is unable to hyperextend the neck.
- When the supine position is used, elevate the patient's trunk on several firm pillows or a suitable pad to allow complete extension of the neck. Flex the patient's knees to relax the abdominal muscles.
- Center the midsagittal plane of the patient's body to the midline of the grid device.

Position of part
- Hyperextend the patient's neck completely so that the IOML is as parallel with the plane of the IR as possible.
- Rest the patient's head on its vertex, and adjust the head so that the midsagittal plane is perpendicular to the plane of the IR (Figs. 20-123 to 20-125).
- *Respiration:* Suspend.

Zygomatic Arches

Central ray

- Perpendicular to the IOML and entering the midsagittal plane of the throat at a level approximately 1 inch (2.5 cm) posterior to the outer canthi
- Center the IR to the central ray.

Collimation

- Adjust to 8 × 10 inches (18 × 24 cm) crosswise on the collimator.

Structures shown

Bilateral symmetric SMV images of the zygomatic arches are shown, projected free of superimposed structures (Fig. 20-126). Unless very flat or traumatically depressed, the arches, being farther from the IR, are projected beyond the prominent parietal eminences by the divergent x-ray beam.

The following should be clearly shown:
- Evidence of proper collimation
- Zygomatic arches free from overlying structures
- No rotation or tilt of head, demonstrated by:
  - ☐ Zygomatic arches symmetric and without foreshortening
- Brightness and contrast demonstrate soft tissue and bony trabecular detail

NOTE: The zygomatic arches are well shown with a decrease in the exposure factors used for this projection of the cranial base.

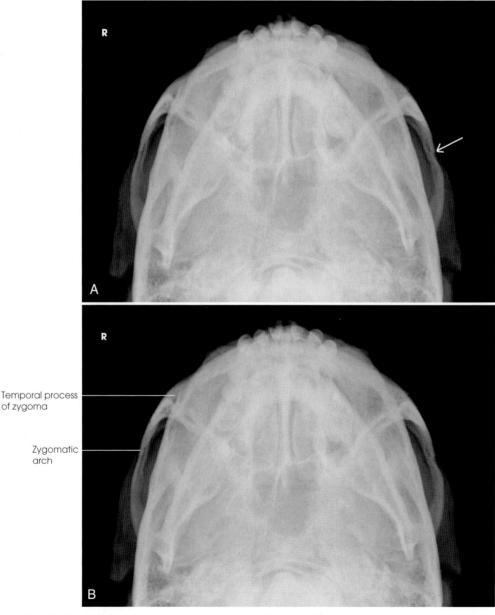

Temporal process of zygoma

Zygomatic arch

Fig. 20-126 A, SMV projection showing normal zygomatic arch (*right*) and fracture (*arrow*) of left zygomatic arch. **B,** SMV zygomatic arches.

(Courtesy of St. Bernard's Medical Center, Jonesboro, AR.)

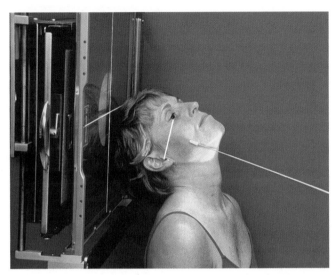

Fig. 20-127 Tangential zygomatic arch, patient upright.

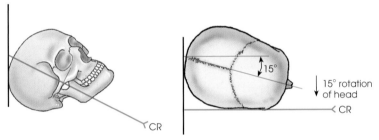

Fig. 20-128 Upright radiography diagram: tangential zygomatic arch.

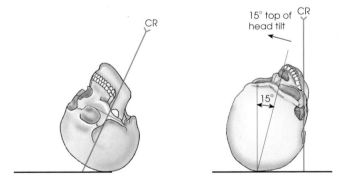

Fig. 20-129 Table radiography diagram: tangential zygomatic arch.

♠ TANGENTIAL PROJECTION

Image receptor: 8 × 10 inch (18 × 24 cm) lengthwise or 10 × 12 inch (24 × 30 cm) lengthwise, depending on availability

Position of patient
- Seat the patient with the back against a vertical grid device, or place the patient in the supine position with the trunk elevated on several firm pillows and the knees flexed to permit complete extension of the neck.

Position of part
Seated position
- Hyperextend the patient's neck, and rest the head on its vertex.
- Adjust the position of the patient's head so that the IOML is as parallel as possible with the plane of the IR.
- Rotate the midsagittal plane of the head approximately 15 degrees toward the side being examined.
- Tilt the top of the head approximately 15 degrees away from the side being examined. This rotation and tilt ensure that the central ray is tangent to the lateral surface of the skull. The central ray skims across the lateral portion of the mandibular angle and the parietal bone to project the zygomatic arch onto the IR.
- Center the zygomatic arch to the IR (Figs. 20-127 to 20-129).

Zygomatic Arches

Supine position

- Rest the patient's head on its vertex.
- Elevate the upper end of the IR on sandbags, or place it on an angled sponge of suitable size.
- Adjust the elevation of the IR and the extension of the patient's neck so that the IOML is placed as nearly parallel with the plane of the IR as possible.
- Rotate and tilt the midsagittal plane of the head approximately 15 degrees toward the side being examined (similar to the upright position).
- If the IOML is parallel with the plane of the IR, center the IR to the zygomatic arch; if not, displace the IR so that the midpoint of the IR coincides with the central ray (see Fig. 20-129).
- Attach a strip of adhesive tape to the inferior surface of the chin; draw the tape upward, and anchor it to the edge of the table or IR stand. This usually affords sufficient support. Do not put the adhesive surface directly on the patient's skin.
- *Respiration:* Suspend.

Central ray

- Perpendicular to the IOML and centered to the zygomatic arch at a point approximately 1 inch (2.5 cm) posterior to the outer canthus
- Centered to the IR

Collimation

- Adjust to 6 × 10 inches (18 × 24 cm) on the collimator.

Structures shown

A tangential image of one zygomatic arch is seen free of superimposition (Fig. 20-130). This projection is particularly useful in patients with depressed fractures or flat cheekbones.

EVALUATION CRITERIA

The following should be clearly shown:
- Evidence of proper collimation
- Zygomatic arch free from overlying structures
- Brightness and contrast demonstrate soft tissue and bony trabecular detail

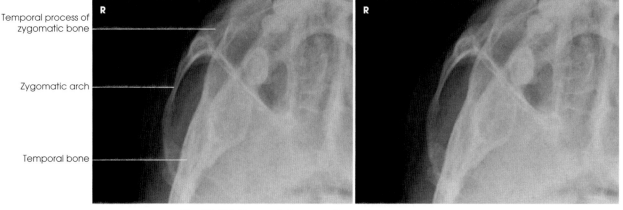

Temporal process of zygomatic bone

Zygomatic arch

Temporal bone

Fig. 20-130 Tangential zygomatic arch.

(Courtesy of St. Bernard's Medical Center, Jonesboro, AR.)

♠ AP AXIAL PROJECTION

MODIFIED TOWNE METHOD

Image receptor: 8 × 10 inch (18 × 24 cm) or 10 × 12 inch (24 × 30 cm) crosswise, depending on availability

Position of patient

- Place the patient in the seated-upright or supine position.
- Center the midsagittal plane of the body to the midline of the grid.

Position of part

- Adjust the patient's head so that the midsagittal plane is perpendicular to the midline of the grid.
- Adjust the flexion of the neck so that the OML is perpendicular to the plane of the IR (Figs. 20-131 to 20-133).
- *Respiration:* Suspend.

Central ray

- Directed to enter the glabella approximately 1 inch (2.5 cm) above the nasion at an angle of 30 degrees caudad
- If the patient is unable to flex the neck sufficiently, adjust the IOML perpendicular with the IR and direct the central ray 37 degrees caudad.
- Center the IR to the central ray.

Collimation

- Adjust to 8 × 10 inches (18 × 24 cm) crosswise on the collimator.

Structures shown

A symmetric AP axial projection of both zygomatic arches is shown. The arches should be projected free of superimposition (Fig. 20-134).

The following should be clearly shown:
- Evidence of proper collimation
- No overlap of zygomatic arches by mandible
- No rotation or tilt, demonstrated by:
  - □ Symmetric arches
  - □ Zygomatic arches projected lateral to mandibular rami
  - □ MSP of head aligned with long axis of collimated field
- Brightness and contrast demonstrate soft tissue and bony trabecular detail

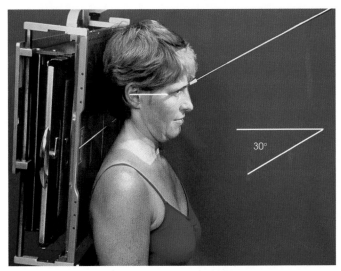

Fig. 20-131 AP axial zygomatic arches: modified Towne method.

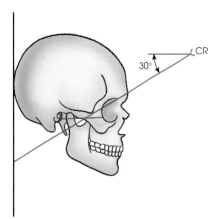

Fig. 20-132 Upright radiography diagram: modified Towne method.

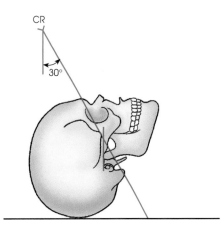

Fig. 20-133 Table radiography diagram: modified Towne method.

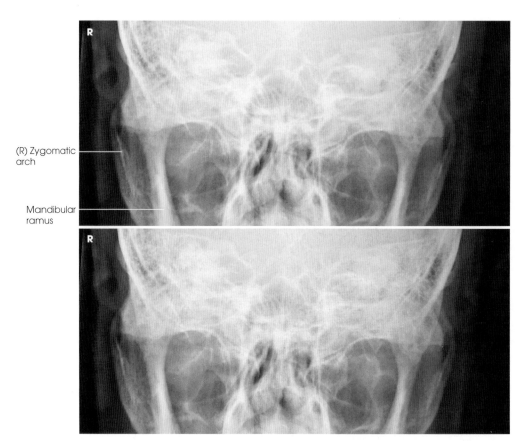

(R) Zygomatic arch

Mandibular ramus

Fig. 20-134 AP axial zygomatic arches: modified Towne method.

♠ PA PROJECTION

Image receptor: 8 × 10 inch (18 × 24 cm) or 10 × 12 inch (24 × 30 cm) lengthwise, depending on availability

Position of patient

- Place the patient in the prone position, or seat the patient before a vertical grid device.

Position of part

- Rest the patient's forehead and nose on the IR. Adjust the OML to be perpendicular to the plane of the IR.
- Adjust the head so that its midsagittal plane is perpendicular to the plane of the IR (Fig. 20-135).
- Immobilize the head.
- *Respiration:* Suspend.

Central ray

- Perpendicular to exit the acanthion
- Center the IR to the central ray.

Collimation

- Adjust to 8 × 10 inches (18 × 24 cm) on the collimator.

Structures shown

PA projection shows the mandibular body and rami (Fig. 20-136). The central part of the body is not well shown because of the superimposed spine. This radiographic approach is usually employed to show medial or lateral displacement of fragments in fractures of the rami.

EVALUATION CRITERIA

The following should be clearly shown:
- Evidence of proper collimation
- Entire mandible
- No rotation or tilt, demonstrated by:
  - Mandibular body and rami symmetric on each side
  - MSP of head aligned with long axis of collimated field
- Brightness and contrast demonstrating soft tissues and bony trabecular detail

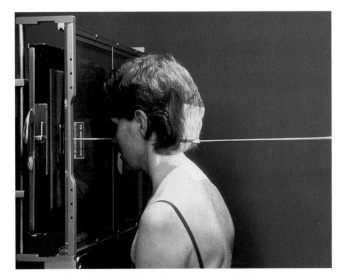

Fig. 20-135 PA mandibular rami.

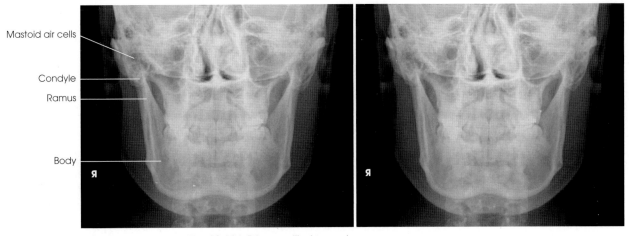

Mastoid air cells

Condyle

Ramus

Body

Fig. 20-136 PA mandibular rami.

(Courtesy of St. Bernard's Medical Center, Jonesboro, AR.)

⚞ PA AXIAL PROJECTION

Image receptor: 8 × 10 inch (18 × 24 cm) or 10 × 12 inch (24 × 30 cm) lengthwise, depending on availability

Position of patient

- Place the patient in the prone position, or seat the patient before a vertical grid device.

Position of part

- Rest the patient's forehead and nose on the IR holder.
- Adjust the OML to be perpendicular to the plane of the IR.
- Adjust the patient's head so that the midsagittal plane is perpendicular to the plane of the IR (Fig. 20-137).
- Immobilize the patient's head.
- *Respiration:* Suspend.

Central ray

- Directed 20 or 25 degrees cephalad to exit at the acanthion
- Center the IR to the central ray.

Collimation

- Adjust to 8 × 10 inches (18 × 24 cm) on the collimator.

Structures shown

PA axial projection shows the mandibular body and rami (Fig. 20-138). The central part of the body is not well shown because of the superimposed spine. This radiographic approach is usually employed to show medial or lateral displacement of fragments in fractures of the rami.

EVALUATION CRITERIA

The following should be clearly shown:
- Evidence of proper collimation
- Entire mandible
- No rotation or tilt, demonstrated by:
  - ☐ Mandibular body and rami symmetric on each side
  - ☐ MSP of head aligned with long axis of collimated field
- Condylar processes
- Brightness and contrast demonstrating soft tissues and bony trabecular detail

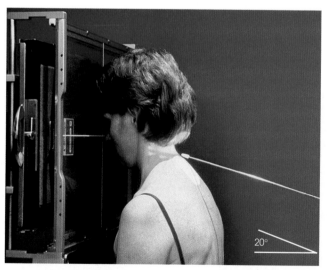

Fig. 20-137 PA axial mandibular rami.

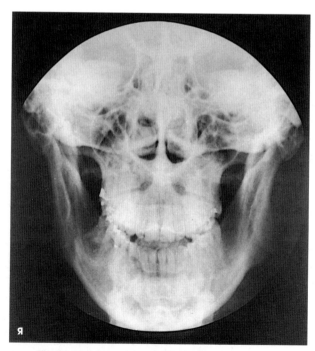

Fig. 20-138 PA axial mandibular body and rami.

Mandibular Body

PA PROJECTION

Image receptor: 8 × 10 inch (18 × 24 cm) or 10 × 12 inch (24 × 30 cm) lengthwise, depending on availability

Position of patient
- Place the patient in the prone position, or seat the patient before a vertical grid device.

Position of part
- With the midsagittal plane of the patient's head centered to the midline of the IR, rest the head on the nose and chin so that the anterior surface of the mandibular symphysis is parallel with the plane of the IR. This position places the acanthiomeatal line (AML) nearly perpendicular to the IR plane.
- Adjust the patient's head so that the midsagittal plane is perpendicular to the plane of the IR (Fig. 20-139).
- *Respiration:* Suspend

Central ray
- Perpendicular to the level of the lips
- Center the IR to the central ray.

Structures shown
This image shows the mandibular body (Fig. 20-140).

EVALUATION CRITERIA
The following should be clearly shown:
- Evidence of proper collimation
- Entire mandible
- No rotation or tilt, demonstrated by:
  - ☐ Mandibular body symmetric on each side
  - ☐ MSP of head aligned with long axis of collimated field
- Brightness and contrast demonstrating soft tissues and bony trabecular detail

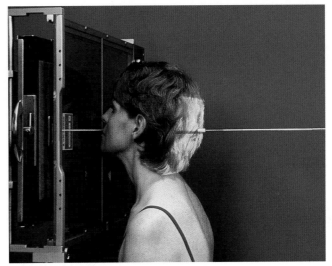

Fig. 20-139 PA mandibular body.

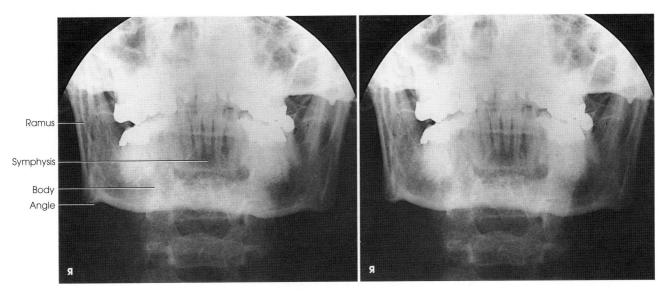

Ramus

Symphysis

Body

Angle

Fig. 20-140 PA mandibular body.

PA AXIAL PROJECTION

Image receptor: 8 × 10 inch (18 × 24 cm) or 10 × 12 inch (24 × 30 cm) lengthwise, depending on availability

Position of patient
- Place the patient in the prone position, or seat the patient before a vertical grid device.

Position of part
- With the midsagittal plane of the patient's head centered to the midline of the IR, rest the head on the nose and chin so that the anterior surface of the mandibular symphysis is parallel with the plane of the IR. This position places the AML nearly perpendicular to the plane of the IR.
- Adjust the patient's head so that the midsagittal plane is perpendicular to the plane of the IR (Fig. 20-141).
- *Respiration:* Suspend.

Central ray
- Directed midway between the temporomandibular joints (TMJs) at an angle of 30 degrees cephalad. Zanelli[1] recommended that better contrast around the TMJs could be obtained if the patient was instructed to fill the mouth with air for this projection.
- Center the IR to the central ray.

Structures shown
This image shows the mandibular body and TMJs (Fig. 20-142).

[1]Zanelli A: Le proiezioni radiografiche dell' articolazione temporomandibolare, *Radiol Med* 16:495, 1929.

The following should be clearly shown:
- Evidence of proper collimation
- Entire mandible
- TMJs just inferior to the mastoid process
- No rotation or tilt, demonstrated by:
  - □ Symmetric rami
  - □ MSP of head aligned with long axis of collimated field

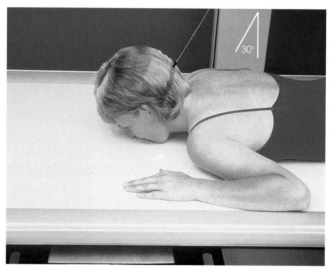

Fig. 20-141 PA axial mandibular body.

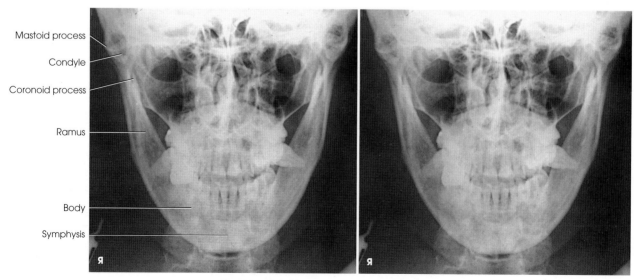

Mastoid process
Condyle
Coronoid process
Ramus
Body
Symphysis

Fig. 20-142 PA axial mandibular body.

♠ AXIOLATERAL AND AXIOLATERAL OBLIQUE PROJECTION

The goal of these projections is to place the desired portion of the mandible parallel with the IR.

Image receptor: 8 × 10 inch (18 × 2 cm) or 10 × 12 inch (24 × 30 cm) lengthwise, depending on availability, placed according to region

Position of patient
- Place the patient in the seated, semiprone, or semi-supine position.

Position of part
- Place the patient's head in a lateral position with the interpupillary line perpendicular to the IR. The mouth should be closed with the teeth together.

- Extend the patient's neck enough that the long axis of the mandibular body is parallel with the transverse axis of the IR to prevent superimposition of the cervical spine.
- If the projection is to be performed on the tabletop, position the IR so that the complete body of the mandible is on the IR.
- Adjust the rotation of the patient's head to place the area of interest parallel to the IR, as follows.

Ramus
- Keep the patient's head in a true lateral position (Fig. 20-143).

Body
- Rotate the patient's head 30 degrees toward the IR (Fig. 20-144).

Symphysis
- Rotate the patient's head 45 degrees toward the IR (Fig. 20-145).

NOTE: When the patient is in the semi-supine position, place the IR on a wedge device or wedge sponge (Fig. 20-146). Ensure that combined CR angle and midsagittal plane tilt equals 25 degrees.

Central ray
- Directed 25 degrees cephalad to pass directly through the mandibular region of interest (see Note on p. 345)
- Center the IR to the central ray for projections done on upright grid units.

Collimation
- Adjust to 8 × 10 inches (18 × 24 cm) on the collimator.

Structures shown
Each axiolateral oblique projection shows the region of the mandible that was parallel with the IR (Figs. 20-147 to 20-149).

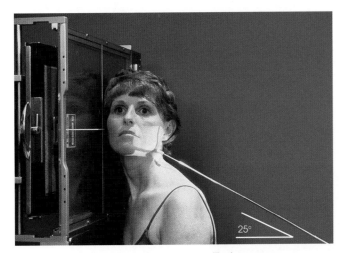

Fig. 20-143 Axiolateral mandibular ramus.

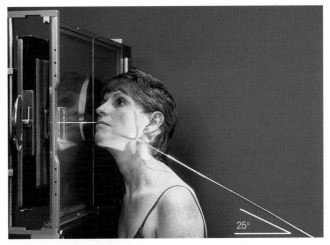

Fig. 20-144 Axiolateral oblique mandibular body.

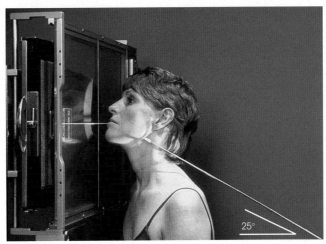

Fig. 20-145 Axiolateral oblique mandibular symphysis.

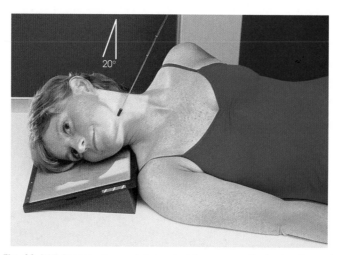

Fig. 20-146 Semi-supine axiolateral oblique mandibular body and symphysis.

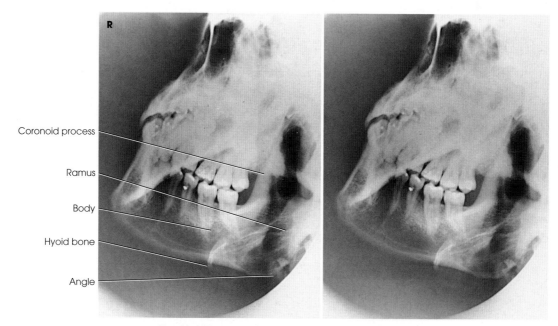

Coronoid process

Ramus

Body

Hyoid bone

Angle

Fig. 20-147 Axiolateral oblique mandibular body.

EVALUATION CRITERIA

The following should be clearly shown:
- Evidence of proper collimation

Ramus and Body
- No overlap of the ramus by the opposite side of the mandible
- No elongation or foreshortening of ramus or body

- No superimposition of the ramus by the cervical spine

Symphysis
- No overlap of the mentum region by the opposite side of the mandible
- No foreshortening of the mentum region

NOTE: To reduce the possibility of projecting the shoulder over the mandible when radiographing muscular or hypersthenic patients, adjust the midsagittal plane of the patient's skull with an approximately 15-degree angle, open inferiorly. The cephalad angulation of 10 degrees of the central ray maintains the optimal 25-degree central ray/part angle relationship.

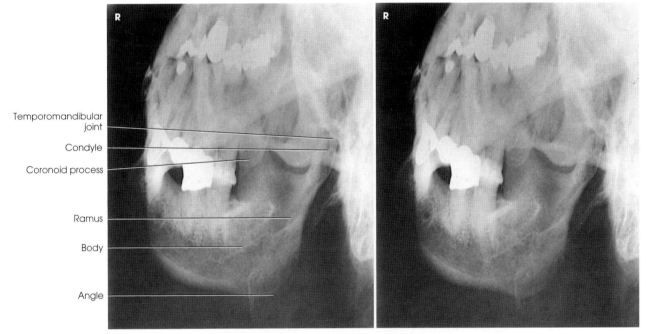

Temporomandibular joint
Condyle
Coronoid process
Ramus
Body
Angle

Fig. 20-148 Axiolateral oblique mandibular ramus.

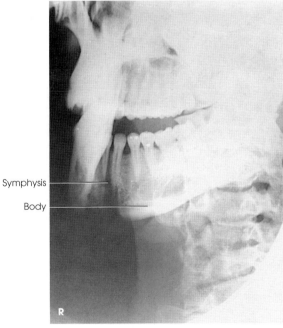

Symphysis
Body

Fig. 20-149 Axiolateral oblique mandibular symphysis.

SUBMENTOVERTICAL PROJECTION

Image receptor: 8 × 10 inch (18 × 24 cm) or 10 × 12 inch (24 × 30 cm) lengthwise, depending on availability

Position of patient

- Place the patient upright in front of a vertical grid device or in the supine position. When the patient is supine, elevate the shoulders on firm pillows to permit complete extension of the neck.
- Flex the patient's knees to relax the abdominal muscles and relieve strain on the neck muscles.
- Center the midsagittal plane of the body to the midline of the grid device.

Position of part

- With the neck fully extended, rest the head on its vertex and adjust the head so that the midsagittal plane is vertical.
- Adjust the IOML as parallel as possible with the plane of the IR (Fig. 20-150).
- When the neck cannot be extended enough that the IOML is parallel with the IR plane, angle the *grid device* and place it parallel to the IOML.
- Immobilize the head.
- *Respiration:* Suspend.

Central ray

- Perpendicular to the IOML and centered midway between the angles of the mandible

Structures shown

SMV projection of the mandibular body shows the coronoid and condyloid processes of the rami (Fig. 20-151).

EVALUATION CRITERIA

The following should be clearly shown:
- Evidence of proper collimation
- No rotation or tilt, demonstrated by:
  - □ Distance between the lateral border of the skull and the mandible equal on both sides
  - □ MSP of head aligned to long axis of collimated field
- Condyles of the mandible anterior to the pars petrosa
- Symphysis extending almost to the anterior border of the face so that the mandible is not foreshortened

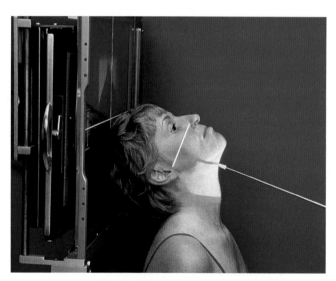

Fig. 20-150 SMV mandible.

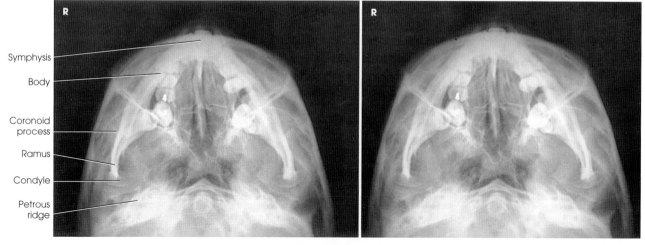

Symphysis
Body
Coronoid process
Ramus
Condyle
Petrous ridge

Fig. 20-151 SMV mandible.

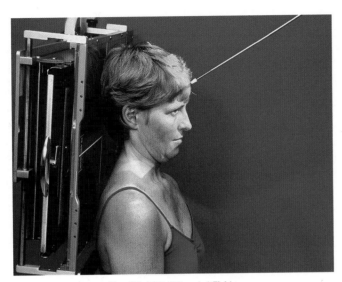

Fig. 20-152 AP axial TMJs.

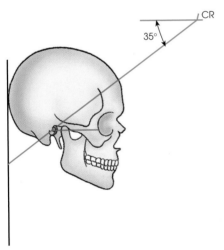

Fig. 20-153 Upright radiography diagram: AP axial TMJs.

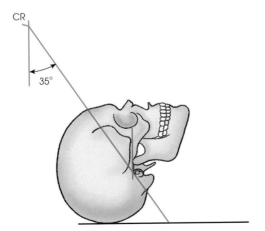

Fig. 20-154 Table radiography diagram: AP axial TMJs.

⚜ AP AXIAL PROJECTION

For radiography of the TMJs in the closed-mouth position, the *posterior teeth,* rather than the incisors, must be in contact. Occlusion of the incisors places the mandible in a position of protrusion, and the condyles are carried out of the mandibular fossae. In the open-mouth position, the mouth should be opened as wide as possible but not with the mandible protruded (jutted forward).

Because of the danger of fragment displacement, the open-mouth position should not be attempted in patients with recent injury. Trauma patients are examined without any stress movement of the mandible. Tomography is particularly useful when a fracture or dislocation is suspected.

> **Image receptor:** 8 × 10 inch (18 × 24 cm) or 10 × 12 inch (24 × 30 cm) lengthwise, depending on availability

Position of patient
- Place the patient in a supine or seated-upright position with the posterior skull in contact with the upright Bucky.

Position of part
- Adjust the patient's head so that the midsagittal plane is perpendicular to the plane of the IR.
- Flex the patient's neck so that the OML is perpendicular to the plane of the IR (Figs. 20-152 to 20-154).
- *Respiration:* Suspend.

Central ray

- Directed 35 degrees caudad, centered midway between the TMJs, and entering at a point approximately 3 inches (7.6 cm) above the nasion
- Expose one image with the mouth closed; when not contraindicated, expose one image with the mouth open.
- Center the IR to the central ray.

Collimation

- Adjust to 8 × 10 inches (18 × 24 cm) on the collimator.

Structures shown

The AP axial projection shows the condyles of the mandible and the mandibular fossae of the temporal bones (Figs. 20-155 and 20-156).

EVALUATION CRITERIA

The following should be clearly shown:

- Evidence of proper collimation
- No rotation of head
- Minimal superimposition of petrosa on the condyle in the closed-mouth examination
- Condyle and temporomandibular articulation below pars petrosa in the open-mouth position

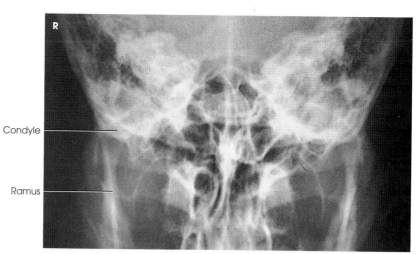

Fig. 20-155 AP axial TMJs: mouth closed.

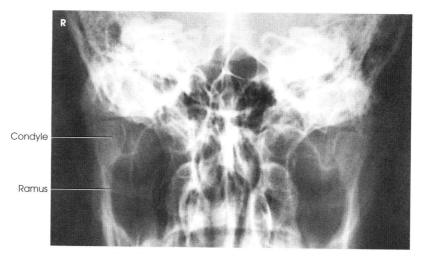

Fig. 20-156 AP axial TMJs: mouth open.

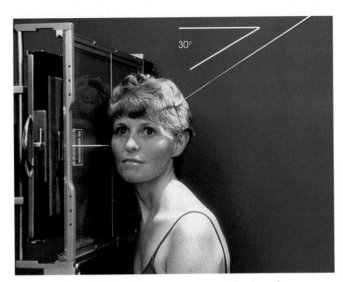

Fig. 20-157 Axiolateral TMJ: mouth closed.

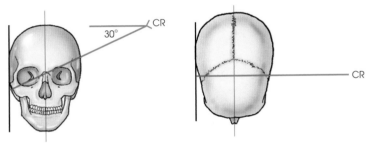

Fig. 20-158 Upright radiography diagram: axiolateral TMJ.

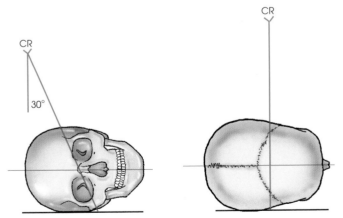

Fig. 20-159 Table radiography diagram: axiolateral TMJ.

AXIOLATERAL PROJECTION
R and L positions

This projection is sometimes called the *Shüller method* because it consists of approximately the same positioning details and CR orientation as the Shüller method for the petromastoid portion of the temporal bone, seen in the tenth edition of *Merrill's Atlas.*

> **Image receptor:** 8 × 10 inch (18 × 24 cm) or 10 × 12 inch (24 × 30 cm) crosswise, depending on availability

Position of patient
- Put a mark on each cheek at a point ½ inch (1.3 cm) anterior to the EAM and 1 inch (2.5 cm) inferior to the EAM to localize the TMJ if needed.
- Place the patient in a semi-prone position, or seat the patient before a vertical grid device.

Position of part
- Center a point ½ inch (1.3 cm) anterior to the EAM to the IR, and place the patient's head in the lateral position with the affected side closest to the IR.
- Adjust the patient's head so that the midsagittal plane is parallel with the plane of the IR and the interpupillary line is perpendicular to the IR plane (Figs. 20-157 to 20-159).
- Immobilize the head.
- *Respiration:* Suspend.
- After making the exposure with the patient's mouth closed, change the IR; then, unless contraindicated, have the patient open the mouth widely (Fig. 20-160).
- Recheck the patient's position, and make the second exposure.

Central ray

- Directed to the midpoint of the IR at an angle of 25 or 30 degrees caudad. The central ray enters about ½ inch (1.3 cm) anterior and 2 inches (5 cm) superior to the upside EAM.

Structures shown

These images show the TMJ when the mouth is open and closed (Figs. 20-161 and 20-162). Examine both sides for comparison.

EVALUATION CRITERIA

The following should be clearly shown:

- Evidence of proper collimation
- TMJ anterior to the EAM
- Condyle in mandibular fossa in the closed-mouth examination
- Condyle inferior to the articular tubercle in the open-mouth examination if the patient is normal and able to open the mouth widely

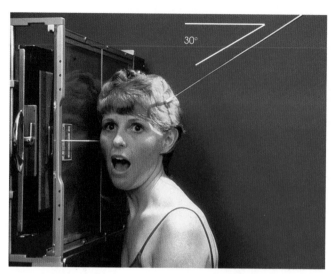

Fig. 20-160 Axiolateral TMJ with mouth open.

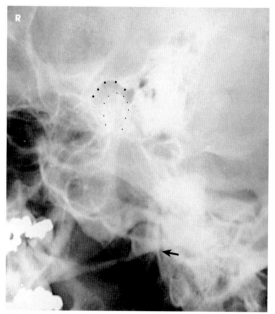

Fig. 20-161 Axiolateral TMJ, mouth closed. Mandibular condyle (*small dots*) and mandibular fossa (*large dots*) are shown. Mandibular condyle of side away from film is also seen (*arrow*).

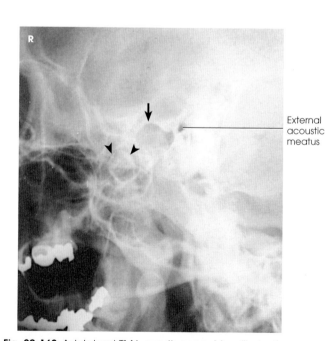

External acoustic meatus

Fig. 20-162 Axiolateral TMJ, mouth open. Mandibular fossa (*arrow*) and mandibular condyle (*arrowheads*) are shown.

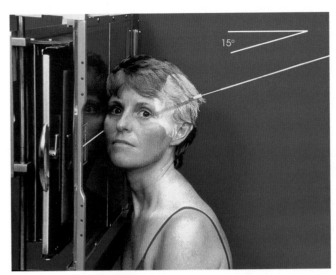

Fig. 20-163 Axiolateral oblique TMJ.

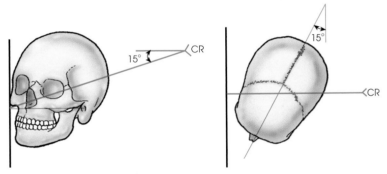

Fig. 20-164 Upright radiography diagram: axiolateral oblique TMJ.

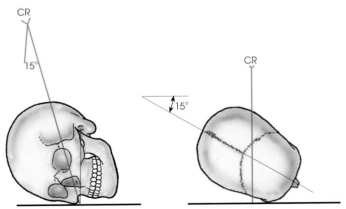

Fig. 20-165 Table radiography diagram: axiolateral oblique TMJ.

▲ AXIOLATERAL OBLIQUE PROJECTION
R and L positions

This projection is sometimes called the *modified Law method* because it consists of approximately the same positioning details and CR orientation as the modified Law method for the petromastoid portion of the temporal bone, seen in the tenth edition of *Merrill's Atlas*.

> **Image receptor:** 8 × 10 inch (18 × 24 cm) or 10 × 12 inch (24 × 30 cm) crosswise, depending on availability

Position of patient
- Place the patient in a semi-prone position, or seat the patient before a vertical grid device.
- In TMJ examinations, make one exposure with the mouth closed, and when not contraindicated, make one exposure with the mouth open.
- Use an IR-changing tunnel or Bucky tray so that the patient's head does not have to be adjusted between the two exposures.
- Examine both sides for comparison.

Position of part
- Center a point ½ inch (1.3 cm) anterior to the EAM to the IR, and rest the patient's cheek on the grid device.
- Rotate the midsagittal plane of the head approximately 15 degrees toward the IR.
- Adjust the interpupillary line perpendicular to the plane of the IR.
- Adjust the flexion of the patient's neck so that the AML is parallel with the transverse axis of the IR (Figs. 20-163 to 20-165).
- Immobilize the head.
- *Respiration:* Suspend.
- After making the exposure with the mouth closed, change the IR and instruct the patient to open the mouth widely.
- Recheck the position of the AML, and make the second exposure.

Central ray
- Directed 15 degrees caudad and exiting through the TMJ closest to the IR. The central ray enters about 1½ inches (3.8 cm) superior to the upside EAM.

Collimation
- Adjust to 8 × 10 inches (18 × 24 cm) on the collimator.

Structures shown

The images in the open-mouth and closed-mouth positions show the condyles and necks of the mandible. The images also show the relationship between the mandibular fossa and the condyle. The open-mouth position shows the mandibular fossa and the inferior and anterior excursion of the condyle. Both sides are examined for comparison (Fig. 20-166). The closed-mouth position shows fractures of the neck and condyle of the ramus.

EVALUATION CRITERIA

The following should be clearly shown:
- Evidence of proper collimation
- Temporomandibular articulation
- Condyle lying in the mandibular fossa in the closed-mouth examination
- Condyle lying inferior to the articular tubercle in the open-mouth projection if the patient is normal and is able to open the mouth widely

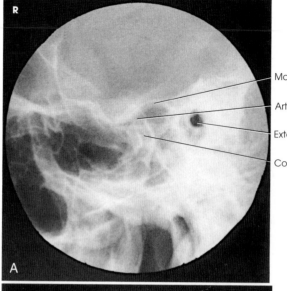

Mandibular fossa

Articular tubercle

External acoustic meatus

Condyle

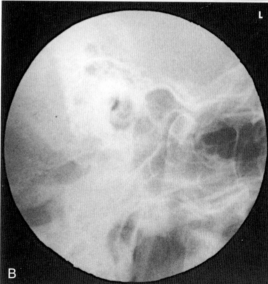

Fig. 20-166 Axiolateral oblique TMJ. **A,** Mouth open, right side. **B,** Mouth open, left side (*same patient*), showing more movement on left side.

Panoramic Tomography of the Mandible

Panoramic tomography, pantomography, and *rotational tomography* are terms used to designate the technique employed to produce tomograms of curved surfaces. This technique of body-section radiography provides a panoramic image of the entire mandible, including the TMJ, and of both dental arches on one long, narrow image. Digital panorex units are capable of providing several images necessary for orthodontic and dental treatments, including three-dimensional images, cephalo-metric analysis, and surgical implant treatment planning.

Two types of equipment are available for pantomography. In the first type, the patient and the IR are rotated before a stationary x-ray tube. This type of machine consists of (1) a specially designed chair mounted on a turntable and (2) a second turntable to support a 4 × 10 inch (10 × 24 cm) IR. The seated and immobilized patient and the film are electronically rotated in opposite directions at coordinated speeds. The x-ray tube remains stationary. In one machine, the exposure is interrupted in the midline.

In the second type of unit, the x-ray tube and the IR rotate in the same direction around the seated and immobilized patient (Fig. 20-167). The x-ray tube and IR drum are attached to an overhead carriage that is supported by the vertical stand assembly. The chair of this unit is fixed to the base but can be removed to accommodate patients in wheelchairs. The attached head holder and radiolucent bite device center and immobilize the patient's head. A scale on the head holder indicates the jaw size. The latest digital technology offers 33 panoramic options.

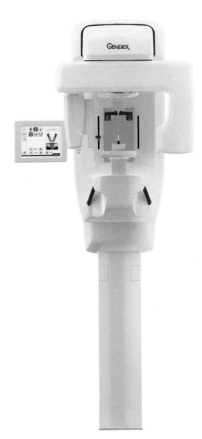

Fig. 20-167 Digital panograph unit. (Courtesy Gendex.)

In both types of equipment, the beam of radiation is sharply collimated at the tube aperture by a lead diaphragm with a narrow vertical slit. A corresponding slit diaphragm is fixed between the patient and the IR so that the patient and the IR (or the tube and the film) rotate. Each narrow area of the part is recorded on the film without overlap and without fogging from scattered and secondary radiation.

The scan (exposure) time varies from 10 to 20 seconds in different makes of equipment. Because of the slit diaphragm, however, radiation exposure to the patient at each fraction of a second is restricted to the skin surface that is passing before the narrow vertical slit aperture.

Panoramic tomography provides a distortion-free lateral image of the entire mandible (Fig. 20-168). It also affords the most comfortable way to position patients who have sustained severe mandibular or TMJ trauma, before and after splint wiring of the teeth. It must be supplemented with an AP, PA, or verticosubmental projection to establish fragment position.

This tomographic technique is useful for general survey studies of various dental and facial bone abnormalities. It is also used to supplement rather than replace conventional periapical images, although digital units are capable of providing standard bitewing images as well as lateral TMJ images.

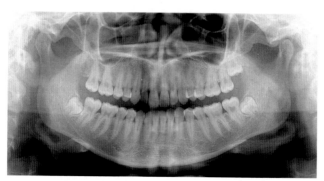

Fig. 20-168 Panoramic digital tomogram.

(Courtesy Gendex.)

Technical Considerations

For digital imaging, the most important technical consideration for demonstration of potential pathology of the paranasal sinuses is to image the patient in the *upright* position whenever possible. The upright position is best for demonstration of air-fluid levels and to differentiate fluid from other pathologic conditions, as shown by the research by Cross[1] and Flecker.[2] An appropriate balance of brightness and contrast is also necessary so that air, fluid, soft tissue, and bony tissues are all well visualized. An appropriate kVp and mAs combination and a well-collimated radiation field will ensure optimum digital image quality at the lowest possible patient dose.

In film-screen radiography, optimum density is perhaps more critical in the sinuses than in any other region of the body. High kVp levels cause overpenetration, which can diminish if not completely obliterate pathology, and low kVp underpenetrates this anatomy, which simulates pathologic conditions that do not exist (Figs. 20-169 to 20-171).

The paranasal sinuses vary not only in size and form but also in position. The cells of one group frequently encroach on and resemble those of another group. This characteristic of the sinuses, together with their proximity to the vital intracranial organs, makes accurate radiographic demonstration of their anatomic structure of prime importance. The patient's head must be carefully placed in a sufficient number of positions so that the projections of each group of cavities are as free of superimposed bony structures as possible. The images must be of such quality that it is possible to distinguish the cells of several groups of sinuses and their relationship to surrounding structures.

[1]Cross KS: Radiography of the nasal accessory sinuses, *Med J Aust* 14:569, 1927.
[2]Flecker H: Roentgenograms of the antrum, *AJR Am J Roentgenol* 20:56, 1928 (letter).

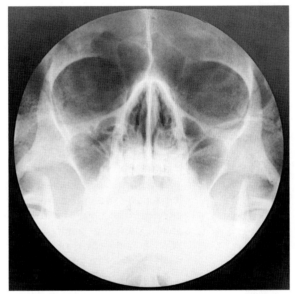

Fig. 20-169 Correctly exposed radiograph of sinuses.

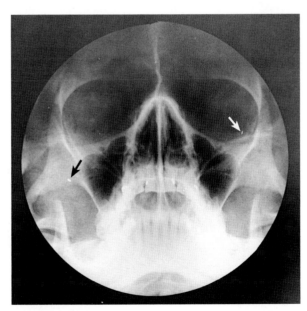

Fig. 20-170 Overexposed radiograph of sinuses showing two artifacts caused by dirt on screens (*arrows*).

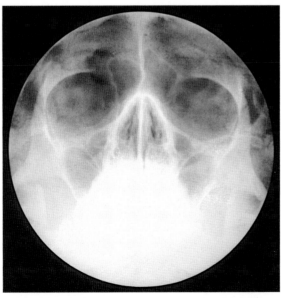

Fig. 20-171 Underexposed radiograph of sinuses.

Technical Considerations

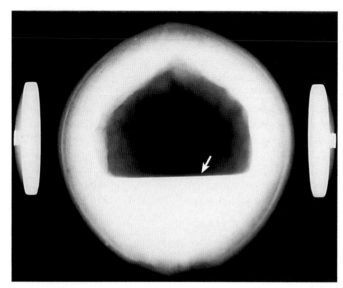

Fig. 20-172 Coconut, vertical position: horizontal central ray. Air-fluid level is shown (*arrow*).

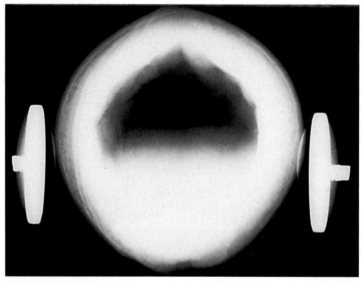

Fig. 20-173 Coconut, vertical position: central ray angled 45 degrees upward. Air-fluid level is not as sharp.

Unless sinus images are almost perfect technically, they are of little diagnostic value. For this reason, a precise technical procedure is necessary in radiography of the paranasal sinuses. The first requirements are a small focal spot and IRs that are free of artifacts. As mentioned previously, the image contrast must markedly distinguish the sinuses from surrounding structures. The head must be carefully positioned and rigidly immobilized, and respiration must be suspended for the exposures.

The effect of body position and central ray angulation is shown in radiographs of a coconut held in position by head clamps. Fig. 20-172 shows a sharply defined air-fluid level. This coconut was placed in the vertical position, and the central ray was directed horizontally. Fig. 20-173 was also taken with the coconut in the vertical position, but the central ray was directed upward at an angle of 45 degrees to show gradual fading of the fluid line when the central ray is *not* horizontal. This effect is much more pronounced in actual practice because of structural irregularities. Fig. 20-174 was made with the coconut in the horizontal position and the central ray directed vertically. The resultant radiograph shows a homogeneous density throughout the cavity of the coconut, with no evidence of an air-fluid level.

Exudate contained in the sinuses is not fluid in the usual sense of the word but is commonly a heavy, semi-gelatinous material. The exudate, rather than flowing freely, clings to the walls of the cavity and takes several minutes, depending on its viscosity, to shift position. For this reason, when the position of a patient is changed or the patient's neck is flexed or extended to position the head for special projections, *several minutes* should be allowed for the exudate to gravitate to the desired location before the exposure is made.

Although numerous sinus projections are possible, with each serving a special purpose, many are used only when required to show a specific lesion. The consensus is that five standard projections adequately show all of the paranasal sinuses in most patients. The following steps are observed in preparing for these projections:

- Use a suitable protractor to check and adjust the position of the patient's head to ensure accurate positioning.
- Have the patient remove dentures, hairpins, and ornaments such as earrings and necklaces before proceeding with the examination.
- Because the patient's face is in contact with the IR holder or the IR itself for many of the images, these items should be cleaned before the patient is positioned.

Even with the most hygienic patients, the hair and face are naturally oily and leave a residue. If a patient is sick, the residue is worse. During positioning of the patient's head, the hair, mouth, nose, and eyes come in direct contact with the vertical grid device, tabletop, or IR. Medical asepsis can be promoted by placing a paper towel or sheet between the imaging surface and the patient. As standard procedure, the contacted area should be cleaned with a disinfectant before and after positioning.

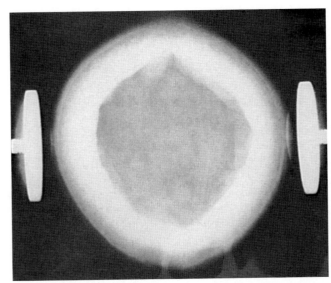

Fig. 20-174 Coconut, horizontal position: vertical central ray. No evidence of air-fluid level is seen.

🪶 LATERAL PROJECTION
R or L position

Image receptor: 8 × 10 inch (18 × 24 cm) or 10 × 12 inch (24 × 30 cm), depending on availability

Position of patient

- Seat the patient before a vertical grid device with the body placed in the RAO or LAO position so that the head can be adjusted in a true lateral position. This is the same basic position that is used for the lateral skull and facial bone positions.

Position of part

- Rest the side of the patient's head on the vertical grid device, and adjust the head in a true lateral position. The midsagittal plane of the head is parallel with the plane of the IR, and the interpupillary line is perpendicular to the plane of the IR.
- The infraorbitomeatal line (IOML) is positioned horizontally to ensure proper extension of the head. This position places the IOML perpendicular to the front edge of the vertical grid device (Fig. 20-175).
- *Respiration:* Suspend.

Central ray

- Directed *horizontal,* enter the patient's head ½ to 1 inch (1.3 to 2.5 cm) posterior to the outer canthus
- Center the IR to the central ray.
- Immobilize the head.

Collimation

- Adjust to 8 × 10 inches (18 × 24 cm) on the collimator.

Structures shown

A lateral projection shows the AP and superoinferior dimensions of the paranasal sinuses, their relationship to surrounding structures, and the thickness of the outer table of the frontal bone (Fig. 20-176).

When the lateral projection is to be used for preoperative measurements, it should be made at a 72-inch (183-cm) source–to–image receptor distance to minimize magnification and distortion.

The following should be clearly shown:
- Evidence of proper collimation; close beam restriction to sinus area
- All four sinus groups, but the sphenoidal sinus is best demonstrated
- No rotation or tilt of sinus anatomy, as demonstrated by:
  □ Sella turcica in profile
  □ Superimposed orbital roofs
  □ Superimposed mandibular rami
- Brightness and contrast sufficient to visualize air-fluid levels, if present

NOTE: If the patient is unable to assume the upright body position, a lateral projection can be obtained using the dorsal decubitus position. The horizontal beam enables fluid levels to be seen. Positioning of the part is the same except for the IOML, which is vertical rather than horizontal.

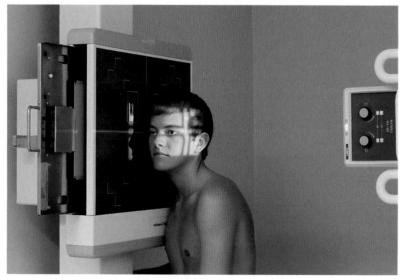

Fig. 20-175 Lateral sinuses.

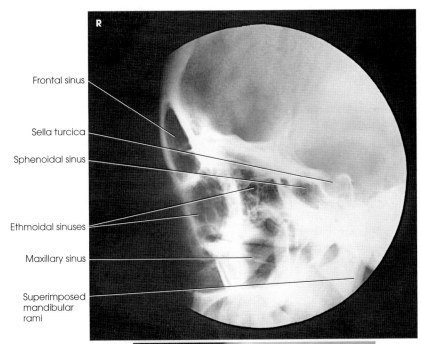

Frontal sinus

Sella turcica

Sphenoidal sinus

Ethmoidal sinuses

Maxillary sinus

Superimposed
mandibular
rami

R

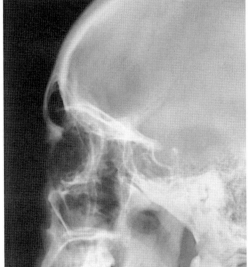

Fig. 20-176 Lateral sinuses.

♠ PA AXIAL PROJECTION
CALDWELL METHOD

Because sinus images should always be obtained with the patient in the upright body position and with a *horizontal* direction of the central ray, the Caldwell method is easily modified when a head unit or other vertical grid device capable of angular adjustment is used. For the modification, all anatomic landmarks and localization planes remain unchanged.

> **Image receptor:** 8 × 10 inch (18 × 24 cm) or 10 × 12 inch (24 × 30 cm) lengthwise, depending on availability

Position of patient

- Seat the patient facing a vertical grid device.
- Center the midsagittal plane of the patient's body to the midline of the grid.

Position of part
Angled grid technique

- Before positioning the patient, tilt the vertical grid device down so that an angle of 15 degrees is obtained (Fig. 20-177, *A*).
- Rest the patient's nose and forehead on the vertical grid device, and center the nasion to the IR.
- Adjust the midsagittal plane and orbito-meatal line (OML) of the patient's head perpendicular to the plane of the IR.
- This positioning places the OML perpendicular to the angled IR and 15 degrees from the horizontal central ray.
- Immobilize the head.
- *Respiration:* Suspend.

Vertical grid technique

- When the vertical grid device cannot be angled, extend the patient's neck slightly, rest the tip of the nose on the grid device, and center the nasion to the IR.
- Position the patient's head so that the OML forms an angle of 15 degrees with the horizontal central ray. For support, place a radiolucent sponge between the forehead and the grid device (see Figs. 20-177, *B,* and 20-178).
- Adjust the midsagittal plane of the patient's head perpendicular to the plane of the IR.
- Immobilize the head.
- *Respiration:* Suspend.

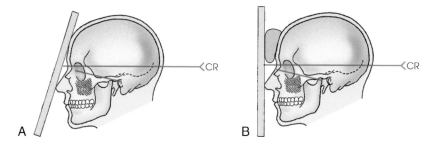

Fig. 20-177 Diagram of PA axial sinuses: Caldwell method. **A,** IR tilted 15 degrees. **B,** Same projection with vertical IR.

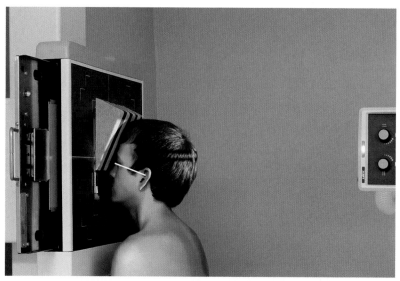

Fig. 20-178 PA axial sinuses: Caldwell method.

Central ray

- Directed *horizontal* to exit the nasion. The 15-degree relationship between the central ray and the OML remains the same for both techniques.
- Center the IR to the central ray.

NOTE: The *angled grid technique* is preferred because it brings the IR closer to the sinuses, increasing resolution. Angulation of the grid device provides a natural position for placement of the patient's nose and forehead.

Collimation

- Adjust to 8 × 10 inches (18 × 24 cm) on the collimator.

Structures shown

The angled grid technique and the vertical grid technique show the frontal sinuses lying superior to the frontonasal suture, the anterior ethmoidal air cells lying on each side of the nasal fossae and immediately inferior to the frontal sinuses, and the sphenoidal sinuses projected through the nasal fossae just inferior to or between the ethmoidal air cells (Fig. 20-179). The dense petrous pyramids extend from the inferior third of the orbit inferiorly to obscure the superior third of the maxillary sinus. This projection is used primarily to show the frontal sinuses and anterior ethmoidal air cells.

The following should be clearly shown:

- Evidence of proper collimation with close beam restriction to the sinus area
- Frontal sinuses lying above the frontonasal suture and the anterior ethmoidal air cells lying above the petrous ridges
- No rotation or tilt, demonstrated by:
  - Equal distance between the lateral border of the skull and the lateral border of the orbits
  - Petrous ridge symmetric on both sides
  - MSP of head aligned with long axis of collimated field
- Petrous ridge lying in the lower third of the orbit
- Brightness and contrast sufficient to visualize air-fluid levels, if present

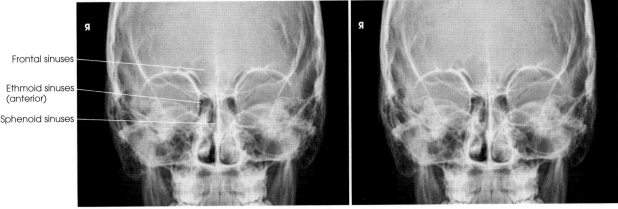

Frontal sinuses

Ethmoid sinuses (anterior)

Sphenoid sinuses

Fig. 20-179 PA axial sinuses.

♠ PARIETOACANTHIAL PROJECTION
WATERS METHOD

Image receptor: 8 × 10 inch (18 × 24 cm) or 10 × 12 inch (24 × 30 cm) lengthwise, depending on availability

For the Waters method,[1,2] the goal is to hyperextend the patient's neck just enough to place the dense petrosae immediately below the maxillary sinus floors (Fig. 20-180). When the neck is extended too little, the petrosae are projected over the inferior portions of the maxillary sinuses and obscure underlying pathologic conditions (Fig. 20-181). When the neck is extended too much, the maxillary sinuses are foreshortened, and the antral floors are not shown.

---

[1]Waters CA: A modification of the occipitofrontal position in the roentgen examination of the accessory nasal sinuses, *Arch Radiol Ther* 20:15, 1915.
[2]Mahoney HO: Head and sinus positions, *Xray Techn* 1:89, 1930.

Position of patient
- Place the patient seated in an upright position, facing the vertical grid device.
- Center the midsagittal plane of the patient's body to the midline of the grid device.

Position of part
- Because this position is uncomfortable for the patient to hold, have the IR and equipment in position so that the examination can be performed quickly.
- Hyperextend the patient's neck to approximately the correct position, and then center the IR to the acanthion.

- Rest the patient's chin on the vertical grid device and adjust it so that the midsagittal plane is perpendicular to the plane of the IR.
- Using a protractor as a guide, adjust the head so that the OML forms an angle of 37 degrees from the plane of the IR (Fig. 20-182; see Fig. 20-180). As a positioning check for the average-shaped skull, the mentomeatal (MML) line should be approximately perpendicular to the IR plane.
- Immobilize the head.
- *Respiration:* Suspend.

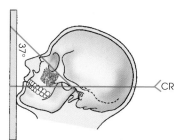

Fig. 20-180 Proper positioning diagram. Petrous ridges are projected below maxillary sinuses.

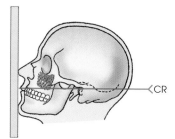

Fig. 20-181 Improper positioning diagram. Petrous ridges are superimposed on maxillary sinuses.

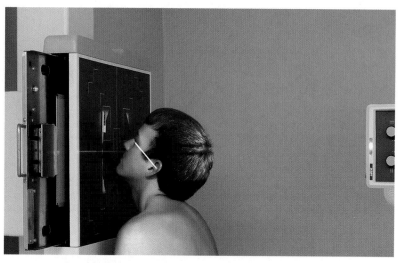

Fig. 20-182 Parietoacanthial sinuses: Waters method.

Central ray

- *Horizontal* to the IR and exiting the acanthion

Collimation

- Adjust to 8 × 10 inches (18 × 24 cm) on the collimator.

Structures shown

The image shows a parietoacanthial projection of the maxillary sinuses, with the petrous ridges lying inferior to the floor of the sinuses (Fig. 20-183). The frontal and ethmoidal air cells are distorted.

The Waters method is also used to show the foramen rotundum. The images of these structures are seen, one on each side, just inferior to the medial aspect of the orbital floor and superior to the roof of the maxillary sinuses.

The following should be clearly shown:

- Evidence of proper collimation with close beam restriction to the sinus area
- Maxillary sinuses
- OML in proper position (sufficient neck extension), as demonstrated by:
  - Petrous pyramids lying immediately *inferior* to the floor of the maxillary sinuses
- No rotation or tilt, demonstrated by:
  - Equal distance between the lateral border of the skull and the lateral border of the orbit on both sides
  - Orbits and maxillary sinuses symmetric on each side
  - MSP of head aligned with long axis of collimated field
- Brightness and contrast sufficient to visualize air-fluid levels, if present

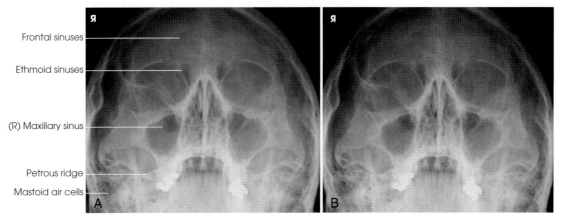

Frontal sinuses

Ethmoid sinuses

(R) Maxillary sinus

Petrous ridge

Mastoid air cells

Fig. 20-183 A, Parietoacanthial sinuses: Waters method. **B,** Same projection.

♠ PARIETOACANTHIAL PROJECTION

OPEN-MOUTH WATERS METHOD

Image receptor: 8 × 10 inch (18 × 24 cm) or 10 × 12 inch (24 × 30 cm) lengthwise, depending on availability

This method provides an excellent demonstration of the sphenoidal sinuses projected through the open mouth. For patients who cannot be placed in position for the submentovertical (SMV) projection, the *open-mouth Waters method* and lateral projections may be the only techniques to show the sphenoidal sinuses. Because the open-mouth position is uncomfortable for the patient to hold, the radiographer must have the IR and equipment in position to perform the examination quickly.

Position of part
- Hyperextend the patient's neck to approximately the correct position, and then position the IR to the acanthion.
- Rest the patient's chin on the vertical grid device, and adjust it so that the midsagittal plane is perpendicular to the plane of the IR.
- Using a protractor as a guide, adjust the patient's head so that the OML forms an angle of 37 degrees from the plane of the IR. The MML would not be perpendicular (Fig. 20-184).
- Have the patient *slowly open the mouth wide open* while holding the position.
- Immobilize the head.
- *Respiration:* Suspend.

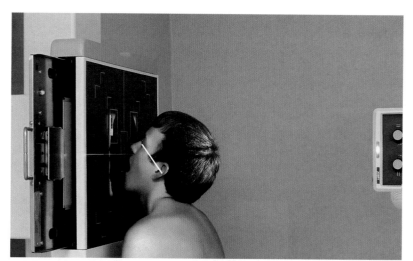

Fig. 20-184 Parietoacanthial sinuses: open-mouth Waters method.

Central ray

- *Horizontal* to the IR and exiting the acanthion

Collimation

- Adjust to 8 × 10 inches (18 × 24 cm) on the collimator.

Structures shown

The open-mouth Waters method shows the sphenoidal sinuses projected through the open mouth along with the maxillary sinuses (Fig. 20-185).

EVALUATION CRITERIA

The following should be clearly shown:

- Evidence of proper collimation with close beam restriction to sinus area
- Sphenoidal sinuses projected through the open mouth
- Maxillary sinuses
- OML in proper position (sufficient neck extension), as demonstrated by:
  - □ Petrous pyramids lying immediately *inferior* to the floor of the maxillary sinuses
- No rotation or tilt, demonstrated by:
  - □ Equal distance between the lateral border of the skull and the lateral border of the orbit on both sides
  - □ Orbits and maxillary sinuses symmetric on each side
  - □ MSP of head aligned with long axis of collimated field
- Brightness and contrast sufficient to visualize air-fluid levels, if present

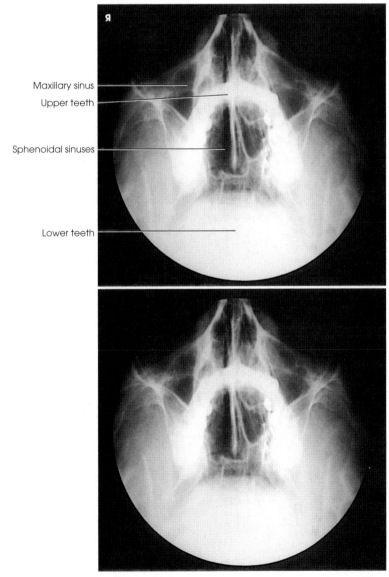

Maxillary sinus
Upper teeth

Sphenoidal sinuses

Lower teeth

Fig. 20-185 Open-mouth Waters modification shows sphenoidal sinuses projected through open mouth along with maxillary sinuses.

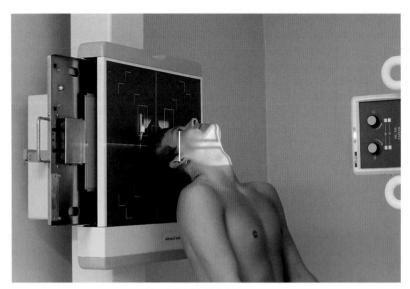

Fig. 20-186 SMV sinuses.

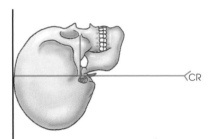

Fig. 20-187 Upright radiography diagram: SMV sinuses, preferred position of skull.

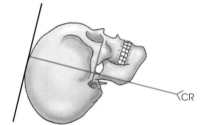

Fig. 20-188 Upright radiography diagram: SMV sinuses.

♠ SUBMENTOVERTICAL PROJECTION

Image receptor: 8 × 10 inch (18 × 24 cm) or 10 × 12 inch (24 × 30 cm) lengthwise, depending on availability

Position of patient

The success of the SMV projection depends on placing the IOML as nearly parallel as possible with the plane of the IR and directing the central ray perpendicular to the IOML. The upright position is recommended for all paranasal sinus images and is more comfortable for the patient. The following steps are observed:

- Use a chair that supports the patient's back to obtain greater freedom in positioning the patient's body to place the IOML parallel with the IR.
- Seat the patient far enough away from the vertical grid device that the head can be fully extended (Figs. 20-186 and 20-187).
- If necessary to examine short-necked or hypersthenic patients, angle the vertical grid device downward to achieve a parallel relationship between the grid and the IOML (Fig. 20-188). The disadvantage of angling the vertical grid device is that the central ray is not horizontal, and air-fluid levels may not be shown as easily as when the central ray is truly horizontal.

Position of part

- Hyperextend the patient's neck as far as possible, and rest the head on its vertex. If the patient's mouth opens during hyperextension, ask the patient to keep the mouth closed to move the mandibular symphysis anteriorly.
- Adjust the patient's head so that the midsagittal plane is perpendicular to the midline of the IR.
- Adjust the tube so that the central ray is perpendicular to the IOML (see Fig. 20-186).
- Immobilize the patient's head. In the absence of a head clamp, place a suitably backed strip of adhesive tape across the tip of the chin and anchor it to the sides of the radiographic unit. Do not put the adhesive surface directly on the patient's skin.
- *Respiration:* Suspend.

Central ray

- *Horizontal* and perpendicular to the IOML through the sella turcica. The central ray enters on the midsagittal plane approximately ¾ inch (1.9 cm) anterior to the level of the external acoustic meatus.

Collimation

- Adjust to 8 × 10 inches (18 × 24 cm) on the collimator.

Structures shown

The SMV projection for the sinuses shows a symmetric image of the anterior portion of the base of the skull. The sphenoidal sinus and ethmoidal air cells are shown (Fig. 20-189).

EVALUATION CRITERIA

The following should be clearly shown:
- Evidence of proper collimation with close beam restriction to sinus area
- Sphenoid and ethmoid sinuses

- No tilt (MSP positioned perpendicular to IR), demonstrated by:
  - □ Equal distance from the lateral border of the skull to the mandibular condyles on both sides
- IOML positioned parallel to IR (sufficient neck extension), demonstrated by:
  - □ Superimposition of anterior frontal bone by mental protuberance
  - □ Insufficient neck extension will cause mandible to superimpose ethmoid sinuses
- Mandibular condyles anterior to petrous pyramids
- Brightness and contrast sufficient to visualize air-fluid levels, if present

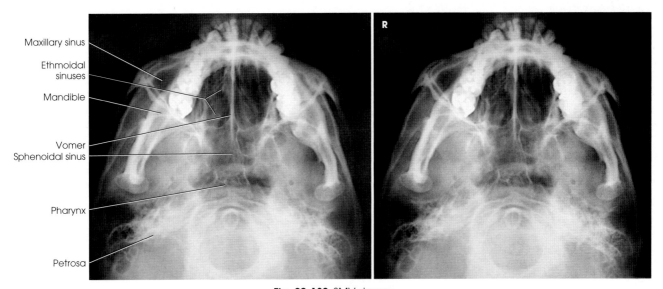

Maxillary sinus
Ethmoidal sinuses
Mandible
Vomer
Sphenoidal sinus
Pharynx
Petrosa

Fig. 20-189 SMV sinuses.

21

MAMMOGRAPHY

VALERIE F. ANDOLINA
JESSICA L. SAUNDERS

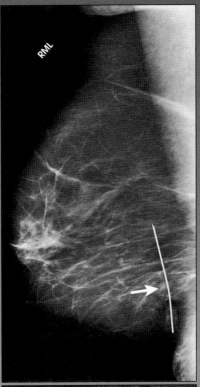

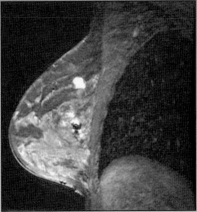

SUMMARY OF PROJECTIONS

PROJECTIONS, POSITIONS, AND METHODS

Page	Essential	Anatomy	Projection	Method
413	♠	Breast	Craniocaudal (CC)	
415	♠	Breast	Mediolateral oblique (MLO)	
420	♠	Breast	Craniocaudal (CC)	IMPLANT
422	♠	Breast	Craniocaudal (CC ID)	IMPLANT DISPLACED
424	♠	Breast	Mediolateral oblique (MLO)	IMPLANT
425	♠	Breast	Mediolateral oblique (MLO ID)	IMPLANT DISPLACED
428		Breast	Variable (M)	MAGNIFICATION
429	♠	Breast	Variable	SPOT COMPRESSION
433	♠	Breast	Mediolateral (ML)	
435		Breast	Lateromedial (LM)	
437	♠	Breast	Exaggerated craniocaudal (XCCL)	
439		Breast	Craniocaudal (CV)	CLEAVAGE
441		Breast	Craniocaudal (RL)	ROLL LATERAL
441		Breast	Craniocaudal (RM)	ROLL MEDIAL
443		Breast	Tangential (TAN)	
445		Breast	Variable (CL)	CAPTURED LESION
448		Breast	Caudocranial (FB)	
450		Breast	Mediolateral oblique (AT)	AXILLARY TAIL
454		Breast	Lateromedial oblique (LMO)	
456		Breast	Superolateral to inferomedial oblique (SIO)	

Icons in the Essential column indicate projections frequently performed in the United States and Canada. Students should be competent in these projections.

Principles of Mammography

INTRODUCTION AND HISTORICAL DEVELOPMENT

The worldwide incidence of breast cancer is increasing. In the United States, one in eight women who live to age 95 years develop breast cancer sometime during their lifetime. Breast cancer is one of the most common malignancies diagnosed in women; only lung cancer has a greater overall mortality in women. Research has failed to reveal the precise etiology of breast cancer, and only a few major factors, such as family history, are known to increase a woman's risk of developing the disease. Most women who develop breast cancer have no family history of the disease, however.

Despite its frequency, breast cancer is one of the most treatable cancers. Because this malignancy is most treatable when it is detected early, efforts have been directed toward developing breast cancer screening and early detection methods. Death rates for breast cancer in the United States have steadily decreased in women since 1989, with larger decreases in younger women; from 2005 to 2009, rates decreased 3.0% per year in women younger than 50 and 2.0% per year in women 50 and older. The decrease in breast cancer death rates represents progress in earlier detection, improved treatment, and possibly decreased incidence as a result of declining use of menopausal hormone therapy (MHT).[a]

[a]American Cancer Society: Cancer Facts and Figures 2013, p9.

Before the radical mastectomy was introduced by Halstead in 1898, breast cancer was considered a fatal disease. Less than 5% of patients survived 4 years after diagnosis, and the local recurrence rate for surgically treated breast cancer was greater than 80%. Radical mastectomy increased the 4-year survival rate to 40% and reduced the rate of local recurrence to approximately 10%. No additional improvement in breast cancer survival rates occurred over the next 60 years. Some of the principles of breast cancer management were developed during this time, however, and these remain valid:

1. Patients in the early stage of the disease respond well to treatment.
2. Patients with advanced disease do poorly.
3. The earlier the diagnosis, the better the chance of survival.

Reflecting these principles, the theory of removing all palpable breast masses in hopes of finding earlier cancers was developed, and it was recognized that careful physical examination of the breast could lead to detection of some early breast cancers. Most patients with breast cancer still were not diagnosed until their disease was advanced, however. This fact, coupled with the dismal breast cancer survival statistics, highlighted the need for a tool for the early detection of breast cancer. Mammography filled that need (Fig. 21-1).

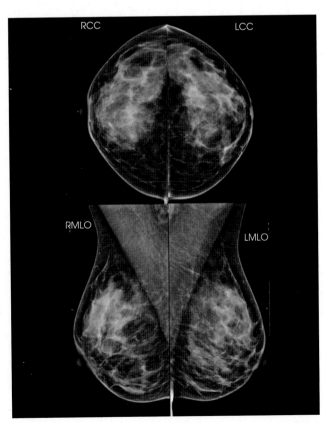

Fig. 21-1 Four-image, bilateral mammogram. Craniocaudal and mediolateral oblique projections show normal, symmetric, heterogeneously dense breast parenchyma.

In 1913, Albert Soloman, a German physician, reported the radiographic appearance of breast cancers. Using radiographic studies of cancerous breasts removed at surgery, he described the mechanism of how breast cancer spread. Stafford Warren of Rochester, New York, noted in 1926 that he was able to see a reasonable image of the female breast during thoracic aortic fluoroscopy and published a report of 119 women, 48 with breast cancer.[b] The first published radiograph of a living person's breast, made by Otto Kleinschmidt, appeared in a 1927 German medical textbook on malignant tumors. Although publications on mammography appeared in South America, the United States, and Europe during the 1930s, the use of mammography for the diagnosis of breast cancer received little clinical interest. A few pioneers, including LeBorgne in Uruguay, Gershon-Cohen in the United States, and Gros in Germany, published excellent comparisons of mammographic and pathologic anatomy and developed some of the clinical techniques of mammography. At that time, the significance of breast microcalcifications was also well understood.

By the mid-1950s, mammography was considered a reliable clinical tool because of such refinements as low-kilovoltage x-ray tubes with molybdenum targets and high-detail, industrial-grade x-ray film. During this time, Egan in the United States and Gros in Germany popularized the use of mammography by utilizing industrial grade x-ray film for diagnosing and evaluating breast cancer. Breast xerography was introduced in the 1960s and was popularized by Wolfe and Ruzicka. Xerography substantially reduced the radiation dose received by the patient compared with the dose received using industrial grade x-ray film (Fig. 21-2). Because many physicians found xerographic images easier to understand and evaluate, xeromammography became widely used for evaluating breast disease. The first attempts at widespread population screening began at this time.

The combination of higher-resolution, faster x-ray film and an intensifying screen was first introduced by the duPont Company. As a result, radiation exposure to the patient was reduced even more. Improved screen-film combinations were developed by Kodak and duPont in 1975. By this time, extremely high-quality mammography images could be produced with very low patient radiation exposures. Since 1975, faster lower-dose films, the magnification technique, and grids for scatter reduction have been introduced.

[b]Thomas AMK, Banerjee AK, Busch U: *Classic papers in modern diagnostic radiology*, Berlin, 2005, Springer, p540.

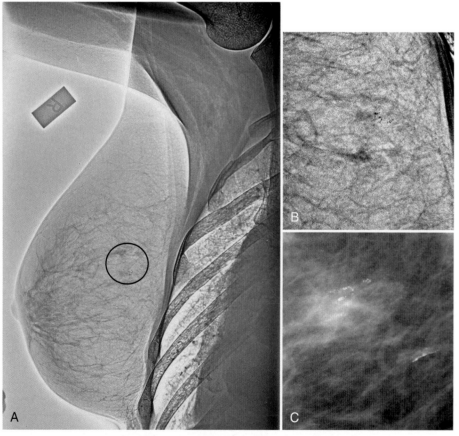

Fig. 21-2 A, Right lateral xeromammogram, circa 1981. **B,** *Circled area* is photographically magnified, showing small area of microcalcifications. **C,** Film-screen magnification study 10 years later shows same calcifications. This was proven to be ductal carcinoma in situ on biopsy.

EVOLUTION OF MAMMOGRAPHY SYSTEMS

Because the breast is composed of tissues with very similar densities and effective atomic numbers, little difference in attenuation is noticed when conventional x-ray equipment and techniques are used. Therefore, manufacturers have developed imaging systems that optimally and consistently produce images with high contrast and resolution.

Diligent research and development began in the 1960s, and the first dedicated mammography unit was introduced in 1967 by CGR (France) (Fig. 21-3). In the 1970s, increased awareness of the elevated radiation doses prevalent in mammography served as the catalyst for the rapid progression of imaging systems. In the 1970s and the early 1980s, xeromammography, named for the Xerox Corporation that developed it, was widely used (see Fig. 21-2). This method used much less radiation than the direct-exposure, silver-based films that were available. Eventually, film manufacturers introduced several generations of mammography film-screen systems that used even less exposure and improved tissue visualization. Each subsequent new system showed improvement in contrast and resolution while minimizing patient dose.

In the 1980s, the American College of Radiology (ACR) accreditation program established quality standards for breast imaging to optimize mammographic equipment, processors, and screen-film systems to ensure the production of high-quality images. This program was expanded in the 1990s to include quality control and personnel qualifications and training. The voluntary ACR program has become the model from which the Mammography Quality Standards Act of 1992 (MQSA) operates, and the ACR has been instrumental in designing clinical practice guidelines for quality mammography in the United States. The evolution of mammography has resulted in the implementation of radiographic systems designed specifically for breast imaging.

MAMMOGRAPHY EQUIPMENT

Over the years, equipment manufacturers have produced dedicated mammography units with high-frequency generators, various tube and filter materials, focal spot sizes that allow tissue magnification, specialized grids to help improve image quality, and streamlined designs with ergonomic patient positioning aids.

The high-frequency generators offer more precise control of kilovolt (peak) (kVp), milliamperes (mA), and exposure time. The linearity and reproducibility of radiographic exposures using high-frequency generators are uniformly excellent. The greatest benefit of these generators may be the efficient waveform output that produces a higher effective energy x-ray beam per set kVp and mA. High-frequency generators are not as bulky, and they can be installed within the single-standing mammography unit operating on single-phase incoming line power, facilitating installation and creating a less intimidating appearance (Fig. 21-4).

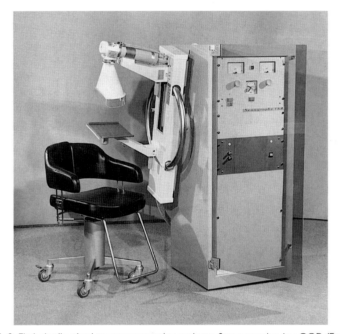

Fig. 21-3 First dedicated mammography system: Senographe by CGR (France).

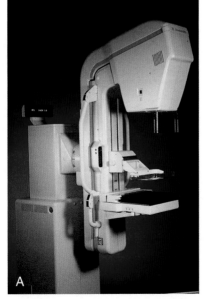 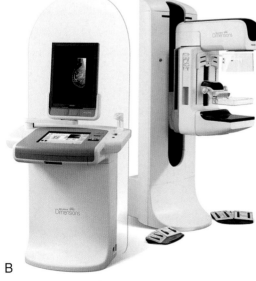

Fig. 21-4 A, Senographe DMR film-screen mammography unit by General Electric (Milwaukee, WI). **B,** Dimensions 3-D digital breast tomosynthesis unit by Hologic (Bedford, MA).

As manufacturers of dedicated mammography equipment have sought to improve image quality, they have tried many different combinations of tube and filter materials. The most widely accepted combinations used at this time are molybdenum target with molybdenum filter (Mo/Mo), molybdenum target with rhodium filter (Mo/Rh), and rhodium target with rhodium filter (Rh/Rh). The Mo/Rh and Rh/Rh combinations are used for better penetration of denser breasts with thick tissues.

Specialized grids were developed for mammography during the 1980s to reduce scatter radiation and increase image contrast in mammography. Many units employ moving linear focused grids, but other manufacturers have developed very specialized grids. The Hologic (Lorad) High Transmission Cellular (HTC) Grid employs a honeycomb-pattern, multidirectional design. All dedicated mammography units today, with the exception of slit-scan digital units, still employ grids.

Manufacturers also knew that technologists and physicians were interested in the comfort of their patients. They worked to make the examination more tolerable for patients, more ergonomically acceptable, and more efficient for the technologist performing the examination, while developing positioning aids to increase visualization of the tissue. Some of these aids include rounded corners on Bucky devices and compression paddles, automatic release of compression after exposure, and foot pedal controls.

The next logical step toward improved breast imaging has been the adoption of full-field digital mammography (FFDM) and digital breast tomosynthesis (DBT), also referred to as 3D breast imaging. To bring mammography into the digital world was no simple task. To achieve the resolution and detail necessary for breast imaging, entire systems, from acquisition to diagnostic review workstations, were developed by competing manufacturers. Each of these included proprietary components that made integration of the units into a current picture archiving and communication system (PACS) network difficult. Integrating the healthcare enterprise has brought together manufacturers of the many components necessary in a full-field digital mammography (FFDM) system to work out problems of compatibility and language, allowing facilities the opportunity to transition more seamlessly into digital mammography.

Full-Field Digital Mammography (FFDM)

Mammography has been the last area in the field of radiography to take advantage of digital technology. In addition to the many technical issues associated with FFDM, the prohibitive cost of the equipment and its maintenance make digital mammography not practical for all facilities. Its many advantages in imaging dense breast tissue have provided the motive, however, for more than 89% of mammography facilities in the United States to transition to this technology over the past 8 years.

FFDM units allow radiologists to manipulate digital images electronically, potentially saving patients from undergoing additional projections and additional radiation. The ability to manipulate digital images improves the sensitivity of mammography, especially in women with dense breast tissue. Results of the ACRIN DMIST study, a multifacility, multiunit study comparing film-screen mammography with digital mammography, were published in September 2005.[1] The authors of this study concluded that FFDM would benefit some patients, specifically women younger than age 50, premenopausal and perimenopausal women, and women of any age with dense breast tissue. If FFDM is not available to women who fall within these benefit guidelines, they should continue having film-screen mammography studies because these have successfully been used as a screening tool for breast cancer for over 35 years.

Digital breast imaging requires much finer resolution than other body imaging. FFDM images are extremely large files that require a great deal of archival space in PACS. Because of regulations safeguarding the image quality of mammography, the images cannot be interpreted on a traditional PACS workstation; they can be interpreted only on high-resolution 5-megapixel or better monitors.

Innovative solutions and approaches to FFDM continue to be developed. Digital breast tomosynthesis (DBT) is a three-dimensional imaging technology that acquires images of a stationary, compressed breast at multiple angles during a short scan. These images are reconstructed into thin, high-resolution slices that can be displayed individually or in a dynamic cine mode. These units can simultaneously acquire the traditional two-dimensional mammogram and the additional exposures necessary to reconstruct a three-dimensional image. DBT was approved for clinical use by the FDA in 2011. It is believed that DBT will reduce the number of patients recalled for additional views, will reduce the number of biopsies performed on benign lesions, and will result in fewer short-interval follow-up examinations.[c]

---

[1]Bassett L: Clinical image evaluation, *Radiol Clin North Am* 33:1027, 1995.

[c]Zuley M et al: Digital breast tomosynthesis versus supplemental diagnostic mammographic views for evaluation of noncalcified breast lesions, *Radiology* 266:89, 2013.

Computer-Aided Detection

When performing mammographic interpretation, the radiologist must locate any suspicious lesions (sensitivity) and then determine the probability that the lesion is malignant or benign (specificity). Even with high-quality mammography, some breast cancers are missed on initial interpretation. Double-reading of screening mammograms by a second radiologist can improve detection rates by approximately 10%.[1] Efforts have been made to develop and apply a computer-aided detection (CAD) system to achieve the same result as double-reading. It has also been found that double-reading plus the use of CAD can increase detection rates by an additional 8%.[2]

CAD is a method by which a radiologist can use computer analysis of digitally acquired images as a "second opinion" before making a final interpretation. CAD works similar to a spell-check on a computer; an area is pointed out for the radiologist to check, but it is up to the radiologist to decide whether the area is suspicious enough to warrant additional procedures. CAD requires that the mammographic image exist in a digital format to facilitate computer input. The use of images directly acquired with full-field digital technology is preferred; however, CAD can also be accomplished on film images with the use of an optical scanner. The computer may detect lesions that are missed by the radiologist, minimizing the possibility of false-negative readings (Fig. 21-5). When a lesion is detected, the computer can be programmed with basic algorithms to estimate the likelihood of malignancy, increasing true-positive rates. Ultimately, the objective of this technology is to improve early detection rates and minimize the number of unnecessary breast biopsies. Another advantage of CAD is that computers are not subject to the bias, fatigue, or distractions to which a radiologist may be subject. Because of the high rates of sensitivity and specificity shown by CAD, it has become a standard of care for many mammography practices.

[1]Kopans DB: Double-reading, *Radiol Clin North Am* 38:719, 2000.

[2]Destounis SV et al: Can computer-aided detection with double reading of screening mammograms help decrease the false-negative rate? Initial experience, *Radiology* 232:578, 2004.

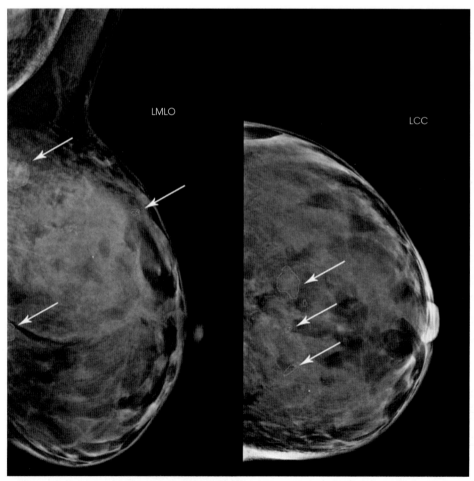

Fig. 21-5 LCC and MLO projections of extremely dense breast with CAD markers indicating areas of suspicion that proved to be cancer.

BREAST CANCER SCREENING

It is now known that high-quality mammography, careful physical examination, and monthly breast self-examination (BSE) can result in the detection of breast cancer at an early stage—when it is most curable.

The 5-year relative survival rate for female invasive breast cancer patients has improved from 75% in the mid-1970s to 90% today. The 5-year relative survival for women diagnosed with localized breast cancer (cancer that has not spread to lymph nodes or other locations outside the breast) is 98%; if the cancer has spread to nearby lymph nodes (regional stage) or distant lymph nodes or organs (distant stage), the survival rate falls to 84% or 24%, respectively.[d]

Mammography must be performed well to be fully effective. The American College of Radiology (ACR) had been a proponent of high standards in breast imaging since 1967 and implemented an optional Mammography Accreditation Program in 1989. In 1992, the Mammography Quality Standards Act (MQSA) was implemented to mandate the maintenance of high-quality breast cancer screening programs. In 1994, mammography became the only radiographic examination to be fully regulated by the federal government. MQSA requires formal training and continuing education for all members of the breast imaging team. In addition, imaging equipment must be inspected regularly, and all quality assurance activities must be documented. Facilities are also required to provide protocols documenting responsibility for communicating mammogram results to the patient and the referring physician, providing follow-up, tracking patients, and monitoring outcomes. The goal of MQSA is for high-quality mammography to be performed by individuals most qualified to do so and by individuals who are willing to accept full responsibility for providing that service with continuity of care.

RISK VERSUS BENEFIT

In the mid-1970s, the media-influenced public perception was that radiation exposure from diagnostic x-rays would induce more breast cancers than would be detected. Although radiation dosage during a mammography examination has decreased dramatically since the 1970s,

fear of radiation exposure still causes some women to refuse mammography, and many women who undergo the examination are concerned about exposure levels and the resultant risk of carcinogenesis. To assuage these fears, the radiographer must understand the relationship between breast irradiation and breast cancer and the relative risks of mammography in light of the natural incidence of breast cancer and the potential benefit of the examination. No direct evidence exists to suggest that the small doses of diagnostic x-rays used in mammography can induce breast cancer. It has been shown, however, that large radiation doses can increase the incidence of breast cancer, and that the risk is dose-dependent. Evidence to support increased risk of breast cancer from breast irradiation comes from studies of three groups of women in whom the incidence of breast cancer increased after they were exposed to large doses of radiation: (1) women exposed to the atomic bombs at Hiroshima and Nagasaki, (2) women with tuberculosis who received multiple fluoroscopic examinations of the chest, and (3) women who were treated with radiation for postpartum mastitis. The radiation dose received by these women (600 to 700 rads) was many times higher, however, than the dose received from mammography.

Mean glandular dose provides the best indicator of radiation risk to a patient. In 1997, the average mean glandular dose for a two-projection screen-film-grid mammogram for all facilities in the United States inspected under MQSA was 320 mrad.[1] If this level is used as a gauge, the lifetime risk of mortality from mammography-induced radiation is 5 deaths per 1 million patients. In other terms, the risk received from an x-ray mammogram that uses a screen-film combination is equivalent to that associated with smoking several cigarettes, driving 60 miles in an automobile, or being a 60-year-old man for 10 minutes.

Fig. 21-6 shows a chart displaying average values for mean glandular dose and estimates of image quality in mammography for the period from the early 1970s to 2005. Doses in mammography have consistently decreased with time, with the most substantial reductions in dose occurring from the early 1970s to the early 1980s. Image quality data are presented from the mid-1980s to the present and show consistent improvement with time.[2]

An important observation in the previously mentioned population studies is that the breast tissue of young women in their teenage years to early 20s seems to be much more sensitive to radiation than the breast tissue of women older than 30 years. Because breast irradiation is a concern, radiologic examinations need to be performed with only the radiation dose that is necessary for providing accurate detection.

[1]Haus AG: Screen-film and digital mammography image quality and radiation dose considerations, *Radiol Clin North Am* 38:871, 2000.
[2]Spelic DC: *FDA updated trends in mammography dose and image quality—related article: dose and image quality in mammography: trends during the first decade of MQSA,* Available at: www.FDA.gov. Accessed August 18, 2009.

[d]American Cancer Society: Cancer Facts & Figures 2013, p11.

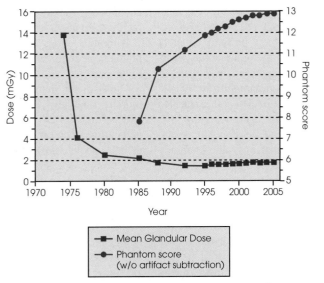

Fig. 21-6 Average values for mean glandular dose and estimates of image quality in mammography for the period from the early 1970s to 2005.

Screening vs diagnostic mammography

The frequency with which women should undergo screening mammography depends on their age and personal risk of developing breast cancer. Current recommendations from the American Cancer Society and the ACR are that all women older than 40 years should undergo annual mammography and should continue yearly mammography for as long as they are in reasonably good health otherwise. A baseline examination performed sometime before the onset of menopause is useful for comparison during subsequent evaluations. High-risk patients should consider beginning screening mammography at an earlier age.

The term *screening mammography* is applied to a procedure performed on an asymptomatic patient or a patient who presents without any known breast problems. For a procedure to be used as a screening method, it must meet the following criteria:

1. It must be simple.
2. It must be acceptable.
3. It must show high sensitivity.
4. It must show high specificity.
5. It must be reproducible.
6. It must be cost-effective.
7. It must have a low risk-to-benefit ratio.

Mammography is a relatively simple procedure that takes only about 15 minutes to complete. The acceptability of mammography, which is the only radiographic procedure used to screen cancer, has been confirmed in numerous studies. Mammography cannot detect all cancerous lesions, however. An annual clinical breast examination is recommended by the American Cancer Society. Many physicians also recommend that women perform monthly BSEs. Even when mammography is performed properly, approximately 10% of cancers remain radiographically occult, particularly in dense breasts and augmented breasts. Even so, mammography has greater sensitivity and specificity for detecting breast tumors than any other currently available noninvasive diagnostic technique. When compared with magnetic resonance imaging (MRI), ultrasonography, and digital techniques, mammography is more cost-effective and more reproducible when quality control standards are maintained. Mammography must be performed properly to maintain these characteristics, however. As with other imaging modalities, high-quality mammography requires an extremely dedicated staff with the appropriate training and expertise.

Breast cancer screening studies have shown that early detection is essential for reducing mortality and that the most effective approach is to combine clinical breast examination with mammography at directed intervals. Although massive screening efforts initially may seem cost-prohibitive, the actual cost of screening in the long-term is much less than the expenses involved in caring for patients with advanced breast disease. To this end, screening patients at high risk for breast cancer with the addition of annual breast MRI has been added to screening recommendations.

The preceding paragraphs describe the screening of patients who do not have significant breast symptoms. All patients with clinical evidence of significant or potentially significant breast disease should undergo a *diagnostic mammogram* and subsequent work-up as necessary. Diagnostic mammograms are problem-solving examinations in which specific projections are obtained to rule out cancer or to show a suspicious area seen on routine screening projections. They are also indicated if a woman presents with a palpable mass or other symptom. The area of interest may be better shown using image enhancement methods, such as spot compression and the magnification technique. Further work-up may be necessary if mammography does not show a correlative mass. Alternative imaging modalities such as ultrasonography are often used to complete a successful work-up. The radiologist and radiographer direct and conduct the diagnostic mammogram to facilitate an accurate interpretation.

Although most diagnostic mammograms conclude with probable benign findings, some women are asked to return for subsequent mammograms in 3 or 6 months to assess for interval changes. Other women must consult with a specialist or surgeon about possible options such as fine-needle aspiration biopsy (FNAB), core biopsy, or excisional biopsy.

Although it is an excellent tool for detecting breast cancer, mammography does *not* permit diagnosis of breast cancer. Some lesions may appear consistent with malignant disease but turn out to be completely benign conditions. Breast cancer can be diagnosed only by a pathologist through evaluation of tissue extracted from the lesion. After interpreting the diagnostic work-up, the radiologist must carefully determine whether core biopsy and/or surgical intervention is warranted.

RISK FACTORS

Assessing a woman's risk for developing breast cancer is complicated. An accurate patient history must be elicited to identify potential individual risk factors. The radiologist considers these known risks after interpreting the mammogram. Other than gender, factors that are known to influence the development of breast cancer include age, hormonal history, and family history.

Besides being female, increasing age is the most important risk factor for breast cancer. Potentially modifiable risk factors include weight gain after age 18, being overweight or obese (for postmenopausal breast cancer), use of menopausal hormone therapy (combined estrogen and progestin), physical inactivity, and alcohol consumption. Medical findings that predict higher risk include high breast tissue density (a mammographic measure of the amount of glandular tissue relative to fatty tissue), high bone mineral density (women with low density are at increased risk for osteoporosis), and biopsy-confirmed hyperplasia (overgrowth of cells), especially atypical hyperplasia (overgrowth of abnormal cells). High-dose radiation to the chest for cancer treatment also increases risk. Reproductive factors that increase risk include a long menstrual history (menstrual periods that start early and/or end later in life), recent use of oral contraceptives, never having children, and having one's first child after age 30.

Risk is also increased by a family history of breast cancer, particularly having one or more first-degree relatives with breast cancer (although most women with breast cancer do not have a family history of the disease). Inherited mutations (alterations) in breast cancer susceptibility genes account for approximately 5% to 10% of all female breast cancers and an estimated 4% to 40% of all male breast cancers but are very rare in the general population (much less than 1%). Most of these mutations are located in *BRCA1* and *BRCA2* genes, although mutations in other known genes have also been identified. Individuals with a strong family history of breast and certain other cancers, such as ovarian and colon cancer, should consider counseling to determine whether genetic testing is appropriate. Prevention measures may be possible for individuals with breast cancer susceptibility mutations. In *BRCA1* and *BRCA2* mutation carriers, studies suggest that prophylactic removal of the ovaries and/or breasts decreases the risk of breast cancer considerably, although not all women who choose this surgery would have developed breast cancer. Women who consider prophylactic surgery should undergo counseling before reaching a decision. The drugs tamoxifen and raloxifene have been approved to reduce breast cancer risk in women at high risk. Raloxifene appears to have a lower risk of certain side effects, such as uterine cancer and blood clots; however, it is approved only for use in postmenopausal women.

Limited but accumulating evidence suggests that long-term heavy smoking increases the risk of breast cancer, particularly among women who began smoking at an early age. The International Agency for Research on Cancer has concluded that limited evidence indicates that shift work, particularly at night, is also associated with an increased risk of breast cancer.[e]

---

[e]American Cancer Society: Cancer Facts and Figures 2013.

Breast

The terms *breast* and *mammary gland* are often used synonymously. Anatomy textbooks tend to use the term *mammary gland,* whereas radiography textbooks tend to use the term *breast.* The breasts (mammary glands) are lobulated glandular structures located within the *superficial fascia* of the anterolateral surface of the thorax of both males and females. The mammary glands divide the superficial fascia into anterior and posterior components. The mammary tissue is completely surrounded by fascia and is enveloped between the anterior and posterior layers of the superficial fascia. In females, the breasts are secondary sex characteristics and function as accessory glands to the reproductive system by producing and secreting milk during lactation. In males, the breasts are rudimentary and without function. Male breasts are subject to abnormalities such as neoplasms that require radiologic evaluation; however this occurs more rarely than in female breasts.

Female breasts vary considerably in size and shape, depending on the amount of fat and glandular tissue and the condition of the suspensory ligaments. Each breast is usually cone-shaped, with the base or posterior surface of the breast overlying the *pectoralis major* and *serratus anterior* muscles. These muscles extend from the second or third rib inferiorly to the sixth or seventh rib, and from near the lateral margin of the sternum laterally toward the anterior axillary plane. An additional portion of breast tissue, the *axillary prolongation* or *axillary tail (AT),* extends from the upper lateral base of the breasts into the *axillary fossa* (Fig. 21-7).

The breast tapers anteriorly from the base, ending in the *nipple,* which is surrounded by a circular area of pigmented skin called the *areola.* The breasts are supported by *Cooper's ligaments,* suspensory ligaments that extend from the posterior layers of the superficial fascia through the anterior fascia into the subcutaneous tissue and skin. It is the condition of these ligaments—not the relative fat content—that gives the breasts their firmness or lack of firmness.

The adult female breast consists of 15 to 20 *lobes,* which are distributed such that more lobes are superior and lateral than inferior and medial. Each lobe is divided into many *lobules,* which are the basic structural units of the breast. The lobules contain the glandular elements, or *acini.* Each lobule consists of several acini, numerous draining ducts, and the interlobular stroma or connective tissue. These elements are part of the breast parenchyma and participate in hormonal changes. By the late teenage years to early 20s, each breast contains several hundred lobules. These lobules tend to decrease in size with increasing age, particularly after pregnancy—a normal process called *involution.*

The openings of each *acinus* join to form *lactiferous ductules* that drain the lobules, which join to form 15 to 20 lactiferous ducts, one for each lobe. Several lactiferous ducts may combine before emptying directly into the nipple. As a result, there are usually fewer duct openings on the nipple than there are breast ducts and lobes. The individual lobes are incompletely separated from each other by Cooper's ligaments. The space between the lobes contains fatty tissue and additional connective tissue. A layer of fatty tissue surrounds the gland, except in the area immediately under the areola and nipple (Fig. 21-8).

The lymphatic vessels of the breast drain laterally into the *axillary lymph nodes* and medially into the chain of *internal mammary lymph nodes* (Fig. 21-9). Approximately 75% of lymph drainage is toward the axilla, and 25% is toward the internal mammary chain. The number of axillary nodes varies from 12 to 30 (sometimes more). The axilla is occasionally radiographed during breast examinations so the axillary nodes can be evaluated. The internal mammary nodes are situated behind the sternum and manubrium and, if enlarged, are occasionally visible on a lateral chest radiograph.

The radiographer must take into account breast anatomy and patient body habitus to successfully image as much breast tissue as possible. Image receptor (IR) size and compression paddles must be appropriate for the breast being imaged. Larger breasts would not be entirely shown on small IRs. Conversely, smaller breasts should not be imaged on larger IRs because (1) other body structures may interfere with the compression device, resulting in an unacceptable image; and (2) the pectoral muscle and the skin are likely to become taut from upward stretching of the arm, preventing the breast tissue from being completely pulled onto the film.

The natural mobility of the breast is another important consideration. The lateral and inferior aspects of the breast are mobile, whereas the medial and superior aspects are fixed. The breast is most effectively positioned by moving the mobile aspects toward the fixed tissues. Likewise, the radiographer should avoid moving the compression paddle against fixed tissues because this would cause less breast tissue to be imaged.

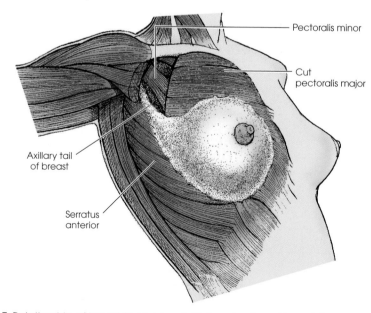

Fig. 21-7 Relationship of breast to chest wall. Note extension of breast tissue posteriorly into axilla.

Pectoralis minor

Cut pectoralis major

Axillary tail of breast

Serratus anterior

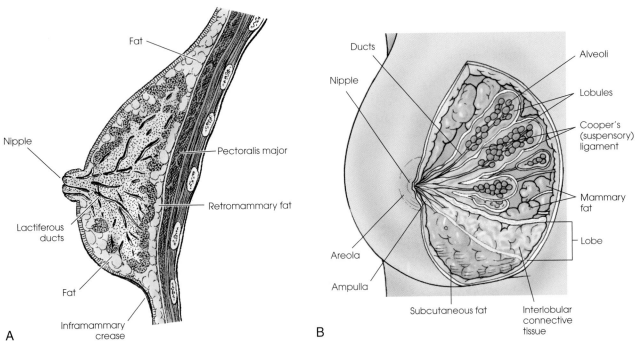

Fig. 21-8 A, Sagittal section through female breast, illustrating structural anatomy. **B,** Breast anterior view.

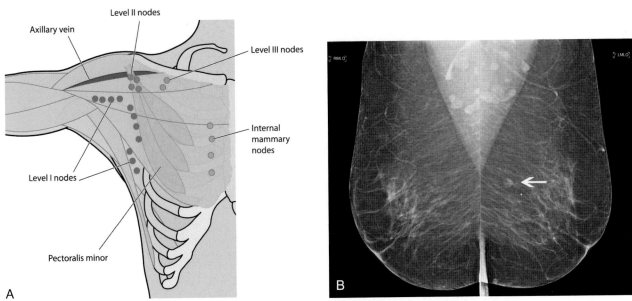

Fig. 21-9 A, Schematic drawing of lymph node system surrounding the breast. **B,** MLO views of the breast often include axillary lymph nodes; occasionally intramammary lymph nodes may also be seen (*arrow*).

Breast

Tissue Variations

The *glandular* and *connective tissues* of the breasts are soft tissue–density structures. The ability to show radiographic detail within the breast depends on the fat within and between the breast lobules and the fat surrounding the breasts. The postpubertal adolescent breast contains primarily dense connective tissue and casts a relatively homogeneous radiographic image with little tissue differentiation. The development of glandular tissue decreases radiographic contrast. During pregnancy, significant hypertrophy of glands and ducts occurs within the breasts. This change causes the breasts to become extremely dense and opaque (Fig. 21-10). After the end of lactation, considerable involution of glandular and parenchymal tissues usually occurs, and these tissues are replaced with increased amounts of *fatty tissue*. Fat accumulation varies markedly among individuals. This normal fat accumulation significantly increases the natural radiographic contrast within the breasts. The breasts of patients with fibrocystic parenchymal conditions may not undergo this involution.

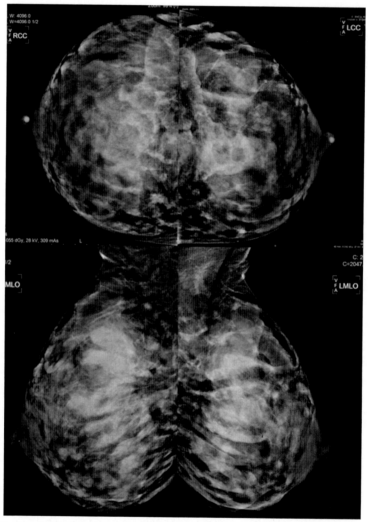

Fig. 21-10 CC and MLO projections of a nursing mother. During lactation, the breasts become very dense and opaque as the ducts and glands become hypertrophic and engorged with milk. If mammography must be performed on a nursing mother, it is best to have the patient nurse or pump her breasts immediately before imaging.

The glandular and connective tissue elements of the breast can regenerate as needed for subsequent pregnancies. After menopause, the glandular and stromal elements undergo gradual atrophy. External factors such as surgical menopause and hormone replacement therapy (HRT) may inhibit this normal process. From puberty through menopause, mammotrophic hormones influence cyclic changes in the breasts. The glandular and connective tissues are in a state of constant change (Fig. 21-11).

Breast tissue density is the ratio of fatty to glandular tissue within the breast. The more glandular tissue, the denser the breast, meaning that it is more difficult for x-rays to penetrate the tissue. Breasts are classified into four density ranges: fatty, scattered, heterogeneously dense, and extremely dense (Fig. 21-12). Breast density has been brought to the forefront recently, with several states mandating that patients are told the composition of their personal breast density and the classification that the radiologist has reported.

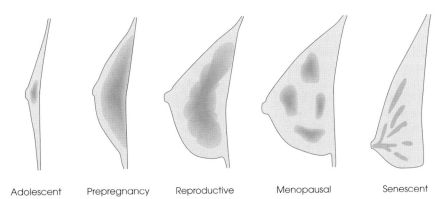

Adolescent   Prepregnancy   Reproductive   Menopausal   Senescent

Fig. 21-11 Diagrammatic profile drawings of breast, illustrating most likely variation and distribution of radiographic density (*shaded areas*) related to the normal life cycle from adolescence to senescence. This normal sequence may be altered by external factors, such as pregnancy, hormone medications, surgical menopause, and fibrocystic breast condition.

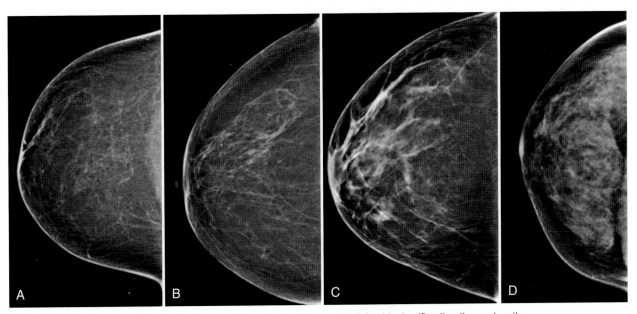

Fig. 21-12 When reading the mammogram, the radiologist classifies the tissue density into one of four categories based on the ratio of fatty to glandular tissue within the breast: **A,** Fatty. **B,** Scattered. **C,** Heterogeneously dense. **D,** Extremely dense.

PATHOLOGIC AND MAMMOGRAPHIC FINDINGS

Numerous radiographic findings, benign or malignant, can be evident within the breast tissue on any mammogram. Distinguishing the characteristics of a finding is the main function of the mammogram. From these characteristics, the radiologist can make a determination of the probability of malignancy. This helps the radiologist determine whether biopsy of the lesion is necessary, if the lesion is most likely benign, or if the area should be followed carefully for indications of change. Characterization of a finding helps the radiologist make these determinations, but it must be kept in mind that cancer is a very tricky disease, and sometimes even the most benign-appearing lesion can be found to be malignant. Therefore, sometimes biopsies are performed on probable benign lesions to ensure that they are benign.

Each breast is a symmetric mirror image of the other. Subtle variations may normally occur from one breast to the other, but an asymmetric variation that is new or enlarging can be cause for concern and can lead to a more thorough work-up. These variations generally present as a mass or density, calcifications within the tissue, or distortion within the architecture of the breast tissue. When these findings are noted on a screening mammogram, the radiologist will often request additional diagnostic mammography views or specialized imaging such as ultrasonography for a more clear view of the area of concern.

Masses

A mass is generally categorized by its shape, by the margins of the mass, and by its radiographic density.

- The *shape* of a lesion is described as round, oval, lobular, or irregular. A round or oval mass is more likely to indicate benign pathology such as a cyst (a fluid-filled pocket within the tissue) or a lymph node (depending on its location). An irregularly shaped mass can more likely indicate a malignancy, or it can be an indication of trauma to an area of breast tissue. This illustrates the importance of taking a thorough patient history.
- The *margins,* or borders, of the mass are described as circumscribed (meaning well defined or sharply defined), microlobulated, obscured (meaning that parts are hidden by superimposed tissue), indistinct or ill defined, or spiculated (showing fine spicules radiating from the center of the mass). Margin characteristics help the clinician to predict whether a mass is malignant or benign.

A mass with a well-defined border is more likely to be benign. Masses with obscured, ill-defined, indistinct margins are suspicious, and a spiculated mass is more worrisome. Microlobulated masses have a 50% chance of being malignant. Post-biopsy scarring may appear as a spiculated mass, and an accurate patient history revealing previous breast biopsies can prevent an unnecessary work-up (Fig. 21-13).

- Examples of benign stellate or spiculated lesions include radial scar, fat necrosis, breast abscess, and sclerosing adenosis. Examples of benign circumscribed masses include fibroadenoma (Fig. 21-14), cyst, intramammary lymph node, hematoma, and galactocele.
- *Density* may be described as high density, equal density or isodense, low density, or radiolucent. Breast cancer that forms a visible mass is more likely to be higher in density than the fibroglandular tissue surrounding it, but it can be of equal density. However, breast cancers never contain fatty tissue. Masses that are radiolucent contain fat and are overwhelmingly benign appearing. These include oil cysts, lipomas, galactoceles, and mixed tissue lesions such as hamartomas and fibrolipadenomas (Fig. 21-15).

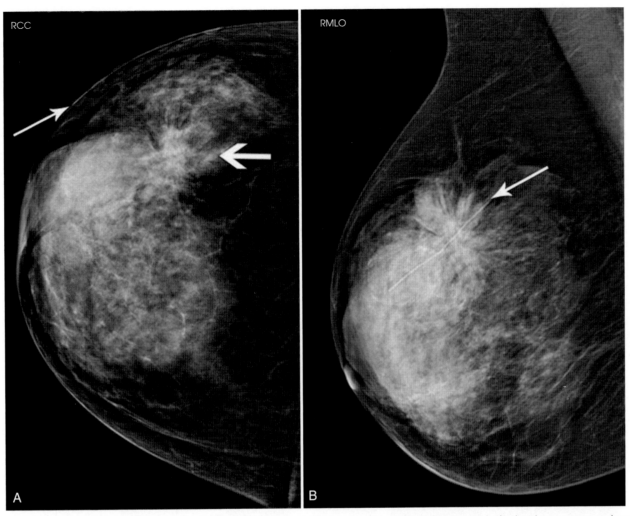

Fig. 21-13 A, RCC projection of a patient who had previously undergone surgical biopsy for removal of a benign mass reveals an area of architectural distortion with spiculated borders. **B,** MLO projection reveals that the area coincides with the surgical scar. Note the radiopaque skin marker that the technologist placed over the site of the scar (*thin arrows*).

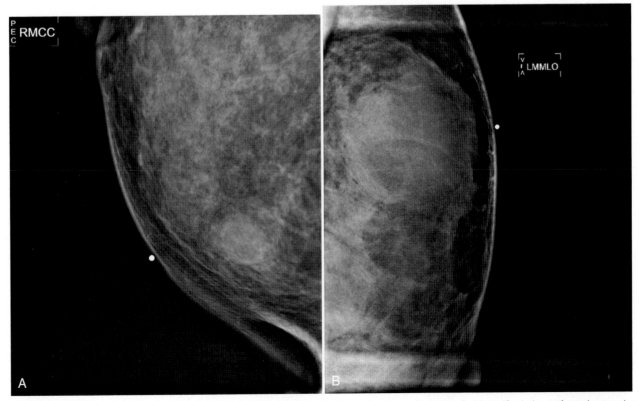

Fig. 21-14 Circumscribed masses are often benign. **A,** TAN MAG projection of a fibroadenoma. **B,** Magnified view of a retroareolar cyst. A mass is determined to be solid or cystic (fluid-filled) on ultrasound.

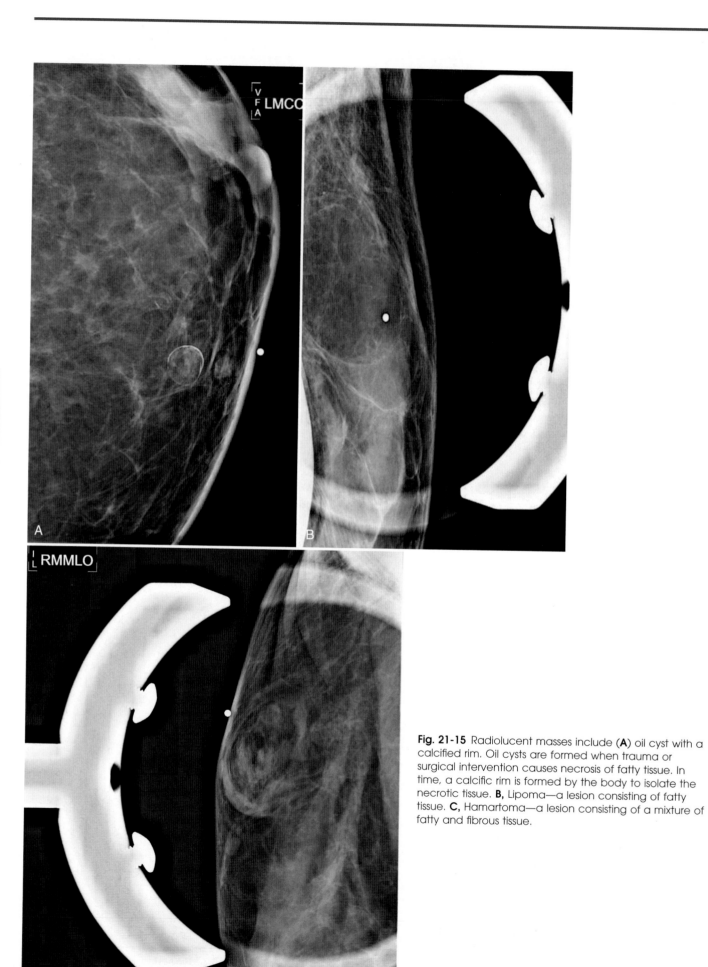

Fig. 21-15 Radiolucent masses include (**A**) oil cyst with a calcified rim. Oil cysts are formed when trauma or surgical intervention causes necrosis of fatty tissue. In time, a calcific rim is formed by the body to isolate the necrotic tissue. **B,** Lipoma—a lesion consisting of fatty tissue. **C,** Hamartoma—a lesion consisting of a mixture of fatty and fibrous tissue.

The malignant or benign nature of a mass cannot be determined on the basis of *location*. Most cancers are detected in the UOQ of the breast; however, most breast lesions—malignant and benign—are found in that quadrant. Cancer can occur in any region of the breast with a certain degree of probability. It is important to determine the location of a lesion for additional diagnostic procedures such as core biopsy or open surgical biopsy.

Interval change may increase the suspicion of malignancy. The radiologist carefully compares current images with previous ones and notes whether the mass is newly apparent, an interval enlargement is present, the borders have become nodular or ill defined, a mass has increased in density, or calcifications have appeared (Fig. 21-16).

Almost all (98%) of the axillary lymph nodes are located in the UOQ. These nodes are well circumscribed, may have a central or peripheral area of fat, and can be kidney bean–shaped (see Fig. 21-9). If the lymph nodes appear normal, they are rarely mentioned in the context of an identifiable mass on the radiology report.

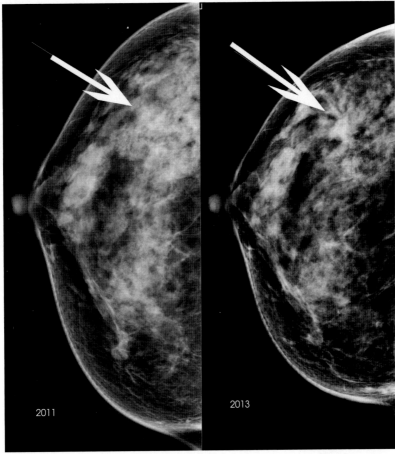

Fig. 21-16 Interval change. A change in tissue architecture and density was noted during a screening mammogram on this 51-year-old woman. Core biopsy of this area was positive for invasive ductal carcinoma.

A *density* that is seen on only one projection is not confirmed three-dimensionally and may represent superimposed structures. These may appear to have scalloped edges or concave borders or both. The radiologist may request spot compression projections, rolled projections, or angled projections to confirm or rule out the presence of a real density. A suspicious density seen on only one projection within the breast is often a summation shadow of superimposed breast parenchyma and disappears when the breast tissue is spread apart (Fig. 21-17).

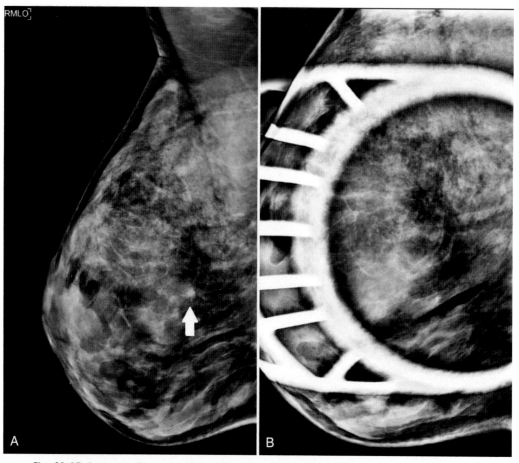

Fig. 21-17 An area of increased density was noted on this MLO projection of the right breast (**A**). Spot compression of this area (**B**), also performed in the MLO position, spreads the tissue out more uniformly. The density was no longer seen, indicating that overlapped tissue was causing a summation shadow.

Calcifications

Calcifications are often normal metabolic occurrences within the breast and are usually benign. Approximately 15% to 25% of microcalcifications found in asymptomatic women are associated with cancer, however. These calcifications can have definitive characteristics. Because of size, some microcalcifications are more difficult to interpret. The most valuable tool for defining microcalcifications is a properly performed image obtained using the magnification technique. Using this image, the radiologist can determine better whether calcifications are suspicious and warrant further work-up.

Calcifications are categorized by size, shape, and distribution. Benign calcifications are generally larger, coarser, rounder, and smoother. Typically, they are easily seen on the mammogram, whereas malignant calcifications are usually very small, often requiring magnification to be seen (Fig. 21-18).

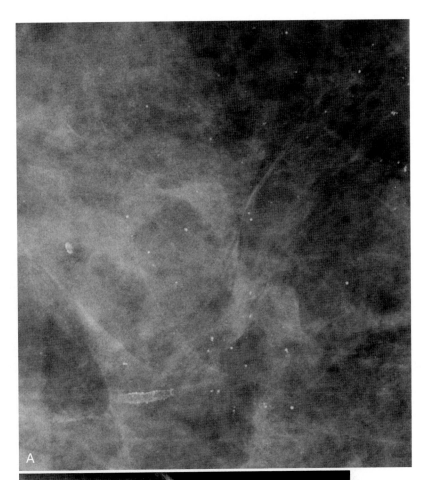

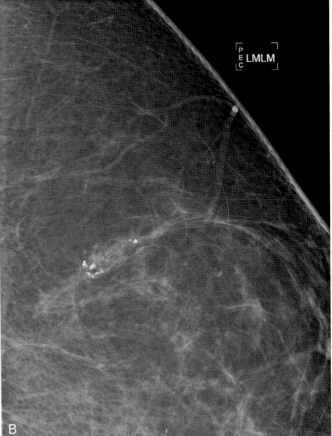

Fig. 21-18 Examples of benign calcifications seen on mammography: **A,** Coarse and round calcification. **B,** Calcifications caused by dystrophic fat necrosis. *Continued*

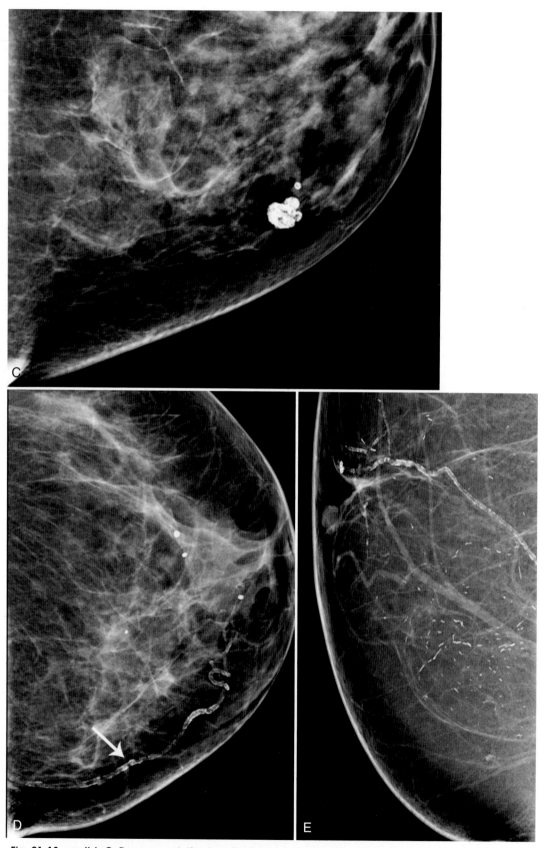

Fig. 21-18, cont'd C, Popcorn calcification. **D,** Vascular calcification. **E,** Rodlike secretory calcifications.

Benign calcifications may have one or more of the following attributes: moderate size, scattered location, round shape, and, usually, bilateral occurrence. In addition, they may be eggshell (lucent center), arterial (parallel tracks), crescent, or sedimented ("teacup" milk of calcium). Calcifications may represent a fibroadenoma ("popcorn"), postsurgical scarring (sheets or large strands of calcium), skin calcifications (which can mimic suspicious microcalcifications within the breast parenchyma), and vascular calcifications. Vascular calcifications are often noted, and studies have indicated that vascular calcifications in women younger than 50 years of age may suggest potential risk for coronary artery disease.

- The projection suggested for better defined sedimented milk of calcium is the 90-degree lateral projection—lateromedial (LM) or mediolateral (ML). If possible, the mammographer should select the lateral projection that places the suspected area closest to the IR. The 90-degree lateral is also used as a triangulation projection before needle localization and to show air-fluid-fat levels (Fig. 21-19).

Calcifications that are suspicious and cause intermediate concern are categorized as amorphous or indistinct, or coarse heterogeneous calcifications. Amorphous or indistinct calcifications appear small and hazy. When diffusely scattered, they can usually be dismissed as benign, but when clustered, they may warrant biopsy. Coarse heterogeneous calcifications are conspicuous and irregularly shaped, are generally larger than 0.5 mm, and can be associated with malignancy, but they also may be present in areas of fibrosis, within fibroadenomas, or in areas of trauma.

Fine pleomorphic calcifications and fine linear or branching calcifications indicate a higher probability of malignancy. The fine linear type suggests filling of the lumen of a duct involved in a breast cancer. Fine pleomorphic forms vary in shape but are generally smaller than 0.5 mm (Fig. 21-20).

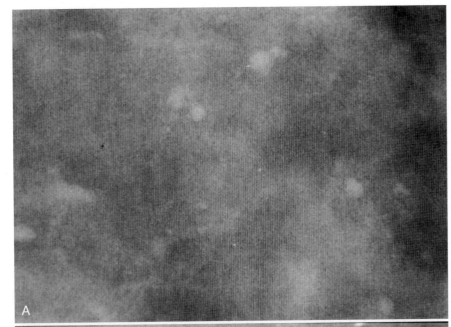
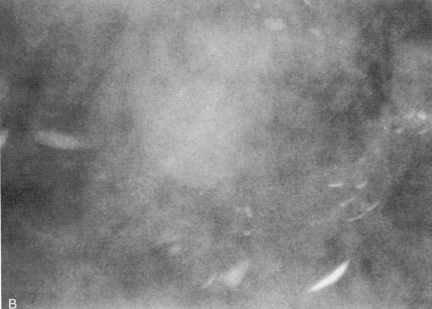

Fig. 21-19 Milk of calcium occurs when residual milk remains in the alveoli following lactation. Over time, the calcium within the milk solidifies into tiny particles that become sediment. On the CC projection, it appears as rounded low-density areas (**A**). On the ML projection, the sediment appears crescent shaped as it settles, in a "teacup" appearance (**B**).

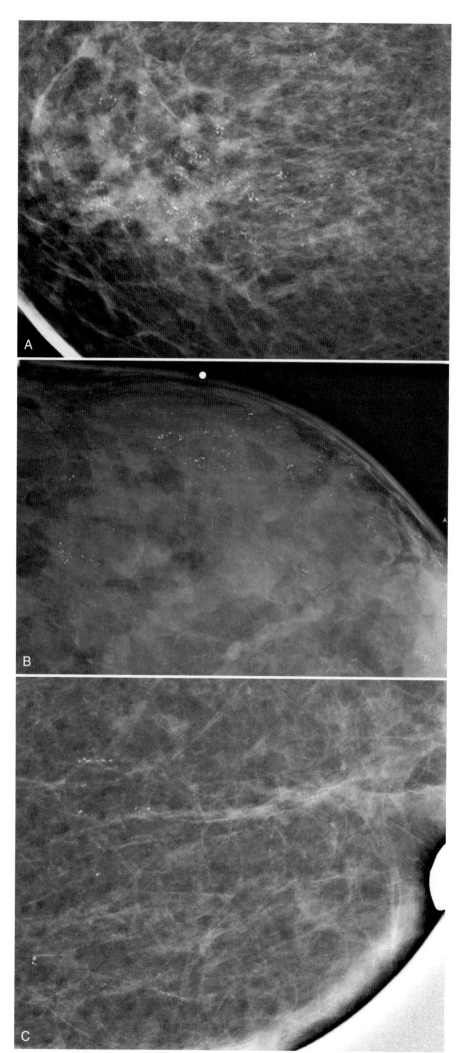

Fig. 21-20 Examples of calcifications seen on mammography that are suspicious or have a high probability of indicating cancer. **A,** These amorphous, diffuse calcifications proved to be ductal carcinoma in situ (DCIS) on biopsy. **B,** These linear, branching calcifications proved to be invasive ductal carcinoma on biopsy. **C,** Pleomorphic linear calcifications proved to be DCIS.

The distribution of the calcifications describes the arrangement of calcifications in the breast. Diffuse or scattered calcifications are usually benign and usually bilateral. Regional distribution of calcifications indicates that a large volume of breast tissue contains calcifications. A group or cluster of calcifications indicates a minimum of five calcifications occupying a small volume of breast tissue. Linear distribution calcifications are arranged in a line, suggesting deposits within a duct. Segmental distribution suggests deposits in ducts and the possibility of extensive or multifocal breast cancer. Although benign causes of segmental calcifications are known, segmental distribution of otherwise benign-appearing calcifications elevates suspicion of carcinoma.

Architectural Distortions

When the normal architecture of the breast tissue is distorted but no definitive mass is visible, this is called *architectural distortion* (AD). AD is seen as a presentation of thin lines or spiculations radiating from a central point. Focal retraction or distortion of the edge of the parenchyma may also be present. Architectural distortion can be associated with a mass or with asymmetry or calcifications. A history of trauma or of prior surgery may present as architectural distortion, but in the absence of this history, AD is suspicious for malignancy or radial scar, and biopsy of the area is appropriate (Fig. 21-21).

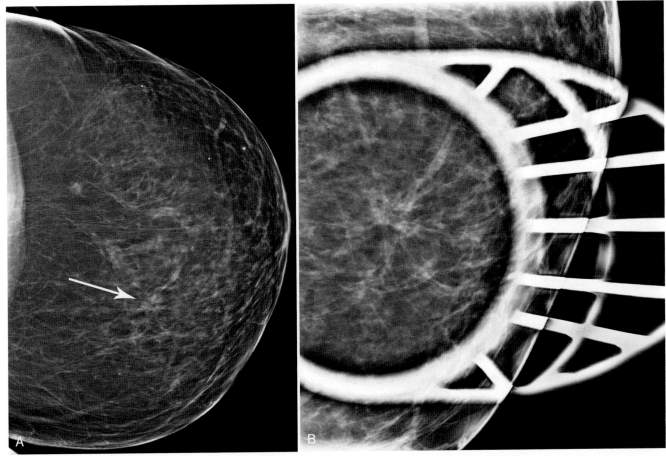

Fig. 21-21 Architectural distortion is seen on this CC projection (**A**). Spot compression view (**B**) of this area confirms that this is a mass, not overlapped tissue. This proved to be invasive ductal carcinoma on biopsy.

FFDM MANUAL TECHNIQUE CHART

Compressed thickness	Target	Fatty breast filter	kVp	mAs	Target	50% fatty–50% dense filter	kVp	mAs	Target	Dense breast filter	kVp	mAs
Amorphous selenium detector												
<3 cm	Mo	Mo	28	70	Mo	Mo	28	80	Mo	Mo	28	90
3-5 cm	Mo	Mo	28	80	Mo	Mo	28	80	Mo	Mo	28	90
5-7 cm	Mo	Rh	29	100	Rh	Rh	29	100	Rh	Rh	29	100
>7 cm	Rh	Rh	30	120	Rh	Rh	30	140	Rh	Rh	30	160
CCD detector												
<3 cm	Mo	Mo	25	32	Mo	Mo	26	28	Mo	Mo	26	36
3-4 cm	Mo	Mo	36	36	Mo	Rh	26	45	Mo	Rh	27	50
4-5 cm	Rh	Rh	28	50	Rh	Rh	29	56	Rh	Rh	29	63
5-6 cm	Rh	Rh	29	56	Rh	Rh	29	63	Rh	Rh	30	71
6-7 cm	Rh	Rh	29	71	Rh	Rh	29	80	Rh	Rh	30	80
7-8 cm	Rh	Rh	29	80	Rh	Rh	30	90	Rh	Rh	31	80
>8 cm	Rh	Rh	30	90	Rh	Rh	30	140	Rh	Rh	31	140

Note: Manual techniques based on use of grid and taut compression.

Mammography

SUMMARY OF ANATOMY

Mammary gland (breast)	Axillary fossa	Axillary lymph nodes
Superficial fascia	Nipple	Internal mammary lymph nodes
Pectoralis major muscle	Areola	Glandular tissue
Serratus anterior muscle	Cooper's ligaments	Connective tissue
Axillary prolongation (axillary tail)	Lobes	Fatty tissue
	Acini	
	Lactiferous ductules	

SUMMARY OF PATHOLOGY

Radiographic Findings	Definition
Masses and Margins	
• Circumscribed	Smooth borders; mostly benign
• Indistinct	Ill-defined borders
• Spiculated	Mass with thin, elongated lines of tissue emerging from its center
Architectural Distortion	The interruption of a regular pattern; when tissue opposes the natural breast pattern flowing from ducts to nipple
Calcifications	
Radiographic description	
• Round or punctate	Benign spherical calcium that can vary in size with well-defined margins
• Amorphous or indistinct	Small or hazy calcium with no clearly defined shape or form
• Course heterogeneous	Large calcium deposits of various sizes clustered together
• Fine heterogeneous	Small calcium deposits of various sizes clustered together. Usually less than 0.5 mm in diameter with a high probability of malignancy

Radiographic Findings	Definition
Benign Calcifications	
• Popcorn-type	Large, thick, dense, popcorn shaped; often result from involuting fibroadenomas
• Rim calcifications	Calcifications residing along the border of benign masses such as cysts, oil cysts, or sebaceous cysts
• Milk of calcium (teacup)	Found in microcysts, which contain radiopaque particles mixed with fluid
• Arterial calcifications	Found within vessels resulting from arterial atherosclerosis
• Skin calcifications	Found within the dermal layer of the breast, usually with smooth outlines and radiolucent centers
Benign Pathologies	
• Cyst	Fluid-filled sac with distinct edges and round or oval in shape
• Galactocele	Milk-filled cyst typically found in lactating women
• Fibroadenoma	Solid benign tumor of glandular and connective tissue with clearly defined margins. Often easy to move
• Lipoma	Growth of fatty cells
• Hamartoma	Typically well-circumscribed lesion comprised of fibrous, glandular, and fatty tissue
• Papilloma	Growth inside the ducts; may cause discharge
• Ductal ectasia	Dilation of milk ducts with thickening of the walls; may cause discharge or fluid blockage
• Hematoma	Collection of blood within the tissue, typically resulting from trauma
• Abscess and inflammation	Accumulation of pus with swelling as a result of infection
• Fat necrosis	Lucent area within the breast resulting from trauma, surgery, or radiation therapy
High-Risk Conditions	
• Lobular carcinoma in situ (LCIS)	Abnormal cell growth within the lobules or milk glands
• Atypical ductal hyperplasia (ADH)	Increased production or growth within breast ducts causing architectural abnormalities
• Atypical lobular hyperplasia	Increased cell growth within breast lobes
• Radial scar	Complex sclerosing lesion. Benign mass with spiculated borders not related to surgery. Caused by abnormal cell growth
• Papilloma with atypia	The presence of atypical hyperplasia within a papilloma
Malignant Pathologies	
• Ductal carcinoma in situ (DCIS)	Abnormal, cancerous cells within the milk ducts
• Invasive/Infiltrating ductal carcinoma	Cancerous cells that started in the milk ducts and have spread to surrounding breast tissue. Most common type of breast cancer
• Invasive lobular carcinoma	Cancerous cells that started within a lobule and have spread to other breast tissue
• Inflammatory carcinoma	Aggressive carcinoma that blocks the lymph vessels in the skin of the breast, causing signs of inflammation such as swelling, reddening of the skin, or an orange peel–like texture to the skin (peau d'orange)
• Paget's disease	Carcinoma in the skin of the nipple causing a sore, reddened appearance of the nipple and areola. Commonly associated with other types of carcinoma within the breast tissue
• Sarcoma	Cancerous cells that begin in the connective tissue supporting the lobules and ducts of the breast

Summary of Pathology Table

METHOD OF EXAMINATION

Both breasts are routinely radiographed obtaining craniocaudal (CC) and mediolateral oblique (MLO) projections. Image enhancement methods, such as spot compression and the magnification technique, are often useful as diagnostic tools. It is sometimes necessary to enhance images or vary projections to better characterize lesions and calcifications. In symptomatic patients, the examination should not be limited to the symptomatic breast. Both breasts should be examined for comparison purposes and because significant radiographic findings may be shown in a clinically normal breast.

Patient preparation

No specific patient preparations are needed before a mammographic examination to enhance image quality. However, during the mammography procedure, the breasts will be compressed, and this may cause some discomfort to the patient. To help alleviate the discomfort and solicit patient cooperation, some practices recommend that the patient refrain from or reduce caffeine intake for 2 weeks before the examination, or take ibuprofen approximately an hour before the examination.

Artifacts are common in mammography because of the sensitivity of the imaging techniques and the design of the equipment used for mammography (Fig 21-22). To prevent artifacts caused by objects protruding into the image, you may need to ask the patient to remove eyeglasses, earrings, and necklaces. Some hairstyles may need to be pulled or clipped back to prevent the hair from falling forward into the image. It is advisable to dress patients in open-front gowns because the breast must be bared for the examination. The technologist needs to ensure before each exposure that all of the above items, as well as chins, fingers, and other body parts, are outside of the field of radiation.

Some radiology practices require that patients remove any deodorant and powder from the axillary and inframammary regions because these substances can resemble calcifications on the resultant image (Fig. 21-23). Before the breast is radiographed, a complete history is taken, and a careful physical assessment is performed, noting all biopsy scars, palpable masses, suspicious thickenings, skin abnormalities, and nipple alterations (Fig. 21-24).

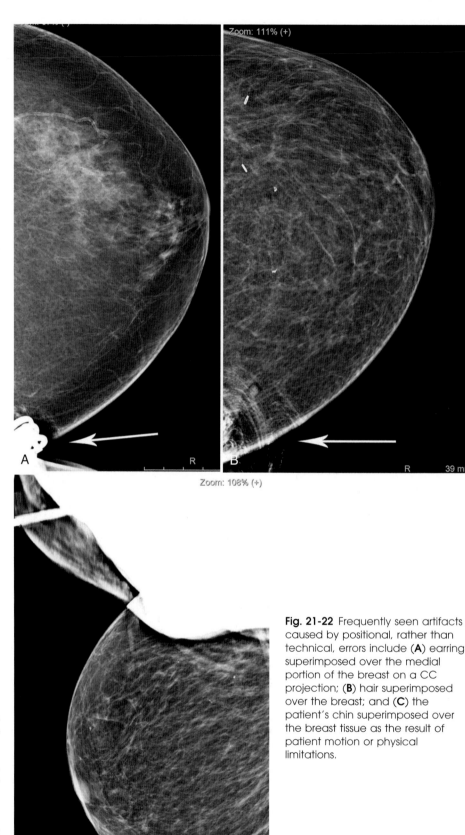

Fig. 21-22 Frequently seen artifacts caused by positional, rather than technical, errors include (**A**) earring superimposed over the medial portion of the breast on a CC projection; (**B**) hair superimposed over the breast; and (**C**) the patient's chin superimposed over the breast tissue as the result of patient motion or physical limitations.

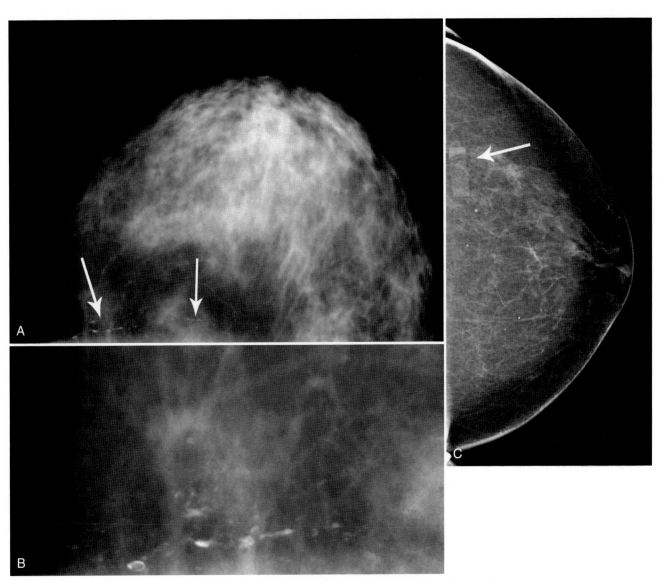

Fig. 21-23 Artifacts are often the result of poor patient preparation. Figures **A** and **B** show pseudocalcifications along the inframammary crease—the result of caked powder. Figure **C** shows a band-aid applied by the patient on the posterior aspect of the breast that was not noticed by the technologist until it was seen on the mammogram.

EWBC MEDICAL HISTORY FORM   M.R.#_____

— *please remember to* **sign the back** *of this form* AND **only use ink** *to fill out this form*—

1. Purpose of today's visit? _____

2. Do you use:

							If discontinued

a. Hormones?   Yes   No   Brand _____ Dosage _____ How long? _____ when? _____

b. Oral Contraceptive?   Yes   No   Brand _____

c. Anti-Estrogen/Breast Cancer Prevention?   Yes   No   Brand _____

3. Do you have breast implants?   Yes   No   *(type)*   Silicone Gel   Saline   Combination   Unknown

4. Are you taking aspirin or blood thinners? Yes   No

5. Are you allergic to any of the following?

a. Medicine(s)?   Yes   No   *(type)* _____

b. Adhesive Tape?   Yes   No

c. Lidocaine?   Yes   No

d. Iodine Contrast Material? Yes   No

e. Latex?   Yes   No

f. Others? _____

6. Do you currently have any of the following? – *please check only those that apply to you and explain below:*

☐ Fever/Chills	☐ Weakness	☐ Leg Swelling	☐ Seasonal Allergies
☐ Eye Problems	☐ Depression	☐ Joint Aches	☐ Stomach Problems
☐ Kidney Problems	Explanation _____		

OFFICE USE ONLY   ☐ All other systems negative

7. Questions for female patients: *(please circle your answers)*

1. How many months since your physician examined your breasts? _____ months

2. Your age at birth of your 1st child.   _____   No biological children ☐

3. Your age at time of 1st menstrual cycle. _____

   a. Are your periods regular?   Yes   No   *if no, date of your last period* _____

4. Age you entered menopause. _____ (If you are no longer having periods for at least one year).

5. Are you pregnant?   Yes   No

6. Are you breastfeeding?   Yes   No

7. Do you have your ovaries?   Yes   No

8. Do you have your uterus?   Yes   No

9. Have you had breast surgery?   Yes   No

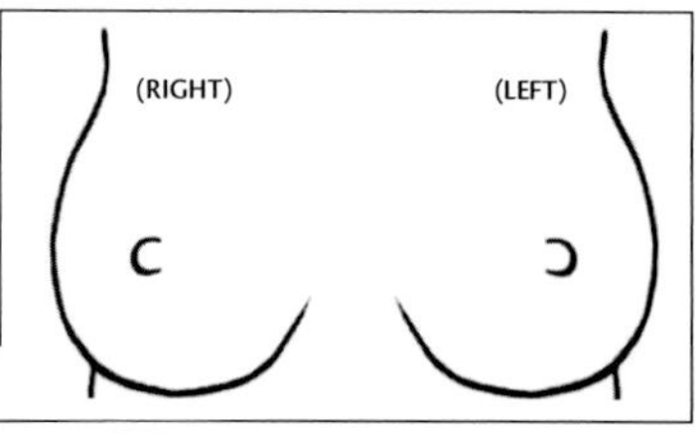

(RIGHT)   (LEFT)

If yes, please mark the area of surgery with the year it was done.

10. Have you ever had radiation therapy to your breast/chest area? ☐ Yes ☐ No if yes, when? _____

11. Have you ever had chemotherapy? ☐ Yes ☐ No   if yes, when? _____ for what? _____

8. Social History: ☐ Male ☐ Female

Marital Status: ☐ Single ☐ Married ☐ Divorced ☐ Partner ☐ Widowed

Occupation: _____

Do you drink alcohol? ☐ Yes ☐ No **if yes,** how often?_____

Do you smoke? check one: ☐ Daily ☐ Occasional ☐ Never Smoked ☐ Former Smoker ☐ Unknown

Race: ☐ American Indian ☐ Alaska Native ☐ Asian ☐ Black or African American

☐ Native Hawaiian or Pacific Islander ☐ White

Ethnicity: ☐ Hispanic or Latino ☐ Not Hispanic or Latino

Preferred Language: ☐ English ☐ Other _____

Please list medications *(include non-prescription medications and birth control pills, write "none" if no medications are used)*

_____ _____ _____
_____ _____ _____
_____ _____ _____
_____ _____ _____

(over)

Fig. 21-24 Sample mammography patient history questionnaire. Note that a good amount of emphasis is placed on patient and family history to determine risk and inclusion for *BRCA* testing and breast MRI.

(Courtesy Elizabeth Wende Breast Care, LLC, Rochester, NY.)

Mammography

9. Medical/Family History: Directions-Check "None" if neither you nor anyone in your family has had this problem. Check "Self" if this is true for you. Check "Family" if a member of your family has had this problem.

	NONE	SELF	FAMILY	
Breast Cysts	☐	☐		
Breast Pain	☐	☐		
Nipple Changes				
Inversion: ☐ Left ☐ Right				
Discharge: ☐ Left ☐ Right				
Rash: ☐ Left ☐ Right				
HIV	☐	☐		
Heart Valve Replacement	☐	☐		
High Blood Pressure	☐	☐		
Pacemaker/Cardiac Stent	☐	☐		
Heart Attack	☐	☐		
Stroke	☐	☐		
Hepatitis/Liver Problems	☐	☐		type: _____
Asthma	☐	☐		
Diabetes	☐	☐	☐	
Arthritis	☐	☐	☐	type: _____
Hives	☐	☐	☐	
Pancreatic Cancer	☐	☐	☐	
Melanoma	☐	☐	☐	
Lymphoma	☐	☐	☐	type: _____
Leukemia	☐	☐	☐	type: _____
Other Cancers	☐	☐	☐	type: _____

(Please list breast and ovarian history below)

Have you ever been tested for BRCA1/BRCA2 Mutations?

☐ **NO** ☐ **YES** If yes, were the results: ☐ **Positive** ☐ **Negative** ☐ **Uncertain Variant**

Are you of Ashkenazi Jewish Ancestry? ☐ **NO** ☐ **YES**

HISTORY OF BREAST CANCER:

☐ **NO** ☐ **YES**

	Age at diagnosis	Age if diagnosed with a second NEW Breast Cancer		Mother *or* Father's side (PLEASE CIRCLE)
Self				
Mother				
Sister				
Daughter				
Brother				
Father				
Son				
Niece				
Nephew				
Grandmother				M F
Grandfather				M F
Aunt				M F
Uncle				M F
Cousin				M F

HISTORY OF OVARIAN CANCER:

☐ **NO** ☐ **YES**

	Age at diagnosis		Mother *or* Father's side (PLEASE CIRCLE)
Self			
Mother			
Sister			
Daughter			
Niece			
Grandmother			M F
Cousin			M F
Aunt			M F

If we may contact you by email, please list your email address: _____

Print Name: _____ Date of birth: _____ Date: _____

Signature: _____ Date: _____

Patient Review: _____ Date: _____ Patient Review: _____ Date: _____

OFFICE USE ONLY	MD Review: _____ Date: _____	MD Review: _____ Date: _____	MD Review: _____ Date: _____

The above information is accurate and any unanswered questions are considered not applicable or negative.   May 3.12

Fig. 21-24, cont'd

EXAMINATION PROCEDURES

This section describes procedures for conducting mammographic examinations. Only dedicated breast imaging equipment should be used to perform mammography. The following steps should be taken:

- If possible, examine previous mammographic studies of patients who are undergoing subsequent mammography screening. These images should be evaluated for positioning, compression, and exposure factors to determine whether any improvement in image quality can be obtained with the current study. Position the breast consistently so that any lesion can be accurately localized and a valid comparison with prior studies can be made.

- Determine the correct image receptor (IR) and compression paddle size for the patient, and use the smallest possible size to image all of the breast tissue fully. Positioning the breast on a surface and detector that is too large causes the skin and muscles to overextend, reducing the amount of posterior tissue imaged, and may compromise the technical image quality. Occasionally, a patient may present with oversized breasts that do not fit completely on the largest IR. When this happens, overlapping images are taken to visualize all of the breast tissue. This is referred to as "mosaic" imaging or tiling, as image tiles are fitted together to form a complete picture (Fig. 21-25).

- Explain the procedure simply and completely to the patient before beginning the examination. It should never be assumed that the patient is fully aware of what the mammographer is about to do, even if the patient has had prior examinations.

- In many cases, routine projections do not sufficiently show all of the breast tissue, and additional projections may be necessary. To allay patient concerns, the mammographer should explain to the patient, before beginning the procedure, why additional projections are sometimes needed and that they do not indicate a potential problem.

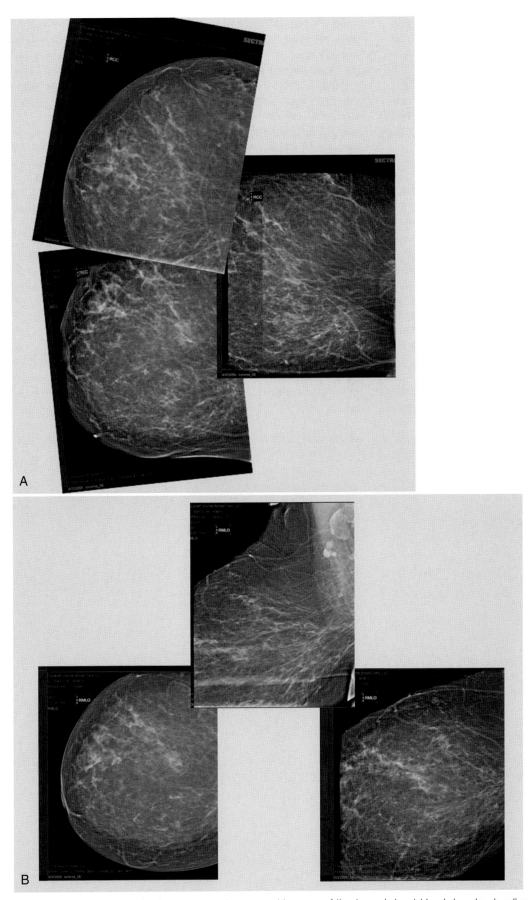

Fig. 21-25 When the breast is larger than the image receptor, several images of the breast should be taken to visualize all of the tissue. **A,** Three mosaic images of the CC projection, taken to image anteromedial, anterolateral, and posterior tissue. **B,** Mosaic images of the MLO view, imaging inferoposterior, anterior, and posteroaxillary tissue.

(Reprinted with permission from Andolina V, Lille S: *Mammographic imaging, a practical guide,* ed 3, Baltimore, 2011, Wolters Kluwer Health/Lippincott Williams & Wilkins.)

- Before positioning the patient's breast and applying compression, consider the natural mobility of the breast, so that patient discomfort can be minimized. The inferior and lateral portions of the breast are mobile, whereas the superior and medial portions are fixed. When possible, the mobile tissues should be moved toward the fixed tissues.

- For each of the two basic breast projections, ensure that the breast is firmly supported and adjusted, so that the nipple is directed forward.

- Profile the nipple, if possible. Obtaining an image of the posterior breast tissue should be the primary consideration, but positioning of the nipple in profile is not always possible. An additional projection can be obtained to profile the nipple, if necessary. Alternatively, a marker may be used to locate clearly the nipple that is not in profile, in which case an additional image may not be needed.

- Apply adequate compression to the breast. Compression is an important factor in achieving a high-quality mammogram. The primary objective of compression is to produce uniform breast thickness from the nipple to the most posterior aspect of the breast. Properly applied compression spreads the breast so that the tissue thickness is more evenly distributed over the image and better separation of the glandular elements is achieved. A rigid, radiolucent mammography compression paddle facilitates breast compression. Generally, compression is applied initially using a hands-free control and is applied manually during the final phase of compression. The compression should be taut but not painful. The skin of a properly compressed breast should feel tight when lightly tapped with the fingertips. When evaluating images, compare the degree of compression with that of previous mammograms, and note any variations. If a patient is unable to tolerate an adequate amount of compression, document this information on the patient history form for the radiologist. Use only as much compression as the patient can tolerate.

- Be sure that standard identification information is included on the image. For FFDM images, all of the pertinent information should be included in the DICOM header. The information should also be seen on the processed and printed image. Often, this DICOM overlay can be turned on or off as needed by the radiologist to prevent interference during interpretation of the image. For film-screen images, the American College of Radiology recommends the following standard conventions (Fig. 21-26):

A. Before processing, photographically expose a permanent identification label that includes on the image the facility's name and address; the date of the examination; and the patient's name, age, date of birth, and medical number. Include the initials of the person performing the examination on the identification label (C).

B. On the IR near the patient's axilla, place a radiopaque marker indicating the side examined and the projection used (Table 21-1).

C. Label the mammography cassette with an identification number (an Arabic numeral is suggested by the ACR).

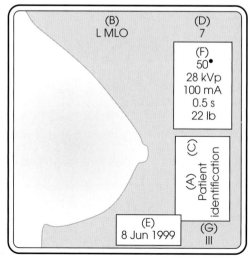

Fig. 21-26 Correct labeling of mammography image: MLO projection.

TABLE 21-1

Labeling codes and uses for mammographic positioning

View	ACR ID	Suggested ID	Projection	C-arm angle	Image receptor placement	Tissue best visualized	Applications
Cranial-Caudal	CC		Sup-Inf	0 degrees	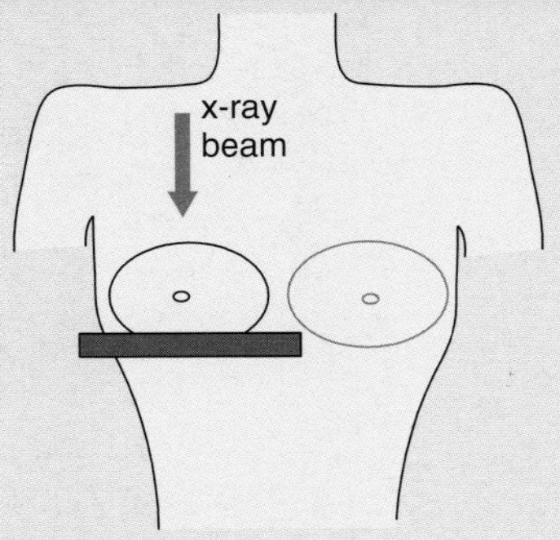	Subareolar, central, medial, and posteromedial tissue	Routine
Exaggerated Cranial-Caudal	XCCL		Sup-Inf	0 degrees	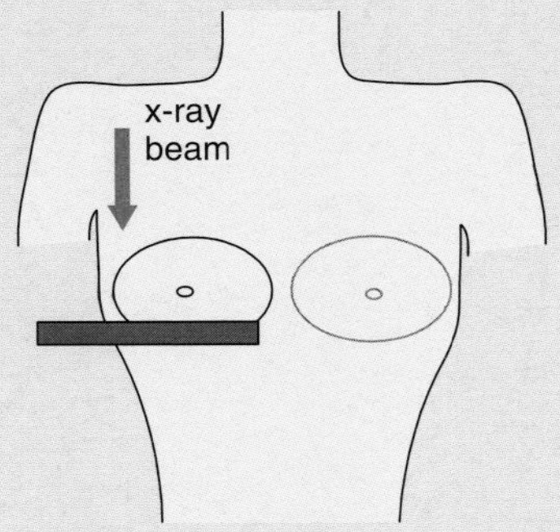	Posterolateral	"Wrap-around" breast
Elevated Cranial-Caudal or Pushed-Up CC	None	ECC	Sup-Inf	0 degrees	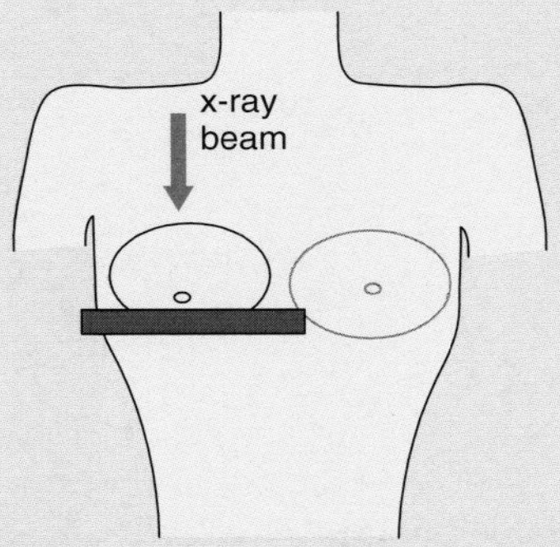	Central and medial, high on chest wall	Superior lesion not seen on CC

Continued

TABLE 21-1

Labeling codes and uses for mammographic positioning—cont'd

View	ACR ID	Suggested ID	Projection	C-arm angle	Image receptor placement	Tissue best visualized	Applications
Caudal-Cranial	FB	Inf-Sup	0 degrees	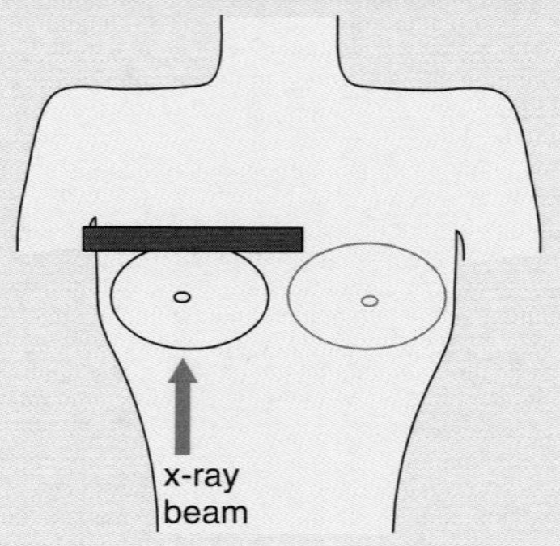	Central and medial, high on chest wall	Non-conforming pt, superior lesion not seen on CC
Mediolateral Lateral	ML	Med-Lat	90 degrees	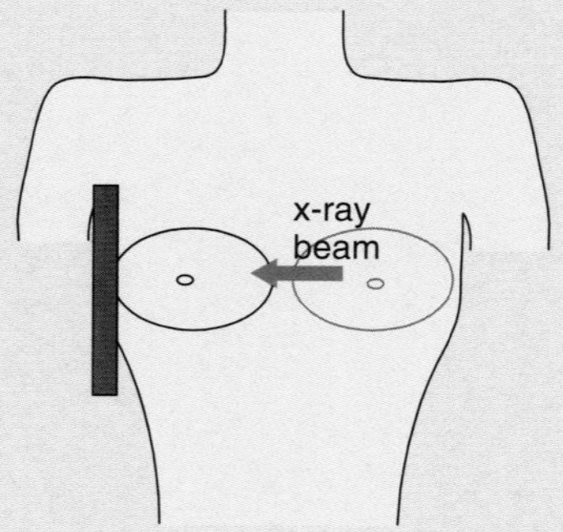	Lateral, central, superior, and inferior	True orthogonal to CC for lesion localization, opens tissue for structural overlap
Lateromedial Lateral	LM	Lat-Med	90 degrees	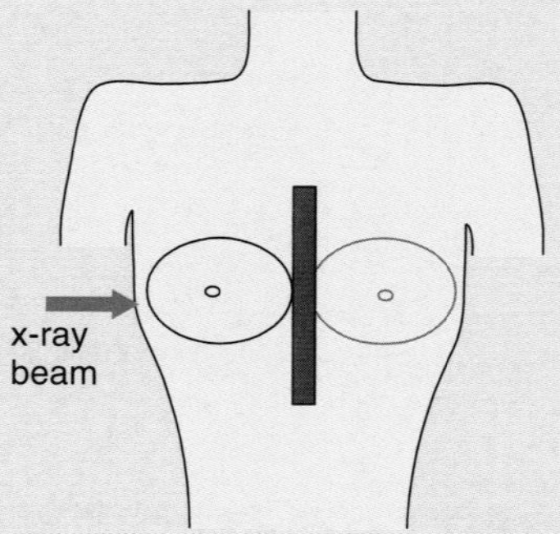	Medial, central, superior, and inferior	True orthogonal to CC for lesion localization, opens tissue for structural overlap

Medial-Lateral Oblique	MLO	30-60 degrees	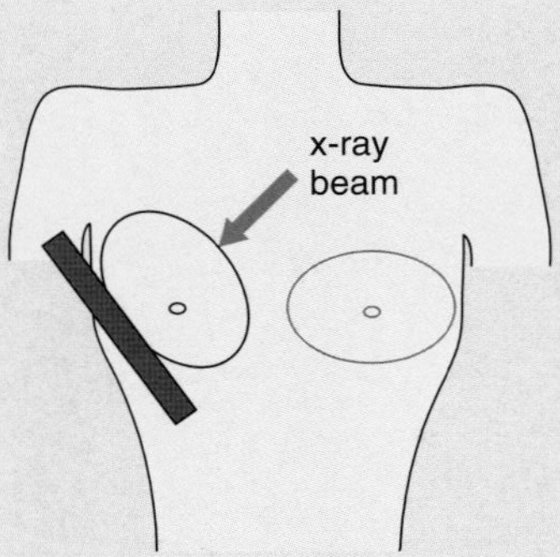	Posterior, upper outer quadrant, axillary tail, lower inner quadrant	Routine
Superolateral-Inferomedial Oblique	SIO	1-90 degrees	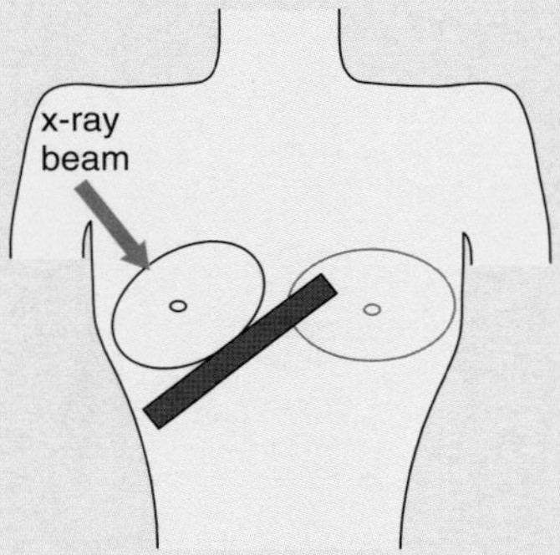	Posterior, medial, upper inner quadrant, lower outer quadrant	Additional view for encapsulated implants, non-conforming pt, orthogonal to MLO for localization
Inferolateral-Superomedial Oblique	LMO	90-180 degrees	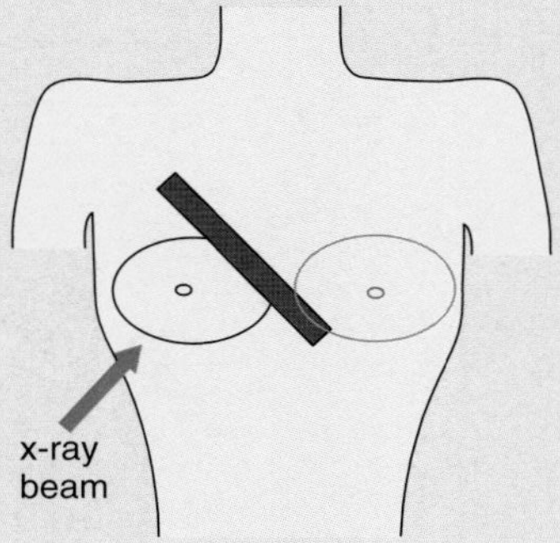	Posterior, medial, upper outer quadrant, lower inner quadrant	Can replace MLO in pts with pacemakers, open heart surgical scars

Continued

405

Mammography

TABLE 21-1
Labeling codes and uses for mammographic positioning—cont'd

View	ACR ID	Suggested ID	Projection	C-arm angle	Image receptor placement	Tissue best visualized	Applications
Inferomedial-Superolateral Oblique	None	ISO	IM-SL	90-180 degrees	x-ray beam	Lateral, upper inner quadrant, lower outer quadrant	Stereotactic positioning
Axillary Tail	AT		SM-IL	60-80 degrees	x-ray beam	Posterior-lateral, axillary tail	
Axilla	None	AX	SM-IL	70-90 degrees	x-ray beam	Axillary content	Additional view for cancer patients on affected side, suspected inflammatory ca, lymphadenopathy, search for primary ca

View	Abbr.	Angle	Projection	Diagram	Region	Purpose
Cleavage View	CV	0 degrees	Sup-Inf		Medial	Extreme medial tissue, slippery medial lesions
Rolled Lateral	RL	0 degrees	Sup-Inf		Subareolar, central, medial, and posteromedial tissue	Separation of superimposed glandular tissue
Rolled Medial	RM	0 degrees	Sup-Inf		Subareolar, central, medial, and posteromedial tissue	Separation of superimposed glandular tissue

Continued

TABLE 21-1

Labeling codes and uses for mammographic positioning—cont'd

View	ACR ID	Suggested ID	Projection	C-arm angle	Image receptor placement	Tissue best visualized	Applications
Captured Lesion (Coat-Hanger View)	None	CL	All	0-90 degrees		Posterior	Palpable abnormality near chest wall or implant, often performed with magnification
Tangential View	TAN		All	0-90 degrees		All	Palpable abnormality, to visualize borders with better detail; often used in conjunction with magnification
TECHNIQUES							
Magnification	M						Improved resolution; better shows calcifications and borders of lesions
Implant Displacement	ID					Tissue anterior to subpectoral implants	Patients with implants
Nipple In Profile	NIP					Subareolar	
Spot Compression		S					Palpable abnormality, to visualize borders with better detail; often used in conjunction with magnification

From Andolina V, Lille S: *Mammographic imaging: a practical guide,* ed 3, Baltimore, MD, 2011, Lippincott Williams & Wilkins.

- Mammography film labeling may also include the following:
  - D. A separate date sticker or perforation
  - E. A label indicating the technical factors used: kVp, milliampere-seconds (mAs), target material, degree of obliquity, density setting, exposure time, and compression thickness. This is often included on the automatic identification labeling system that most manufacturers offer with their units.
  - F. Facilities with more than one unit must identify the mammographic unit used (Roman numerals are suggested by the ACR).
  - G. For FFDM images, all of the aforementioned pertinent information should be included in the DICOM header. This information should also be seen on the processed image or, if possible, used in a DICOM overlay that can be turned on or off as needed by the radiologist, to prevent interference during interpretation of the image.
- For patients with palpable masses, a radiopaque (BB or X-spot) marker may be used to identify the location of the mass. A different type of radiopaque marker may be used to identify skin lesions, scars, or moles. This is determined by the policy of the facility, at the discretion of the reading radiologists.
- When using automatic exposure control (AEC), position the variable-position detector at the chest wall, the mid-breast, or the anterior breast, depending on breast composition and size. The appropriate location of the AEC detector must be determined for each individual patient. If possible, the detector should be placed under the most glandular portion of the breast, usually just posterior to the nipple. Most FFDM units will automatically determine these settings based on the technology used by the manufacturer.
- When reviewing images, assess contrast and density for optimal differentiation of breast tissues. Anatomic markers should be visible. The projections of one breast should be compared with the same projections of the contralateral breast so that symmetry and consistency of positioning can be evaluated. All images should be absent of motion blur, artifacts, and skin folds. Images must be evaluated for potentially suspicious lesions and calcifications that may require image enhancement methods.
- To evaluate whether sufficient breast tissue is shown, the radiographer should measure the depth of the breast from the nipple to the chest wall on the CC and MLO projections. The posterior nipple line (PNL) is an imaginary line that is "drawn" obliquely from the nipple to the pectoralis muscle or the edge of the image, whichever comes first on the MLO projection. On the CC projection, the PNL is "drawn" from the nipple to the chest wall or to the edge of the image, whichever comes first. The PNL on the CC should be within $\frac{1}{3}$ inch (1 cm) of depth of the PNL on the MLO projection (Fig. 21-27).
- Between examinations, use a disinfectant to clean the breast tray surface, compression paddle, patient handle grips, and face guard.
- If practical, a heating pad or a commercially available mammography image receptor cover may be used to warm the image receptor tray surface and to enhance patient comfort. Breast cushions available through several manufacturers provide a warmer and more comfortable examination for the patient (Fig. 21-28). Check with the unit's manufacturer before implementing any patient comfort modifications.
- Mammography is a team effort involving the patient and the mammographer. Acknowledge the individual needs of each patient to facilitate the cooperation and trust necessary to complete the procedure successfully. The nature of the interaction between the radiographer and the patient is likely to determine whether the patient chooses to have subsequent mammograms.

Respiration

- To avoid patient motion and image blurring, the patient may be asked to suspend respiration during the exposure. The preferred method is to ask the patient to simply "stop breathing" rather than "hold your breath." Saying "hold your breath" often implies to the patient that she will need to take a deep breath in, this may result in an unintentional movement of the ribs and therefore the breast tissue, causing blurring or a change in the position of the breast. Alternatively, some mammographers prefer to avoid suspending respiration and simply ask the patient to remain still throughout the exposure. Once the breast is vigorously compressed, the patient is not liable to take deep breaths, especially if she is concentrating on not moving.

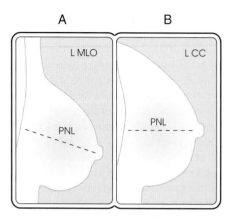

A B

L MLO L CC

PNL PNL

Fig. 21-27 A, Schematic MLO projection with PNL drawn. **B,** Schematic CC projection with PNL drawn. PNL of CC projection should be within 1 cm of PNL of MLO projection, as noted on the MLO (**C**) and CC (**D**) projections of this mammogram.

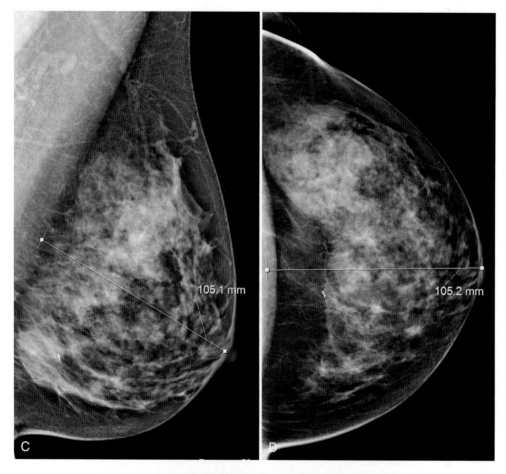

105.1 mm   105.2 mm

C   D

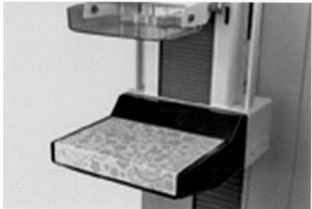

Fig. 21-28 Breast cushions are sometimes used to provide a more comfortable environment and examination for the patient.

(Image courtesy of Beekley Corp., Bristol, CT.)

Summary of Mammography Projections

Before beginning to learn mammography projections, the student of radiography should carefully study the illustrative summary of mammography projections shown in the box. Familiarity with the different projection names and abbreviations would enhance the student's understanding of the detailed discussions of the projections presented in this chapter.

DESCRIPTIVE TERMINOLOGY FOR LESION LOCATION

Descriptive terminology has been developed for the referring physician, the technologist, and the radiologist to communicate efficiently regarding an area of concern within a breast. When describing an area of concern, the laterality (right or left) must accompany the description (Fig. 21-29).

Each breast is divided into four quadrants: the upper outer quadrant (UOQ), the lower outer quadrant (LOQ), the upper inner quadrant (UIQ), and the lower inner quadrant (LIQ). Clock time is also used to describe the location of a specific area of concern within the breast, but it changes from the right to the left breast, that is, 2:00 in the right breast is in the UIQ, whereas 2:00 in the left breast is in the UOQ. This opposite labeling applies to all clock times; therefore it is important to identify the correct breast, clock time, and quadrant. The distance of the abnormality from the nipple, which is the only fixed point of reference in the breast, is also noted. The terms *subareolar* and *periareolar* describe the area directly beneath the nipple and near (or around) the nipple area. Central describes a lesion located directly behind the nipple in both radiographic projections.

The location of a lesion seen on the mammogram is described using the clinical orientation (described above) extrapolated from the image location. The location of an imaged lesion is described by its laterality, quadrant, clock location, and depth, thus providing a consistency check for possible right-left confusion.[f] Depth of a lesion on the mammogram is described as anterior (nipple), middle, or posterior.

[f]American College of Radiology (ACR): ACR BI-RADS-mammography, 4th edition. In: *ACR breast imaging reporting and data system, breast imaging atlas*, Reston, VA, 2003, American College of Radiology.

Illustrative summary of mammography projections

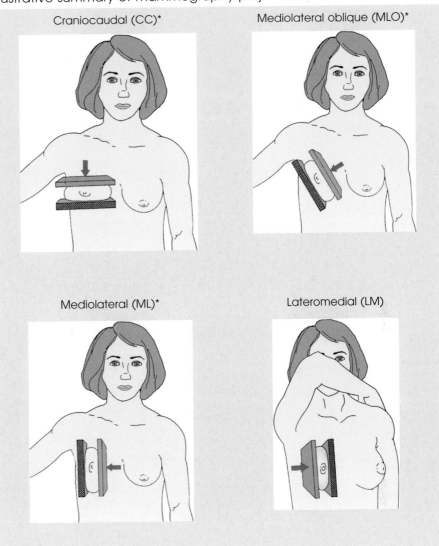

Craniocaudal (CC)*

Mediolateral oblique (MLO)*

Mediolateral (ML)*

Lateromedial (LM)

Routine Projections of the Breast

Mammography is routinely performed using the CC and MLO projections. The combination of these two views best allows visualization of the greatest amount of breast tissue for screening purposes. When diagnostic examinations are performed for specific areas of concern, additional views may be indicated as desired by the radiologist.

Illustrative summary of mammography projections—cont'd

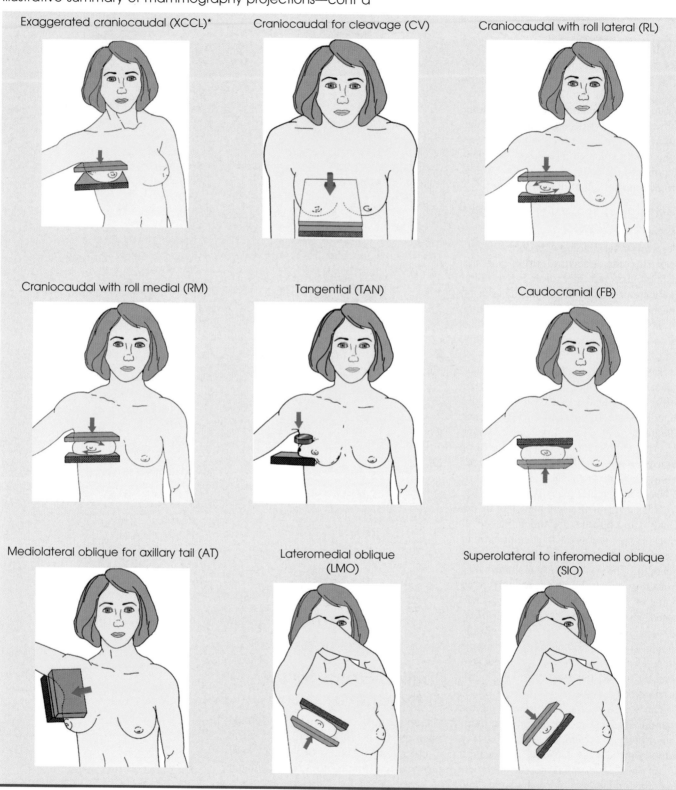

Exaggerated craniocaudal (XCCL)*

Craniocaudal for cleavage (CV)

Craniocaudal with roll lateral (RL)

Craniocaudal with roll medial (RM)

Tangential (TAN)

Caudocranial (FB)

Mediolateral oblique for axillary tail (AT)

Lateromedial oblique (LMO)

Superolateral to inferomedial oblique (SIO)

*Essential projection.

♠ CRANIOCAUDAL (CC) PROJECTION

Image receptor: 8 × 10 inch (18 × 24 cm) or 10 × 12 inch (24 × 30 cm)

Position of patient
- Have the patient stand facing the image receptor, or seat the patient on an adjustable stool facing the unit.

Position of part
- While standing on the medial side of the breast to be imaged, elevate the inframammary fold to its maximal height.
- Adjust the height of the C-arm to the level of the inferior surface of the patient's breast.
- Have the patient lean slightly forward from the waist. Use both hands to pull the breast gently onto the image receptor holder, while instructing the patient to press the thorax against the image receptor.
- Drape the opposite breast over the corner of the image receptor. This maneuver improves demonstration of the medial tissue.
- Have the patient hold onto the grab bar with the contralateral hand; this helps steady the patient as you continue positioning.
- Keep the breast perpendicular to the chest wall. The technologist should use his or her fingertips to pull the inferior posterior tissue gently forward onto the IR.
- Center the breast over the AEC detector, with the nipple in profile if possible.

- Immobilize the breast with one hand, while taking care not to remove this hand until compression begins.
- While placing your arm against the patient's back with your hand on the shoulder of the affected side, make certain the patient's shoulder is relaxed and in external rotation.
- Rotate the patient's head away from the affected side, and rest the patient's head against the face guard.
- Make certain that no other objects such as jewelry or hair obstruct the path of the beam.
- With your hand on the patient's shoulder, gently slide the skin up over the clavicle.
- Using the hand that is anchoring the patient's breast, pull the lateral tissue onto the image receptor without sacrificing medial tissue.
- Inform the patient that compression of the breast will begin. Using foot pedal compression controls, bring the compression paddle into contact with the breast while sliding the hand toward the nipple.
- Slowly apply compression manually until the breast feels taut.
- Check the medial and lateral aspects of the breast for adequate compression.
- Instruct the patient to indicate whether the compression becomes uncomfortable.
- After full compression is achieved and checked, instruct the patient to stop breathing (Fig. 21-30).
- Make the exposure.
- Release breast compression immediately.

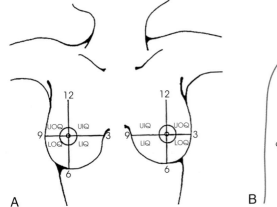 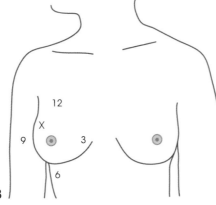

Fig. 21-29 A, Each breast is viewed as a clock and is divided into four quadrants to describe the location of a lesion: upper outer quadrant (UOQ), upper inner quadrant (UIQ), lower outer quadrant (LOQ), and lower inner quadrant (LIQ). **B,** An abnormality should always be described in a consistent manner. For example, the location of the abnormality denoted by the *x* would be described as "right breast UOQ at approximately 10:30 position."

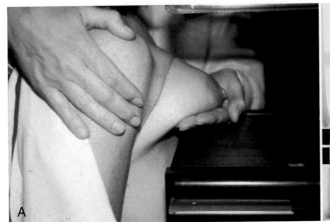 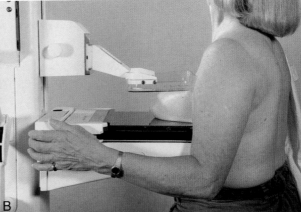

Fig. 21-30 A, Lift breast to adjust level of C-arm to elevated inframammary fold. **B,** CC projection.

Central ray

• Perpendicular to the base of the breast

Structures shown

The CC projection shows the central, sub-areolar, and medial fibroglandular breast tissue. The pectoral muscle is shown in approximately 30% of all CC images.[1]

---

[1]Bassett L, Heinlein R: Good positioning key to imaging of breast, *Diagn Imaging* 9:69, 1993.

The following should be clearly shown:
■ The PNL extending posteriorly to the edge of the image and measuring within ⅓ inch (1 cm) of the depth of the PNL on MLO projection (Fig. 21-31)
■ All medial tissue, as shown by visualization of medial retroglandular fat and the absence of fibroglandular tissue extending to the posteromedial edge of the image

■ Nipple in profile (if possible) and at midline, indicating no exaggeration of positioning
■ For emphasis of medial tissue, some lateral tissue may be excluded
■ Pectoral muscle seen posterior to medial retroglandular fat in about 30% of properly positioned CC images
■ Slight medial skin reflection at the cleavage, ensuring adequate inclusion of posterior medial tissue
■ Uniform tissue exposure if compression is adequate

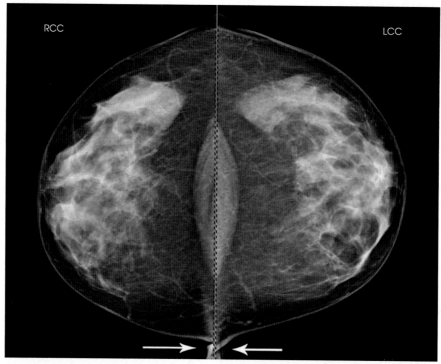

Fig. 21-31 Bilateral CC projections show proper positioning and compression. The CC projection should include maximal medial breast tissue (*arrows*) with the nipple centered and in profile. As much lateral and inferior tissue as possible should be pulled onto the image receptor without compromising visualization of medial tissue. Note that pectoral muscle is seen posteriorly on these images, but this may not be possible to achieve on most CC projections.

⚘ MEDIOLATERAL OBLIQUE (*MLO*) PROJECTION

Image receptor: 8 × 10 inch (18 × 24 cm) or 10 × 12 inch (24 × 30 cm)

Position of patient
- Have the patient stand facing the image receptor with her feet pointed forward, or seat the patient on an adjustable stool facing the unit.

Position of part
- Determine the degree of obliquity of the C-arm. The degree of obliquity should be approximately 45 degrees but will vary from 30 to 60 degrees, depending on the patient's body habitus. Draw an imaginary line from the patient's shoulder to midsternum, and angle the C-arm to parallel this line.
- Adjust the height of the C-arm so that the superior border of the IR is level with the axilla.
  - Instruct the patient to lean slightly forward from the waist.
- Elevate the arm of the affected side over the corner of the image receptor, and rest the hand on the adjacent handgrip. The patient's elbow should be flexed and resting posterior to the image receptor.
- Place the upper corner of the image receptor as high as possible into the patient's axilla between the pectoral and latissimus dorsi muscles, so that the image receptor is behind the pectoral fold.

- Ensure that the patient's affected shoulder is relaxed and leaning slightly anterior. While placing the flat surface of the hand along the lateral aspect of the breast, gently pull the patient's breast and pectoral muscle anteriorly and medially.
- Holding the breast between the thumb and fingers, gently lift it up, out, and away from the chest wall.
- Center the breast on the IR with the nipple in profile, if possible, and hold the breast in position.
- Hold the breast up and out from the body by rotating the hand so that the base of the thumb and the heel of the hand support the breast.
  - Inform the patient that compression of the breast will begin. Continue to hold the breast up and out while sliding the hand toward the nipple as the compression paddle is brought into contact with the breast. Loosen the skin at the clavicle with the opposite hand to ensure that posterior tissue is imaged while preventing injury to the shoulder. Roll the contralateral shoulder toward the unit to ensure that medial tissue is visualized.

- Slowly apply compression until the breast feels taut. The corner of the compression paddle should be inferior to the clavicle.
- Check the superior and inferior aspects of the breast for adequate compression.
- Instruct the patient to indicate whether the compression becomes uncomfortable.
- Gently pull down on the patient's abdominal tissue to open the inframammary fold.
- Instruct the patient to hold the opposite breast away from the path of the beam if necessary.
- After full compression is achieved, instruct the patient to stop breathing (Fig. 21-32).
- Make the exposure.
- Release breast compression immediately.

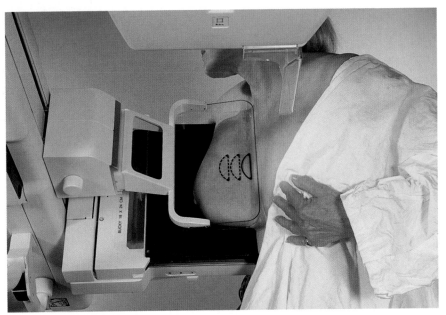

Fig. 21-32 MLO projection.

Central ray

- Perpendicular to the base of the breast
- The C-arm apparatus is positioned at an angle determined by the slope of the patient's pectoral muscle (30 to 60 degrees). The actual angle is determined by the patient's body habitus: Tall, thin patients require steep angulation, whereas short, stout patients require shallow angulation.

Structures shown

The MLO projection usually shows most of the breast tissue, with emphasis on the lateral aspect and axillary tail.

EVALUATION CRITERIA

The following should be clearly shown:

- PNL measuring within ⅓ inch (1 cm) of the depth of the PNL on CC projection[1]
  - □ While drawing the imaginary PNL obliquely following the orientation of breast tissue toward the pectoral muscle, use the fingers to measure its depth from nipple to pectoral muscle or to the edge of the image, whichever comes first (Fig. 21-33).
- Inferior aspect of the pectoral muscle extending to the PNL or below it if possible

[1]Bassett L: Clinical image evaluation, *Radiol Clin North Am* 33:1027, 1995.

- Pectoral muscle showing anterior convexity to ensure relaxed shoulder and axilla
- Nipple in profile if possible
- Open inframammary fold
- Deep and superficial breast tissues well separated when breast is adequately maneuvered up and out from the chest wall
- Retroglandular fat well visualized to ensure inclusion of deep fibroglandular breast tissue
- Uniform tissue exposure if compression is adequate

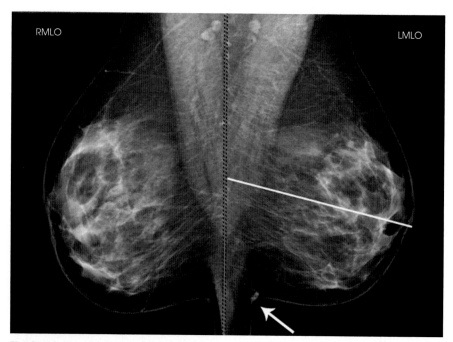

Fig. 21-33 Bilateral MLO projections show proper positioning. Images should include pectoral muscle to level of nipple (*white line*), posterior breast tissue; and junction of inframammary fold and abdominal skin (*arrow*).

Routine Projections of the Augmented Breast

Mammography has an 80% to 90% true-positive rate for detecting cancer in breasts that do not contain implants. For the millions of women in the United States who have undergone augmentation mammoplasty for cosmetic or reconstructive purposes, the true-positive (pathologic-mammographic) breast cancer detection rate decreases to approximately 60% because implants can obscure 85% of the breast's structures, potentially hiding a small cancer that could normally be detected with mammography at an early and curable stage.

Successful radiography of an augmented breast requires a highly skilled mammographer. During the examination, precautions must be taken to avoid rupture of the augmentation device.

Mammography of the augmented breast presents a challenge that cannot be met with the standard two-view examination of each breast. An eight-radiograph examination (four views of each breast) is preferred when possible. The tissue within the posterior and superior aspects of the augmented breast can be satisfactorily evaluated using the standard CC and MLO projections. However, these four images do not adequately show the surrounding breast parenchyma. The addition of a second set of images utilizing the implant displacement technique (ID), also known as the Eklund method or maneuver, improves compression of the breast tissue and visualization of breast structures. For the Eklund method, the implant is pushed posteriorly against the chest wall so that it is excluded from the image, and the breast tissue surrounding the implant is pulled anteriorly and compressed. This technique is most effective when used on patients with implants that have been placed posterior to the pectoral muscle. It can be used when the implant is placed anterior to the pectoral muscle, but notably less tissue will be able to be pulled onto the IR (Fig. 21-34).

Complications frequently associated with breast augmentation include fibrosis, increased fibrous tissue surrounding the implant, shrinking, hardening, leakage, and pain. Breast augmentation does not increase the risk of developing a cancer in the breast; however the presence of the implant may make detection of a cancer on a screening mammogram more difficult.[g] Because mammography alone cannot fully show all complications, ultrasonography and MRI are also used for breast examinations in symptomatic patients. Whether ultrasonography or MRI is used as the adjunct imaging after

[g]McIntosh SA, Horgan K: Augmentation mammoplasty: effect on diagnosis of breast cancer, *J Plastic Reconstr Aesthet Surg* 61:124, 2008.

mammography for patients with suspected implant rupture varies from practice to practice.

Ultrasonography of the breast has proved useful in identifying implant leakage when implant rupture is suggested by mammographic findings and clinical examination, and occasionally when leakage is not suspected. It has also

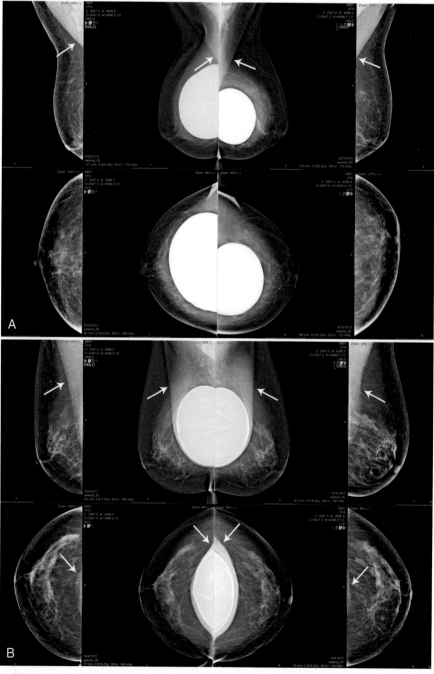

Fig. 21-34 A, Eight-view mammogram of a patient with implants placed anterior to the pectoralis muscle (*arrow*). **B,** Eight-view mammogram of a patient with implants placed posterior to the pectoralis muscle (*arrow*). Note that more pectoral muscle and breast tissue are seen when the implant is placed posterior to the muscle.

successfully identified leakage that has migrated to the axillary lymph nodes. Although ultrasonography is not yet recommended as a screening modality for implant leakage, it does enhance the mammographic examination.

MRI is also commonly used for diagnostic evaluation of augmented breasts, but there is disagreement over the appropriateness of guidelines for its use.[h]

Although MRI offers several diagnostic advantages, the cost and time-consuming nature of the procedure inhibit its use as a screening modality for patients who have undergone augmentation. It may be used as a screening tool for women who have undergone reconstruction after breast cancer surgery. MRI has proved useful as a preoperative tool in locating the position of an implant, identifying the contour of the deformity, and confirming rupture and leakage migration patterns.[1]

---

[h]Stoblen F et al: Imaging in patients with breast implants: results of the First International Breast (implant) Conference 2009, *Insights Imaging* 1:93, 2010.

---

[1]Orel SG: MR imaging of the breast, *Radiol Clin North Am* 38:899, 2000.

♠ CRANIOCAUDAL (CC) PROJECTION WITH FULL IMPLANT

Image receptor: 8 × 10 inch (18 × 24 cm) or 10 × 12 inch (24 × 30 cm)

Position of patient

- Have the patient stand facing the image receptor, or seat the patient on an adjustable stool facing the unit.

Position of part

- Turn the AEC *off,* and preselect a *manual* technique. For FFDM units, be sure that Implant View processing settings are chosen if applicable.
- Follow the same positioning sequence as for the standard CC projection.
- Inform the patient that minimal compression of the breast will be used. Bring the compression paddle into contact with the breast, and slowly apply only enough compression to immobilize the breast. Compression should be *minimal.* The anterior breast tissue should still feel soft.
- Select the appropriate exposure factors, and instruct the patient to stop breathing.
- Make the exposure.
- Release compression immediately.

Central ray

• Perpendicular to the base of the breast

Structures shown

The image should show the entire implant and surrounding posterior breast tissue with suboptimal compression of the anterior fibroglandular breast tissue (Fig. 21-35).

The following should be clearly shown:

■ Implant projected over fibroglandular tissue, extending to posterior edge of image

■ Posterior breast tissue on medial and lateral aspects extending to chest wall

■ Nipple in profile, if possible, and at midline, indicating no exaggeration of positioning

■ Nonuniform compression of anterior breast tissue

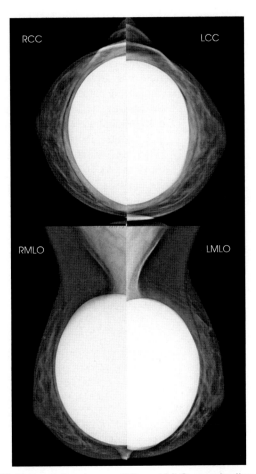

Fig. 21-35 Bilateral, four-image CC and MLO examination of augmented breasts. Implants have been surgically placed behind the pectoral muscle. Additional radiographs should be obtained using the Eklund (ID) technique to complete the eight-radiograph study (see Fig. 21-37).

CRANIOCAUDAL PROJECTION WITH IMPLANT DISPLACED (*CC ID*)

Image receptor: 8 × 10 inch (18 × 24 cm) or 10 × 12 inch (24 × 30 cm)

Position of patient

- Have the patient stand facing the image receptor, or seat the patient on an adjustable stool facing the unit. Select an AEC technique. For FFDM units, be sure that Implant View processing settings are chosen if applicable.

Position of part

- While standing on the medial side of the breast to be imaged, elevate the inframammary fold to its maximal height.
- Adjust the height of the C-arm to the level of the inferior surface of the breast.
- Standing behind the patient, place both arms around the patient and locate the anterior border of the implant by walking the fingers back from the nipple toward the chest wall, or
  - Stand beside the patient lateral to the breast being imaged. Have the patient hold the grip with the opposite hand to retain her balance. Locate the anterior border of the implant by walking the fingers back from the nipple toward the chest wall.

- When the anterior border of the implant has been located, gently pull the anterior breast tissue forward onto the image receptor (Fig. 21-36). Use the hands and the edge of the image receptor to keep the implant displaced posteriorly.
- Center the breast over the AEC detector with the nipple in profile if possible.
- Hold the implant back against the chest wall. Slowly apply compression to the anterior skin surface, being careful not to allow the implant to slip under the compression paddle. As compression continues, the implant should be seen bulging behind the compression paddle.
- Apply compression until the anterior breast tissue is taut. Compared with the full-implant projection, an additional ¾ to 2 inches (2 to 5 cm) of compression should be achieved with the implant displaced.
- Instruct the patient to indicate if the compression becomes too uncomfortable or intolerable.
- When full compression is achieved, move the AEC detector to the appropriate position and instruct the patient to stop breathing.
- Make the exposure.
- Release breast compression immediately.

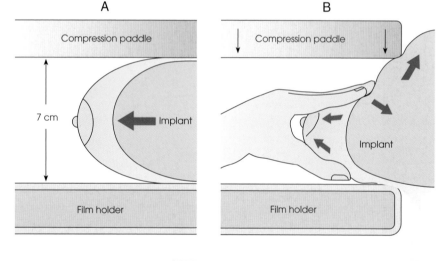

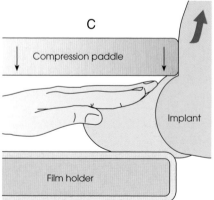
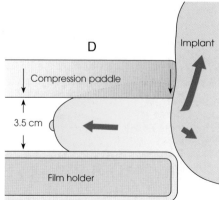

Fig. 21-36 A, Breast with implant and normal positioning techniques. **B-D,** Eklund technique of pushing implant posteriorly against chest wall, pulling breast anteriorly, and compressing tissue.

(From Eklund GW et al: Improved imaging of the augmented breast, *AJR Am J Roentgenol* 151:469, 1988.)

Central ray

• Perpendicular to the base of the breast

Structures shown

This projection shows the anterior and central breast tissue projected free of superimposition with uniform compression and improved tissue differentiation. The implant is displaced posteriorly and should not be visualized on the image (Fig. 21-37).

The following should be clearly shown:

■ Breast tissue superior and inferior to the implant pulled forward with the anterior breast tissue projected free of the implant

■ PNL extending posteriorly to edge of implant, measuring within $\frac{1}{3}$ inch (1 cm) of depth of PNL on MLO projection with implant displaced

■ Implant along posterior edge of image, flattened against chest wall, should not be visualized on the image, but often remnants of the implant may be seen.

■ Image sharpness is enhanced by increased compression of the breast tissue and reduced scatter due to removal of the implant from the path of the beam.

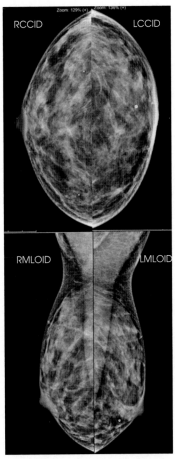

Fig. 21-37 Bilateral, four-image CC and MLO projections with implant displacement (ID) of the same patient as in Fig. 21-35, using Eklund (ID) technique. Implants are pushed back for better visualization of surrounding breast tissue.

MEDIOLATERAL OBLIQUE (*MLO*) PROJECTION WITH FULL IMPLANT

Image receptor: 8 × 10 inch (18 × 24 cm) or 10 × 12 inch (24 × 30 cm)

Position of patient
- Have the patient stand facing the image receptor, or seat the patient on an adjustable stool facing the unit.

Position of part
- Turn the AEC *off,* and preselect a *manual* technique. For FFDM units, be sure that Implant View processing settings are chosen if applicable.
- Follow the same positioning sequence as for the standard MLO projection.
- Inform the patient that minimal compression of the breast will be used. Continue to hold the breast up and out while sliding the hand toward the nipple as the compression paddle is brought into contact with the breast.

- Slowly apply only enough compression to immobilize the breast. Compression should be minimal, and the anterior breast tissue should still feel soft.
- Pull down on the patient's abdominal tissue to open the inframammary fold.
- Select the appropriate exposure factors, and instruct the patient to stop breathing.
- Make the exposure.
- Release breast compression immediately.

Central ray
- Perpendicular to the image receptor
- The C-arm apparatus is positioned at an angle determined by the slope of the patient's pectoral muscle (30 to 60 degrees). The actual angle is determined by the patient's body habitus: Tall, thin patients require steep angulation, whereas short, stout patients require shallow angulation.

Structures shown
The image shows the entire implant and surrounding posterior breast tissue as well as axillary tissue and pectoral muscle, with suboptimal compression of the anterior fibroglandular breast tissue (see Fig. 21-35).

EVALUATION CRITERIA
The following should be clearly shown:
- Implant projected over fibroglandular tissue, extending to posterior edge of image
- Posterior breast tissue on the inferior aspect, extending to chest wall
- Nipple in profile if possible
- Open inframammary fold
- Breast adequately maneuvered up and out from chest wall
- Nonuniform compression of anterior breast tissue

MEDIOLATERAL OBLIQUE PROJECTION WITH IMPLANT DISPLACED (*MLO ID*)

Image receptor: 8 × 10 inch (18 × 24 cm) or 10 × 12 inch (24 × 30 cm)

Position of patient
- Have the patient stand facing the image receptor, or seat the patient on an adjustable stool facing the unit.
- Select an AEC technique. For FFDM units, be sure that Implant View processing settings are chosen if applicable.

Position of part
- Determine the degree of obliquity of the C-arm apparatus by rotating the tube until the long edge of the image receptor is parallel to the upper third of the pectoral muscle of the affected side. The degree of obliquity should be between 30 degrees and 60 degrees, depending on the patient's body habitus.
- Adjust the height of the C-arm so that the superior border is level with the axilla.
- Instruct the patient to elevate the arm of the affected side over the corner of the image receptor and to rest the hand on the adjacent handgrip. The patient's elbow should be flexed.
- Standing in front of the patient, locate the anterior border of the implant by walking the fingers back from the patient's nipple toward the chest wall.
- After locating the anterior border of the implant, gently pull the anterior breast tissue forward onto the image receptor. Use the edge of the image receptor and the hands to keep the implant displaced posteriorly.
- Center the breast tissue over the AEC detector with the nipple in profile if possible.

- Hold the anterior breast tissue up and out so that the base of the thumb and the heel of the hand support the breast.
- Hold the implant back against the chest wall while using fingers to bring the anterior breast tissue forward onto the IR. Slowly apply compression to the anterior skin surface, taking care not to allow the implant to slip under the compression paddle. As compression continues, the implant should be seen bulging behind the compression paddle.
- Apply compression until the anterior breast tissue is taut. Compared with the full-implant projection, an additional ¾ to 2 inches (2 to 5 cm) of tissue should be adequately visualized with the implant displaced.
- Instruct the patient to indicate if the compression becomes uncomfortable or intolerable.
- Pull down on the patient's abdominal tissue to open the inframammary fold.
- Instruct the patient to hold the opposite breast away from the path of the beam, as necessary.
- When full compression is achieved, move the AEC detector to the appropriate position if necessary and instruct the patient to stop breathing.
- Make the exposure.
- Release breast compression immediately.

Central ray
- Perpendicular to the image receptor
- The C-arm apparatus is positioned at an angle determined by the slope of the patient's pectoral muscle (30 to 60 degrees). The actual angle is determined by the patient's body habitus: Tall, thin patients require steep angulation, whereas short, stout patients require shallow angulation.

Structures shown
This image shows the anterior and central breast tissue projected free of superimposition of the implant, with uniform compression and improved tissue differentiation (see Fig. 21-37).

EVALUATION CRITERIA
The following should be clearly shown:
- Breast tissue superomedial and inferolateral to the implant with anterior breast tissue projected free of the implant
- Pectoral muscle showing anterior convexity to ensure relaxed shoulder and axilla
- PNL extending obliquely to edge of implant, measuring within ⅓ inch (1 cm) of depth of PNL on CC projection with implant displaced
- Implant should not be visualized on the image, but often some remnants of the implant may be seen posteriorly.
- Posterior breast tissue on inferior aspect of breast, extending to chest wall
- Nipple in profile if possible
- Open inframammary fold
- Breast adequately maneuvered up and out from chest wall
- Image sharpness is enhanced by increased compression of the breast tissue and reduced scatter due to removal of the implant from the path of the beam.

Male Mammography
EPIDEMIOLOGY OF MALE BREAST DISEASE

In the United States, more than 2200 men develop invasive breast cancer every year, and nearly 20% of these men die of the disease.[i] Although most men who develop breast cancer are 60 years of age and older, juvenile cases have been reported. Nearly all male breast cancers are primary tumors. An estimated 4% to 40% of male breast cancers are due to inherited mutations. Men typically have significantly less breast tissue; therefore smaller breast lesions are palpable and diagnosed at early stages. Other symptoms of breast cancer in men include nipple retraction, crusting, discharge, and ulceration.

Gynecomastia, a benign excessive development of the male mammary gland, can make malignant breast lesions more elusive to palpation. Gynecomastia occurs in 40% of male breast cancer patients; however a histologic relationship between gynecomastia and male breast cancer has not been definitively established. Because gynecomastia is caused by a hormonal imbalance, it is believed that abnormal hormonal function may increase the risk of male breast cancer.[j] Other associated risk factors for male breast cancer include increasing age, positive family history, *BRCA1* and *BRCA2* gene mutations, and Klinefelter syndrome.[1,2]

Breast cancer treatment options are limited among male patients. Because men have less breast tissue, lumpectomy is not considered practical. Most of the male glandular tissue is located directly posterior to the nipple. Therefore, a modified radical mastectomy including dissection of the nipple is usually the preferred surgical procedure.[k,l] Radiation and systemic therapy are considered when the tumor is located near the chest wall or when indicated by lymph node analysis. Similar to female breast cancer, the prognosis for male breast cancer is directly related to the stage of the disease at diagnosis. An early diagnosis indicates a better chance of survival. Survival rates among male patients with localized breast carcinomas are positive: 97% survive for 5 years.

Routine Projections of the Male Breast

Male breast anatomy varies significantly from female breast anatomy. The pectoral muscle is more highly developed in men, and most of the glandular breast tissue is located directly posterior to the nipple. The radiographer must take this variance into consideration. The standard CC and MLO projections may be applied with success in most male patients (Figs. 21-38 to 21-40). For men (or women) with large pectoral muscles, the radiographer may perform the caudocranial (FB) projection instead of the standard CC because it may be easier to compress the inferior portion of the breast. In addition, the lateromedial oblique (LMO) projection may replace the standard MLO.

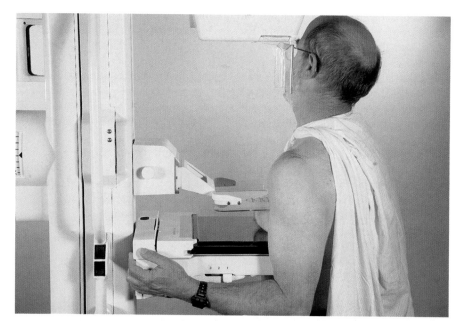

Fig. 21-38 Positioning for CC projection of male breast.

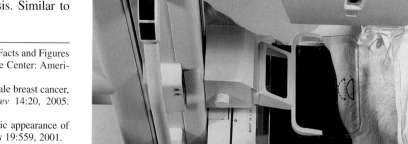

Fig. 21-39 Positioning for MLO projections of male breast.

[i]American Cancer Society: Cancer Facts and Figures 2013, Atlanta, GA, 2013, Corporate Center: American Cancer Society Inc., p9.

[j]Weiss JR et al: Epidemiology of male breast cancer, *Cancer Epidemiol Biomarkers Prev* 14:20, 2005. Published online January 24, 2005.

[1]Appelbaum A et al: Mammographic appearance of male breast disease, *RadioGraphics* 19:559, 2001.

[2]National Cancer Institute Factsheet. Available at: www.cancer.gov. Accessed August 14, 2009.

[k]Camus C et al: Ductal carcinoma in situ of the male breast, *Cancer* 74:1289, 1994.

[l]Hill T et al: Comparison of male and female breast cancer incidence trend, tumor characteristics, and survival, *Ann Epidemiol* 15:773, 2005.

Keep in mind that these unconventional views are rarely necessary but are viable alternatives in extreme cases. These projections may allow the radiographer to accommodate more successfully a patient with prominent pectoral muscles. Some facilities also use narrower quadrant compression paddles (3 inches [8 cm] wide) to compress the male breast or the extremely small female breast.[1] The smaller paddle permits the radiographer to hold the breast in position while applying final compression. A wooden spoon or a plastic spatula can be used to hold the breast in place, then can be slowly removed as the compression paddle replaces it.

Because most men who undergo mammography present with outward symptoms, mammography of the male breast is

---

[1]Eklund GW, Cardenosa G: The art of mammographic positioning, *Radiol Clin North Am* 30:21, 1992.

---

usually considered a diagnostic examination. It can be considered a screening examination for men who know they carry the *BRCA1* or *BRCA2* gene, or who have a history of breast cancer. The radiographer should work closely with the radiologist to achieve a thorough demonstration of the potential abnormality. In the male breast, most tumors are located in the subareolar region. Careful attention should be given to positioning the nipple in profile and to providing adequate compression of this area to allow the best visualization of this tissue.

Calcifications are rare in male breast cancer cases. When present, they are usually larger, rounder, and more scattered than the calcifications associated with female breast cancer. Spot compression and the magnification technique are common image enhancement methods for showing the morphology of calcifications.

Procedures other than mammography are used to diagnose male breast cancer.

Fine-needle aspiration biopsy (FNAB) and excisional biopsy of palpable lesions are standard methods of diagnosis. Histologically, most breast cancers in men are ductal, and most are infiltrating ductal carcinomas. Very few in situ cancers are found in male patients.

Because breast cancer is traditionally considered a "woman's disease," the radiographer should remain sensitive to the feelings of the male patient by offering not only physical comfort but also psychological and emotional support during the procedure.

Image Enhancement Methods

The spot compression technique and the magnification technique are designed to enhance the image of the area under investigation.

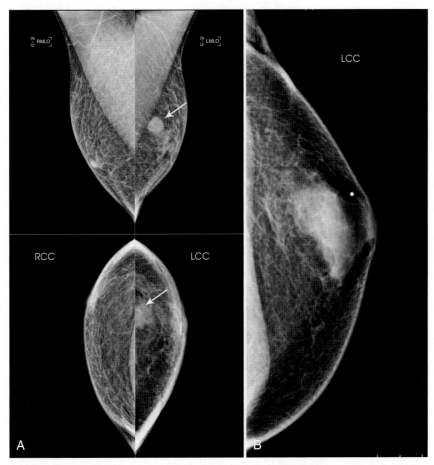

Fig. 21-40 A, Four-view mammogram of a 55-year-old man with a new palpable lump (*arrow*). This proved to be cancer on biopsy. **B,** Left CC view of a 49-year-old male with a new lump. This proved to be gynecomastia, a benign process, on biopsy.

MAGNIFICATION TECHNIQUE (*M* USED AS PREFIX)

Image receptor: 8 × 10 inch (18 × 24 cm)

Position of patient

• Have the patient stand facing the image receptor, or seat the patient on an adjustable stool facing the unit.
• Use only equipment designed to be used for magnification mammography to perform this maneuver, and use the equipment according to the manufacturer's directions.

Position of part

• Attach the firm, radiolucent magnification platform to the unit. The patient's breast is positioned on the platform between the compression device and a nongrid IR.
• Select the smallest focal spot target size (≤0.1 mm is preferred). Most units allow magnification images to be exposed only when the correct focal spot size is used.

• Select the appropriate compression paddle (regular, quadrant, or spot compression). Collimate according to the size of the compression paddle.
• Position the patient's breast to obtain the projection that best shows the area of interest. The angle of the C-arm can be adjusted to accommodate any projection normally performed using a traditional grid technique.
• When full compression is achieved, move the AEC detector to the chest wall position (if necessary) and instruct the patient to stop breathing (Fig. 21-41).
• Make the exposure.
• Release breast compression immediately.

Central ray

• Perpendicular to the area of interest

Structures shown

This technique magnifies the compressed area of interest with improved detail, facilitating determination of the characteristics of microcalcifications[m] (Fig. 21-42) and the margins (or lack of definitive margins) of suspected lesions (Fig. 21-43).

---

[m]Kim HH et al: Comparison of calcification specificity in digital mammography using soft-copy display versus screen-film mammography, *AJR Am J Roentgenol* 187:47, 2006.

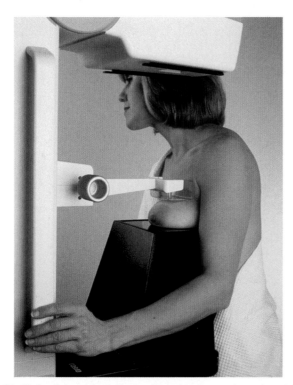

Fig. 21-41 Radiolucent platform placed between breast and film holder causes breast image to be enlarged.

(Courtesy Lorad Corp.)

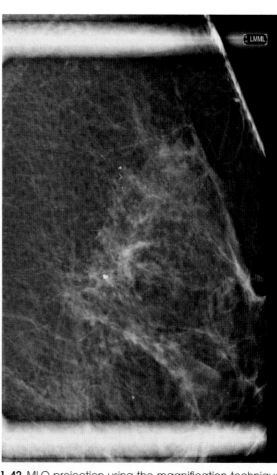

Fig. 21-42 MLO projection using the magnification technique and a quad paddle to better visualize microcalcifications.

EVALUATION CRITERIA

The following should be clearly shown:

- Area of interest within collimated and compressed margins
- Improved delineation of number, distribution, and morphology of microcalcifications
- Enhanced architectural characteristics of focal density or mass
- Uniform tissue exposure if compression is adequate

SPOT COMPRESSION TECHNIQUE

Image receptor: 8 × 10 inch (18 × 24 cm)

Position of patient

- Have the patient stand facing the image receptor, or seat the patient on an adjustable stool facing the unit.
- This technique is often performed in conjunction with the magnification technique, especially for determination of number, distribution, and morphology of microcalcifications.

Position of part
In conjunction with magnification technique

- Place a firm, radiolucent magnification platform, designed for use with the dedicated mammography equipment on the unit, between the patient's breast and a nongrid image receptor.
- Select the smallest focal spot target size (≤0.1 mm is preferred).

For palpable masses

A TAN projection combined with spot compression and the magnification technique is most often used to image a palpable mass; however the spot compression technique in a previously imaged projection is also requested by many radiologists.

- Select the appropriate spot compression device.
- Mark the location of the palpable mass with a felt-tip pen or with a radiopaque beebee marker placed on the lump, according to the policy of the facility.
- Center the area of interest under the compression device in the position indicated by the radiologist.
- Inform the patient that compression of the breast will be used and may be uncomfortable. Bring the compression paddle into contact with the breast, and slowly apply compression until the breast feels taut.

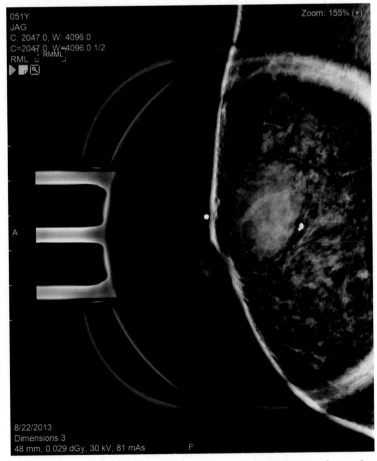

Fig. 21-43 Right MLO projection using the magnification technique and a spot paddle to perform a tangential view of a palpable mass. This proved that the mass was smoothly outlined with uniform edges and was shown to be a cyst on ultrasound.

- Instruct the patient to indicate if the compression becomes too uncomfortable.
- When full compression is achieved, move the AEC detector to the chest wall position if necessary, and instruct the patient to stop breathing (Fig. 21-44).
- Make the exposure.
- Release breast compression immediately.

For nonpalpable masses

- While viewing the routine mammogram, measure the location of the area of interest from a reference point (the nipple), using a tape measure or the fingertips (Fig. 21-45).
- Select the appropriate spot compression device.
- Reposition the patient's breast to obtain the projection from which the measurements were taken.
- Using the same reference point, transfer onto the patient the measurements taken from the mammogram.
- Mark the area of interest with a felt-tip pen, or mentally note the location on the breast.
- Center the area of interest under the compression device in the requested view, which may be different from the original projection.
- Inform the patient that compression of the breast will be used. Bring the compression paddle into contact with the breast, and slowly apply compression until the breast feels taut. Adequate compression is especially important for spot views of nonpalpable masses, as the objective is to use targeted compression to separate tissue islands that may be overlapped, causing an area of suspicious density.
- Instruct the patient to indicate if the compression becomes too uncomfortable.
- When full compression is achieved, move the AEC detector to the appropriate position if necessary, and instruct the patient to stop breathing.
- Make the exposure.
- Release breast compression immediately.

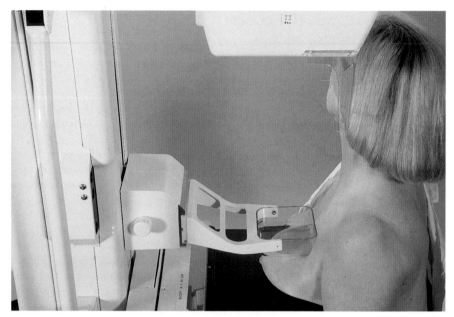

Fig. 21-44 Spot compression used with CC projection.

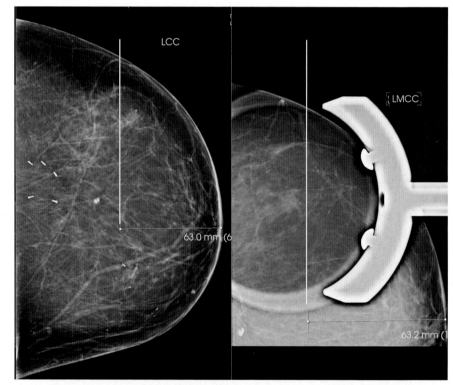

Fig. 21-45 To find the area of interest in the breast for a spot view, measure how far posterior the area is by using the nipple as a reference point. This image illustrates how measurement of the lesion from the nipple on the CC view approximates measurement of the lesion from the nipple on the magnified spot view.

Central ray

• Perpendicular to the area of interest

Structures shown

The spot compression technique resolves superimposed structures seen on only one projection, better visualizes small lesions located in the extreme posterior breast, separates superimposed ductal structures in the subareolar region, and improves visualization in areas of dense tissue through localized compression (Fig. 21-46).

The following should be clearly shown:
■ Area of interest clearly seen within compressed margins
■ Close collimation to the area of interest unless contraindicated by radiologist
■ Improved recorded detail through the use of close collimation and the magnification technique employing a spot compression device
■ Uniform tissue exposure if compression is adequate

NOTE: Densities caused by the superimposition of normal breast parenchyma disappear on spot compression images.

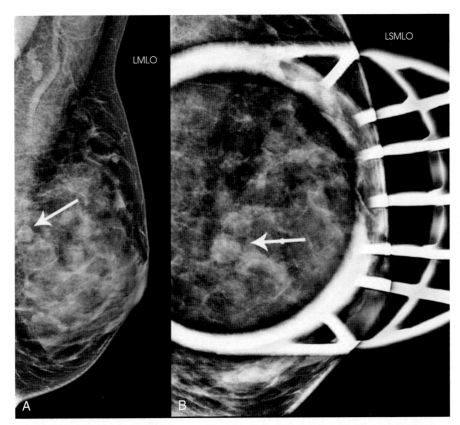

Fig. 21-46 A, This 45-year-old woman with extremely dense tissue was recalled for a questionable mass (*arrow*) in the left breast on screening mammography. **B,** A spot view was performed to spread the tissue and more clearly delineate the borders of the mass. This proved to be a fibroadenoma on biopsy.

Supplemental Projections

The routine projections are not always adequate in completely showing a patient's breast tissue, or a specific area may require clearer delineation. Supplemental projections complement the routine projections and have distinct applications (Table 21-2). The mammographer should fully understand the value of each projection and its potential to show significant findings in the breast. This section provides a brief overview of significant mammographic findings in their most common radiographic presentation and provides suggested correlative supplemental projections. The language related to mammographic findings must be appreciated for the mammographer and the radiologist to work collaboratively toward a successful diagnostic examination.

The mass is the most common presentation of a potential abnormality in the breast.

It is identified on two projections of the affected breast. A mass has a convex shape or an outward contour to its margins. If a suspected mass is identified on only one projection, the mammographer must strive to position the breast so that the area in question is shown on at least two projections. If the suspected mass is seen only on the MLO projection in the deep medial aspect of the breast, a CC projection for cleavage may complement the standard CC projection. Conversely, if the mass is seen in the extreme lateral aspect, an exaggerated craniocaudal (XCCL) projection laterally would be the projection of choice. In a sense, the radiographer is collecting evidence to prove whether the mass is real or is merely a summation shadow of superimposed breast parenchyma.

Other supplemental projections are intended to offer alternative methods for tailoring the mammographic procedure to the specific abilities of the patient and the requirements of the interpreting physi-

cian. Often the need for additional projections is determined only after careful examination of the standard projections. Throughout mammographic procedures, the radiographer should consistently evaluate the images, keeping foremost in mind the optimal demonstration of possible findings. For example, when performing lateral projections, the mammographer should place the area of interest closest to the image receptor. The mammographer may develop the expertise to predict and perform supplemental projections that confirm or rule out suspected breast abnormalities. As with all radiographic procedures, image evaluation is a crucial component of high-quality imaging. In evaluating images, the mammographer becomes an integral member of the breast imaging team, actively participating in the work-up of an asymptomatic patient.

TABLE 21-2

Supplemental projections or methods and their suggested applications

Projection or method	Application
Spot compression	Defines lesion or area through focal compression; separates overlying parenchyma
Magnification (M)	Combines with spot compression to show margins of lesion; delineates microcalcifications
Mediolateral (ML)	Localization; shows air-fluid-fat levels; defines lesion located in lateral aspect of breast; complements mediolateral oblique (MLO) projection
Lateromedial (LM)	Localization; shows air-fluid-fat levels; defines lesion located in medial aspect of breast
Exaggerated craniocaudal (XCCL)	Visualizes lesions in deep outer aspect of breast that are not seen on standard CC
CC for cleavage (CV)	Visualizes deep medial breast tissue; shows medial lesion in true transverse or axial plane
CC with roll (RL, RM)	Triangulates lesion seen only on CC projection; defines location of lesion as in superior or inferior aspect of breast
Tangential (TAN)	Confirms dermal vs. breast calcifications; shows obscure palpable lump over subcutaneous fat
Captured lesion	Shows palpable lump in posterior tissue that is difficult to immobilize with conventional techniques
Caudocranial (FB)	Visualizes superior breast tissue; defines lesion located in superior aspect of breast; replaces standard CC for patients with kyphosis or prominent pectoral muscles
MLO for axillary tail (AT)	Focal compression projection of AT
Lateromedial oblique (LMO)	Shows medial breast tissue; replaces standard MLO for patients with pectus excavatum, prominent pacemakers, prominent pectoral muscles, Hickman catheters, and postoperative open heart surgery
Superolateral to inferomedial oblique (SIO)	Visualizes upper-inner quadrant and lower-outer quadrant, which normally are superimposed on MLO and LMO projections

▲ 90-DEGREE MEDIOLATERAL (*ML*) PROJECTION

Image receptor: 8 × 10 inch (18 × 24 cm) or 10 × 12 inch (24 × 30 cm)

Position of patient

- Have the patient stand facing the image receptor, or seat the patient on an adjustable stool facing the unit.

Position of part

- Rotate the C-arm assembly 90 degrees, with the x-ray tube placed on the medial side of the patient's breast.
- Have the patient bend slightly forward from the waist. Position the superior corner of the image receptor high into the axilla, with the patient's elbow flexed and the affected arm resting behind the image receptor.

- Ask the patient to relax the affected shoulder.
- Pull the breast tissue and the pectoral muscle superiorly and anteriorly, ensuring that the lateral rib margin is pressed firmly against the edge of the image receptor.
- Rotate the patient slightly laterally to help bring the medial tissue forward.
- Gently pull the medial breast tissue forward from the sternum, and position the nipple in profile.
- Hold the patient's breast up and out by rotating the hand so that the base of the thumb and the heel of the hand support the breast.
- Inform the patient that compression of the breast will be used. Continue to hold the patient's breast up and out while sliding the hand toward the nipple as the compression paddle is brought into contact with the breast. Do not allow the breast to droop (Fig. 21-47).
- Slowly apply compression until the breast feels taut.
- Instruct the patient to indicate if compression becomes too uncomfortable.
- Ask the patient to hold the opposite breast away from the path of the beam.
- When full compression is achieved, move the AEC detector to the appropriate position if necessary, and instruct the patient to stop breathing (Fig. 21-48).
- Make the exposure.
- Release breast compression immediately.

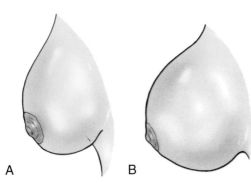

Fig. 21-47 A, Lateral profile of breast showing inadequate compression and drooping breast. **B,** Lateral profile of properly compressed breast. Note how compression has overcome the effect of gravity and how the breast is spread out over a greater area.

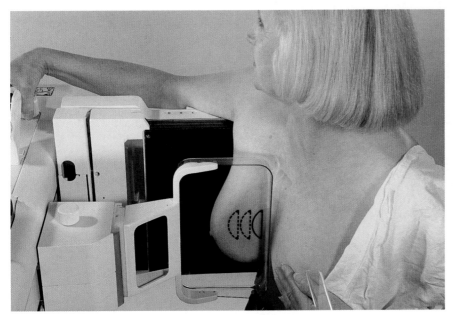

Fig. 21-48 ML projection.

Central ray

• Perpendicular to the base of the breast

Structures shown

This projection shows lesions on the lateral aspect of the breast in the superior and inferior aspects. It resolves superimposed structures seen on the MLO projection, localizes a lesion seen on one (or both) of the initial projections, and shows air-fluid and fat-fluid levels in breast structures (e.g., milk of calcium, galactoceles) and in pneumocystography (a rarely performed procedure involving injection of air into an aspirated cyst to image the cyst lining for intracystic lesions). The ML view is an orthogonal view to the CC and is often used to localize the depth of breast lesions.

The following should be clearly shown:

■ Nipple in profile
■ Open inframammary fold
■ Deep and superficial breast tissues well separated when breast is adequately maneuvered up and out from chest wall (Fig. 21-49)
■ Retroglandular fat well visualized to ensure inclusion of deep fibroglandular breast tissue
■ Uniform tissue exposure if compression is adequate

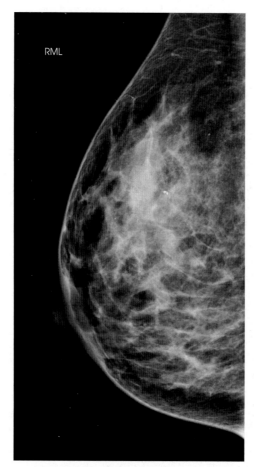

Fig. 21-49 ML projection

90-DEGREE LATEROMEDIAL (*LM*) PROJECTION

Image receptor: 8 × 10 inch (18 × 24 cm) or 10 × 12 inch (24 × 30 cm)

Position of patient
- Have the patient stand facing the image receptor, or seat the patient on an adjustable stool facing the unit.

Position of part
- Rotate the C-arm assembly 90 degrees, with the x-ray tube placed on the lateral side of the patient's breast.
- Position the superior corner of the image receptor at the level of the jugular notch.
- Have the patient flex the neck slightly forward.
- Have the patient relax the affected shoulder, raise her arm on the affected side and flex the elbow, then rest the affected arm over the top of the image receptor.
- Pull the breast tissue and pectoral muscle superiorly and anteriorly, ensuring that the patient's sternum is pressed firmly against the edge of the image receptor.
- Rotate the patient slightly medially to help bring the lateral tissue forward.
- Have the patient rest the chin on the top edge of the image receptor to help loosen the skin in the medial aspect of the breast.
- Position the nipple in profile.
- Hold the patient's breast up and out. Do not let it droop.
- Inform the patient that compression of the breast will be used. Bring the compression paddle past the latissimus dorsi muscle and into contact with the breast. Slowly apply compression while sliding the hand out toward the nipple until the patient's breast feels taut.
- Instruct the patient to indicate whether the compression becomes uncomfortable.
- When full compression is achieved, move the AEC detector to the appropriate position if necessary, and instruct the patient to stop breathing (Fig. 21-50).
- Make the exposure.
- Release breast compression immediately.

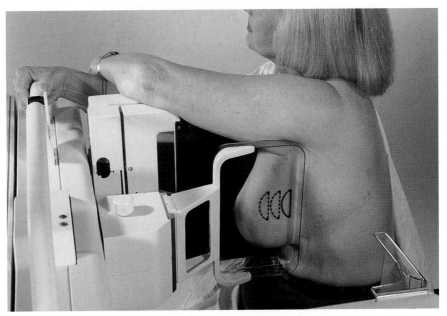

Fig. 21-50 LM projection.

Central ray

• Perpendicular to the base of the breast

Structures shown

This projection shows lesions on the medial aspect of the breast in the superior or inferior aspects (Fig. 21-51). It resolves superimposed structures seen on the MLO projection, localizes a lesion seen on one (or both) of the initial projections, and shows air-fluid and fat-fluid levels in breast structures (e.g., milk of calcium, galactoceles) and in pneumocystography (a rarely performed procedure involving injection of air into an aspirated cyst to image the cyst lining for intracystic lesions). The LM view is an orthogonal view to the CC and is often used to localize the depth of breast lesions.

EVALUATION CRITERIA

The following should be clearly shown:
■ Nipple in profile
■ Open inframammary fold
■ Deep and superficial breast tissues well separated when breast is adequately maneuvered up and out from chest wall
■ Retroglandular fat well visualized to ensure inclusion of deep fibroglandular breast tissue
■ Uniform tissue exposure if compression is adequate

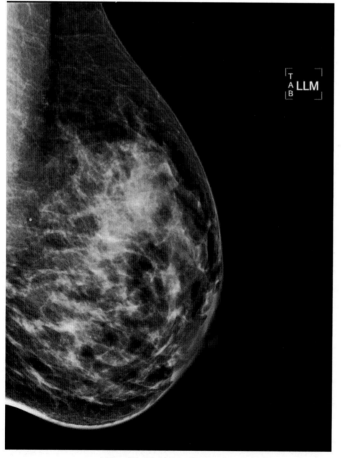

Fig. 21-51 LM projection.

Mammography

⋏ EXAGGERATED CRANIOCAUDAL (*XCCL*) PROJECTION

Image receptor: 8 × 10 inch (18 × 24 cm) or 10 × 12 inch (24 × 30 cm)

Position of patient

- Have the patient stand facing the image receptor, or seat the patient on an adjustable stool facing the unit.

Position of part

- Elevate the inframammary fold to its maximal height.
- Adjust the height of the C-arm accordingly.
- Use one hand to scoop the inferior and posterior breast tissue up from the inframammary fold and place the breast onto the image receptor.
  - This should be done with the technologist's right hand when the left breast is positioned, and with the left hand when the right breast is positioned.

- Use both hands to pull the breast gently onto the image receptor while instructing the patient to press the thorax against the breast tray.
- Slightly rotate the patient medially to place the lateral aspect of the breast on the image receptor.
- Place an arm against the patient's back with the hand on the shoulder of the affected side, ensuring that the shoulder is relaxed in external rotation.
- Slightly rotate the patient's head away from the affected side.
- Have the patient lean toward the machine and rest the head against the face guard.
- Rotate the C-arm assembly mediolaterally approximately 5 degrees if necessary to eliminate overlapping of the humeral head.
- Inform the patient that compression of the breast will be used. Smooth and flatten the breast tissue toward the nipple while bringing the compression paddle into contact with the breast.
- Slowly apply compression until the breast feels taut.
- Instruct the patient to indicate if the compression becomes uncomfortable.
- When full compression is achieved, move the AEC detector to the appropriate position if necessary, and instruct the patient to stop breathing (Figs. 21-52 and 21-53).
- Make the exposure.
- Release breast compression immediately.

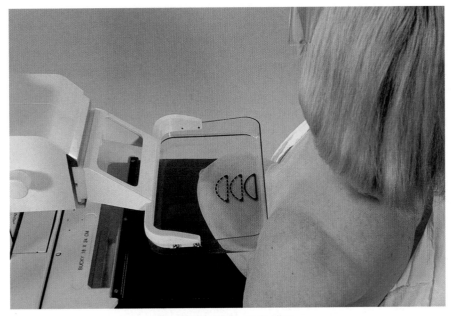

Fig. 21-52 XCCL projection.

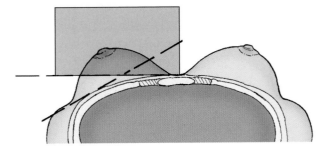

Fig. 21-53 Superior profile illustrates how placement of flat edge of image receptor against curved chest wall excludes a portion of breast tissue (*shaded area*). *Dashed line* indicates placement of image receptor for exaggerated position.

Supplemental Projections

Central ray

- Angled 5 degrees mediolaterally to the base of the breast, if necessary

Structures shown

This projection shows a superoinferior projection of the lateral fibroglandular breast tissue and posterior aspect of the pectoral muscle. It also shows a sagittal orientation of a lateral lesion located in the axillary tail of the breast.

The following should be clearly shown:

- Retroglandular fat well visualized to ensure inclusion of deep fibroglandular breast tissue on lateral aspect of breast and lower axillary region
- Pectoral muscle visualized over lateral chest wall (Fig. 21-54)
- Humeral head projected clear of image with use of a 5-degree ML angle
- Uniform tissue exposure if compression is adequate

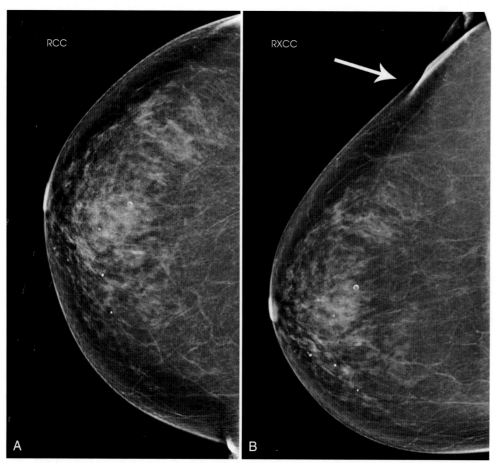

Fig. 21-54 A, CC projection of right breast. **B,** XCCL projection of right breast. This projection is exaggerated laterally to show AT (*arrow*). Note also some visualization of pectoral muscle.

CRANIOCAUDAL PROJECTION FOR CLEAVAGE (CV)

Image receptor: 8 × 10 inch (18 × 24 cm) or 10 × 12 inch (24 × 30 cm)

Position of patient

- Have the patient stand facing the image receptor, or seat the patient on an adjustable stool facing the unit

Position of part

- Turn the AEC *off*, and preselect a *manual* technique. The radiographer may use AEC only if enough breast tissue is positioned over the AEC detector. The cleavage may be intentionally offset for this purpose.
- Determine the proper height of the breast tray by elevating the inframammary fold to its maximal height.
- Adjust the height of the C-arm accordingly.

- Lift and pull both breasts gently forward onto the image receptor while instructing the patient to press the thorax against the image receptor.
- Pull as much medial breast tissue as possible onto the image receptor.
- Slightly rotate the patient's head away from the affected side.
- Have the patient lean toward the machine and rest the head against the face guard.
- Ask the patient to hold the grip bars with both hands to keep in position on the image receptor.
    - Raise the height of the image receptor slightly to loosen the superior tissue.
- Place one hand at the level of the patient's jugular notch, and then slide the hand down the patient's chest while pulling forward as much deep medial tissue as possible.
- Inform the patient that compression of the breast will be used. Bring the compression paddle into contact with the breasts, and slowly apply compression until the medial tissue feels taut. Using a quadrant compression paddle allows better compression of the cleavage area and allows more of the area of interest to be pulled into the imaging area. If a quadrant paddle is used, collimate to the area of compression to better visualize the detail of the tissue.
- Instruct the patient to indicate if the compression becomes uncomfortable.
- When full compression is achieved, move the AEC detector to the appropriate position if AEC is used, and instruct the patient to stop breathing (Fig. 21-55).
- Make the exposure.
- Release breast compression immediately.

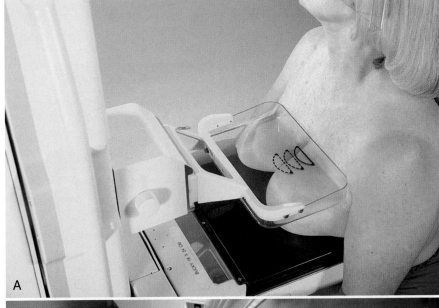

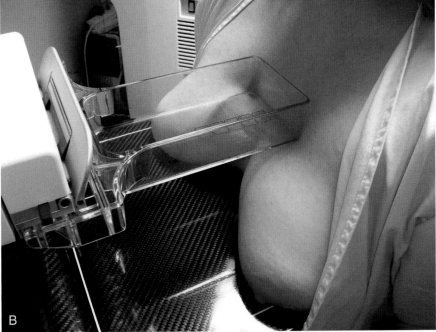

Fig. 21-55 A, Craniocaudal projection for cleavage. Cleavage is slightly off-center, so that AEC is under breast tissue. **B,** Craniocaudal projection for cleavage using a smaller-quadrant paddle for maximum posterior visualization.

Central ray

• Perpendicular to the area of interest or the centered cleavage

Structures shown

This projection shows lesions located in the deep posteromedial aspect of the breast.

The following should be clearly shown:

■ Area of interest over the central portion of the image receptor (over the AEC detector if possible) with cleavage slightly off-centered or with cleavage centered to the image receptor and manual technique selected (Fig. 21-56)

■ Deep medial tissue of affected breast

■ All medial tissue included, as shown by visualization of medial retroglandular fat and the absence of any fibroglandular tissue extending to the posteromedial edge of imaged breasts

■ Uniform tissue exposure. It is not necessary to image all of the breast tissue on this projection.

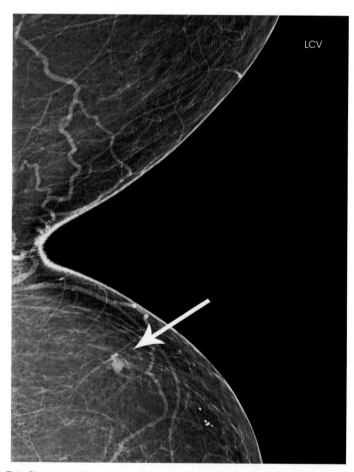

Fig. 21-56 This Cleavage View was off-center to the left (LCV) but was performed to view the medial aspect of the right breast. A mass was seen on the RMLO but was not visualized on the standard RCC view. This extremely medial mass (*arrow*) proved to be invasive carcinoma on biopsy.

CRANIOCAUDAL PROJECTION WITH ROLL LATERAL OR ROLL MEDIAL (*RL* OR *RM* USED AS SUFFIX)

Image receptor: 8 × 10 inch (18 × 24 cm) or 10 × 12 inch (24 × 30 cm)

Position of patient

- Have the patient stand facing the image receptor, or seat the patient on an adjustable stool facing the unit.

Position of part

- Reposition the patient's breast in the CC projection.
- Place the hands on opposite surfaces of the patient's breast (superior/inferior), and roll the surfaces in opposite directions. The direction of the roll is not important as long as the mammographer rolls the superior surface in one direction and the inferior surface in the other direction. In a sense, the mammographer is very gently rotating the breast approximately 10 to 15 degrees (Fig. 21-57).

- Place the patient's breast onto the image receptor surface with the lower hand while holding the rolled position with the upper hand.
- Note the direction of the superior surface roll (lateral or medial), and label the image accordingly. If the superior aspect of the breast is rolled medially, the image should be labeled RM.
- Inform the patient that compression of the breast will be used. Bring the compression paddle into contact with the breast, and slide the hand out while rolling the breast tissue.
- Slowly apply compression until the breast feels taut.
- Instruct the patient to indicate if the compression becomes uncomfortable.
- When full compression is achieved, move the AEC detector to the appropriate position if necessary and instruct the patient to stop breathing (Fig. 21-58).
- Make the exposure.
- Release breast compression immediately.

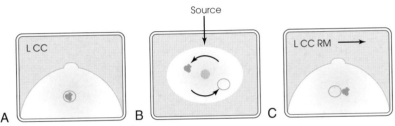

Fig. 21-57 A, CC projection showing lesion that may represent superimposition of two structures. If spot compression fails to resolve these structures, CC projection with the roll position may be performed. **B,** Anterior view of CC projection, with *arrows* indicating rolling of superior and inferior breast surfaces in opposite directions to separate superimposed structures. **C,** CC projection with RM, showing resolution of two lesions. *Arrow* indicates direction of roll of superior surface of breast.

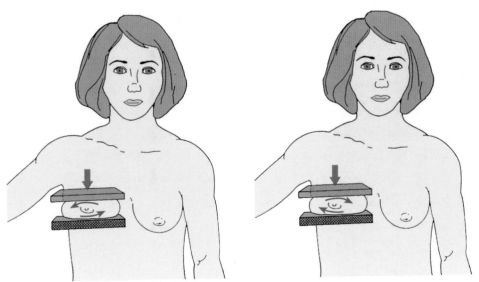

Fig. 21-58 CC projection with lateral and medial roll.

Central ray
• Perpendicular to the base of the breast

Structures shown
This position shows separation of superimposed breast tissues (also known as *summation shadow*), particularly those seen only on the CC projection. The position also helps determine whether a lesion is located in the superior or inferior aspect of the breast (Fig. 21-59). Alternatively, the standard CC projection may be performed using the spot compression technique, or with the C-arm assembly rotated 10 to 15 degrees mediolaterally or lateromedially to eliminate superimposition of breast tissue. These methods are often preferred because they allow for easier duplication of the projection during subsequent examinations.

The following should be clearly shown:
- Suspected superimposition adequately resolved
- Suspected lesion in superior or inferior aspect of breast
- All medial tissue included, as shown by visualization of medial retroglandular fat and the absence of fibroglandular tissue extending to posteromedial edge of image
- Nipple in profile and at midline, indicating no exaggeration of positioning. The nipple is used as a point of reference to distinguish the location of the suspected lesion, if it exists.
- Some lateral tissue possibly excluded to emphasize medial tissue visualized
- Slight medial skin reflection at cleavage, ensuring that posterior medial tissue is adequately included
- Uniform tissue exposure if compression is adequate

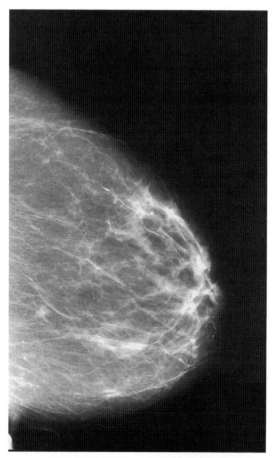

Fig. 21-59 CC projection with RL.

TANGENTIAL (*TAN*) PROJECTION

Image receptor: 8 × 10 inch (18 × 24 cm)

Position of patient
- Have the patient stand facing the image receptor, or seat the patient on an adjustable stool facing the unit.

Position of part
For a palpable mass
The TAN projection is most often performed with use of the magnification technique.
- Select a standard, quadrant, or spot compression paddle, as appropriate.
  - Place the AEC detector at the chest wall.
- Locate the area of interest by palpating the patient's breast.
- Place a radiopaque marker or BB on the mass, or have the patient place the BB on the area of concern.
- Using the imaginary line between the nipple and the BB as the angle reference (Fig. 21-60), rotate the C-arm apparatus parallel to this line. The central ray is directed tangential to the breast at the point identified by the BB marker.
- Place the breast on the image receptor or magnification stand with the area of interest marked by the BB on the edge of the skin.
  - The "shadow" of the BB will be projected onto the image receptor surface.
- Using the appropriate compression paddle, compress the breast while ensuring that enough breast tissue covers the AEC detector area.
- Slowly apply compression until the breast feels taut.
- Instruct the patient to indicate if the compression becomes uncomfortable.
- When full compression is achieved, instruct the patient to stop breathing (Figs. 21-61 and 21-62).
- Make the exposure.
- Release breast compression immediately.

Central ray
- Perpendicular to the area of interest

Structures shown
This projection shows superficial lesions close to the skin surface with minimal parenchymal overlapping. It also shows skin calcifications or palpable lesions projected over subcutaneous fat (Fig. 21-63).

EVALUATION CRITERIA
The following should be clearly shown:
- Palpable lesion visualized over subcutaneous fat
- Tangential radiopaque marker or BB marker accurately correlated with palpable lesion
- Minimal overlapping of adjacent parenchyma
- Calcification in parenchyma or skin
- Uniform tissue exposure if compression is adequate

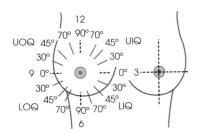
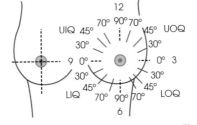

Fig. 21-60 Degree of angle for TAN projection. Correlation of location of abnormality with degree of rotation of C-arm; an angle of the C-arm shows upper quadrant and lower quadrant abnormality tangentially.

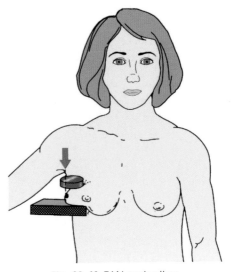

Fig. 21-61 TAN projection.

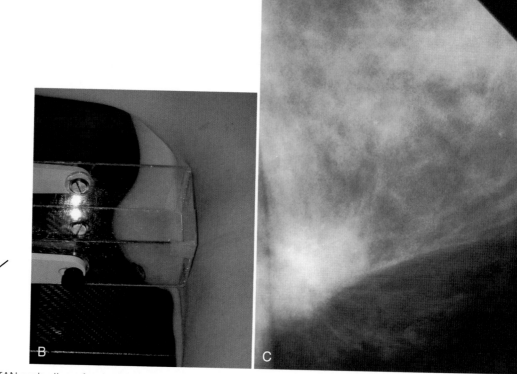

Fig. 21-62 TAN projection of palpable mass in LOQ. **A,** IR is angled parallel to nipple-to-mass line. **B,** The mass, marked by *BB,* is positioned on edge of skin line. **C,** Radiograph of mass imaged in tangent using the magnification technique. Spiculated borders indicate cancer.

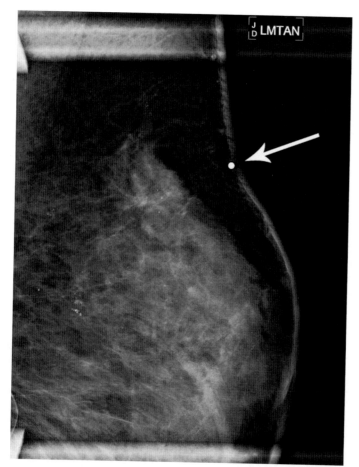

Fig. 21-63 Left magnified tangential view of a palpable mass with a BB placed on it shows the area of interest in the subdermal fatty tissue. The magnified view showed an area of architectural distortion with scattered clusters of coarse calcifications. This proved to be a cancer on biopsy.

CAPTURED LESION OR COAT-HANGER PROJECTION (CL)

This specialized positioning is seldom used but is very useful when a palpable lesion located in the extreme posterior or lateral breast tissue is imaged. Sometimes lesions in these areas tether themselves to the chest wall and resist being pulled forward to be visualized on a routine projection. This procedure is a variation of the TAN projection and should be labeled as such. It is generally performed using magnification and tight collimation. The captured lesion or coat-hanger projection captures and isolates the palpable lump for imaging (Figs. 21-64 and 21-65).

Image receptor: 8 × 10 inch (18 × 24 cm)

Position of patient

- Have the patient stand facing the image receptor, or seat the patient on an adjustable stool facing the unit.

Position of part

- Place the magnification platform designed for use with the dedicated mammography unit on the equipment.
- Place a lead BB over the palpable mass.
- Using your hands, determine the projection most likely to image the lump with no superimposition of other tissue. Place the area of clinical concern at the edge of the breast in a tangent plane to the film.
- The palpable area of clinical concern is captured with a corner of a wire coat-hanger or an inverted spot compression device. No additional compression is needed.

- It may be necessary to use a manual technique if the amount of tissue captured within the coat-hanger or inverted compression device does not cover the AEC detector.

Central ray

- Perpendicular to the film

Structures shown

The area of clinical concern is positively identified and visualized with the advantages of magnification mammography.

EVALUATION CRITERIA

The following should be clearly shown:
- Area of interest within collimated and self-compressed margins

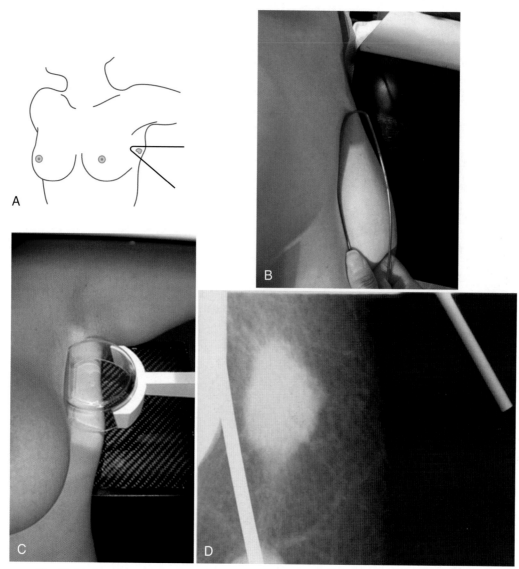

Fig. 21-64 Coat-hanger projection. **A** and **B,** A slippery lesion is captured for imaging by the angle of a wire coat-hanger. **C,** Inverted spot compression device can sometimes achieve the same results. **D,** Radiograph of lesion imaged using coat-hanger projection. This lesion could not be viewed on routine projections because of its position within the breast and the elastic nature of the lesion, which was determined to be a cancer on biopsy.

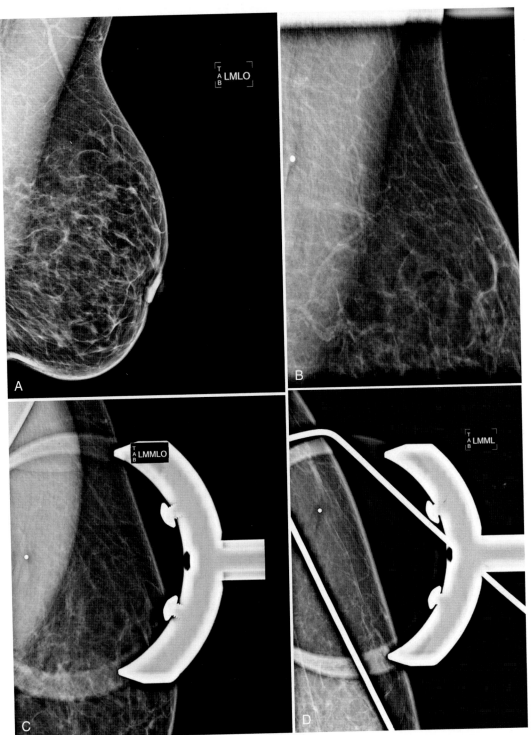

Fig. 21-65 This 40-year-old patient presented with a palpable lump on the left breast extremely posterior at 1:00. A BB was placed on the lump before imaging. The area was not visualized on the standard MLO view (**A**). Subsequent tangential imaging was unsuccessful because of the proximity of the pectoral muscle (**B** and **C**). A CL view was performed (**D**) to stabilize the lump within the imaged area. This proved to be a lipoma.

CAUDOCRANIAL (*FB*) PROJECTION

Image receptor: 8 × 10 inch (18 × 24 cm) or 10 × 12 inch (24 × 30 cm)

Position of patient
- Have the patient stand facing the image receptor.

Position of part
- Rotate the C-arm apparatus 180 degrees from the rotation used for a routine CC projection. The tube head will be near the floor and the image receptor will be above the patient's breast.
- Standing on the medial side of the breast to be imaged, elevate the inframammary fold to its maximal height.

- Adjust the height of the C-arm so that the image receptor is in contact with the superior breast tissue.
- Lean the patient slightly forward while gently pulling the elevated breast out and perpendicular to the chest wall. Hold the breast in position.
- Have the patient rest the affected arm over the top of the image receptor.
- Inform the patient that compression of the breast will be used. Bring the compression paddle from below into contact with the patient's breast while sliding the hand toward the nipple.
- Slowly apply compression until the breast feels taut.

- Instruct the patient to indicate if the compression becomes uncomfortable.
- To ensure that the patient's abdomen is not superimposed over the path of the beam, have the patient pull in the abdomen or move the hips back slightly.
- When full compression is achieved, move the AEC detector to the appropriate position, and instruct the patient to stop breathing (Fig. 21-66).
- Make the exposure.
- Release breast compression immediately.

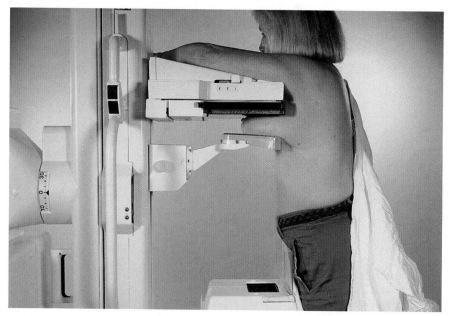

Fig. 21-66 FB projection.

Central ray

- Perpendicular to the base of the breast

Structures shown

This projection shows an inferosuperior projection of the breast for improved visualization of lesions located in the superior aspect as a result of reduced object–to–image receptor distance. The FB projection may facilitate a shorter route for needle-wire insertion to localize an inferior lesion (Fig. 21-67) or during prone stereotactic core biopsy. The projection may also be used as a replacement for the standard CC projection in patients with prominent pectoral muscles or kyphosis.

The following should be clearly shown:

- Superior breast tissue and lesions clearly visualized
- For needle localization images, inferior lesion visualized within specialized fenestrated compression plate
- Patient's abdomen projected clear of image
- Inclusion of fixed posterior tissue of superior aspect of breast
- PNL extending posteriorly to edge of image, measuring within ⅓ inch (1 cm) of depth of PNL on MLO projection
- All medial tissue included as shown by visualization of medial retroglandular fat and absence of fibroglandular tissue extending to posteromedial edge of image
- Nipple in profile, if possible, and at midline, indicating no exaggeration of positioning
- Some lateral tissue possibly excluded to emphasize medial tissue
- Slight medial skin reflection at cleavage, ensuring that posterior medial tissue is adequately included
- Uniform tissue exposure if compression is adequate

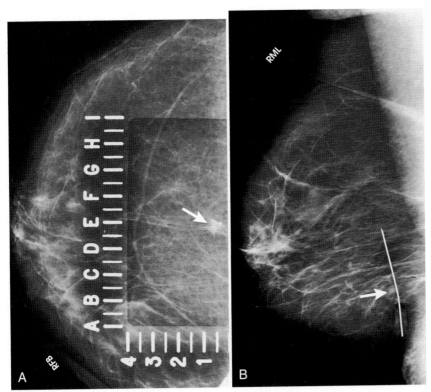

Fig. 21-67 A, FB projection performed in a 57-year-old woman to access the shortest route for localizing lesions identified in the inferior aspect of the breast (*arrow*). **B,** Orthogonal 90-degree ML projection of the same patient, showing successful placement of needle-wire system within lesion (*arrow*). The lesion was found to be a 9-mm infiltrating ductal carcinoma.

Supplemental Projections

MEDIOLATERAL OBLIQUE PROJECTION FOR AXILLARY TAIL (*AT*)

Image receptor: 8 × 10 inch (18 × 24 cm) or 10 × 12 inch (24 × 30 cm)

Position of patient
- Have the patient stand facing the image receptor, or seat the patient on an adjustable stool facing the unit.

Position of part
- Determine the degree of obliquity of the C-arm apparatus by rotating the tube until the long edge of the image receptor is parallel with the AT of the affected side. The degree of obliquity varies between 10 degrees and 35 degrees.
- Adjust the height of the C-arm so that the superior border of the image receptor is just under the axilla.

- Instruct the patient to elevate the arm of the affected side over the corner of the image receptor and to rest the hand on the adjacent handgrip. The patient's elbow should be flexed.
- Have the patient relax the affected shoulder and lean it slightly anterior. Using the flat surface of the hand, gently pull the tail of the breast anteriorly and medially onto the image receptor, keeping the skin and tissue smooth and free of wrinkles.
- Ask the patient to turn the head away from the side being examined and to rest the head against the face guard.
- Inform the patient that compression of the breast will be used. Continue to hold the breast in position while sliding the hand toward the nipple as the compression paddle is brought into contact with the AT (Fig. 21-68).

- Slowly apply compression until the breast feels taut. The corner of the compression paddle should be inferior to the clavicle. To avoid patient discomfort caused by the corner of the paddle and to facilitate even compression, remind the patient to keep the shoulder relaxed.
- Instruct the patient to indicate if the compression becomes uncomfortable.
- When full compression is achieved, move the AEC detector to the appropriate position, and instruct the patient to stop breathing. It may be necessary to increase exposure factors if compression is not as taut as in the routine projections.
- Make the exposure.
- Release breast compression immediately.

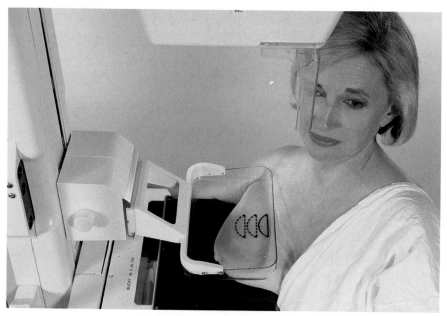

Fig. 21-68 MLO projection for AT.

Central ray

- Perpendicular to the image receptor
- The angle of the C-arm apparatus is determined by the slope of the patient's AT.

Structures shown

This projection shows the AT of the breast, with emphasis on its lateral aspect.

EVALUATION CRITERIA

The following should be clearly shown:
- AT with inclusion of axillary lymph nodes under focal compression (Fig. 21-69)
- Uniform tissue exposure if compression is adequate
- Slight skin reflection of affected arm on superior border of image

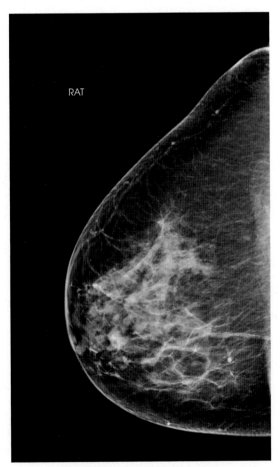

Fig. 21-69 Right AT projection.

AXILLA PROJECTION FOR AXILLARY TAIL (*AT*)

Image receptor: 8 × 10 inch (18 × 24 cm)

Position of patient

- Have the patient stand facing the image receptor, or seat the patient on an adjustable stool facing the unit.

Position of part

- Rotate the c-arm to approximately 70 degrees.
- Adjust the height of the C-arm so that the superior edge of the image receptor is even with the top of the patient's shoulder.
- Select the appropriate compression device. A quadrant paddle will capture more deep axillary tissue; a standard 18 × 24-cm compression paddle will capture additional lateral tissue and axillary tail.

- Instruct the patient to elevate the arm of the affected side so that it is perpendicular to the body.
- Place the arm against the image receptor so that the posterior aspect of the shoulder is resting against the IR. The patient's arm is draped across the IR with the forearm resting on the grip bar.
- Have the patient relax the affected shoulder and lean slightly anterior. Using the flat surface of the hand placed under the axillary region, gently pull the tail of the breast anteriorly and medially onto the image receptor, keeping the skin and tissue smooth and free of wrinkles.
- Inform the patient that compression of the breast will be used. Slowly bring compression down along the patient's ribs, with the top edge of the compression paddle skimming the lower edge of the patient's upper arm.

- Slowly apply compression until the axillary tissue feels taut. The corner of the compression paddle should be inferior to the clavicle. To avoid patient discomfort caused by the corner of the paddle and to facilitate even compression, remind the patient to keep the shoulder relaxed.
- Instruct the patient to indicate if the compression becomes uncomfortable. Vigorous compression is not necessary for this view (Fig. 21-70).
- When full compression is achieved, move the AEC detector to the appropriate position, and instruct the patient to stop breathing. It may be necessary to increase exposure factors if compression is not as taut as in the routine projections.
- Make the exposure.
- Release breast compression immediately

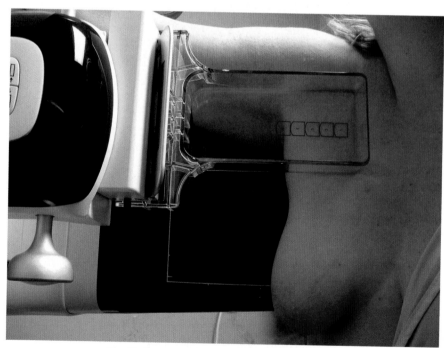

Fig. 21-70 Axilla projection for axillary tail (AT).

Structures shown

This projection shows the axilla and the AT of the breast, with emphasis on its lateral aspect.

The following should be clearly shown:

- AT with inclusion of axillary lymph nodes under focal compression (Fig. 21-71)
- Uniform tissue exposure if compression is adequate
- Slight skin reflection of affected arm on superior border of image

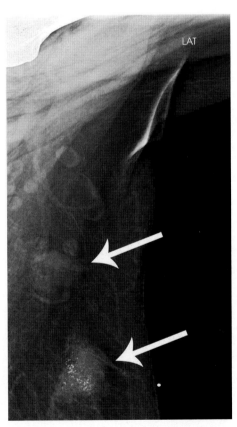

Fig. 21-71 Left AT projection demonstrating the axilla and its contents. Note ductal carcinoma and metastasized lymph nodes (*arrows*).

LATEROMEDIAL OBLIQUE (*LMO*) PROJECTION

Image receptor: 8 × 10 inch (18 × 24 cm) or 10 × 12 inch (24 × 30 cm)

Position of patient
• Have the patient stand facing the image receptor, or seat the patient on an adjustable stool facing the unit.

Position of part
• Determine the degree of obliquity of the C-arm apparatus by rotating the assembly until the long edge of the image receptor is parallel with the upper third of the pectoral muscle of the affected side. The central ray enters the inferior aspect of the breast from the lateral side. The degree of obliquity should be between 30 degrees and 60 degrees, depending on the body habitus of the patient.

• Adjust the height of the C-arm so that the superior border of the image receptor is level with the jugular notch.
• Ask the patient to place the opposite hand on the C-arm. The patient's elbow should be flexed.
• Lean the patient toward the C-arm apparatus, and press the sternum against the edge of the image receptor, which is slightly off-center toward the opposite breast.
• Have the patient relax the affected shoulder and lean it slightly anterior. Gently pull the patient's breast and pectoral muscle anteriorly and medially, with the flat surface of the hand positioned along the lateral aspect of the breast.
• Scoop breast tissue up with the hand, gently grasping the breast between fingers and thumb.
• Center the breast with the nipple in profile, if possible, and hold the breast in position.

• Inform the patient that compression of the breast will be used. Continue to hold the patient's breast up and out while sliding the hand toward the nipple as the compression paddle is brought into contact with the LOQ of the breast.
• Slowly apply compression until the breast feels taut.
• Instruct the patient to indicate if the compression becomes uncomfortable.
• Pull down on the patient's abdominal tissue to open the inframammary fold.
• Ask the patient to rest the affected elbow on the top edge of the image receptor.
• When full compression is achieved, move the AEC detector to the appropriate position, and instruct the patient to stop breathing (Fig. 21-72).
• Make the exposure.
• Release breast compression immediately.

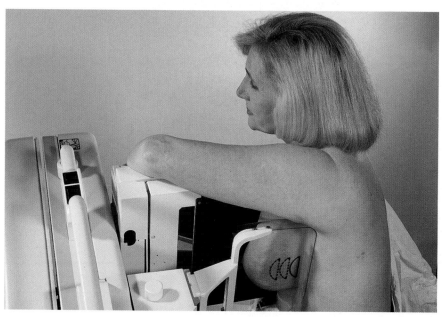

Fig. 21-72 LMO projection.

Central ray

- Perpendicular to the image receptor
- The C-arm apparatus is positioned at an angle determined by the slope of the patient's pectoral muscle (30 to 60 degrees). The actual angle is determined by the patient's body habitus: Tall, thin patients require steep angulation, whereas short, stout patients require shallow angulation.

Structures shown

This projection shows a true reverse projection of the routine MLO projection and is typically performed to better show the medial breast tissue. It is also performed if the routine MLO cannot be completed because of one or more of the following conditions: pectus excavatum, extreme kyphosis, post open-heart surgery, prominent pacemaker, men or women with prominent pectoralis muscles, or Port-A-Cath/MediPort (Hickman catheters).

EVALUATION CRITERIA

The following should be clearly shown:
- Medial breast tissue clearly visualized (Fig. 21-73)
- PNL measuring within $\frac{1}{3}$ inch (1 cm) of the depth of the PNL on the CC projection. (While drawing the PNL obliquely, following the orientation of the breast tissue toward the pectoral muscle, measure its depth from nipple to pectoral muscle or to the edge of the image, whichever comes first.)
- Inferior aspect of the pectoral muscle extending to nipple line or below it if possible
- Pectoral muscle with anterior convexity to ensure a relaxed shoulder and axilla
- Nipple in profile if possible
- Open inframammary fold
- Deep and superficial breast tissues well separated when breast is adequately maneuvered up and out from chest wall
- Retroglandular fat well visualized to ensure inclusion of deep fibroglandular breast tissue
- Uniform tissue exposure if compression is adequate

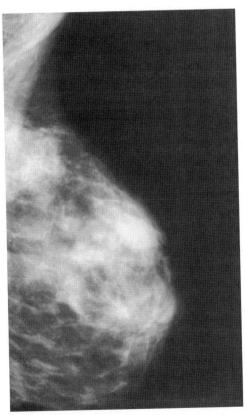

Fig. 21-73 LMO projection.

(From Svane G: *Screening mammography*, St Louis, 1993, Mosby.)

SUPEROLATERAL TO INFEROMEDIAL OBLIQUE (*SIO*) PROJECTION

Image receptor: 8 × 10 inch (18 × 24 cm) or 10 × 12 inch (24 × 30 cm)

Position of patient

- Have the patient stand facing the image receptor, or seat the patient on an adjustable stool facing the unit.

Position of part

- Rotate the C-arm apparatus so that the central ray is directed at an angle to enter the superior and lateral aspect of the affected breast. The LIQ is adjacent to the image receptor.
- Adjust the degree of C-arm obliquity according to the body habitus of the patient, or, when the SIO projection is being used as an additional projection to image an area of the tissue more clearly without superimposition of surrounding tissue, adjust the C-arm to the degree of angulation required by the radiologist, generally a 20- to 30-degree angle.

- Adjust the height of the C-arm to position the patient's breast over the center of the image receptor.
- Instruct the patient to rest the hand of the affected side on the handgrip adjacent to the image receptor holder. The patient's elbow should be flexed. For shallow-angled SIO projections, the arm on the affected side should lie straight against the patient's side. The handgrip is held by the hand on the contralateral side.
- Place the upper corner of the image receptor along the sternal edge adjacent to the upper inner aspect of the patient's breast.
- With the patient leaning slightly forward, gently pull as much medial tissue as possible away from the sternal edge while holding the breast up and out. The breast should not droop. Ensure that the patient's back remains straight during positioning, and that the patient does not lean to the side or toward the image receptor.
- Inform the patient that compression of the breast will be used. Continue to hold the breast up and out.
- Bring the compression paddle under the affected arm and into contact with the patient's breast while sliding the hand toward the patient's nipple. For shallow-angled SIO, the affected arm at the patient's side should be bent at the elbow to avoid superimposition of the humeral head over the breast tissue.
- Slowly apply compression until the breast feels taut. The upper corner of the compression paddle should be in the axilla for the standard SIO projection.
- Instruct the patient to indicate if the compression becomes uncomfortable.
- When full compression is achieved on the standard SIO, help the patient bring the arm up and over with the flexed elbow resting on top of the image receptor.
- Gently pull down on the patient's abdominal tissue to smooth out any skin folds.
- Move the AEC detector to the appropriate position, and instruct the patient to stop breathing (Fig. 21-74).
- Make the exposure.
- Release breast compression immediately.

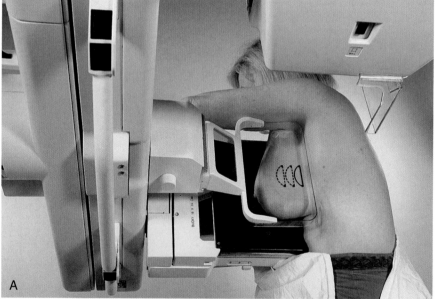

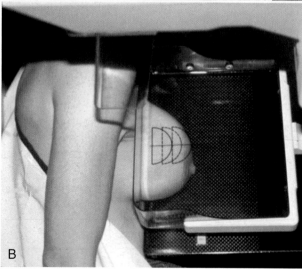

Fig. 21-74 A, SIO projection. **B,** Shallow-angled SIO with arm down.

Central ray

- Perpendicular to the image receptor
- The C-arm apparatus is positioned at an angle determined by the patient's body habitus or tissue composition.

Structures shown

This projection shows the UIQ and LOQ of the breast free of superimposition. In addition, lesions located in the lower inner aspect of the breast are shown with better recorded detail. This projection may also be used to replace the MLO ID projection in patients with encapsulated implants (Fig. 21-75).

The following should be clearly shown:

- UIQ and LOQ free of superimposition (these quadrants are superimposed on MLO and LMO projections)
- Lower inner aspect of breast visualized with greater detail
- Nipple in profile if possible
- Deep and superficial breast tissues well separated when breast is adequately maneuvered up and out from chest wall
- Retroglandular fat well visualized to ensure inclusion of deep fibroglandular breast tissue
- Uniform tissue exposure if compression is adequate.

Supplemental Projections

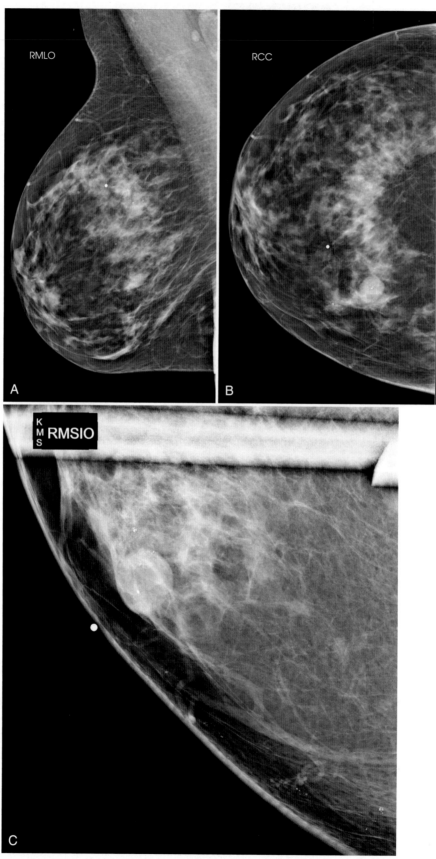

Fig. 21-75 Patient presented with a palpable mass at 1:00 in the right breast. A BB was placed on the skin over the lump, and standard MLO and CC projections were taken (**A** and **B**). A tangential view taken in an SIO projection (**C**) places the palpable lump within the dermis for best visualization. This proved to be invasive ductal carcinoma on biopsy.

Ductography (Examination of Milk Ducts)

Ductography is indicated in a patient who presents with a unilateral spontaneous discharge from the nipple that is either bloody or clear and watery. This type of discharge can be associated with a ductal carcinoma that is mammographically occult. More often, nipple discharge is the product of a papilloma within the duct. The ductogram can help the radiologist determine the cause and location of the origin of the discharge by injecting an opaque contrast medium into the duct. These patients can often be biopsied immediately using stereotactic methods with contrast-enhanced ducts (Fig. 21-76).

Equipment and supplies for the examination include a sterile hypodermic syringe (usually 1 to 3 mL); a 30-gauge ductography cannula with a smooth, round tip; a skin cleansing agent; sterile gauze sponges or cotton balls; paper tape; a waste basin; and an organic, water-soluble, iodinated contrast medium.

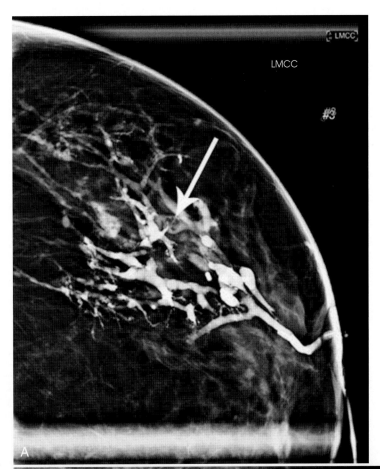

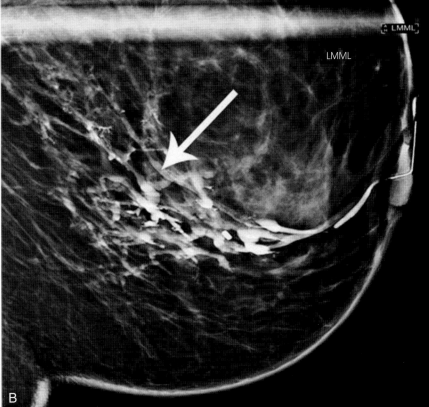

Fig. 21-76 This 55-year-old patient presented with a spontaneous brown discharge from the left nipple. Ductography was performed for visualization of the ducts. A probable papilloma was noted as an area of lucency (*arrow*) on CC (**A**) and ML (**B**) views. This patient was sent for stereotactic core biopsy (**C**, pre-fire images) where the area was excised. It proved to be a papilloma. *Continued*

Ductography

After the nipple is cleaned, a small amount of discharge is expressed to identify the correct ductal opening. The cannula is inserted into the orifice of the duct, and undiluted iothalamate meglumine or iopamidol is gently injected. So that the patient does not experience unnecessary discomfort and extravasation does not occur, the injection is terminated as soon as the patient experiences a sense of fullness, pressure, or pain. The cannula is taped in place before the patient is positioned for the radiographs. If cannulation is unsuccessful, a sterile local anesthetic gel or warm compress may be applied to the nipple and areola, and the procedure is reattempted. If ductography is unsuccessful after several attempts, the procedure may be rescheduled in 7 to 14 days. On successful injection, the following guidelines are observed:

- Immediately obtain radiographs with the patient positioned for the CC and lateral projections of the subareolar region using the magnification technique (see Fig. 21-76, *A* and *B*). If needed, MLO or rolled CC and rolled MLO magnification projections may be obtained to resolve superimposed ducts.
- Employ the exposure techniques used in general mammography.
- Leave the cannula in the duct to minimize leakage of contrast material during compression and to facilitate reinjection of the contrast medium without the need for recannulation.
- If the cannula is removed for the images, do not apply vigorous compression because this would cause the contrast medium to be expelled.

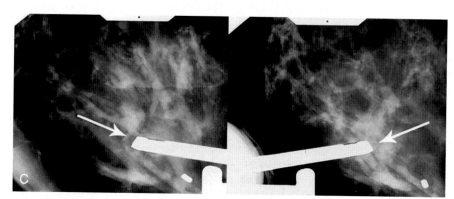

Fig. 21-76, cont'd

Localization and Biopsy of Suspicious Lesions

Approximately 80% of nonpalpable lesions identified by mammography are not malignant. Nonetheless, a breast lesion cannot be definitively judged benign until it has been microscopically evaluated. When mammography identifies a nonpalpable lesion that warrants biopsy, the abnormality must be accurately located so that the smallest amount of breast tissue is removed for microscopic evaluation, minimizing trauma to the breast. This technique conserves the maximal amount of normal breast tissue unless extensive surgery is indicated by pathologic findings.

Suspicious breast lesions can be biopsied using three techniques: (1) fine-needle aspiration biopsy (FNAB), (2) large-core needle biopsy (LCNB), and (3) open surgical biopsy. FNAB uses a hollow small-gauge needle to extract tissue cells from a suspicious lesion. The location of the lesion is identified by the doctor using palpation, ultrasonography, or stereotactic guidance. FNAB can potentially decrease the need for surgical excisional biopsy by identifying benign lesions and by diagnosing malignant lesions that require extensive surgery rather than excisional biopsy.

LCNB obtains small samples of breast tissue by means of a larger-gauge (generally sized between 9-gauge and 14-gauge) hollow needle with a trough adjacent to the tip of the needle. A vacuum suction system is frequently employed during this procedure to pull the target tissue through the trough into a collecting chamber. Once the tissue sample has been obtained, a titanium clip is often placed in the breast through the needle to mark the exact location of the biopsy. This clip can be used by the surgeon to locate the areola during an open surgical excision, or to indicate the area of prior LCNB during subsequent mammography. Because larger tissue samples are obtained with LCNB, and because results are very accurate, clinical support is available for use of this technique instead of surgical excisional biopsy to diagnose pathology of a lesion. LCNB may be used with clinical, ultrasound, stereotactic, and MRI guidance. The method used depends on the preference of the radiologist and the surgeon and is typically determined by the modality with which the lesion is most visible.

When a patient is a candidate for an open surgical biopsy, needle-wire localization is a predominant method for localizing nonpalpable lesions before surgery. Needle-wire localization uses a long needle containing a hooked guidewire, which is inserted into the breast to lead the surgeon directly to the lesion. The location of the nonpalpable lesion can be initially located using ultrasound or stereotactic imaging, but it is primarily calculated using a standard mammography unit with specialized compression plates. The four most common needle-wire localization systems are the Kopans, Homer (18-gauge), Frank (21-gauge), and Hawkins (20-gauge) biopsy guides. A small incision (1 to 2 mm) at the entry site may be necessary to facilitate insertion of a larger-gauge needle. With each system, a long needle containing a hooked wire is inserted into the breast until the needle's tip is adjacent to the lesion. When the needle and wire are in place, the needle is withdrawn over the wire. The hook on the end of the wire anchors the wire within the breast tissue. Some radiologists also inject a small amount of methylene blue dye to label the proper biopsy site visually. After needle-wire localization, the patient is bandaged and taken to the surgical area for excisional biopsy (Fig. 21-77). The surgeon then cuts along the guidewire and removes the breast tissue around the wire's hooked end. Alternatively, the surgeon may choose an incision site that intercepts the anchored wire distant from the point of wire entry. Ideally, the radiologist and the surgeon should review the localization images together before the excisional biopsy is performed.

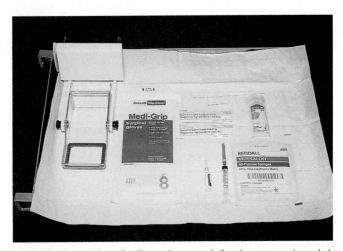

Fig. 21-77 Material for breast localization using specialized compression plate: alphanumeric localization compression plate, sterile gloves, topical antiseptic, alcohol wipe, local anesthetic, 5-mL syringe, 25-gauge needle, scalpel blade, sterile gauze, tape, and needle-wire localization system.

BREAST LESION LOCALIZATION WITH A SPECIALIZED COMPRESSION PLATE

Most breast cancers that are surgically removed are nonpalpable lesions that have been found during mammography. Preoperative localization of these lesions is often performed to aid the surgeon in locating the area of concern to ensure excision of the lesion. Most mammography units are adaptable with specialized compression plates with openings that can be positioned over a breast lesion. Through the opening, a specialized localizing needle-wire set can be introduced into the breast. The initial mammogram and a 90-degree lateral projection are usually reviewed together to determine the shortest distance from the skin to the breast lesion. A lesion in the inferior aspect of the breast may be best approached from the medial, lateral, or inferior surface of the breast but not from the superior surface.

Two styles of fenestrated localization compression paddles are currently in use: a rectangular cutout with radiopaque alphanumeric grid markings along at least two adjacent sides, and a device in which the plate may be fenestrated with several rows of holes, each large enough to accommodate insertion of a localization needle (Fig. 21-78). There are proponents for each of the paddles, and which one is used is usually decided by the radiologist performing the localization procedure. The device with fenestrated holes allows the breast tissue to be more firmly fixed and compressed; this in turn allows the area to be localized, making it more discernible from the surrounding tissue.

Needle-localization procedures vary from radiologist to radiologist. As a result, no standardized procedure is known. The following steps are typically taken:

- Perform preliminary routine full-breast projections to confirm the existence of the lesion (Figs. 21-79 and 21-80). Orthogonal views will be more helpful in visualizing the exact location of the lesion; therefore the MLO projection may be replaced by a 90-degree lateral projection.
- Obtain informed consent after discussing the following topics with the patient:
  1. Full explanation of the procedure
  2. Full description of potential problems per facility policy: These may include vasovagal reaction, excessive bleeding, allergic reaction to lidocaine, and possible failure of the procedure (failure rate of 0% to 20%).[n,o,p]
  3. Answers to patient's preliminary questions

[n]Jackman RJ, Marzoni FA Jr: Needle-localized breast biopsy: why do we fail? *Radiology* 204(3):677, 1997.

[o]Abrahamson PE et al: Factors predicting successful needle-localized breast biopsy, *Acad Radiol* 10(6):601, 2003.

[p]Kouskos E et al: Wire localisation biopsy of nonpalpable breast lesions: reasons for unsuccessful excision, *Eur J Gynaecol Oncol* 27(3):262, 2006.

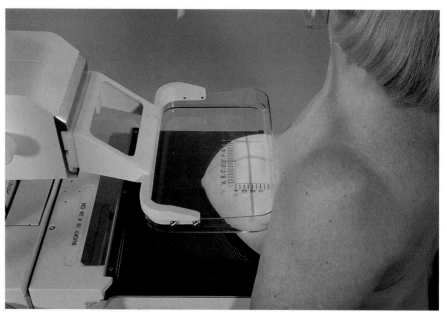

Fig. 21-79 CC projection shown with specialized open-hole compression plate.

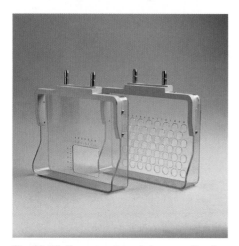

Fig. 21-78 Compression plates specifically designed for breast localization procedure.

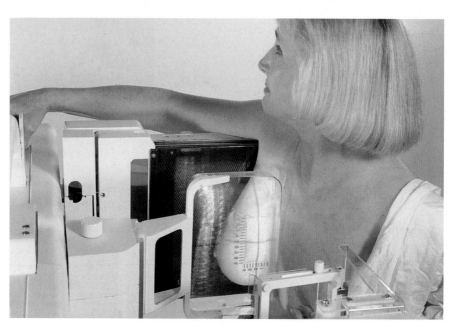

Fig. 21-80 ML projection shown with specialized open-hole compression plate.

- Position the patient so that the compression plate is against the skin surface closest to the lesion as determined from preliminary images.
- Tell the patient that compression will not be released until the needle has been successfully placed and that the patient is to hold as still as possible.
- Disable the automatic release of the compression paddle.
- Make a preliminary exposure using compression. Ink marks may be placed at the corners of the paddle window or in several of the concentric holes away from the area to be localized to determine whether the patient moves during the procedure.

- Process the image without removing compression. The resultant image shows where the lesion lies in relation to the compression plate openings (Fig. 21-81). If using the circularly fenestrated paddle, count the holes visible on the image to determine the correct entry point of the needle. If using the rectangular hole, use the alphanumeric marker system supplied with the paddle to determine the location of the lesion and the needle entry point.
- Clean the skin of the breast over the entry site with a topical antiseptic. Some radiologists may prefer to do this before compression.
- Apply a topical anesthetic if necessary.

- Insert the localizing needle and guidewire into the breast perpendicular to the compression plate and parallel to the chest wall, moving the needle directly toward the underlying lesion. Advance the needle to the estimated depth of the lesion. Because the breast is compressed in the direction of the needle's insertion, it is better to pass beyond the lesion than to be short of the lesion. Do not advance the guidewire into the tissue until the depth of the lesion has been determined by the orthogonal view.
- With the needle in position, make an exposure. Be sure that the shadow of the hub of the needle projects directly over the insertion point of the needle during the exposure to precisely indicate the location of the tip. Slowly release the compression plate, leaving the needle-wire system in place. Obtain an additional projection after the C-arm apparatus has been shifted 90 degrees. (These two orthogonal radiographs are used to determine the position of the end of the needle-wire relative to the depth of the lesion.)
- If the needle is not located adjacent to or within the area of interest, reposition the needle-wire, and repeat the exposures.
- When the needle is accurately placed within the lesion, withdraw the needle, but leave the hooked guidewire in place.
- Place a gauze bandage over the breast.
- Transport the patient to surgery along with the final localization images.

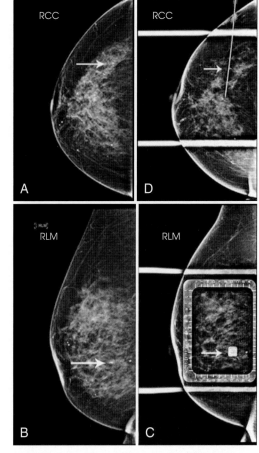

Fig. 21-81 CC and ML projections (**A** and **B**) taken to verify area to be excised. Clips from prior core biopsy (*arrows*) indicate correct area for wire localization. These images show that inserting the localization needle from the lateral aspect of the breast uses the closest route, thereby minimizing trauma and scarring from surgery. The breast is positioned in the LM projection using the alphanumeric fenestrated paddle. The needle is inserted, and an image is taken to verify that it has been inserted over the lesion (**C**). The arrow indicates the hub of the needle. A final image (**D**) is taken in the CC projection to affirm that the needle passes through the area to be biopsied.

Localization of dermal calcifications

For localization of nonpalpable dermal calcifications, two projections are necessary: (1) a localization projection (which depends on the area of interest) and (2) a TAN projection.

- From the routine CC and MLO projections, determine the quadrant in which the area of interest is located.
- Determine which projection would best localize the area of interest—the CC or 90-degree lateral projection.
- Turn off the automatic compression release, and inform the patient that compression will be continued while the first image is processed.
- Using a localization compression paddle, position the C-arm and breast so that the paddle opening is positioned over the quadrant of interest.
- Slowly apply compression until the breast feels taut.
- Instruct the patient to indicate if the compression becomes uncomfortable.
- When full compression is achieved, move the AEC detector to the appropriate position, and instruct the patient to stop breathing.
- Make the exposure.
- *Do not release compression.* Keep the breast compressed while the initial image is processed.

Tangential projection

- Check the initial image, and locate the area of interest using the alphanumeric identifiers.
- With the patient's breast still under compression, locate the corresponding area on the breast and place a radiopaque marker or BB over the area.
- Release breast compression, and replace the localization compression paddle with a regular or spot compression paddle.
- Rotate the C-arm apparatus until the central ray is directed tangential to the breast at the point identified by the BB marker (the "shadow" of the BB is projected onto the image receptor surface).
- Compress the area while ensuring that enough breast tissue covers the AEC detector area.
- Slowly apply compression until the breast feels taut.
- Instruct the patient to indicate whether the compression becomes uncomfortable.
- When full compression is achieved, move the AEC detector to the appropriate position, and instruct the patient to stop breathing.
- Make the exposure.
- Release breast compression immediately.

Central ray

- Perpendicular to the area of interest

Structures shown

This projection shows superficial lesions close to the skin surface with minimal parenchymal overlapping. It also shows skin calcifications or palpable lesions projected over subcutaneous fat (see Fig. 21-63).

EVALUATION CRITERIA

The following should be clearly shown:

- Palpable lesion visualized over subcutaneous fat
- Tangential radiopaque marker or BB marker accurately correlated with palpable lesion
- Minimal overlapping of adjacent parenchyma
- Calcification in parenchyma or skin
- Uniform tissue exposure if compression is adequate

STEREOTACTIC IMAGING AND BIOPSY PROCEDURES

Stereotactic imaging, or *stereotaxis,* is a method of calculating the exact location of a specific lesion in the breast using mammographic imaging. Stereotaxis uses three-dimensional triangulation to identify the exact location of a breast lesion by taking two *stereo images* 30 degrees apart (Fig. 21-82). Once the lesion has been identified in a perpendicular *scout image,* the x-ray tube is rotated +15 degrees for the first stereo exposure, then −15 for the second. At a computer workstation, the lesion is marked in each stereo image, and a digitizer calculates *X, Y,* and *Z* coordinates (Fig. 21-83).

The *X, Y,* and *Z* coordinates allow the physician to calculate the exact location of the breast lesion in three dimensions. The *X* coordinate identifies the transverse location, right to left, or the inferior breast versus the lateral breast. The *Y* coordinate designates depth, front to back, or anterior versus posterior breast. The *Z* coordinate identifies the height of the lesion, top to bottom, or superficial to the skin versus the center of the breast (Fig. 21-84). Different stereotactic systems have different methods for calculating a *Z* value depending on the location of the center reference point. The operator should be familiar with the system in use so that accurate adjustments of the localization device can be made.

Imaging with stereotactic units is available as conventional screen-film or small-field (2 × 2 inch [5 × 5 cm]) digital imaging. Although conventional screen-film systems are considerably less expensive, digital imaging is preferred because of its shorter acquisition time. This is important, as the breast is held in compression throughout the procedure. Any slight movement changes the *X, Y,* and *Z* values.

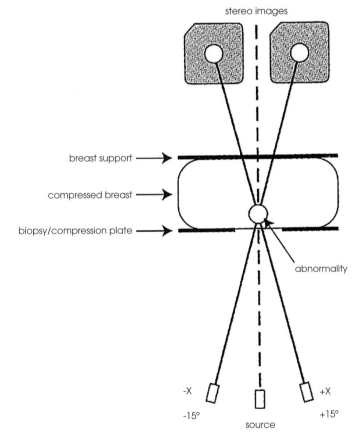

Fig. 21-82 Three-dimensional localization. Acquisition of two planar images from different source positions provides the means for 3D localization.

(Reprinted with permission from Willison KM: Fundamentals of stereotactic breast biopsy. In: Fajardo LL, Willison KM, Pizzutello RJ, eds: *A comprehensive approach to stereotactic breast biopsy,* Cambridge, 1996, Blackwell Science, p14.)

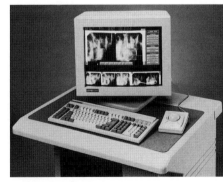

Fig. 21-83 Digitizer calculates and transmits *X, Y,* and *Z* coordinates to stage, or "brain," of biopsy system, where biopsy gun is attached. This information is used to determine placement of biopsy needle.

(Courtesy Trex Medical Corp., LORAD Division, Danbury, CT.)

Once the lesion is localized using stereotaxis, three general methods can be used to biopsy a breast lesion. The physician's preference generally determines the procedure that is performed. The lesion can be mapped with hooked guidewire in needle-wire localization for subsequent surgery, or it can be biopsied through FNAB or LCNB. In FNAB, cells are extracted from a suspicious lesion with a thin needle. For large-core needle biopsies, core samples of tissue are obtained by means of a larger needle with a trough adjacent to its tip. Samples are then evaluated to determine the benign or malignant nature of the suspicious breast lesion. Given that LCNB using stereotactic imaging is a minor outpatient procedure and the preferred biopsy method, it is discussed in depth in this chapter.

The benefits of *stereotactic core needle biopsy* over open surgical biopsy include less pain, less scarring, shorter recovery time, less patient anxiety, and lower cost. Most women with a mammographic or clinical breast abnormality are candidates for stereotactic core needle biopsy. The only exceptions are patients who cannot cooperate for the procedure, patients with physical limitations prohibiting use of the equipment, patients who have mammographic findings at the limits of perception, and patients with lesions of potentially ambiguous histology.

Stereotactic biopsies are generally quicker and easier to schedule than conventional surgery. This can expedite pathology results, so potential surgical decisions regarding lumpectomy or mastectomy can be made with minimal delay. When operating on the basis of a core biopsy diagnosis of cancer, surgeons are more likely to obtain clean (negative) lumpectomy margins with the first excision. Axillary lymph nodes, which are evaluated to ascertain metastases, are also sampled at the time of the initial surgery. A woman with a known diagnosis of breast cancer may avoid a second operation.

Two types of mammographic equipment are commercially available for stereotactic biopsy procedures: prone biopsy tables and upright add-on devices. Disadvantages of the upright add-on system include a limited working space, increased potential for patient motion, and greater potential for vasovagal reactions, as the patient can watch the biopsy procedure (Fig. 21-85). The dedicated prone system allows the patient to lie face down with the breast hanging pendulous through a hole in the table (Figs. 21-86 and 21-87). This gives the technologists and doctors more work space underneath the raised table, and the procedure is out of sight of the patient. The prone table is more expensive than the add-on system, requires a larger space, and should not be used for conventional mammography. It can be more difficult to locate suspicious lesions close to the chest wall with the prone table versus the upright add-on system. But the success or failure of core needle breast biopsy ultimately depends more on the experience and interest of the diagnostic team, including a radiologist, a mammographer, a pathologist, and a specially trained nurse or technologist, than on the particulars of the system that is used.

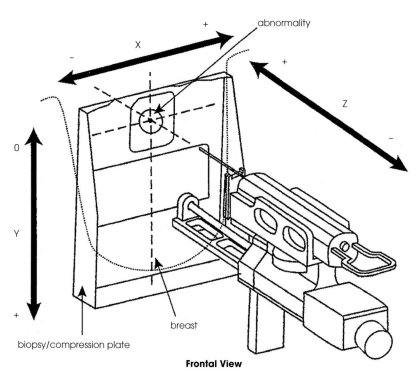

Fig. 21-84 Cartesian coordinates. A Cartesian system identifies the location of a unique point by three axes intersecting at right angles.

(Reprinted with permission from Willison KM: Fundamentals of stereotactic breast biopsy. In: Fajardo LL, Willison KM, Pizzutello RJ, eds: *A comprehensive approach to stereotactic breast biopsy*, Cambridge, 1996, Blackwell Science, p16.)

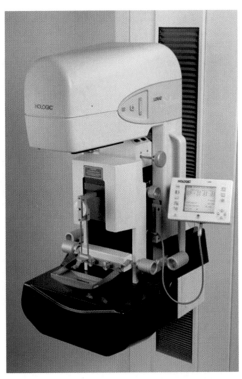

Fig. 21-85 Upright stereotactic system attached to dedicated mammography unit.

(Courtesy Hologic, Bedford, MA.)

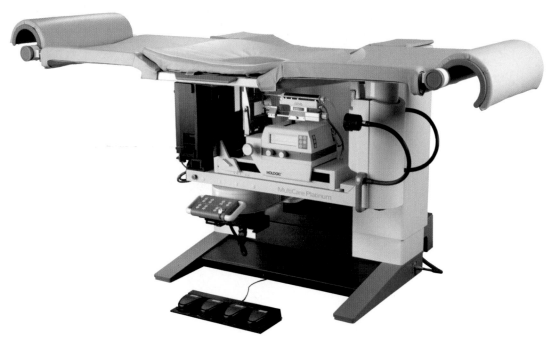

Fig. 21-86 Prone stereotactic biopsy system with digital imaging.

(Courtesy Hologic, Bedford, MA.)

Before beginning the procedure, the physician reviews the initial mammographic images to determine the best approach and projection of the breast to allow for the shortest distance from the surface of the skin to the breast lesion. The biopsy needle should be inserted through the least amount of tissue, limiting the amount of trauma to the breast. A lesion located in the lateral aspect of the UOQ is approached from the lateral aspect, whereas a lesion located in the medial and superior portion of the breast is approached from above. After the best approach to the lesion has been determined, the affected breast is positioned and compressed with an open compression paddle for a scout image to localize the breast lesion. Once the breast lesion has been localized, stereo images are taken to triangulate the lesion and measure its X, Y, and Z coordinates (Fig. 21-88).

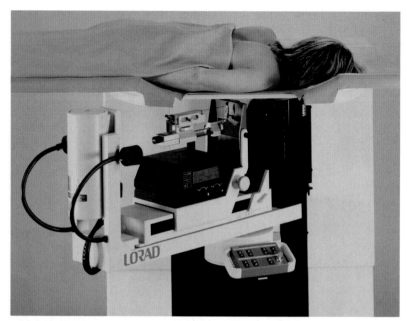

Fig. 21-87 Open aperture in table for prone biopsy system allows breast to be positioned beneath table.

(Courtesy Trex Medical Corp., LORAD Division, Danbury, CT.)

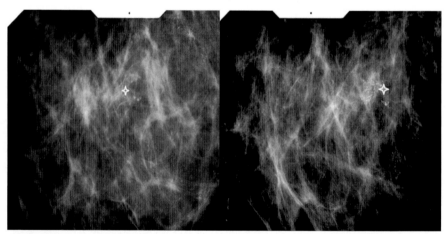

Fig. 21-88 Stereo images showing three-dimensional view of breast lesion before intervention.

At the computer workstation, the physician reads the two side-by-side stereotactic images and identifies the center of the lesion on each image. The computer is then used to calculate the exact X, Y, and Z coordinates. At this point the physician must determine whether the Z value, or depth of the lesion, is within range for the biopsy. If the lesion is very deep within the breast with a high Z value, it may be appropriate to change the approach and positioning of the breast to minimize trauma. If the Z value is too low, the lesion is very shallow and close to the surface of the skin; there may not be enough breast tissue to cover the trough and tip of the biopsy needle. In this case, another approach would be justified. Once an appropriate Z value is found, the physician transmits the coordinates from the computer workstation to the biopsy table stage (Fig. 21-89).

At the biopsy table, the breast is aseptically cleansed to minimize infection, and the skin is anesthetized at the area where the biopsy needle enters. The physician can effectively manage the pain associated with the procedure by anesthetizing the tissue within the breast at the biopsy site. The biopsy needle is then placed on the *stage,* which holds it in place and interprets the coordinates sent by the computer. Next, the tip of the needle must be *zeroed* by aligning it with the center reference point. The needle is then moved into position within the opening of the compression plate based on the appropriate X and Y values sent from the workstation. A small incision is made with a scalpel to facilitate entry of the needle into the breast and proper positioning of the Z axis. Before the needle enters the lesion at the exact Z axis, the needle is "dialed back," and "pre-fire" images are obtained with stereotaxis to ensure proper positioning (Fig. 21-90).

Swift firing of the needle into place and capturing of specimens from the lesion are dependent on the type of needle and retrieval device selected by the physician. The physician may use a spring-loaded biopsy device to power the needle back and forth through the target. After the pre-fire images verify the needle's tip adjacent to the lesion, the needle is fired into the lesion quickly to penetrate the tissue without pushing it deeper within the breast. Once the first pass is made, stereotactic "post-fire" images confirm correct needle placement. This image determines the course of subsequent passes. Redigitization (use of a digitizer to repeat the steps needed to calculate the new triangulation coordinates) can be performed to obtain additional samples. Alternatively, the physician can estimate where to move the biopsy needle based on the initial needle location within the breast. With the needle located inside the lesion, a sheath, or needle cover, slides over the trough of the needle. The sheath cuts the tissue sample within the trough and holds the sample in place while the needle is withdrawn. When the needle is outside the breast, the sheath is pulled back, exposing the tissue sample for collection.

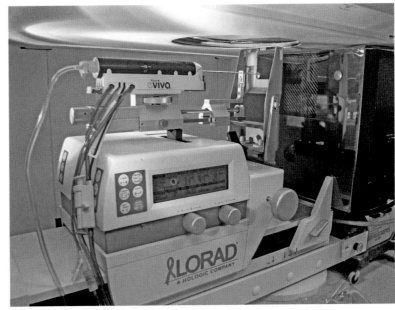

Fig. 21-89 Stage of biopsy system supports biopsy gun. X, Y, and Z coordinates are displayed.

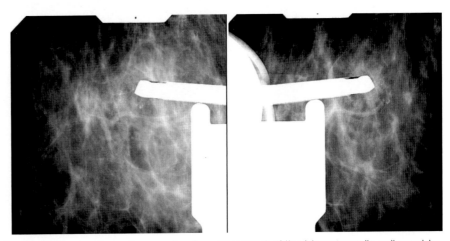

Fig. 21-90 Pre-fire stereo images showing placement of the biopsy needle adjacent to calcium to be biopsied.

An alternative technique is vacuum-assisted core biopsy. The probe is fired quickly into the lesion with the use of air pressure. After post-fire images are acquired, the tissue is gently vacuum-aspirated through a trough in a rotating cutter into the probe's aperture and collected in a basket. With the probe in the center of the lesion, the cutter can be spun in a circle to move the trough and collect samples from every direction without multiple insertions. When the biopsy is complete, the cutter is removed, and a radiopaque clip can be deployed through the probe and into the biopsy site to mark the area for future reference.

Radiopaque clips are placed following most large-core needle biopsies, using both spring-loaded and vacuum-assisted devices. The titanium clip serves as a marker, allowing radiologists to know the location of past biopsies for subsequent

mammograms or for surgical guidance. Immediately after the clip is seeded, "post-clip" images are obtained to ensure proper deployment and placement (Fig. 21-91). After this is done, the patient is released from compression and is given follow-up care. The time required to perform a stereotactic procedure is approximately 40 to 50 minutes.

With each technique, a minimum of 5 to a maximum of 20 tissue samples are obtained to ensure proper sampling of the abnormality. If the abnormality contains radiopaque calcium, the radiologist may choose to x-ray the sample to guarantee the presence of calcium for accurate diagnosis. Following this image, the tissue samples are transferred into a formalin specimen container for transportation to the pathology laboratory. For vacuum-assisted biopsies, a larger amount of tissue sample is obtained; this has been reported

to improve accuracy in diagnosing atypical ductal hyperplasia and ductal carcinoma in situ lesions.[1]

After the LCNB procedure is completed, the breast is cleaned and bandaged using sterile technique. Compression to the biopsy site is necessary to prevent excessive bleeding, and a cold compress is applied to minimize discomfort and swelling of related tissues. The patient should limit strenuous activity and keep the affected breast immobilized for at least 8 hours to prevent future bleeding or excessive bruising. The patient may be asked to return within 24 to 48 hours, so the breast can be examined to ensure that no bleeding or infection has occurred. The physician who performed the biopsy discusses the biopsy results and subsequent treatment options, if applicable, with the patient.

[1]Dershaw DD: Equipment, technique, quality assurance, and accreditation for image-guided breast biopsy procedures, *Radiol Clin North Am* 38:773, 2000.

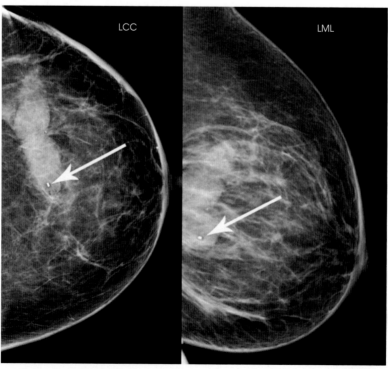

Fig 21-91 Post-biopsy images in standard CC and lateral projections to document accuracy of biopsy site and marker clip placement.

Breast Specimen Radiography

When open surgical biopsy is performed, the suspected lesion must be contained in its entirety in the tissue removed during the biopsy. Very small lesions that are characterized by tissue irregularity or microcalcifications on a mammographic image and that are nonpalpable in the excised specimen may be undetectable on visual inspection; a radiographic image of the biopsied tissue may be necessary to determine that the entire lesion has been removed. Compression of the specimen is necessary to identify lesions, especially lesions that do not contain calcifications. Magnification imaging is used to better visualize microcalcifications. Specimen radiography is often performed as an immediate post-excision procedure while the patient is still under anesthesia. Speed is essential.

The procedure for handling the specimen must be established before the procedure is started. Cooperation among radiologist, mammographer, surgeon, and pathologist is imperative. Together, a system of identifying the orientation of the tissue sample to the patient's breast (anterior, posterior, medial, or lateral aspect of the sample) can be applied to help the clinician confirm that the lesion has been completely removed.[q]

[q]Britton SE et al: Breast surgical specimen radiographs: How reliable are they? *Eur J Radiol* 79:245, 2011.

The specimen may be imaged using the magnification technique, with or without compression, as ordained by the policy of the facility. As patient radiation exposure and patient motion are no longer factors, imaging for high resolution regardless of dose is appropriate. Exposure factors depend on the thickness of the specimen and the imaging modality that is used (Fig. 21-92). Alternatively, radiographic equipment is manufactured specifically for imaging tissue specimens. These units are self-contained, are often portable, and allow specimens to be imaged directly in the operating suite. Digital technology allows the image to be seen by the surgeon and the radiologist and the pathologist in remote locations, almost immediately and simultaneously.[r,s]

[r]Kim SH et al: An evaluation of intraoperative digital specimen mammography versus conventional specimen radiography for the excision of nonpalpable breast lesions, *Am J Surg* S0002-9610(13)00081-0, 2013.
[s]Layfield DM et al: The effect of introducing an in-theatre intra-operative specimen radiography (IOSR) system on the management of palpable breast cancer within a single unit, *The Breast* 21:459, 2012.

The pathologist often uses the specimen radiograph to precisely locate the area of concern, so a copy of the image should be sent with the specimen. The next step is to match the actual specimen to the specimen radiograph before the specimen is dissected. Marking the area of concern within the specimen by placing a radiopaque object, such as a 1- or 2-inch (2.5- or 5-cm) needle, directly at the area of concern helps the pathologist locate the abnormality more accurately.

Specimens of tissue from large-core needle biopsies (LCNBs) are frequently radiographed, particularly when the biopsy is performed for calcifications. Radiographing tissue specimens can confirm that the area of interest has been sampled and is included within the tissue sent for examination by the pathologist (Fig. 21-93).

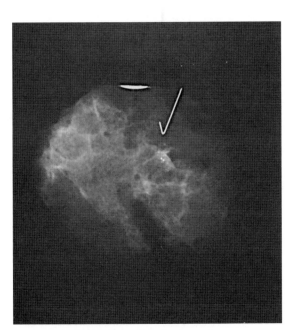

Fig. 21-92 Radiograph of surgical specimen containing suspicious microcalcifications.

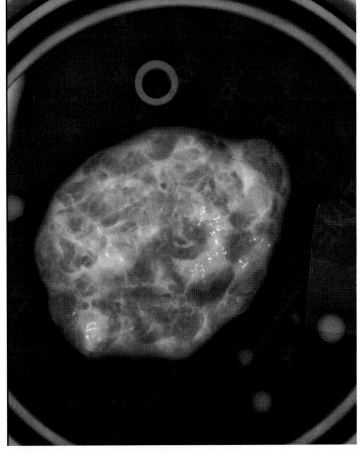

Fig 21-93 Magnified radiograph of specimen obtained from core biopsy shown in Figs. 21-88, 21-90, and 21-91. Note calcium indicating successful biopsy.

Breast Magnetic Resonance Imaging

Breast MRI has proved most useful in patients with proven breast cancer or at high risk for breast cancer, to assess for multifocal or multicentric disease, chest wall involvement, chemotherapy response, or tumor recurrence, or to identify the primary site in patients with occult breast disease.

INDICATIONS

Assessment of extent of disease and residual disease

MRI can be helpful for patients who have had a lumpectomy and have positive margins and no evidence of residual disease on conventional imaging (mammography, ultrasound). Postoperative mammography can help detect residual calcifications but is limited for residual mass. MRI is very sensitive for detection of residual mass and identifies other potentially suspicious sites seen only on MRI.

Assessment of tumor recurrence

Assessment of tumor recurrence on MRI can be very complicated because scars can become enhanced for 1 to 2 years after surgery. Suggestion of recurrence can be made by MRI, yet the cost of the procedure should be weighed against a less expensive needle biopsy of the area.

Occult primary breast cancer

Patients with axillary metastases suspicious for primary breast cancer with a negative physical examination, mammogram, and ultrasound are good candidates for MRI because of its high sensitivity for invasive cancers. MRI has been shown to detect 90% to 100% of cancers if tumor is present in the breast. If the primary site is detected, the patient may be spared a mastectomy, and MRI can influence patient surgical management.

Neoadjuvant chemotherapy response

In patients with advanced breast cancer, MRI may be used to predict earlier which patients are responding to chemotherapy. Mammography and physical examination can sometimes be limited by fibrosis. Studies suggest that MRI may be better for assessing patients' response to treatment.[1]

---

[1]Yeh E et al: Prospective comparison of mammography, sonography, and MRI in patients undergoing neoadjuvant chemotherapy for palpable breast cancer, *AJR Am J Roentgenol* 184:868, 2005.

High-risk screening

Breast MRI is recommended as an annual screening examination for patients at high risk for developing breast cancer.[1] These include women

1. Who have a first-degree relative (parent, sibling, child) with a *BRCA1* or *BRCA2* mutation, even if they have yet to be tested themselves.
2. Whose lifetime risk of breast cancer has been scored at 20% to 25% or greater, based on one of several accepted risk assessment tools that look at family history and other factors.
3. Who have received radiation to the chest between 10 and 30 years of age.
4. Who have Li-Fraumeni syndrome, Cowden syndrome, or Bannayan-Riley-Ruvalcaba syndrome, or who may have one of these syndromes based on history in a first-degree relative.

A study published in the *New England Journal of Medicine* concluded that MRI is "more sensitive than mammography in detecting tumors in women with an inherited susceptibility of breast cancer."[2] At the present time, not all insurance companies cover breast MRI in these high-risk women.

Breast MRI is recommended for women at high risk to be used as an adjunct to mammography. The most beneficial method for screening is to schedule 6-month intervals alternating MRI with mammography. Women who are found to have MRI-detected foci suspicious of cancer need to have these verified by biopsy. Often these areas are reexamined with mammography and directed ultrasound for potential biopsy. If these lesions are not found by conventional imaging, confirmation with MRI-guided biopsy would be necessary before the patient is committed to potential lumpectomy or mastectomy or both.

---

[1]American Cancer Society, March 2007.
[2]Kriege M et al: Efficacy of MRI and mammography for breast cancer screening in women with a familial or genetic predisposition, *N Engl J Med* 351:427, 2004.

Thermography and Diaphanography

Beginning in the 1950s, thermography and diaphanography were actively investigated in the hope that breast cancer and other abnormalities could be diagnosed using nonionizing forms of radiation. These two diagnostic tools are seldom used today.

Thermography is the photographic recording of the infrared radiation emanating from a patient's body surface. The resulting thermogram shows areas of increased temperature, with a temperature increase often suggesting increased metabolism. (More complete information on this technique is provided in the fourth through eighth editions of this atlas.)

Diaphanography is an examination in which a body part is transilluminated using selected light wavelengths and special imaging equipment. With this technique, the interior of the breast is inspected using light directed through its exterior wall. The light exiting the patient's body is recorded and interpreted. Rapid advances in mammography have essentially eliminated the use of this technique for evaluating breast disease. (More complete information on diaphanography is given in this chapter in the fourth through eighth editions of this atlas.)

Conclusion

Radiographic examination of the breast is a technically demanding procedure. Success depends in large part on the skills of the mammographer—more so than in most other areas of radiology. In addition to skill, the mammographer must have a strong desire to perform high-quality mammography and must be willing to work with the patient to allay qualms and to obtain cooperation. In the course of taking the patient's history and physically assessing and radiographing the breasts, the mammographer may be asked questions about breast disease, BSE, screening guidelines, and breast radiography that the patient has been reluctant to ask other health care professionals. The knowledge, skill, and attitude of the mammographer may be lifesaving for the patient. Although most patients do not have significant breast disease when first examined, statistics show that approximately 12% of patients develop breast cancer at some time during their lifetime. An early positive mammography encounter may make the patient more willing to undergo mammography in the future. When properly performed, breast radiography is safe, and presently, it offers the best hope for significantly reducing the mortality of breast cancer.

Suggested reading

Adler D, Wahl R: New methods for imaging the breast: techniques, findings and potential, *AJR Am J Roentgenol* 164:19, 1995.

American Cancer Society: *Breast cancer facts and figures 2013*, Available at: www.cancer.org. Accessed February 2013.

Andolina V, Lille S: *Mammographic imaging, a practical guide*, ed 3, Philadelphia, 2011, Lippincott, Williams & Wilkins.

Appelbaum A et al: Mammographic appearance of male breast disease, *RadioGraphics* 19:559, 2001.

Bassett L: Imaging of breast masses, *Radiol Clin North Am* 38:669, 2000.

Bassett L et al, editors: *Quality determinants of mammography*, AHCPR Pub No 95-0632, Rockville, MD, 1994, U.S. Department of Health and Human Services.

Burbank F: Stereotactic breast biopsy of atypical hyperplasia and ductal carcinoma in situ lesions: improved accuracy with directional, vacuum-assisted biopsy, *Radiology* 202:843, 1997.

Carr J et al: Stereotactic localization of breast lesions: how it works and methods to improve accuracy, *RadioGraphics* 21:463, 2001.

Dershaw DD: Equipment, technique, quality assurance, and accreditation for image-guided breast biopsy procedures, *Radiol Clin North Am* 38:773, 2000.

Dershaw DD et al: Mammographic findings in men with breast cancer, *AJR Am J Roentgenol* 160:267, 1993.

Eklund GW, Cardenosa G: The art of mammographic positioning, *Radiol Clin North Am* 30:21, 1992.

Eklund GW et al: Improved imaging of the augmented breast, *AJR Am J Roentgenol* 151:469, 1988.

F-D-C Reports, Inc: ImageChecker unanimously endorsed by radiology panel. *Medical devices, diagnostics, and instrumentation: "the gray sheet,"* 24:20, 1998.

Feig S: Breast masses: mammographic and sonographic evaluation, *Radiol Clin North Am* 30:67, 1992.

Haus A, Yaffe M: Screen-film and digital mammography image quality and radiation dose considerations, *Radiol Clin North Am* 38:871, 2000.

Healy B: BRCA genes: bookmarking, fortune-telling, and medical care, *N Engl J Med* 336:1448, 1997 (editorial).

Henderson IC: Breast cancer. In Murphy GP, Lawrence WL, Lenhard RE, editors: *Clinical oncology,* Atlanta, 1997, American Cancer Society.

Jackson V: The status of mammographically guided fine needle aspiration biopsy of non-palpable breast lesions, *Radiol Clin North Am* 30:155, 1992.

Kopans DB: Double reading, *Radiol Clin North Am* 38:719, 2000.

Krainer M et al: Differential contributions of *BRCA1* and *BRCA2* to early-onset breast cancer, *N Engl J Med* 336:1416, 1997.

Liberman L: Clinical management issues in percutaneous core breast biopsy, *Radiol Clin North Am* 38:791, 2000.

Logan-Young W et al: The cost effectiveness of fine-needle aspiration cytology and 14-gauge core needle biopsy compared with open surgical biopsy in the diagnosis of breast cancer, *Cancer* 82:1867, 1998.

Mammography quality control manual, rev ed, Chicago, 1999, American College of Radiology.

National Cancer Institute CancerNet, Available at: www.cancernet.nci.nih.gov. Accessed April 2001.

Nishikawa R et al: Computerized detection of clustered microcalcifications: evaluation of performance on mammograms from multiple centers, *RadioGraphics* 15:443, 1995.

Orel SG: MR imaging of the breast, *Radiol Clin North Am* 38:899, 2000.

Parker SL, Burbank F: A practical approach to minimally invasive breast biopsy, *Radiology* 200:11, 1996.

Parker SL et al: Percutaneous large-core breast biopsy: a multi-institutional study, *Radiology* 193:359, 1994.

Prechtel K, Pretchel V: Breast carcinoma in the man: current results from the viewpoint of clinic and pathology, *Pathologe* 18:45, 1997.

Rozenberg S et al: Principal cancers among women: breast, lung, and colorectal, *Int J Fertil* 41:166, 1996.

Schmidt R et al: Computer-aided diagnosis in mammography. In: *RSNA categorical course in breast imaging* [syllabus], Oak Park, IL, 1995, RSNA.

Skolnick AA: Ultrasound may help detect breast implant leaks, *JAMA* 267:786, 1992.

Slawson SH et al: Ductography: how to and what if? *RadioGraphics* 21:133, 2001.

Vyborny CJ: Computer-aided detection and computer-aided diagnosis of breast cancer, *Radiol Clin North Am* 38:725, 2000.

Mammography

ADDENDUM B
SUMMARY OF ABBREVIATIONS, VOLUME TWO

AAA	abdominal aortic aneurysm	GML	glabellomeatal line	OID	object–to–image receptor (IR) distance
ACR	American College of Radiology	GSW	gunshot wound		
AML	acanthiomeatal line	HSG	hysterosalpingography	OML	orbitomeatal line
AP	anteroposterior	IAM	internal acoustic meatus	PA	posteroanterior
ASRT	American Society of Radiologic Technologists	IOML	infraorbitomeatal line	PTC	percutaneous transhepatic cholangiography
		IPL	interpupillary line		
BE	barium enema	IR	image receptor	RUQ	right upper quadrant
BPH	benign prostatic hyperplasia	IUD	intrauterine device	SID	source–to–image receptor (IR) distance
BUN	blood urea nitrogen	IV	intravenous		
CDC	Centers for Disease Control and Prevention	IVP	intravenous pyelogram	SMV	submentovertical
		IVU	intravenous urography	TEA	top of ear attachment
CPR	cardiopulmonary resuscitation	KUB	kidneys, ureters, and bladder	TMJ	temporomandibular joint
CR	central ray	MML	mentomeatal line	UGI	upper gastrointestinal
CT	computed tomography	MPR	multiplanar reconstruction	UPJ	ureteropelvic junction
CTC	CT colonography	MRI	magnetic resonance imaging	UVJ	ureterovesical junction
CVA	cerebrovascular accident	MVA	motor vehicle accident	VC	virtual colonoscopy
EAM	external acoustic meatus	NPO	nil per os (nothing by mouth)	VCUG	voiding cystourethrogram
ED	emergency department				
ERCP	endoscopic retrograde cholangiopancreatography				

INDEX

Page numbers followed by "f" indicate figures, "t" indicate tables, and "b" indicate boxes.

I-1

Bloch, Felix, **3:**342
Blood, handling of, **1:**16, 16b
Blood oxygen level dependent (BOLD) imaging, **3:**366
Blood pool agents for MRI, **3:**355
Blood-brain barrier, **3:**417, 437
Blood-vascular system, **3:**22-26, 22f
   arteries in, **3:**22f, 23
      coronary, **3:**25, 25f
      pulmonary, **3:**22f, 23
      systemic, **3:**23
   arterioles in, **3:**23
   capillaries in, **3:**23-24
   complete circulation of blood through, **3:**24
   defined, **3:**96
   heart in, **3:**23-24, 25f
   main trunk vessels in, **3:**23
   portal system in, **3:**23, 23f
   pulmonary circulation in, **3:**23, 23f
   systemic circulation in, **3:**23, 23f
   veins in, **3:**22f, 23
      coronary, **3:**25, 25f
      pulmonary, **3:**22f, 23
      systemic, **3:**24
   velocity of blood circulation in, **3:**26
   venules in, **3:**23
Blowout fracture, **2:**46f, 282t, 313, 313f
Blunt trauma, **2:**19
BMC (bone mineral content), **3:**442, 476
BMD (bone mineral density), **3:**442, 476
   calculation of, **3:**453
BMI (body mass index), **1:**44
B-mode acquisition technology (BAT), **3:**497
Body cavities, **1:**68-69, 69f
Body composition dual energy x-ray absorptiometry, **3:**442f, 471, 472f, 476
Body fluids, handling of, **1:**16, 16b
Body habitus, **1:**72-74, 72f, 73b, 74f
   and body position for skull radiography
      in horizontal sagittal plane, **2:**289f
      in perpendicular sagittal plane, **2:**290f
   and gallbladder, **2:**106, 106f
   and stomach and duodenum, **2:**99, 99f
      PA projection of, **2:**124, 125f
   and thoracic viscera, **1:**479, 479f
Body mass index (BMI), **1:**44
Body movement, **1:**96-97
   abduct or abduction as, **1:**96, 96f
   adduct or adduction as, **1:**96, 96f
   circumduction as, **1:**97, 97f
   deviation as, **1:**97, 97f
   dorsiflexion as, **1:**97, 97f
   evert/eversion as, **1:**96, 96f
   extension as, **1:**96, 96f
   flexion as, **1:**96, 96f
   hyperextension as, **1:**96, 96f
   hyperflexion as, **1:**96, 96f
   invert/inversion as, **1:**96f
   plantar flexion as, **1:**97, 97f
   pronate/pronation as, **1:**97, 97f
   rotate/rotation as, **1:**97, 97f
   supinate/supination as, **1:**97, 97f
   tilt as, **1:**97, 97f
Body planes, **1:**66-67
   coronal, **1:**66, 66f-67f
   in CT and MRI, **1:**67, 67f
   horizontal (transverse, axial, cross-sectional), **1:**66, 66f-67f
   imaging in several, **1:**67, 68f
   interiliac, **1:**68, 69f
   midcoronal (midaxillary), **1:**66, 66f
   midsagittal, **1:**66, 66f
   oblique, **1:**66f-67f, 67
   occlusal, **1:**68, 69f
   sagittal, **1:**66, 66f-67f
   special, **1:**68, 69f

Body rotation method for PA oblique projection of sternoclavicular articulations, **1:**465, 465f
Bohr atomic number, **3:**403, 403f
BOLD (blood oxygen level dependent) imaging, **3:**366
Bolus chase method for digital subtraction angiography, **3:**30-31
Bolus in CT angiography, **3:**324, 339
Bone(s), **1:**75-79
   appendicular skeleton of, **1:**75, 75f, 75t
   axial skeleton of, **1:**75, 75f, 75t
   biology of, **3:**445-446
   classification of, **1:**79, 79f
   compact (cortical), **1:**76, 76f
      and bone densitometry, **3:**445, 445t
      defined, **3:**476
   development of, **1:**77-78, 77f-78f
   flat, **1:**79, 79f
   fractures of. *See* Fracture(s).
   functions of, **1:**75
   general features of, **1:**76, 76f
   irregular, **1:**79, 79f
   long, **1:**79, 79f
   markings and features of, **1:**84
   sesamoid, **1:**79, 79f
   short, **1:**79, 79f
   spongy, **1:**76, 76f
   trabecular (cancellous)
      and bone densitometry, **3:**445, 445t
      defined, **3:**477
      in osteoporosis, **3:**446f
   vessels and nerves of, **1:**77, 77f
Bone cyst, **1:**109t, 240t
   aneurysmal, **3:**149, 149f
Bone densitometry, **3:**441-478
   bone biology and remodeling and, **3:**445-446, 445f-446f, 445t
   central (or axial) skeletal measurements in, **3:**469-471, 469f-471f
   defined, **3:**442, 476
   definition of terms for, **3:**476b-477b
   dual photon absorptiometry (DPA) for, **3:**444, 476
   DXA for. *See* Dual energy x-ray absorptiometry (DXA).
   fracture risk models in, **3:**475
   history of, **3:**443-444, 444f
   and osteoporosis, **3:**442, 447-450, 448t
      bone health recommendations for, **3:**450, 450t
      defined, **3:**477
      fractures and falls due to, **3:**449, 449f
   pediatric, **3:**473-474, 473f
   peripheral skeletal measurements in, **3:**474-475, 474f-475f
   principles of, **3:**442-443, 442f
   quantitative computed tomography (QCT) for, **3:**444, 469, 469f, 477
   radiogrammetry for, **3:**443, 477
   radiographic absorptiometry for, **3:**443, 477
   single photon absorptiometry (SPA) for, **3:**444, 444f, 477
   vertebral fracture assessment in, **3:**469-470, 470f-471f, 477
Bone formation, **3:**445, 445f
Bone health, recommendations for, **3:**450, 450t
Bone marrow
   red, **1:**76, 76f
   yellow, **1:**76, 76f
Bone marrow dose, **1:**35, 35t
Bone mass
   defined, **3:**476
   low, **3:**447, 457, 476-477
   peak, **3:**446, 477

Bone mineral content (BMC), **3:**442, 476
Bone mineral density (BMD), **3:**442, 476
   calculation of, **3:**453
Bone remodeling, **3:**445-446, 445f, 476
Bone resorption, **3:**445, 445f
Bone scan, **3:**415-416
Bone scintigraphy, **3:**415-416
Bone studies, **3:**416
Bone turnover, biochemical markers of, **3:**448, 476
Bone windows, **3:**11, 11f
Bony labyrinth, **2:**271
Bony thorax, **1:**445-476
   anatomy of, **1:**447-453
      anterior aspect of, **1:**447f
      anterolateral oblique aspect of, **1:**447f
      articulations in, **1:**449-453, 449t, 450f
      lateral aspect of, **1:**448f
      ribs in, **1:**447f-449f, 448
      sternum in, **1:**447-448, 447f
      summary of, **1:**453b
   body position for, **1:**453
   function of, **1:**447
   respiratory movement of, **1:**451, 451f
      diaphragm in, **1:**452, 452f
   ribs in. *See* Ribs.
   sample exposure technique chart essential projections for, **1:**455t
   sternoclavicular articulations of
      anatomy of, **1:**449, 449t
      PA oblique projection of
         body rotation method for, **1:**465, 465f
         central ray angulation method for, **1:**466, 466f-467f
      PA projection of, **1:**464, 464f
   sternum in. *See* Sternum.
   summary of pathology of, **1:**454t
   summary of projections for, **1:**446
   in trauma patients, **1:**453
Boomerang contact filter
   applications of, **1:**60t, 63-64, 63f
   composition of, **1:**57
   example of, **1:**56f
   placement of, **1:**58, 58f
   shape of, **1:**57
Bowel obstruction, **2:**84t
Bowel preparation, **1:**18
Bowing fractures, **3:**130
Bowman capsule, **2:**185, 185f
Bowtie filters for CT, **3:**329-330, 329f
Boxer fracture, **1:**109t
BPD (biparietal diameter), **3:**390, 390f, 397
BPH (benign prostatic hyperplasia), **2:**188t
   in older adults, **3:**173, 174t
Bq (becquerel), **3:**405, 437
Brachial artery
   anatomy of, **3:**22f, 49f
   arteriography of, **3:**46f
Brachiocephalic artery, **3:**96
   anatomy of, **3:**49f, 50
   arteriography of, **3:**40f
   sectional anatomy of, **3:**270-271, 273-275, 274f, 280-281, 281f
Brachiocephalic vein
   sectional anatomy of, **3:**271
      on axial (transverse) plane, **3:**273-275, 273f-274f
      on coronal plane, **3:**280-281, 281f
   venography of, **3:**60f
Brachycephalic skull, **2:**286, 286f
Brachytherapy, **3:**485, 506
Bradyarrhythmia, **3:**96
Bradycardia, **3:**96
Bragg peak, **3:**505

Brain
  anatomy of, **3:**2, 2f
  CT angiography of, **3:**10f, 324-326, 325f
    perfusion study for, **3:**324-326, 326f
  CT of, **3:**10, 10f-11f, 315f
  defined, **3:**18
  magnetic resonance spectroscopy for, **3:**365,
    365f
  MRI of, **3:**12, 13f, 357, 357f
  PET of, **3:**432f, 434
  plain radiographic examination of, **3:**5
  sectional anatomy of, **3:**254
  SPECT study of, **3:**411f, 417
  vascular and interventional procedures of,
    3:14-16, 14f-15f
  ventricular system of, **3:**2, 4, 4f
Brain perfusion imaging, **3:**417
Brain stem
  anatomy of, **3:**2, 2f
  sectional anatomy of, **3:**255, 264
Brain tissue scanner, **3:**305
BRCA1 gene, **2:**378-379, **3:**482
BRCA2 gene, **2:**378-379, **3:**482
Breast(s)
  anatomy of, **2:**380, 380f-381f, 394b
  axillary tail of
    anatomy of, **2:**380f, 437f
    axillary projection of, **2:**452-453,
      452f-453f
    mediolateral oblique projection of, **2:**412f,
      432t, 450-451, 450f-451f
  connective tissue of, **2:**381f, 382
  density of, **2:**383, 383f
  digital breast tomosynthesis (3D imaging) of,
    2:374-375
  ductography of, **2:**459-460, 459f-460f
  fatty tissue of, **2:**381f, 382
  glandular tissue of, **2:**382
  involution of, **2:**380
  localization and biopsy of suspicious lesions of,
    2:461-470
    breast specimen radiography in, **2:**471, 471f
    for dermal calcifications, **2:**464
    material for, **2:**461, 461f
    stereotactic imaging and biopsy procedures
      for, **2:**465-470
      calculation of X, Y, and Z coordinates in,
        2:465, 465f-466f, 469, 469f
      equipment for, **2:**466, 467f-468f
      images using, **2:**468, 468f-470f
      three-dimensional localization with, **2:**465,
        465f
    tangential projection for, **2:**464
  MRI of, **2:**418-419, 472, **3:**358, 359f
  oversized, **2:**400, 401f
  pathology of, **2:**384-393
    architectural distortions as, **2:**393, 393f,
      394t-395t
    calcifications as, **2:**389-393, 389f-392f
    masses as, **2:**384-388, 394t-395t
      circumscribed, **2:**384, 385f, 394
      density of, **2:**384, 386f
      indistinct, **2:**384, 394
      interval change in, **2:**387, 387f
      location of, **2:**387
      margins of, **2:**384, 394t-395t
      palpable, **2:**409, 429-430, 443
      radiolucent, **2:**384, 386f
      seen on only one projection, **2:**388,
        388f
      shape of, **2:**384
      spiculated, **2:**384, 385f, 394
    summary of, **2:**394t-395t
  during pregnancy and lactation, **2:**382,
    382f
  radiography of. *See* Mammography.

Breast(s) *(Continued)*
  in radiography of sternum, **1:**456
  thermography and diaphanography of, **2:**473
  tissue variations in, **2:**382-393, 382f-383f
  ultrasonography of, **2:**418-419, **3:**375f, 383, 384f
  xerography of, **2:**372, 372f
Breast abscess, **2:**395
Breast augmentation
  complications of, **2:**418
  mammography with, **2:**417-419, 418f
    craniocaudal (CC) projection of
      with full implant, **2:**420-421, 421f
      with implant displaced, **2:**422-423,
        422f-423f
      with implant displacement (ID), **2:**403t-408t
    mediolateral oblique (MLO) projection of
      with full implant, **2:**424
      with implant displaced, **2:**425
  MRI with, **2:**418-419
  ultrasonography with, **2:**418-419
Breast cancer
  architectural distortion due to, **2:**393f
  calcifications in, **2:**392f
  genetic factors in, **3:**482
  in men, **2:**426
  prophylactic surgery for, **3:**482, 507
  radiation oncology for, **3:**504, 504f
  risk factors for, **2:**378-379
  ultrasonography of, **3:**375f
Breast cancer screening, **2:**377
  vs. diagnostic mammography, **2:**378
  high-risk, **2:**472
  risk vs. benefit of, **2:**377-378, 377f
Breast specimen radiography, **2:**471, 471f
Breastbone. *See* Sternum.
Breathing, **1:**451, 451f
  for chest radiographs, **1:**490, 490f
  diaphragm in, **1:**452, 452f
  in radiography of ribs, **1:**468
  in radiography of sternum, **1:**456, 457f
  for trauma radiography, **2:**30
Breathing technique, **1:**41
Bregma, **2:**258f-259f, 259
Bridge of nose, **2:**272
Bridgeman method for superoinferior axial inlet
    projection of anterior pelvic bones, **1:**359,
    359f
Broad ligaments, **3:**284
Broadband ultrasound attenuation (BUA), **3:**475
Bronchial tree, **1:**480, 480b, 480f
Bronchiectasis, **1:**486t
Bronchioles, **1:**480, 480f
  terminal, **1:**480, 480f
Bronchitis, **1:**486t
  chronic, in older adults, **3:**172
Bronchomediastinal trunk, **3:**26
Bronchopneumonia, **1:**486t
Bronchopulmonary segments, **1:**482
Bronchoscopy, **3:**226
Bronchus(i)
  mainstem, **1:**480f
  primary, **1:**480, 480f
  secondary, **1:**480, 480f
  sectional anatomy of, **3:**270, 275-277, 276f, 279,
    280f-281f
  tertiary, **1:**480, 480f
BUA (broadband ultrasound attenuation), **3:**475
Buckle fracture, **1:**109t
Bucky grid with obese patients, **1:**51
Built-in DR flat-panel IR detector position, **1:**28f
Bulbourethral glands, **2:**242
"Bunny" technique
  for gastrointestinal and genitourinary studies,
    3:116f
  for limb radiography, **3:**127, 127f
  for skull radiography, **3:**132, 133f

Burman method for first CMC joint of thumb,
    1:120-121, 120f-121f
Bursae, **1:**82, 82f, 178
  of shoulder, **1:**178, 178f
Bursitis, **1:**109t, 182t
Butterfly sets, **2:**228f, 229
Byte, **3:**437

C
^{11}C (carbon-11) in PET, **3:**425f, 426t
CAD (computer-aided detection) systems for
    mammography, **2:**376-379, 376f
Cadaveric sections, **3:**252
Calcaneal sulcus, **1:**229, 229f
Calcaneocuboid articulation, **1:**236f-237f, 236t,
    238
Calcaneus
  anatomy of, **1:**228f-229f, 229
  axial projection of
    dorsoplantar, **1:**272, 272f-273f
    plantodorsal, **1:**271, 271f
    weight-bearing coalition (Harris-Beath)
      method for, **1:**273, 273f
  lateromedial oblique projection
    (weight-bearing) of, **1:**275, 275f
  mediolateral projection of, **1:**274, 274f
Calcifications of breast, **2:**389-393, 389f-392f,
    394t-395t
  amorphous or indistinct, **2:**391, 392f, 394
  arterial (vascular), **2:**389f-390f, 395
  coarse heterogeneous, **2:**389f-390f, 391,
    394
  fine heterogeneous, **2:**391, 392f, 394
  linear branching, **2:**392f
  male, **2:**427
  milk of calcium as, **2:**391, 391f, 395
  pleomorphic linear, **2:**392f
  popcorn-type, **2:**389f-390f, 395
  rim, **2:**395
  rodlike secretory, **2:**389f-390f
  round or punctate, **2:**389f-390f, 394
  skin (dermal), **2:**395, 464
Calcitonin for osteoporosis, **3:**448t
Calcium and osteoporosis, **3:**447, 450, 450t
Calculus, **2:**62t
  renal, **2:**188t, 190f
Caldwell method
  for PA axial projection of facial bones,
    2:329-330, 329f-330f
  for PA axial projection of frontal and anterior
    ethmoidal sinuses, **2:**360-361, 360f-361f
    in children, **3:**136, 136f
  for PA axial projection of skull, **2:**296-300
    evaluation criteria for, **2:**299b
    position of part for, **2:**296, 297f
    position of patient for, **2:**296
    structures shown on, **2:**298f, 299
Calvaria, **2:**257
Camp-Coventry method for PA axial projection of
    intercondylar fossa, **1:**308, 308f-309f
Canadian Association of Medical Radiation
    Technologists (CAMRT)
  Code of Ethics of, **1:**2-3
  positioning terminology used by, **1:**85-95
Cancellous bone
  and bone densitometry, **3:**445, 445t
  defined, **3:**477
  in osteoporosis, **3:**446f
Cancer, **3:**481-483
  defined, **3:**481, 506
  epidemiology of, **3:**481
  metastasis of, **3:**481, 507
  most common types of, **3:**482, 482t
  PET imaging of, **3:**433, 433f
  radiation oncology for. *See* Radiation
    oncology.

Index

Index

Index

Index

Index